Interprofessional Perspectives for Community Practice

Promoting Health, Well-Being, and Quality of Life

Interprofessional Perspectives for Community Practice

Promoting Health, Well-Being, and Quality of Life

Editors

Michael A. Pizzi, PhD, OTR/L, FAOTA
Co-Owner, Clear Function Rehab
Health and Wellness Consultant
New York, New York

Mark Amir, PT, DPT, MPH, DipMDT
Director of Clinical Education
Doctor of Physical Therapy Program
Dominican University New York
Orangeburg, New York
Residency Director
JAG Physical Therapy
Bridgewater, New Jersey

Routledge
Taylor & Francis Group
NEW YORK AND LONDON

Instructors: *Interprofessional Perspectives for Community Practice: Promoting Health, Well-Being, and Quality of Life* includes ancillary materials specifically available for faculty use. Included are a Test Bank, PowerPoint Slides, and the Pizzi Health and Wellness Assessment. Please visit www.routledge.com/9781032957340 to obtain access.

Bonus chapters are available online for this book. Please visit www.routledge.com/9781032957340 to obtain access.

First published in hardback 2024

First published in 2024 SLACK Incorporated

Published 2024 by Routledge
605 Third Avenue, New York, NY 10158

and by Routledge
4 Park Square, Milton Park, Abingdon, Oxon OX14 4RN

Routledge is an imprint of the Taylor & Francis Group, an informa business

Publisher's Note
The publisher has gone to great lengths to ensure the quality of this reprint but points out that some imperfections in the original copies may be apparent.

Cover Artist: Tinhouse Design

Library of Congress Cataloging-in-Publication Data

Names: Pizzi, Michael, editor. | Amir, Mark, editor.
Title: Interprofessional perspectives for community practice : Promoting health, well-being, and quality of life / editors, Michael Pizzi, Mark Amir.
Description: Thorofare, NJ : SLACK Incorporated, [2023] | Includes bibliographical references and index.
Identifiers: LCCN 2023036393 (print) | ISBN 9781638220572 (paperback)
Subjects: MESH: Community Health Services | Preventive Health Services | Interprofessional Relations | Health Promotion--methods | Quality of Life
Classification: LCC RA418 (print) | NLM WA 546.1 | DDC 362.1--dc23/eng/20231004
LC record available at https://lccn.loc.gov/2023036393

ISBN: 978-1-03-295734-0 (hbk)
ISBN: 978-1-63822-057-2 (pbk)
ISBN: 978-1-00-352464-9 (ebk)

DOI: 10.4324/9781003524649

Dedication

This book is dedicated to my mom, whose short life living with diabetes, and who lived full out, taught me about promoting health, well-being, and quality of life and how to live fully every moment. I also dedicate this book to the memory of both my parents, who taught me the lesson of what it is to be your authentic self, and to face life's obstacles with grace, dignity, and compassion.

—Michael A. Pizzi, PhD, OTR/L, FAOTA

It is impossible to overstate the importance of great parents, family, and role models. My late father, may his memory always be a blessing, and mother taught me family values, commitment to work ethics, and faith in Hashem (G-d). My brothers are role models of living life with purpose. My wife is my best friend and has demonstrated a level of commitment and family values beyond what I could imagine. Our three boys give us "nachas," meaning calmness and pride, since they have become grown adults who are kind, thoughtful, and compassionate. My extended family, from in-laws to cousins, and lifelong friends are my source of strength. Finally, I am grateful to my physical therapy community, teachers, colleagues, and especially patients, for allowing me to thrive in a great healing profession.

—Mark Amir, PT, DPT, MPH, DipMDT

Contents

Bonus Chapters Available Online

Bonus chapters are available online for this book. Please visit www.routledge.com/9781032957340 to obtain access.

Instructors: *Interprofessional Perspectives for Community Practice: Promoting Health, Well-Being, and Quality of Life* includes ancillary materials specifically available for faculty use. Included are a Test Bank, PowerPoint Slides, and the Pizzi Health and Wellness Assessment. Please visit www.routledge.com/9781032957340 to obtain access.

Acknowledgments

I am very excited having developed this textbook that presents new and innovative ideas for practice for our students, and it is they who I wish to acknowledge with sincere gratitude. They have taught me so much. I wish to acknowledge my colleagues, starting with Dr. Mary Lou Galantino, PT, with whom I had the pleasure of collaborating many years ago, who taught me teamwork can be a joyful experience and that caring for clients and patients from an interprofessional perspective is the best way to care. Mark Amir, it has been an interprofessional journey, and I am grateful for your teamwork. Many thanks to those colleagues who forge ahead and are unafraid of creating new and innovative paths in practice, in order to further expand the possibilities for occupational therapy, despite the naysayers. Finally, I thank my friend, primary cheerleader, and husband, who teaches me daily what is the most meaningful thing in life that supports our own health, well-being, and quality of life.

—Michael A. Pizzi, PhD, OTR/L, FAOTA

This textbook was only possible because of the expertise of the authors, their diligent work, and collaboration. They deserve credit for being innovative and implementing the ideas in this book within their practice and teaching, which gives them credibility and expertise. My co-editor, Michael Pizzi, deserves all the credit for coordinating and organizing the book, teaching me the ins and outs of editing, and pushing me to exceed my self-perceived limitations. I learned more from Michael than I could ever thank him for. Lastly, I am always grateful that God blessed me with an amazing wife, three kind and respectful boys, and a wonderful immediate family that is always supportive and encouraging in all my endeavors, big and small.

—Mark Amir, PT, DPT, MPH, DipMDT

About the Editors

Michael A. Pizzi, PhD, OTR/L, FAOTA, has been an occupational therapist since 1981. He has published over 70 peer-reviewed articles and 25 book chapters, and is co-editor of a health promotion and wellness textbook. His research has focused on hospice, HIV/AIDS, wellness, and childhood obesity, and he is the only occupational therapist to guest edit the *American Journal of Occupational Therapy* on three different topics (AIDS, wellness, and childhood obesity). In occupational therapy, he has created clinical pathways in all of these areas. Dr. Pizzi created the first health and wellness interprofessional conference in 1993 and since then has focused on health, well-being, and quality of life in community practice. Dr. Pizzi developed the first valid and reliable wellness tool that could be used interprofessionally called the Pizzi Health and Wellness Assessment (PHWA), as well as a health and wellness model called the Environment–Health–Occupation–Well-Being (E-HOW) Model. He created Touching Humanity, a not-for-profit whose motto is "given opportunity, always able." Dr. Pizzi combines his musical theater/acting career with his occupational therapy career and created the Special Broadway Camp for children with autism and other disabilities, to provide equity and inclusion in the performing arts. The interprofessional collaboration among health professionals, actors, dancers, and musicians has been very rewarding.

Mark Amir, PT, DPT, MPH, DipMDT, is currently the Director of Clinical Education at DUNY – DPT and Residency Director at JAG Physical Therapy. His passion is to help students integrate newly acquired didactic skills that match their innate strengths to their clinical setting, which can positively impact the lives of their clients, themselves, and their community. Matching clinical experiences with a student-centered focus allows graduates and experienced clinicians to thrive in their chosen physical therapy career. Dr. Amir has hired, trained, and mentored hundreds of clinicians and aspiring clinicians during his 30+ years of experience as a physical therapist, business owner, teacher, and advocate of the physical therapy and health care profession. He uses his passion of learning topics related to leadership, management, professionalism, and customer service to educate new student professionals who are ready to tackle the challenges of their new career.

Dr. Amir was a private practice, multi-state outpatient physical therapy owner for over 20 years. He managed several clinic mergers and acquisitions and consulted with several clinicians through the same process. Dr. Amir was a managing partner of a company that provides innovative workplace injury prevention services to large and midsize companies in New York State. From 2010 to 2015, Dr. Amir was a contractor to APTA's Payment & Policy Department, advising members and staff on regional and national health care policy issues with a focus on improving payment models for physical therapists.

Being a lifelong learner, Dr. Amir is completing his dissertation toward a PhD with a special interest in higher education administration, leadership, and clinical education. Dr. Amir continues to enjoy hobbies of boating, running, biking, boxing, and martial arts training. He was a Krav Maga martial arts instructor, a high school football coach, and coached his own kids in flag football.

Contributing Authors

Laurel D. Abbruzzese, PT, EdD, FNAP (Chapter 15)
Director
Diversity, Equity & Inclusion
Director
Performing Arts Fellowship
Associate Professor
Department of Rehabilitation and Regenerative Medicine
Programs in Physical Therapy
Vagelos College of Physicians & Surgeons
Columbia University Irving Medical Center
New York, New York

Lucinda Acquaye-Doyle, PhD, MSW (Chapter 8)
Program Director and Associate Professor of Social Work
Dominican University New York
Orangeburg, New York

Ashleigh Augello, MOT, OTR/L (Chapter 5)
Occupational Therapist
LINK Home Therapy
Atco, New Jersey

Holly Putnam Bacasa, PT (Chapter 17)
Co-Owner and Pediatric Physical Therapist
Wellness For Life, Inc.
Pittsburgh, Pennsylvania

Kerryn Bagley, PhD, B. Social Work (Hons) (Chapter 3)
Lecturer in Social Work and Social Policy
La Trobe Rural Health School
La Trobe University, Bendigo
Victoria, Australia

Andrew Bailey, D Psych (Clinical) (Chapter 22)
Director Research & Knowledge Translation
Mid North Coast Local Health District
New South Wales, Australia

Pamela Bartlo, PT, DPT, CCS (Chapter 6)
Assistant Professor
Physical Therapy Department
College of Health Professions
Daemen University
Buffalo, New York

Catherine Cavaliere, PhD, OTR/L (Chapter 13)
Associate Professor of Occupational Therapy
Dominican University New York
Orangeburg, New York

Tina Champagne, OT, OTD, OTR, FAOTA (Chapter 13)
Chief Executive Officer
Cutchins Programs for Children and Families, Inc.
Northampton, Massachusetts

Jennifer Crews, MA, CCC-SLP (Chapter 7)
Speech-Language Pathologist
Summit Center for Child Development
Chehalis, Washington

Ann Marie Dale, PhD, OTR/L (Chapter 11)
Washington University in St. Louis
St. Louis, Missouri

Deirdre Daley, PT, DPT, MSHPE (Chapter 11)
WorkWell Prevention & Care
New Ipswich, New Hampshire

Priscilla Denham, MDiv, D.Min (Chapter 21)
Retired

Joy Doll, OTD, OTR/L, FNAP (Chapter 23)
Program Director, Health Informatics
Associate Professor
Creighton University
Omaha, Nebraska

Ayse Ozcan Edeer, PT, MSc, PhD (Chapter 2)
Tenured Associate Professor
Dominican University New York
Doctor of Physical Therapy Program
Orangeburg, New York

Jane Evans, MSc (Chapter 22)
Adjunct Senior Lecturer
Charles Sturt University, Port Macquarie
New South Wales Australia

Nicole A. Fidanza, OTD, OTR/L (Chapter 9)
Clinical Assistant Professor of Occupational Therapy
Quinnipiac University
Hamden, Connecticut

Kelle DeBoth Foust, PhD, OTR/L (Chapters 10 and 16)
Associate Professor
Cleveland State University
Cleveland, Ohio

Avi Friedman, DPT (Chapter 5)
Co-Founder & COO
LINK Home Therapy
Howell, New Jersey

Katie J. Galezniak, MS, OTR/L (Chapter 5)
Occupational Therapist
Director of Rehabilitation
Certified Fall Prevention Specialist
LINK Home Therapy
Atco, New Jersey

Cheryl A. Hall, PT, DHSc, MBA (Chapter 4)
Associate Professor and Program Chair
New York Insitute of Technology
Old Westbury, New York

Lisa Hanson, PhD, MBA, B. Physio (Hons), Grad Cert Higher Ed (Chapter 3)
Associate Professor
Rural Health
La Trobe Rural Health School
La Trobe University, Bendigo
Victoria, Australia

Brad Hodge, PhD, B. Psychological Science (with Hons) (Chapter 3)
Project Coordinator
Rural Health Innovation Lab
La Trobe Rural Health School
La Trobe University, Bendigo
Victoria, Australia

Sharon Holt, MHS, OTRL (Chapter 12)
Full-Time Lecturer III
Health Sciences
Eastern Michigan University
Ypsilanti, Michigan

Tamera Keiter Humbert, DEd, OTR/L, FAOTA (Chapters 19, 20, and 21)
Dean
School of Human and Health Professions
Professor, Occupational Therapy
Elizabethtown College
Elizabethtown, Pennsylvania

Nerida Hyett, PhD, MHSc, BOT, Grad Cert Higher Ed (Chapter 3)
Adjunct Lecturer
La Trobe Rural Health School
La Trobe University, Bendigo
Victoria, Australia

Michele Karnes, EdD, OTR (Chapter 6)
Retired

Jacqueline Kendona, OTD, OTR/L (Chapter 8)
Adjunct Assistant Professor
New York Institute of Technology
Old Westbury, New York

Julie Kugel, OTD, OTR/L (Chapter 7)
Professor
Loma Linda University
Loma Linda, California

Alexander Lopez, JD, OT/L, FAOTA (Chapter 4)
Associate Professor
New York Insitute of Technology
Old Westbury, New York

Melissa Neagles, OTR/L (Chapter 5)
Occupational Therapist
Certified Hand Therapist
The Orthopaedic Institute
Gainesville, Florida

Sandra M. Ribeiro, PT, DPT, MSEd (Chapter 4)
Associate Professor,
CUNY-LaGuardia C.C.
Queens, New York

Nadia Rust, OT, OTD (Chapter 2)
Tenured Associate Professor
Dominican University New York
Occupational Therapy Program
Orangeburg, New York

Amy Sawyer, B.Bus; B.Soc.Sc (Chapter 22)
Mid North Coast Local Health District, Health Promotion
New South Wales, Australia

John M. Schaefer, PhD, BCBA-D (Chapters 10 and 16)
Associate Professor
Cleveland State University
Cleveland, Ohio

Elizabeth Oates Schuster, MSW, PhD (Chapter 18)
Professor Emeritus, Social Work
Eastern Michigan University
Ypsilanti, Michigan

Phyllis Simon, OTD, OTR/L, FNAP (Chapter 15)
Department of Rehabilitation and Regenerative Medicine
Programs in Occupational Therapy
Vagelos College of Physicians and Surgeons
Columbia University
New York, New York

Kathleen Tithof, LMSW, LCSW, LICSW (Chapter 12)

Christine Urish, PhD, OTR/L, BCMH, FAOTA, CCAP (Chapter 14)
Professor of Occupational Therapy and
Doctoral Capstone Coordinator
Drake University
Des Moines, Iowa

Emmy Vadnais, OTR/L (Chapters 19, 20, and 21)
Director
Holistic OT Community
Occupational Therapist
St. Paul, Minnesota

Deanna Waggy, OTR, MSA (Chapter 19)
Owner
DW Healing Arts LLC
South Bend, Indiana

Madalynn Wendland, PT, DPT, ATP, Board-Certified Pediatric Clinical Specialist (Chapters 10 and 16)
Associate Dean for Curriculum and Operations
College of Health
Cleveland State University
Cleveland, Ohio

Erica K. Wentzel, OTD, OTR/L (Chapter 17)
Assistant Professor
Occupational Therapy Program
Elizabethtown College
Elizabethtown, Pennsylvania

Gail Whiteford, PhD (Chapter 22)
Emeritus Professor
Charles Sturt University
New South Wales, Australia

Andrea Gossett Zakrajsek, OTD, OTRL, FNAP (Chapters 12 and 18)
Professor
Health Sciences
Eastern Michigan University
Ypsilanti, Michigan

Introduction

Shifting the Health Care Paradigm: Interprofessionalism, Community Practice, and the Promotion of Health, Well-Being, and Quality of Life

Adolph Meyer, a psychiatrist, stated, "Our conception of man is that of an organism that maintains and balances itself in the world of reality and actuality by being in active life and active use. . . . It is the use that we make of ourselves that gives the ultimate stamp to our every organ" (1922, p. 1). Thus, engagement in the world and viewing health and well-being from a holistic perspective is directly related to being useful, active, and productive (Pizzi & Richards, 2017). According to the *Ottawa Charter for Health Promotion*:

> Health is created and lived by people within the settings of their everyday life; where they work, learn, play and love.... Health is created by caring for oneself and others, by being able to make decisions and have control over one's life circumstances. (World Health Organization, 1986, p. 4)

The constant health care policies and changes in the provision of service delivery creates optimal opportunity for interprofessional teams to rise to the occasion and meet the growing need for promoting and maintaining healthier living, preventing disease, and minimizing and preventing disability. Health professionals of any discipline need to create opportunities, environments, and conditions wherein health, well-being, and quality of life can be realized. The imperative is here to develop plans of action for individuals, communities, and organizations; devise strategies for implementation; and develop actions for sustainability.

Unlike most countries of the world, health care in the United States is crisis oriented. A loved one falls over a rug and fractures a hip, unhealthy habits and sedentary behaviors helped to create the obesity epidemic, or barriers for wheelchair mobility continuing to impede community engagement are some examples of health and well-being crises. A focus on prevention strategies to promote health and well-being and targeting improved quality of life for all should be the primary focus of health care.

This book was designed with the intention to shift the paradigm from medical models of care and rehabilitation after disease, illness, or disability to prevention and health promotion for individuals, communities, and organizations. We are not minimizing the need for medical and rehabilitation interventions, but rather shifting the emphasis. In several chapters of this book, there are strategies for integrating principles of health promotion and wellness into rehabilitation as well as during medical intervention. For example, when a client presents symptoms of stroke or a transient ischemic attack, any medical professional can have a conversation about possible etiology that is within the individual's control, such as smoking, weight, and sedentary behaviors, just to increase health awareness to possibly prevent a reoccurrence.

This 21st century paradigm shift, across disciplines, is needed as the U.S. health care system struggles with the lack of preventive care and self-care needed to promote healthier living. Anyone reading this text has responsibility to best serve our clients, patients, and ourselves.

The book is divided into two distinct parts, with the thread of interprofessionalism throughout. Part I are topics related to all disciplines and all areas of health care that are written from interprofessional perspectives and focus on the various needs of all populations. Diversity, equity, justice, and inclusion is a topic very recently brought into greater focus. While there is one chapter solely dedicated to those issues, several chapters dedicate sections to highlight how addressing those issues improve the quality of life, not just of individuals, but also for entire communities.

Parts II through VII are focused on six areas of health: physical, social, occupational/productivity, mental/emotional, family, and spiritual. The chapters for each of those health areas are written to provide readers with a developmental perspective on prevention and health promotion. Within each chapter are sections on interprofessionalism, community practice, assessment, and interventions, with most chapters illustrating the points made through a case study.

Most chapters are written by authors with practical experience of interprofessionalism from various parts of the world. The authors represent a diversity of experiences in academia, research, and clinical practice. Each chapter in the well-being and prevention section of the book contains case studies so students can best learn how to apply the basic principles discussed within each chapter. This in and of itself makes this textbook unique and innovative. The book is also intended to educate all health professionals and students on the importance of teaching and learning about prevention and how best to create healthy individuals, communities, and organizations.

Our hope is that the paradigm shift discussed in this textbook can be incorporated into current and future academic programs and inspire students in all health care disciplines to learn about, implement, and integrate prevention and health promotion to best serve individuals, communities, and organizations. It is our distinct pleasure and privilege to create this bold and innovative textbook to shift our thinking about health and health care service delivery.

—Michael A. Pizzi, PhD, OTR/L, FAOTA
Mark Amir, PT, DPT, MPH, DipMDT

References

Meyer, A. (1922). The philosophy of occupation therapy. *Archives of Occupational Therapy, 1*, 1-10.

Pizzi, M. A. & Richards, L. G. (2017). Guest editorial—Promoting health, well-being, and quality of life in occupational therapy: A commitment to a paradigm shift for the next 100 years. *American Journal of Occupational Therapy, 71*, 7104170010. https://doi.org/10.5014/ajot.2017.028456

World Health Organization. (1986). *The Ottawa Charter for Health Promotion.* http://www.euro.who.int/__data/assets/pdf_file/0004/129532/Ottawa_Charter.pdf?ua51

Part I

PRINCIPLES FOR COMMUNITY PRACTICE TO PROMOTE HEALTH, WELL-BEING, AND QUALITY OF LIFE

CHAPTER 1

Promoting Health, Well-Being, and Quality of Life

Shifting the Paradigm of Health Care

Michael A. Pizzi, PhD, OTR/L, FAOTA

Learning Objectives

At the end of this chapter, the reader will:

1. Understand and discuss how health, well-being, and quality of life is addressed from an interprofessional perspective for individuals, communities, and populations (ACOTE B.4.8, B.4.23)
2. Design programs utilizing the concept of prevention of secondary conditions for people with disabilities (ACOTE B.3.4, B.4.3)
3. Acknowledge and integrate social determinants of health when creating interventions that promote health, well-being, and quality of life (ACOTE B.1.3)
4. Understand the concepts of the E-HOW Model and its use in supporting health promoting interventions and health programming in communities (ACOTE B.3.4, B.2.1)
5. Explore the use of three major health assessments to help determine health and well-being needs of individuals, communities, and populations (ACOTE B.4.4, B.4.5)

The ACOTE Standards used are those from 2018.

Key Words

Capacity Assessment, Client-Centered Care, Environment–Health–Occupation–Well-Being Model, Evidence Informed Practice, Health, Health Behaviors, Health Promotion, Health Risk Appraisal/Assessment, Healthy People 2030, Interprofessional Education Collaborative, Interprofessional team, MAP-IT Framework, Ottawa Charter for Health Promotion, PATCH Framework, People with Disabilities Social Determinants of Health, Pizzi Health and Wellness Assessment, Prevention, WHOQOL-BREF

Pizzi, M. A., & Amir, M. (Eds.). *Interprofessional Perspectives for Community Practice: Promoting Health, Well-Being, and Quality of Life* (pp. 3-17).

Introduction

Health and the promotion of such has been defined in numerous ways by many organizations, philosophers, and medical practitioners. Over time, views of health and the myriad ways to improve health and prevent illness and disease have evolved, as new scientific knowledge provides information that also changes practice and practitioners' views about health. One of the earliest definitions of health was provided by the Greek statesman Pericles (c. 495 to 429 BC) who described **health** as the "state of moral, mental and physical well-being that enables a person to face any crisis in life with the utmost grace and facility" (Wilcock & Hocking, 2015, citing Burn, 1956, p. 3). This is a definition whose major concepts have lasted through time and have been adapted over time. The World Health Organization (WHO) definition of health is the following:

> To reach a state of complete physical, mental and social well-being, an individual or group must be able to identify and to realize aspirations, to satisfy needs, and to change or cope with the environment. Health is, therefore, seen as a resource for everyday life, not the objective of living. Health is a positive concept emphasizing social and personal resources, as well as physical capacities. (WHO, 1986, para. 3)

As health is a resource of everyday living emphasizing resources and capacities, the promotion of health, and by extension well-being and quality of life (QOL), requires practitioners to account for and be more inclusive of more than simply one aspect of the definition of health. The WHO definition emphasizes a strengths-based approach, alerting practitioners to explore a clients' capacities and viewing health as a resource for life and living.

Being a practitioner who embraces all aspects of one's being is quintessential to best practice when working with any individual, community, organization, or population in promoting health and preventing disease or disability. It often considers the need for interprofessional teams, while using discipline-specific tools, to work in tandem to provide best practice. This chapter will focus on the concepts of health, well-being, QOL, and promoting health as well as interprofessional work, assessments, and intervention principles needed for community practice.

Social Determinants of Health

As practitioners committed to promoting the health and well-being of individuals, communities, and populations, one of the most important concepts to embrace is that of being a facilitator of health. Health professionals can best accomplish that by gaining knowledge and subsequent expertise in the factors that determine health and well-being. One of the most important factors is understanding and incorporating the **social determinants of health** (SDH) into assessment and intervention.

> The SDH are the non-medical factors that influence health outcomes. They are the conditions in which people are born, grow, work, live, and age, and the wider set of forces and systems shaping the conditions of daily life. These forces and systems include economic policies and systems, development agendas, social norms, social policies and political systems. (WHO, Social Determinants of Health, 2019b, para. 1)

Under the Ottawa Charter for Health Promotion (OCHP), the fundamental conditions and resources for health that expands the social determinants of health include:

- Peace
- Shelter
- Education
- Food
- Income
- A stable eco-system
- Sustainable resources
- Social justice and equity

These conditions for health speak to the need to examine and explore issues of global health and well-being, and not just those of a particular community or even a nation. However, on a micro-level, they also speak to the need for being holistic practitioners. Considering these conditions for health during assessment and intervention promotes best practice. An example of this is provided (Professional Reasoning Box A).

The Ottawa Charter for Health Promotion

The first conference on health promotion was held in Ottawa Canada in 1986 from which the OCHP was conceived. The intention of the Charter was to create an international movement to improve the health and well-being of all people. The participants in this conference pledged:

- To move into the arena of healthy public policy, and to advocate a clear political commitment to health and equity in all sectors
- To counteract the pressures toward harmful products, resource depletion, unhealthy living conditions and environments, and bad nutrition; and to focus attention on public health issues such as pollution, occupational hazards, housing, and settlements
- To respond to the health gap within and between societies, and to tackle the inequities in health produced by the rules and practices of these societies

Professional Reasoning Box A

Bill and Mary are both social work students. They both aspire to help victims of domestic violence. Bill comes from a neighborhood with high rates of drugs and violence. His dad is a single parent who must work two full-time jobs to provide for his three children. Bill comes from a marginalized population and is often anxious and stressed each day over his living situation, including being concerned about having sufficient food to eat. Along with being a student, Bill works a full-time job. Mary lives in a spacious five-bedroom home in a safe and resource-affluent neighborhood. She is the only child getting full-time attention from two parents. She went to a boarding school and does not have to work while attending school.

Discuss the social determinants of health related to Bill and Mary, and the potential impacts on their academics and lives in general.

If you were to assess Bill and Mary, would an assessment of their health and well-being yield different or the same outcomes? How and why?

- To acknowledge people as the main health resource; to support and enable them to keep themselves, their families, and friends healthy through financial and other means, and to accept the community as the essential voice in matters of its health, living conditions, and well-being
- To reorient health services and their resources toward the promotion of health; and to share power with other sectors, other disciplines, and, most importantly, with people themselves
- To recognize health and its maintenance as a major social investment and challenge; and to address the overall ecological issue of our ways of living (WHO, OCHP, 1986, para. 1)

While there is still more work to be done, the Charter provided a template for promoting health and well-being for individuals, communities, and populations that health professionals today can continue to follow. The above commitments speak to changing policies, understanding how environment(s) influence health, addressing health disparities, and recognizing the social determinants of health as a primary factor in the health of individuals and communities.

> .... health and well-being are intimately connected with societal and environmental factors: what people do throughout their lives and day by day; how they experience and feel about what they do and how they plan ahead, legislate or dream; how they interact with others and belong to families, communities and places through what they do; and how collectively and individually they are in a state of continual transformation through what they do. (Wilcock & Hocking, 2015, p. 140)

Health Promotion

Health promotion is defined by the WHO as "the process of enabling people to increase control over, and to improve, their health" (n.d., para. 1). Thus, as stated earlier, health professionals who truly practice health promotion enable others by being the facilitator of health, or by being a health change agent. This is a client-centered and client-driven process, as the health professional, while having expert knowledge, does not dictate what is to be done, which is currently practiced in the medical model. Rather, those committed to the promotion of health, well-being, and QOL, educate, advocate, and offer opportunities for people, young and old, to take control of their health using the available resources in one's personal life and community and proposing opportunities for growth.

Health, as defined earlier, includes such factors as realizing one's own aspirations, satisfying one's needs, and adapting, changing, and coping with environmental demands. When a person can adapt to demands of social, cultural, and physical environments, their health is concomitantly adapting in a positive way. However, the reverse is also true, and ill health—mental, physical, social, and spiritual—can occur if one is unable to cope or adapt. Health is also determined by one's attitudes, emotions, and the meaning one attributes to the activities engaged in; thus it is a personal phenomenon that is not the same for each person (Professional Reasoning Box B).

Health promotion also encompasses prevention of disease. **Prevention** can be defined as "anticipatory action taken to reduce the possibility of an event or condition from occurring or developing, or to minimize the damage that may result from the event or condition if it does occur" (Pickett & Hanlon, 1990, p. 81). There are three levels of prevention that are defined as primary, secondary, and tertiary (Table 1-1).

Wilma West, an occupational therapy pioneer who focused much of her work advocating for rehabilitation professionals to take more of a public health approach, including work in the prevention of illness and disability, proposed the following:

- Function as health agents (rather than therapists) with responsibility to help ensure normal growth and development
- Encourage occupation (meaningful life activity) focused programs aimed toward maintaining optimum health rather than ... intermittent treatment of acute disease and disability

Professional Reasoning Box B

Shania, who has diabetes, is anxious about having low blood sugar when she goes out, causing her to not socialize with friends who want to socialize after school, resulting in poor social participation, loneliness, and depression. If she was able to better cope with her diabetes, and understand how best to manage it, she would participate more fully with others, and likely experience more happiness and joy in her life. Her level of adaptation and coping with her social environment and medical status requires intervention.

Discuss how her mental, physical, and social health are impacted by her diabetes and anxiety.

What is needed and how might you intervene specifically with Shania to promote improved participation and mental, social, and physical well-being?

Table 1-1

Three Levels of Prevention

LEVEL OF PREVENTION	DESCRIPTION	EXAMPLES
Primary	Focus on healthy individuals to decrease susceptibility to illness or disease; intervening before ill health, disease, injury occurs	• Vaccinations • Altering risky behaviors • Educating about good nutrition or physical activity • Maintaining safe playgrounds
Secondary	Focus on those at risk; mitigating further progression of disease, illness, or disability	• Regular blood pressure testing • Safe needle sharing for substance users • Proper food intake to maintain a healthy weight
Tertiary	Focus on persons with disease or disability and attempts to prevent further complications	• Rehabilitation services • Cardiac programs for post-stroke survivors • Chronic disease management programs in the community • Removal of architectural and attitudinal barriers to social participation

Data source: Centers for Disease Control and Prevention. (n.d.). *Patch: Its origin, basic concepts, and links to contemporary public health policy.* https://wonder.cdc.gov

- Consider more fully, and in a new mold, the socio-economic and cultural, as well as biological, causes of disease and dysfunction
- Develop a HEALTH (author emphasis) model of practice with the assumption that health care would be as concerned with prevention as with rehabilitation
- Find more effective methods to enhance and enrich development of physical, mental, emotional, social, and vocational abilities
- Make a timely translation from a long time focus on activities of daily living for the disabled to advocacy of the balanced regimen of age-appropriate work/play activities for [people] in the predisease/disability phase
- Revisit their underlying philosophy and facilitate a broader application of existing knowledge about the effects of activity, or its absence, on health (West, 1967, 1968, 1969, 1970 as cited in Wilcock & Hocking, 2015, p. 427)

West's words ring true for today's health care landscape. No matter one's professional role, often practiced in a silo, the call and need for promoting health and well-being and preventing social, physical, mental, and spiritual health care crises should be emphasized as "traditional" programming for all health-related programs, particularly when working as an interprofessional team (Pizzi & Richards, 2017; Pizzi [in press]). For example, if an occupational, physical, and speech therapy team implemented their professional evaluations and included a health and wellness assessment, that health and wellness assessment would provide the interprofessional team with a client's own perceptions of their health and help the team develop a more comprehensive plan of care (Professional Reasoning Box C).

Professional Reasoning Box C

Mike the occupational therapist and Mark the physical therapist are working as an interprofessional team with Shira who recovered from a stroke. She is being seen on the stroke unit. Shira was a three-pack-a-day smoker and is obese. She lives alone and has few hobbies. While working with stroke protocols set up by the rehabilitation department, Peter and Paul also develop health promotion strategies to discuss and implement with Shira. Utilizing the rest periods during her neurodevelopmental and exercise interventions, they discuss how smoking and diet routines and habits contributed to her stroke. Once she acknowledged understanding of this, Shira told Mike and Mark about her daily routines (e.g., watching TV 12 hours every day), which also include an absence of much in the way of physical activity or leisure pursuits. They provided interventions that included doing something active during commercials (stand, walk around, engage in sit-stand for 10 repetitions). They also discussed slowly reducing the number of cigarettes smoked each day and having her develop an hourly schedule. These client-centered activities in client-devised routines were intended to promote healthier living for Shira, and help to prevent another stroke, all the while engaging her in a "traditional" rehabilitation program.

What are some other prevention-related and health-promoting interventions an interprofessional team can implement? Why and how would those strategies help Shira?

Healthy People 2030

Healthy People 2030 (HP2030) was released in 2020, identifying the goals for the next decade. The overarching goals of HP2030 include:

- Attain healthy, thriving lives and well-being, free of preventable disease, disability, injury, and premature death.
- Eliminate health disparities, achieve health equity, and attain health literacy to improve the health and well-being of all.
- Create social, physical, and economic environments that promote attaining full potential for health and well-being for all.
- Promote healthy development, healthy behaviors, and well-being across all life stages.
- Engage leadership, key constituents, and the public across multiple sectors to take action and design policies that improve the health and well-being of all (USDHHS, 2019a, 2019b).

Health professionals can review the current version at http://healthypeople.gov, which will help develop community programming and intervention strategies to address documented unmet health needs of people with and without disabilities.

HP2030 established health indicators that needed primary focus. Those included:

- Access to health services
- Clinical preventive services
- Environmental quality
- Injury and violence
- Maternal, infant, and child health
- Mental health
- Nutrition, physical activity, and obesity
- Oral health
- Reproductive and sexual health
- Social determinants
- Substance abuse
- Tobacco (USDHHS, 2019a, 2019b).

These indicators, or areas of health, on which to focus are expected to promote health and well-being for individuals and make communities safer, healthier, and accessible. Promoting health and well-being, as well as preventing illness and disability, needs to be a primary focus for all health professionals. Those students and professionals in the rehab sciences can incorporate principles of health promotion and well-being as part of their rehabilitation protocols. Focusing on individual components of humans—be it the mind, body, or spirit—diminishes the very being of the client and does not promote client-centered care, but rather focuses on reductionistic thinking. Understanding that each professional is part of an interprofessional team who can better view the person holistically, is part of best practice for all health care professions (Professional Reasoning Box D).

Health Behaviors

The outcomes of well-being and QOL are directly influenced by one's **health behaviors**. Health behaviors, also known as health-related behaviors, are an individual's actions taken that can either promote and improve one's health status or be detrimental to one's health and well-being (Short & Mollborn, 2015). Health professionals' understanding of health behaviors, the dynamic interplay of health behaviors, and the factors that influence health behaviors of individuals, communities, and populations is important to successfully create programs that promote health and well-being. Smoking, sedentary lifestyles, eating habits leading to obesity, or overweight and risky sexual activities are some examples of health behaviors. For a person who is obese, there may be leading drivers of obesity such as loneliness, anxiety, and depression. Poverty can also be a driver of poor eating habits when the only affordable options to eating are foods that are high in calories and inexpensive, which may lead

Professional Reasoning Box D

Mark is a physical therapist working in an acute rehabilitation setting, where he sees many orthopedic clients. As he is treating Phyllis, a person who has fallen numerous times and is being treated for a hip replacement, Mark, through having Phyllis discuss her life history, learns she has low vision, has slight cognitive decline, and is a hoarder. Knowing this information, Mark is able to be the expert in treating her hip, but also refers to the social workers for the hoarding issue and the occupational therapist for low vision and cognitive interventions. He also recognizes the safety and mobility issues are clearly due to all of these issues, thus best practice includes work with an interprofessional team and being able to holistically treat Phyllis so she can return to her community day program she attends every day.

What might be other referrals to other team members? Why would you refer to them? Where might there be potential overlap of services and how would you address that overlap?

to unhealthy weight gain. All of these create a dynamic and constant interplay, concurrent with environmental influences and demands, which impact healthy living and influence healthy weight management.

Equally important is for interprofessional teams to acknowledge how all actions taken by individuals impact their health in some way—mentally, physically, socially, spiritually—and how those behaviors can also impact the health of others. Thus, no matter the profession, any action or activity undertaken by an individual, community, or population can be deemed a health behavior. For example, bathing is a health behavior. It is an action undertaken by one that is self-chosen to promote proper hygiene. If a person chooses not to engage in bathing, it becomes a maladaptive behavior and impacts one's hygiene, thus impacting one's physical and social health. Exercise or physical activity is another health behavior. When people exercise, it promotes positive mental and physical health; if not, one's physical health may deteriorate, necessitating interventions.

Both examples incorporate routines and habits of daily living. The development of routines and habits rely on motivation, structure, and organization. Thus, health behaviors always have both a physical and mental/emotional component. Conceptually, viewing all things people do as behaviors that promote health and well-being, in some way, we can then use the health behavior lens to be facilitators of health. This common language for health promotion programming can be useful no matter the profession. This common language can also assist in the development of communications that are open, transparent, and understandable through health care partnering with other professions, deemed interprofessional teaming.

Interprofessional Practice to Promote Health, Well-Being, and Quality of Life

Prior to working as an **interprofessional team**, it is important to build and establish a team that, together, speak the language of promoting health and well-being or at least have an understanding related to the concepts of health promotion and prevention (see Health Behaviors earlier in this chapter). It is also important that team members work within an evidence-based framework to support the assessments and interventions used for promoting the health and well-being of individuals and communities. Benz and Finch-Guthrie (2016) propose the following definition of being an interprofessional team:

> ….a group of individuals from various disciplines who have unique and complementary expertise important to the interprofessional evidence-based practice process, as well as have the team skills of working interdependently and establishing mutual accountability. (p. 64)

The **Interprofessional Education Collaborative** (IPEC; 2021) created several core competencies to enable best practice in interprofessional collaborations for community and population health programming and to enhance outcomes of service provision. The competencies include the following:

- Work with individuals of other professions to maintain a climate of mutual respect and shared values
- Use the knowledge of one's own role and those of other professions to appropriately assess and address the health care needs of patients and to promote and advance the health of populations
- Communicate with patients, families, communities, and professionals in health and other fields in a responsive and responsible manner that supports a team approach to the promotion and maintenance of health and the prevention and treatment of disease
- Apply relationship-building values and the principles of team dynamics to perform effectively in different team roles to plan, deliver, and evaluate patient/population-centered care and population health programs and policies that are safe, timely, efficient, effective, and equitable (IPEC, 2021, p. 10)

These competencies can be applicable to all health professions and academic programs that are committed to the enhancement of health outcomes for all individuals, communities, and populations. One of the areas of emphasis in these competencies is in the area of communication, both across professions and for clients served by those professions.

Using a common language to speak with each other, but also with clients and families, creates a unified approach to health service delivery in the area of promoting health and well-being and prevention within the ever-evolving health care environment. These competencies can be realized best when one considers a theoretical framework that can be utilized by any profession

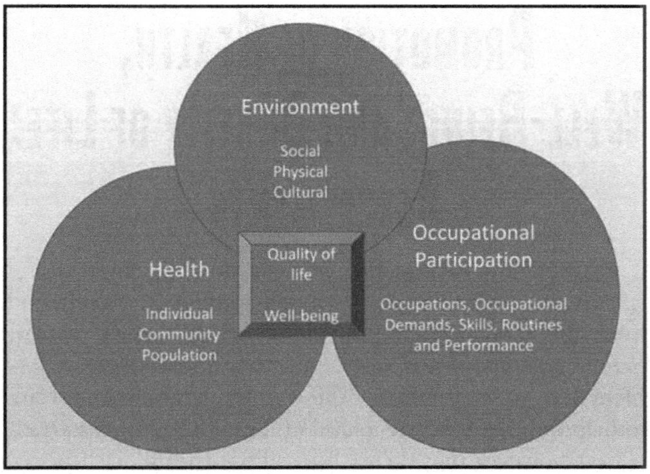

Figure 1-1. E-HOW Model. (Reproduced with permission from Michael A. Pizzi.)

Environment–Health–Occupation–Well-Being Model for Practice

Many models of practice diminish well-being and QOL as ultimate outcomes of practice. Instead, they focus on performance of a skill, increased function, or improvements in one's medical status. The ultimate outcome of service delivery in the area of promoting health and well-being, as well as prevention, is improvements in one's overall state of well-being and QOL. For example, even if one improves in a skill such as dressing or walking, or their diabetes is better controlled, it does not necessarily translate into an overall improvement in one's sense of well-being or QOL. These are very profession-specific areas of health and health behaviors, and thus, taken unto themselves, translate to a reductionistic approach to health. A more specific example is that of a person who experiences a traumatic brain injury (TBI), resulting in being medically stable, but whose function and overall state of being is disrupted for life. This TBI will influence the performance of meaningful daily tasks, mobility, and communication; however, it may not necessarily influence his ability to meaningfully participate. The definition of meaningful participation, though, is client-dependent and can change over time.

Participation in activity that is important and meaningful needs to be addressed over the performance of skill, as that participation promotes well-being for the person (Pizzi & Richards, 2017). In our current health care system, performance is the standard by which one is deemed to be "making progress" and is the factor that enables rehabilitation professionals to get paid for their work. It is time to re-examine the importance of well-being and QOL as the ultimate outcomes of all health care service provisions that are influenced and can influence participation in life.

One clinical model that emphasizes participation over performance is the **Environment–Health–Occupation–Well-Being Model (E-HOW) Model**, developed by the author and can be utilized by all professions (Figure 1-1). In this model, there is a dynamic interaction between the health status of a person, community, or population; the physical, social, or cultural environments in which daily activity (occupation) is engaged; and the participation in activities, meeting activity demands, skill performance, and engaging in routines and roles. The level at which this interaction occurs is the level of well-being and QOL as the outcome of that interaction. Well-being and QOL are the true outcomes any health professional desires for clients, be it a healthier individual, community, or population. An opportunity we have to expand on the triple aim of health care in this ever-changing health care system is to focus on those important issues that matter to all human beings. QOL and well-being are those important issues.

The following assumptions support the E-HOW Model:

- Individuals, communities, and populations strive to optimize their health, well-being, and QOL.
- Health, environments, and participation have a dynamic influence on QOL and well-being.
- Health behavior change can occur when clients become aware of a need for such change.
- Participation in daily activities that are meaningful promotes a positive health trajectory for daily living.
- Health is a resource used daily to pursue and participate in important and meaningful activity in life.
- Use of time for an individual, community, or population in meaningful, culturally relevant, and socially appropriate daily activities can be health promoting.

A final assumption that is foundational for the E-HOW Model is "interprofessional collaboration facilitates clients' health, well-being, and QOL" (Pizzi & Richards, 2017, p. 3). The model recognizes the need to look outside the silo of a single profession for the benefit of those being served and to develop collaborative partnerships to most fully be effective as health behavior change agents.

Promotion of Health, Well-Being, and Quality of Life: Assessments

Currently, in the fields of occupational, physical and speech therapy, social work, nursing, athletic training, and medicine, practitioners utilize profession-specific assessments mostly to assess a person with a disability or impairment of mind and/or body. These assessments are important to help the client restore a level of function, skill, or participation; however, they do not fully address health, well-being, or QOL. They are also not applicable to people who do not have a disability or impairment—people who, in communities and various populations, could benefit from health promoting and prevention programs to maintain and promote health and well-being, which is the thrust of this book. Programming and interventions can be individual or group/community oriented.

Throughout this book, readers will find numerous health- and QOL-related assessments in different areas of health for diverse populations. Following are three primary tools that can be used by all professions to effectively utilize for individuals, communities, and both disabled and nondisabled/well populations. To fully assess the state of health and well-being, and for a more complete evaluation that is client-centered, health professionals should use these to complement traditional profession-specific assessments. People with disabilities or any level of impairment also deserve interventions that promote health and well-being, thus should also be provided a health and wellness assessment.

Health Risk Appraisals/Assessments

Health risk appraisals (HRA), also known as **health risk assessments**, are assessments for individuals to evaluate health risks and lifestyle factors. Data is often collected by computerized questionnaires, which enable organizations and health managers easier and faster access to health data for community and population programming.

> In health promotion, most observers agree that HRAs involve more than the collection of health information. HRAs are techniques or processes of gathering information to develop health profiles, using the profiles to estimate future risks of adverse health outcomes, and providing persons with feedback on means of reducing their health risks. (Oremus et al., 2011, p. 1)

Once the data is collected, the information can be used to educate individuals, communities, and populations about their health status and motivate people to change any maladaptive health behaviors. Like the Pizzi Health and Wellness Assessment (PHWA) discussed next, the act of taking an HRA increases one's level of awareness of health status and possible maladaptive health-related behaviors about which the individual was unaware.

From a community and population level, HRAs have been utilized with health maintenance organizations, at the university level and, most often, are used at worksites (CDC, 2021; Oremus et al., 2011; Wellsource, 2021).

HRAs allow population health managers to collect important data to influence the success of their intervention efforts. This data can help identify and segment individuals who are at greater risk for chronic disease. HRA data can also be viewed in aggregate, helping population health managers identify trends and predict risks before they arise. For example, noticing that individuals are maintaining unhealthy nutrition habits suggests that future health conditions may surface. Population health managers can act by enrolling individuals into coaching programs or lifestyle mediation before it becomes a problem (Wellsource 2021, para. 2).

Health behaviors can also be viewed through the lens of social determinants of health. Utilizing this lens minimizes, but doesn't exclude, personal responsibility for health and one's personal well-being.

> [A social determinants approach] approach shifts the lens from individual attribution and responsibility for health behaviors—to societal organization and the myriad institutions, structures, inequalities, and ideologies that undergird observed variation in health behaviors. (Short & Mollborn, 2015, p. 82)

As mentioned before, there are several factors practitioners must recognize when assessing health behaviors, but also when creating individual, community, or population-based approaches for health behavior change.

World Health Organization Quality of Life Assessment

QOL is a social construct that differs among individuals and groups, as it is subjective and multidimensional. One's physical, mental, and social health can impact one's QOL, as can one's values and beliefs, work, family life, social life, and sense of spirituality. Health-related QOL is all those factors, including social determinants of health, that impact one's health status, and impact one's participation in meaningful life activity. According to the CDC:

- On the individual level, HRQOL includes physical and mental health perceptions (e.g., energy level, mood) and their correlates—including health risks and conditions, functional status, social support, and socioeconomic status.

- On the community level, HRQOL includes community-level resources, conditions, policies, and practices that influence a population's health perceptions and functional status.
- Based on a synthesis of the scientific literature and advice from its public health partners, CDC has defined HRQOL as "an individual's or group's perceived physical and mental health over time" (2018, para. 2).

The **World Health Organization Quality of Life (WHOQOL-BREF) assessment** is one of many assessments of health-related QOL. It is a scientific measure of the impact of health on QOL. While there is a 100-item QOL original assessment (CDC, 2018), the BREF is a shorter and quicker version with 27 questions. Both versions cover domains of physical health, psychological health, level of independence, social relations, environment, and spirituality/religion/personal beliefs. They were developed across cultures and populations and have been used in paper and pencil and computer formats, with good reliability and validity in both (Frank-Stromberg & Olsen, 2004). To obtain a copy of the WHOQOL-BREF, refer to https://depts.washington.edu/seaqol/WHOQOL-BREF (University of Washington, n.d.).

Pizzi Health and Wellness Assessment

The **PHWA** is the first valid and reliable assessment that focuses on having a clear client-centered approach that links participation in life with their perceived status of health, well-being, and QOL (Pizzi, 2001; Pizzi & Richards, 2017; Serwe et al., 2019). It can be administered as a self-assessment or used by a health professional during the client evaluation process. Different than most assessments used by health professionals, it is driven by a client's self-perceptions of their health status, using a Likert scale of 1 to 10 in six different areas of health: physical, social, mental/emotional, family, occupational/productivity, and spiritual. Once this section is complete and based on the client's initial rating, the client reflects upon each rating and answers standardized questions about their daily living and participation in their meaningful daily activity for each area of health. Clients are also asked for their level of wishing to change their participation level (from 1 to 10) and readiness for change in those health behaviors.

The subjectivity of this assessment promotes more of a client-centered approach, vs. those commonly used that are "expert" driven by health professionals. No health provider knows the person's life or what and how they feel about that life better than the person living that life. Too often health providers evaluate a person, then dictate what is right or good for that person based on their impairments, challenges, or the professional's opinion. This hearkens back to the medical model of care. Incorporating and using data that is client driven, related to their own self-perceptions of their health status and participation in life activity, there is a much clearer picture of who the person is as a human being, how they function, what is meaningful and important to them, and if they truly wish to engage in changing any level of participation for improved health. For those professionals that write health care goals, those goals are already written by the client who is provided the PHWA and interventions are created directly from the client responses.

It should also be noted that like HRAs, just having the PHWA administered alerts the person to potential areas for health behavior improvement by having the client reflect upon those areas of health that are likely not contemplated daily. Applying the Stages of Change Theory (Prochaska & DiClemente, 1982), one of the foundational theories used to develop the assessment, the client automatically shifts from pre-contemplation (e.g., I wasn't aware) to contemplation (e.g., maybe I should think about this). The health professional can then facilitate moving the person further along the spectrum of preparing to change, then to action or activities that promote change, and finally to developing habits and other strategies that help the client maintain a healthier lifestyle.

The PHWA can also be utilized to create healthier groups, communities, and populations. When working at the community level, the concept of **capacity assessment** is important to acknowledge.

> Capacity assessment is based upon the capacities, skills and assets of community members, agencies, and organizations … community members at all levels need to be involved in decisions that affect them; they should help plan programs where they are expected to be participants. (Nieto et al., 1997, para. 2)

Capacity assessment is very similar to participatory action research (PAR), wherein researchers and community members take part in problem solving a community need, form a research question, and then take action steps to solve the problem, and mitigate, in the case of health promotion, the health problems and prevent future problems. The main thrust of PAR is to identify and manage issues of social change, inequality, and to help communities take corrective action they might not otherwise have taken (Institute of Development Studies, n.d.).

The PHWA can be administered to all community members to determine health priorities among the majority of community members. The readiness to change question along with the aggregated data can lead to group decisions about which interventions might work best for the community regarding areas of health and well-being. For example, the aggregate data may show a majority of members wish to implement a community-wide weight reduction program. Group and community leaders would institute such a program based on the PHWA data. Program evaluation after a specific amount of time could then be implemented to see if

Professional Reasoning Box E

Ken is a 66-year-old man who is administered the PHWA. He scores himself a "6" in physical health due to being not very active during the day (he is a rabbi who sits to prepare services or watches TV). He is overweight and has some rheumatic pain. He also scores a "6" in mental/emotional health that he states is directly related to how he physically feels, which interferes with his perceived motivation. Ken does want to change his physical and mental health status but requires some coaching to improve his perceived health status and well-being.

What might be some interventions you would suggest? Why and how would they be implemented? How would you approach Ken to improve his motivation and change his health behaviors? How might you incorporate healthy habits to help Ken?

there is a change in both individual and community health and well-being.

Throughout this book, there are many chapters that address community programs and assessments. Other community assessments that directly or indirectly promote health, well-being, and QOL include the Walkability Checklist, which explores community safety (National Highway Traffic Safety Administration [NHTSA], U.S. Department of Transportation, 2021) and can be found at https://www.nhtsa.gov/document/walkability-checklist. This checklist is utilized to promote safe community mobility.

The **Planned Approach to Community Health** (PATCH) is a model for effective community health education and programming.

From its inception, the primary goal of PATCH was to create a practical mechanism through which effective community health education action could be targeted to address local-level health priorities. A secondary goal was to offer a practical, skills-based program of technical assistance wherein health education leaders in state health agencies would work with their local level counterparts to establish community health education programs (Centers for Disease Control and Prevention, n.d.).

Ensuring success for community health programming is essential. The **Mobilize, Assess, Plan, Implement and Track** (MAP-IT) strategy is one such strategy. MAP-IT helps communities plan and evaluate public health strategies (Community Toolbox, n.d.). There are many reasons MAP-IT can be an effective tool:

- It involves all stakeholders, making for a widely supported and community-owned effort.
- It assesses assets as well as needs and looks for ways to use them.
- Assessment means that the effort will start from the reality of the community, rather than from some preconceived idea of what's necessary or what resources are available.
- It produces a comprehensive and specific plan, with reasonable timelines, assigned responsibility, clear objectives, and well-defined action steps related to an overall strategy.
- It incorporates evaluation from the beginning, allowing adjustment when necessary (Community Toolbox, n.d.).

MAP-IT can be found at https://ctb.ku.edu/en/table-of-contents/overview/models-for-community-health-and-development/map-it/main.

There are many other assessments of well-being and those that relate to promoting health, well-being, and QOL (Professional Reasoning Box E). Utilization of these assessments on a regular basis will ensure that they become essential tools in the interprofessional toolbox (see Table 1-2).

Promotion of Health, Well-Being and Quality of Life: Interventions

In each chapter of this book, there are several interventions that are detailed for individuals, communities, and populations. Before interventions are created, there are certain basic principles that should be followed by all health professionals working collaboratively to support and promote health and well-being. These include being client-centered, evidence-based, and understanding the dynamic between the person/community/population and the environment.

Promoting Client-Centered Care

Throughout this chapter, the concept of client-centered care has been noted numerous times. It has been noted in the assessments described as well as the E-HOW Model. That is because the client—which can be an individual, community, organization, or population—makes the decisions, based on the information provided or known, to improve their health. A **client-centered practice** is "an approach to service that embraces a philosophy of respect for, and partnership with, people receiving services" (Law et al., 1995, p. 253) while

Table 1-2

Assessments of Well-Being and Related Constructs

ASSESSMENT	CONSTRUCT ASSESSED	DESCRIPTION AND REFERENCE	WHERE IT CAN BE OBTAINED
Basic Psychological Needs Scale—General	Well-being	A 21-item assessment of the basic psychological needs for autonomy, competence, and relatedness.	https://selfdeterminationtheory.org/questionnaires
Boredom Proneness Scale (Short Form)	Boredom	A brief 12-item assessment of boredom proneness composed of 2 components: internal and external stimulation.	https://scales.arabpsychology.com/s/boredom-proneness-scale/
COPE (complete and abbreviated versions)	Coping	Assesses a broad range of coping responses with either a 60-item version, or less burdensome 28-item version.	associationforpsychologyteachers.com/uploads/4/5/6/6/4566919/brief_cope.pdf
Swinburne University Emotional Intelligence Test	Emotional intelligence	A 64-item assessment of 5 forms of emotional intelligence including emotional recognition and expression, understanding emotions, emotional management, and emotional control.	www.researchbank.swinburne.edu.au
Meaning in Life Questionnaire	Meaning in life	A 10-item assessment of the presence of meaning in life and the search for meaning in life.	www.michaelfsteger.com/?page_id=13
Medical Outcome Health Survey Short Form (SF-36) Version 2	HRQOL	A 36-item survey which broadly assesses 2 aspects of HRQOL: physical and mental health.	www.qualitymetric.com
Positive and Negative Affect Schedule	Emotion (affect)	A 20-item assessment of affect, including descriptors of positive (e.g., interested, enthusiastic, inspired) and negative (e.g., upset, scared, afraid) emotions.	https://ogg.osu.edu/media/documents/MB%20Stream/PANAS.pdf
Purpose in Life Test	Meaning in life	A 20-item assessment reflecting Victor Frankl's conception of life purpose and meaning.	https://scales.arabpsychology.com/s/purpose-in-life-test/
Sense of Coherence Scale	Meaning in life	A 29-item assessment of personal resources for managing stress comprised of comprehensibility, manageability, and meaningfulness.	https://positivepsychology.com/sense-of-coherence-scale/#scale
Ryff Scales of Psychological Well-Being (long and medium forms)	Well-being	Assesses 6 dimensions of well-being with either 84 or 54 items, including self-acceptance, positive relations with others, autonomy, environmental mastery, purpose in life, and personal growth.	https://centerofinquiry.org/uncategorized/ryff-scales-of-psychological-well-being/
Ways of Coping Questionnaire	Coping	A 66-item questionnaire that assesses thoughts and actions that individuals use to cope with the stressful encounters of everyday living.	www.mindgarden.com

Reproduced with permission from Eakman, A. M. (2015). Person factors: Meaning, sensemaking, and spirituality. In C. H. Christiansen, C. M. Baum, & J. D. Bass (Eds.), *Occupational therapy: Performance, participation, and well-being* (4th ed., pp. 313-331). SLACK Incorporated.

focusing on the meaning and importance of, in the case of promoting health, the health and well-being needs of the client. As discussed previously, incorporating and allowing client perceptions about their own health (e.g., using an HRA or the PHWA) for creating community health promotion interventions (e.g., using capacity assessments or PAR) is critical to motivate, engage, and enable optimal participation of the client in promoting health, well-being, and ultimately, QOL.

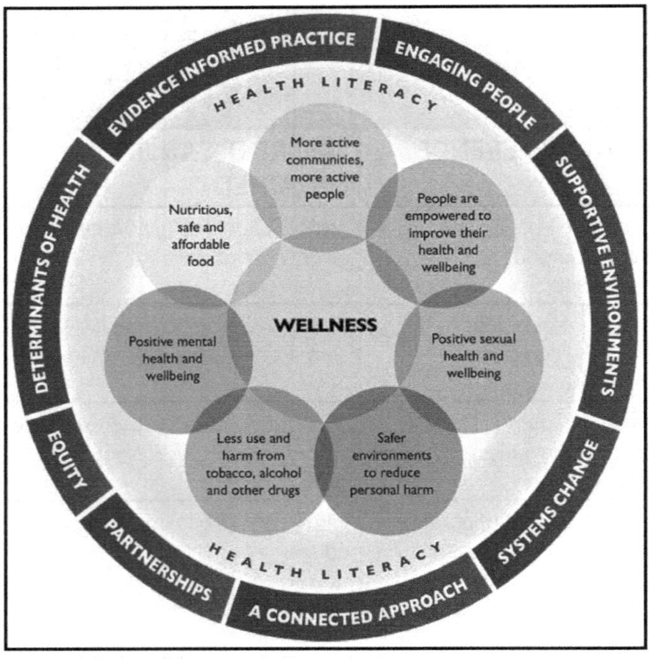

Figure 1-2. Welcome to working in health promoting ways. (Reproduced with permission from Department of Health, Tasmania, Australia, 2015.)

Using and Creating an Evidence Base: Evidence-Informed Practice

To state that a particular assessment or intervention is effective, health care practitioners also need evidence that the assessment or intervention works. This is becoming more critical, especially for increased funding through grants or even private donors and to continue to justify why a program should continue, even though you "know" your program is meeting the needs of the community. While thinking a program is effective because people and communities "seem" healthier, it is the evidence that supports one's opinion.

Bennett (2015), citing the Evidence-Based Medicine Working Group (Sackett et al., 1997), describes, briefly, the process of gathering evidence:

1. Forming clinical questions reflecting the information needed.
2. Searching for the best research evidence most appropriate for answering the clinical question.
3. Critically appraising evidence for its validity or rigor, impact (size or effect), and applicability (usefulness).
4. Integrating the research evidence with clinical experience, client's values, and circumstances (and information from the practice context).
5. Evaluating the effectiveness and efficiency with which the previous steps were carried out and how it might be improved in future (p. 95).

The Tasmanian government (TSA) has proposed that, for health promotion practice, one would:

- Consider the best data available from reliable and high-quality sources.
- Use the evidence to plan and implement actions.
- Consider both short-term and long-term effective outcomes.
- Take into account the capacity of the individual, organization, or community.
- Be sensitive to the specific context in which the health issue occurs (e.g., setting, culture, history and available resources).
- Recognize that moral, ethical, cultural, and spiritual values may affect actions to improve health, as a client or a practitioner.
- Be applied in a systematic way for high-quality evaluation.
- Use different measures such as quantitative data (e.g., the number of people affected) and qualitative data (e.g., information gathered from interviews or open-ended questions; TSA, n.d.b, Evidence informed practice, para. 4).

For health promotion practice to be realized, the TSA looks at eight factors described in Figure 1-2. While **evidence-informed practice** is one of eight factors, it is the driving force that supports sustainability efforts for community health promotion programs.

While exploring the literature for evidence, it is also critical to examine the need to create evidence. This is accomplished by developing research studies around health, well-being, and QOL and publishing them in peer-reviewed journals. Studies can be quantitative, qualitative, or both (mixed methods). It behooves all health professionals, especially as interprofessional teams, to develop these studies to provide clear evidence for improving health and well-being of individuals, communities, and populations. Other evidence that can be produced is program effectiveness. Once a program supporting the health of a community is developed, assessing the efficacy of the program before and after implementation provides the team (and researchers) evidence for future implementation, modifications, and sustainability.

Dynamic Interplay Between Client and Environment

As demonstrated by the E-HOW Model, it is crucial that interventions be understood in the context of environmental supports and barriers. A health intervention for an individual or community (e.g., a smoking cessation program) cannot be optimally effective if there are billboards in the community that advertise cigarettes or organizations that permit smoking within its premises. It is vital that communities create empowering and health-promoting environments where being able to make healthy choices is facilitated. Examples of this include:

- Direct action to create policies, such as tobacco control legislation
- Providing financial incentives or disincentives (e.g., sponsoring alcohol-free events)
- Advocacy for change (e.g., supporting community groups to advocate for banning junk food advertising to children)
- Providing education and empowerment (e.g., teaching people in a disadvantaged community the skills to research local health needs)
- Strengthening links between health and environmental strategies (e.g., implementing walking or cycling programs)
- Ensuring equitable access to supportive environments by mediating between conflicting interests in society (e.g., promoting sexual health and wellbeing for people with disabilities)
- Being inclusive in planning (e.g., consulting community members to identify the best approaches to health and well-being)
- Creating supportive settings for people using health services (e.g., making waiting rooms feel welcoming)
- Promoting health in the workplace (e.g., helping staff quit smoking; TSA, n.d.c, Supportive environments, para. 3)

Creating supportive environments includes understanding the impact of social determinants of health (e.g., food deserts in areas of high poverty), as well as promoting and advocating for health equity. Health equity is defined as everyone having a fair and just opportunity to be as healthy as possible.

> When everyone in the community has the necessary knowledge, skills and resources to achieve and maintain good health and wellbeing we will have health equity. It is having the right services provided in the right ways and in the right places. This is achieved by removing unfair and avoidable barriers that compromise health and wellbeing and by supporting fair access, fair chances and fair resource distribution to alleviate any disadvantage experienced by some people. (TSA, n.d.a, para. 1-2)

Understanding these basic principles for interventions will enable practitioners in all disciplines to create the most effective interventions for individuals, communities, and populations.

Promotion of Health, Well-Being, and Quality of Life: People With Disabilities

As defined above, there needs to be a health equity perspective, or opportunity to be as healthy as possible for everyone, regarding promoting health, well-being, and QOL. This perspective includes **people with disabilities** (PWD). According to Okoro et al. (2018), 25% of the U.S. population is experiencing a disability. PWD also deserve more equitable access to services that are affordable.

> In addition, people with disabilities may have trouble finding a job, going to school, or getting around outside their homes. And they may experience daily stress related to these challenges. Efforts to make homes, schools, workplaces, and public places easier to access can help improve quality of life and overall well-being for people with disabilities. (USDHHS, n.d., para. 3)

Under HP2030, there are many health objectives listed to focus on for the decade 2020 to 2030 (USDHHS, 2019b, para. 4). The following are some examples:

- Increase the proportion of adults with TBI who can do at least half of preinjury activities 5 years after rehabilitation
- Increase the proportion of students with disabilities who are usually in regular education programs
- Reduce the proportion of adults with provider-diagnosed arthritis who experience a limitation in activity due to arthritis or joint symptoms
- Increase the proportion of occupied homes and residential buildings that have a no-step entrance as a visitable feature
- Reduce the proportion of adults with disabilities who delay preventive care because of cost
- Increase the proportion of older adults with physical or cognitive health problems who get physical activity
- Increase the proportion of state and DC health departments with programs aimed at improving health in people with disabilities (USDHHS, 2019b, para. 4)

While those working rehabilitation provide interventions related to improving skills or function, it is now vital that we recognize how those improvements yield health and well-being benefits, and how they enhance one's QOL. For example, when a home assessment reveals the need for a ramp, the person utilizing that newly installed ramp has accessibility they didn't have before, which improves participation in

Professional Reasoning Box F

Sharma is a 22-year-old adult and a wheelchair user since her car accident when she was 20. Since then, she has had numerous decubiti, painful hands, and has been anxious and occasionally withdrawn. She has had a very difficult time coping with going from being a vital young college student to identifying as a "cripple." Her family values independence and creating your own life. These issues have impacted her participation in daily life activities, many of which were meaningful and important to her.

What might be some physical, social, emotional, and cultural issues that should be considered secondary conditions for Sharma? How might you use a prevention framework to help guide her toward recovery?

one's community and enhances one's sense of well-being and QOL, despite any level of disability.

> Health status is critically important to experiencing QOL, maintaining independence and participating fully in society...maintaining health and wellness is essential to reduce the impact of impairment on functioning and to foster positive development. (Pizzi, 2010, p. 392)

Prevention and the promotion of health also includes the prevention of secondary conditions. **Secondary conditions** can be defined as "those physical, medical, cognitive, emotional, or psychosocial consequences to which persons with disabilities are more susceptible by virtue of an underlying impairment, including adverse outcomes in health, wellness, participation and quality of life" (Hough, 1999, p. 162). Mitigating secondary conditions for PWD requires a paradigm shift from solely medical intervention to promoting and incorporating healthier living and giving control over one's health and well-being to the client. A prevention framework is required for implementation of this paradigm shift (Professional Reasoning Box F).

> Therefore, having a disability is viewed as increasing one's risk for a variety of preventable problems that can limit health, functional capacity, participation in life activities and independence. A prevention framework that incorporates rehabilitation interventions and themes of consumer empowerment can be offered using a public health orientation. (Frey et al., 2000, p. 362)

Conclusion

There is a slow but steady transformation in health care toward more emphasis on prevention and the promotion of healthier living. Health professionals and students have an opportunity to be health agents and facilitators of healthy living, working together in interprofessional teams for the health of individual clients, but also to help create healthy communities. Using a prevention framework that is also supported by the E-HOW Model, health and well-being assessments can be used and interventions can be created for clients who can defined as individuals, communities, organizations, or populations.

All people deserve the right to an optimal, equitable, fair, and just health care delivery, without bias, discrimination, or artificial barriers. That includes PWD and those in marginalized communities who have disproportionately poor health outcomes. We all must strive to develop holistic approaches to health service delivery, often best delivered by interprofessional teams, with a framework of prevention, in the service of all clients.

Health is created and lived by people within the settings of their everyday life: where they work, learn, play, and love. Health is created for oneself and others by being able to make decisions and have control over one's life circumstances. Caring, holism, and ecology are essential issues in developing strategies for health promotion and wellness (WHO, OCHP, 1986, p. 1).

References

Bennett, S. (2015). Using evidence to guide practice. In C. H. Christiansen, C. M. Baum, & J. D. Bass (Eds.). *Occupational therapy: Performance, participation and well-being* (4th ed., pp. 93-109). SLACK Incorporated.

Benz, J. & Finch-Guthrie, P. L. (2016) Forming interprofessional teams and clarifying roles. In P. Moyers & P. L. Finch-Guthrie (Eds.), *Interprofessional evidence-based practice: A workbook for health professionals* (pp. 63-78). SLACK Incorporated.

Burn, A. (1956). *Pericles and Athens*. English University Press.

Centers for Disease Control and Prevention. (2018). What is health related quality of life? https://www.cdc.gov/hrqol/concept.htm

Centers for Disease Control and Prevention. (2021). Workplace health promotion. https://www.cdc.gov/workplacehealthpromotion/tools-resources/pdfs/HRA-Decision-Makers-Guide-508.pdf

Centers for Disease Control and Prevention. (n.d.). Patch: Its origin, basic concepts, and links to contemporary public health policy. https://wonder.cdc.gov

Community Toolbox. (n.d.) MAP-IT. https://ctb.ku.edu/en/table-of-contents/overview/models-for-community-health-and-development/map-it/main

Eakman, A. M. (2015). Person factors: Meaning, sensemaking, and spirituality. In C. H. Christiansen, C. M. Baum, & J. D. Bass (Eds.), *Occupational therapy: Performance, participation, and well-being* (4th ed., pp. 313-331). SLACK Incorporated.

Frank-Stromberg, M. & Olsen, S. J. (2004). *Instruments for clinical health research* (3rd ed.). Jones and Bartlett.

Frey, L., Szalda-Petree, A., Traci, M. A., & Seekins, T. (2000). Prevention of secondary health conditions in adults with developmental disabilities: A review of the literature. *Disability and Rehabilitation, 23*(9), 361-369.

Hough, J. (1999). Disability and health: A national public health agenda. In R. J. Simeonsson & D. B. Bailey (Eds.), *Issues in disability and health: The role of secondary conditions and quality of life*. (pp. 161-203). North Carolina Office on Disability and Health.

Institute of Development Studies (n.d.). Participatory Methods. https://www.participatorymethods.org/glossary/participatory-action-research

Interprofessional Education Collaborative. (2021). What Is Interprofessional Education (IPE)? https://www.ipecollaborative.org/about-us

Law, M., Baptiste, S., & Mills, J. (1995). Client-centered practice: What does it mean and does it make a difference? *Canadian Journal of Occupational Therapy, 62*(5), 250-257.

Nieto, R. B., Scaffner, D., & Henderson, J. L. (1997). Examining community needs through a capacity assessment. *Journal of Extension, 35*(3). https://archives.joe.org/joe/1997june/a1.php

Okoro, C. A., Hollis, N. D., Cyrus, A. C., & Griffin-Blake, S. (2018). Prevalence of disabilities and health care access by disability status and type among adults—United States, 2016. *Morbidity and Mortality Weekly Report, 67*(32), 882-887. http://dx.doi.org/10.15585/mmwr.mm6732a3.

Oremus, M., Hammill A., & Raina P. (2011). Health risk appraisals [internet]. Agency for Healthcare Research and Quality, July 6. https://www.ncbi.nlm.nih.gov/books/NBK254034/

Pickett, G. & Hanlon, J. J. (1990). *Public health: Administration and practice*. Times Mirror/Mosby College Pub.

Pizzi, M. (in press). Health promotion, well-being, and quality of life for people with physical disabilities. In H. Pendleton & W. Schultz-Krohn (Eds.), *Pedretti's occupational therapy for physical dysfunction* (9th ed.). Elsevier.

Pizzi, M. (2001). The Pizzi Holistic Wellness Assessment. In B. Velde & P. Wittman (Eds.), *Occupational Therapy in Health Care (special issue on community-based practice). Volume 13*, #3/4, 51-66. Haworth Press.

Pizzi, M. A. (2010). Health promotion for people with disabilities. In, M. E. Scaffa, S. M. Reitz, & M. A. Pizzi (Eds.) *Occupational therapy in the promotion of health and wellness* (pp. 376-396). F.A. Davis.

Pizzi, M. A. & Richards, L. G. (2017). Promoting health, well-being and quality of life in occupational therapy: A commitment to a paradigm shift for the next 100 years. *American Journal of Occupational Therapy, 71*(4), 7104170010p1-7104170010p5.

Prochaska, J. O., & DiClemente, C. C. (1982). Transtheoretical therapy: Toward a more integrative model of change. *Psychotherapy. 19*(3), 276-288. doi:10.1037/h0088437

Sackett, D. L., Richardson, W. S., Rosenberg, W. M., & Haynes, R. B. (1997). *Evidence-based medicine: How to practice and teach EBM*. Churchill Livingstone.

Serwe, K., Walmsley, A., & Pizzi, M. A. (2019). Reliability and responsiveness of the Pizzi health and wellness assessment. *Annals of International Occupational Therapy, 3*(1), 7-13.

Short, S. E. & Mollborn, S. (2015). Social determinants and health behaviors: Conceptual frames and empirical advances. *Current Opinions in Psychology, 5*, 78-84. doi:10.1016/j.copsyc.2015.05.002

Tasmanian Government. (n.d.a). Equity. https://www.health.tas.gov.au/wihpw/principles/equity

Tasmanian Government. (n.d.b). Evidence informed practice. https://www.dhhs.tas.gov.au/wihpw/principles/evidence_informed_practice

Tasmanian Government. (n.d.c). Supportive environments. https://www.health.tas.gov.au/wihpw/principles/supportive_environments

U.S. Department of Health and Human Services. (n.d.). People with disabilities. https://health.gov/healthypeople/objectives-and-data/browse-objectives/people-disabilities

U.S. Department of Health and Human Services. (2019a). Healthy people 2030: about healthy people. https://health.gov/our-work/healthy-people-2030

U.S. Department of Health and Human Services. (2019b). Healthy people 2030: framework. https://www.healthypeople.gov/2020/About-Healthy-People/Development-Healthy-People-2030/Framework

University of Washington. (n.d.). World Health Organization quality of life—BREF (WHOQOL-BREF). https://depts.washington.edu/seaqol/WHOQOL-BREF

Wellsource. (2021). The ultimate guide to health risk assessments. https://www.wellsource.com/health-risk-assessments/

West, W. (1967). The occupational therapists changing responsibilities to the community. *American Journal of Occupational Therapy, 21*, 312.

West, W. (1968). The 1967 Eleanor Clarke Slagle Lecture. Professional responsibility in times of change. *American Journal of Occupational Therapy, 22*(1), 9-15.

West, W. (1969). The growing importance of prevention. *American Journal of Occupational Therapy, 23*, 223-231.

West, W. (1970). The emerging health model of occupational therapy practice. Proceedings of the 5th International Congress of the WFOT, Zurich.

Wilcock, A. A. & Hocking, C. (2015). *An occupational perspective of health* (3rd ed.). SLACK Incorporated.

World Health Organization. (n.d.). Social determinants of health. https://www.who.int/health-topics/social-determinants-of-health#tab=tab_1

World Health Organization. (1986). Health Promotion: Ottawa Charter for Health Promotion. https://www.who.int/teams/health-promotion/enhanced-wellbeing/first-global-conference

CHAPTER 2

Diversity, Equity, Inclusion, and Justice With Community-Oriented Interprofessional Practice

Ayse Ozcan Edeer, PT, MSc, PhD and Nadia Rust, OT, OTD

Learning Objectives

At the end of this chapter, the reader will:

1. Identify the importance of diversity, equity, inclusion, and justice in a community-oriented health care context (ACOTE B.1.2, B.1.3; CAPTE 7D34, 7D8)
2. Understand a client-centered interprofessional approach to community-oriented practice (ACOTE B.5.2; CAPTE 7D28, 7D34, 7D37, 7D39)
3. Recognize the importance of developing cultural humility in health care professionals (ACOTE B.1.2, B.1.3; CAPTE 7D34, 7D8)
4. Apply the occupational and physical therapies' professional associations' missions to community practice (ACOTE B.7.1; CAPTE 7D4)
5. Emphasize and explore an interprofessional community approach to three case studies across the life span (ACOTE B.4.27; CAPTE 7D28, 7D37, 7D39)
6. This chapter will align with the twenty-first-century missions of both the American Occupational Therapy Association (AOTA) and the American Physical Therapy Association (APTA) to foster the long-term sustainability of the occupational and physical therapy professions and to reflect the diversity of current society. The objectives of this chapter will be to discuss the evidence-based concepts of justice, diversity, equity, inclusion, and humility as they relate to community-oriented practice for all disciplines. Additionally, the chapter will describe terms commonly used in the literature and provide examples of case studies that enhance the understanding and awareness of diversity, equity, inclusion, justice, and cultural humility that follow an interprofessional approach to address positive community health outcomes.

The ACOTE Standards used are those from 2018.

Pizzi, M. A., & Amir, M. (Eds.). *Interprofessional Perspectives for Community Practice: Promoting Health, Well-Being, and Quality of Life* (pp. 19-36).

Key Words

Access, Beliefs, Bias, Community-Based, Community Resources, Culture, Cultural Competence, Cultural Humility, Cultural Sensitivity, Customs, Diversity, Equality, Equity, Health Promotion, Inclusion, Interprofessional Approach, Justice, Occupational Justice, Quality Of Life, Stereotype, Wellness

Introduction

Globalization has led to an increased recognition of the world's cultural **diversity**. People within a particular community share customs, habits, and values; however, these individuals may share few, if any, beliefs and practices with people from other cultural groups. The increase of cultural diversity raises questions about ways to deliver appropriate and respectful health care to patients from other **cultures** (Foronda et al., 2016).

To meet the unique and diverse needs of clients in the community, health care practitioners need to understand the importance of cultural differences by valuing, incorporating, and examining their own health-related values and beliefs. In order to provide optimal care within multicultural communities, it is vital that health care practitioners reflect the racial, ethnic, gender, sexual orientation, immigration status, physical ability, and socioeconomic status of the community (Stanford, 2020). Health disparities exist and result in worse health outcomes. Theses disparities may include social factors such as racism, discrimination, and stigma (Subica & Brown, 2020). The health of a community is a shared responsibility of many entities as well as the people of the community (Stoto et al., 1996). Health care practitioners partnering with the community may promote health equality and equity through community involvement and engagement. A culturally relevant workforce and the implementation of a plan of care that is meaningful and compatible with the values and traditions of clients and communities will improve the effectiveness and quality of services (Ekelman et al., 2003).

It is imperative to develop a **community-based** interprofessional health care system that is effective, equitable, and inclusive in order to maintain the highest level of **quality of life (QOL)** and **wellness** in community-based health care (Table 2-1).

Community Health: Justice, Diversity, Equity, Inclusion

Given the growing multicultural and minority population in the United States as well as the shift from hospital to community settings, health care practitioners must understand clients' values, attitudes, beliefs, and behaviors to provide culturally appropriate interventions (Ekelman et al., 2003). The 2020 global pandemic caused by Coronavirus Disease 2019 (COVID-19) has highlighted health inequities within the United States and internationally. COVID-19 unequally affected racial and minority groups placing them at higher risk for illness and death (Centers for Disease Control and Prevention [CDC], 2021).

Equity and **equality** are often used interchangeably without thinking about their difference in meaning. As a result of terminology misinterpretations, health care practitioners may believe they are doing the right thing while actually compounding the problem. Health equality occurs when all people have availability to the same resources or opportunities to be as healthy as possible regardless of their social circumstances (CDC, 2021). Health equity recognizes that individuals have different requirements and resources are allocated accordingly so that equal outcomes are achieved. In order to achieve equity, it is essential to identify, eliminate, or modify health barriers as a just and fair response to health care disparities (Braveman et al., 2017) so that available resources are allocated appropriately. Social determinants of health such as discrimination, health care **access**, occupations, income gaps, education gaps, and housing are some examples of constructs that impact health equity. Public health agencies, policy makers, employers, community and faith-based organizations, and health care systems can play a role in promoting health access (CDC, 2021). It is crucial to develop a definition for community health that reflects the diversity and values of communities and how they make decisions. Goodman et al. (2014) define community health as a multisectoral and multidisciplinary collaborative enterprise committed to improving the health and well-being of citizens within a defined community, using public health science, evidence-based strategies, and other meaningful approaches in a culturally sensitive manner (Goodman et al., 2014, p. 5).

Increased diversity in communities creates opportunities and challenges for health care practitioners to develop and deliver culturally competent care and services that have the potential to reduce inequities in health care. **Cultural competence** includes providing effective health care across diverse cultures by working collaboratively and communicating effectively. Henderson et al. (2018) define attributes of cultural competence as respecting and tailoring care aligned with clients' values, needs, practices and expectations, providing equitable and ethical care, and understanding. Their concept analysis showed that moral reasoning is an important antecedent in cultural competence and has implications

Table 2-1

Terminology as Defined in the Chapter

Culture	An umbrella term that encompasses the thoughts, communications, knowledge, laws, actions, habits, **customs**, **beliefs**, values, institutions, and practices of any racial, ethnic, religious, or social groups (Bjarnason et al., 2009; Erlen, 1998).
Equality	Each individual or group of people is given the same resources or opportunities (GW Online Public Health, 2020. Equity vs. Equality).
Equity	The absence of unfair and avoidable or remediable differences in health among groups of people, whether those groups are defined socially, economically, demographically, or geographically (World Health Organization, 2021, Equity).
Access	Entailing the ability to secure a specified set of health care services, at a specified level of quality, subject to a specified maximum level of personal inconvenience and cost, while in possession of a specified amount of information (Oliver & Mossialos, 2004).
Justice	Equity and fairness for individuals, groups, and communities regarding resources and opportunities for their engagement in diverse populations (Farrer et al., 2015).
Cultural sensitivity	Employing one's knowledge, consideration, understanding, respect, and tailoring these attributes for an individual or group. **Cultural sensitivity** involves awareness of self and others when encountering a diverse group or individual (Foronda, 2008).
Cultural competence	A process involving the attributes of cultural awareness, the attitudes, knowledge, desire, and skills necessary for providing quality care to diverse populations (Swihart et al., 2021).
Cultural humility	Ability to maintain an interpersonal stance that is other-oriented (or open to the other) in relation to aspects of cultural identity that are most important to the person (Hook et al., 2013).

for health care practitioners if health care disparities are to be reduced and better health outcomes are to be achieved for culturally diverse communities. An optimal cross-cultural caregiving model needs to include an **interprofessional approach** with community members and health care practitioners.

Moving From Cultural Competency to Cultural Humility in Practice

Although the relationship between lifestyle behaviors and health has been well-established, health care practitioners' skills in changing health behavior have tended to lag behind other clinical skills (Stanford, 2020). The health care systems and health care practitioners must offer clients a holistic healing experience as whole persons, including their mind, body, and spirit. As a part of current efforts and programs, health care practitioners may receive cultural competency training; however, this may be creating a false sense of security for them. They may believe sufficiently competent after completion of training sessions since the term competency indicates mastery or successful acquisition of a skill set but should be mindful of remaining cultural competency gaps. Cultural competency training itself may also include **stereotypes** and **biases** that cause health care providers to make incorrect assumptions about persons from different cultures. Additionally, use of the term competence would indicate that health care practitioners have a prior understanding of the person's culture before engaging with the patient and meet the requirement to care for all cultures. These false assumptions can lead to misunderstandings, which can have negative effects on the delivery of health care services (Isaacson, 2014). Therefore, the focus of community-based health care should shift from competency to **cultural humility** (Tervalon & Murray-García, 1998).

In health care, "cultural humility is defined as a lifelong commitment to self-evaluation and critique, to redressing the power imbalances in the healthcare practitioner–client dynamic, and to developing mutually beneficial and non-paternalistic partnerships with communities on behalf of individuals and defined populations" (Tervalon & Murray-García, 1998, p. 7). To practice cultural humility, health care practitioners should be aware and humble enough to "say they do not know" when they do not understand a person's culture from their perspective. Green-Moton and Minkler (2020) state that "cultural humility is the ability to maintain an interpersonal stance that is other-oriented (or open to others) while accepting cultural competence as the ability to interact effectively with people of different cultures more of a learned/taught condition" (p. 4). The concept of cultural humility extends beyond the concept of cultural competence, since it is not always possible to know about cultures that are not your own. Foronda et al. (2016) performed a concept analysis of the term cultural humility, which was used in a variety of contexts from individuals having ethnic and racial differences to differences in sexual preference, social status, interprofessional roles, to health care provider-patient relationship. The following attributes of cultural humility were discovered: openness, self-awareness, egoless, supportive interactions, self-reflection, and critique. Although developing cultural humility and leaving the notion of cultural competence behind is in a way a paradigm shift that has long been needed among health care providers, a culture of cultural humility should be developed based on self-reflexivity, appreciation for clients' lay expertise, and openness to sharing power with clients, as well as a commitment to constantly learning from clients. To interact with cultural humility, health care practitioners must listen with interest and curiosity, be aware of their own biases, and seek a nonjudgmental stance when they hear what their clients are saying, as well as accept their inherent privilege as health care providers and be willing to learn from their clients (Khan, 2021).

Opportunities to Grow for the Health Care Practitioners

Promoting cultural competence and cultural humility in health care can be achieved from two perspectives: creating practice environments that support culturally humble and competent care and developing educational programs that foster cultural awareness and sensitivity among students in the health care professions (Purden, 2005). Jongen et al. (2018) emphasize that an increased focus is needed on evaluating the application of knowledge, attitudes, and skills in practice as well as the impact of cultural competence trainings on specific practitioner behaviors and their subsequent impact on health care systems and health outcomes.

There are many cultural competence training interventions that are quite generic in nature, without necessarily focusing on specific skill sets or types of relationships in health care.

There is also a lack of consistency in the measurement instruments used to assess cultural competency training outcomes. Additionally, tests and assessments validated for specific demographics such as the White, middle-class, English-speaking population may not be valid when used with a more culturally diverse population. Cultural bias exists with testing, and health care practitioners should be aware of the many factors that could influence performance and participation and determine the appropriateness of standardized test results and other methods of client and program evaluation (Chang & Richardson, 2020). In most cultural competence trainings, one key problem is the lack of a consensus on terminology and a definition of cultural competence, in addition to its related concepts. Another major problem is that cultural training does not measure changes or predictions in behavior (Bartlett, 2017). In other words, regardless of training or testing, behavior is unpredictable for better or worse.

Despite issues with tests, assessment tools, and the content and efficacy problems with regard to training materials, health care practitioners should seek relevant training opportunities that may improve their awareness, skills, and knowledge to appropriately administer and interpret tests and assessments with an understanding of their limitations. In order to improve overall health care and cultural knowledge in the communities, the health care practitioners should be trained in how to practice cultural humility. As part of cultural humility, health care practitioners must recognize and embrace the complexity of identities—that even within the sameness, there is difference—and that they will never be fully competent to address the ever-evolving and always-changing personal experiences of patients. Therefore, a sense of self is at the core of cultural humility (Khan, 2021). Health care practitioners should choose cultural training opportunities that provide long-term, comprehensive, multistep educational experiences emphasizing cultural humility as a dynamic and lifelong process focusing on self-reflection, criticism, and acknowledgment of one's own biases.

Occupational Justice

The Occupational Therapy Practice Framework: Domain and Process (OTPF; AOTA, 2020) defines occupational justice as "A justice that recognizes occupational rights to inclusive participation in everyday occupations for all persons in society regardless of age, ability, gender, social class, or other differences" (Nilsson & Townsend, 2014, p. 58; Townsend & Wilcock, 2004). Fundamental to this definition are the core concepts of social justice that embrace the broader interprofessional influence (Braveman & Suarez-Balcazar, 2009). In the field of occupational therapy, the concept of occupational justice is central to the key values and beliefs of occupational therapy practice and has an influence on but is not limited to client-centered practice, cultural humility, ethics, interprofessional collaborations, micro and macro systems knowledge, and occupational-based practice (AOTA, 2020).

It is important to adopt an occupational justice lens when working with client's thereby addressing concerns such as social inclusion that could be experienced by marginalized groups of people such as people with disabilities, those who are homeless, or have experienced trauma (Nilsson & Townsend, 2014). Understanding the cause of occupational injustices is critical to justice-related outcomes. Injustices relate to social policies that govern communities and populations that are structured to allow some people the experience of privilege and social inclusions while others may not have the benefit of full participation and inclusion (Nilsson & Townsend, 2014). The Occupational-based Community Development Framework (ObCD) is a framework developed by the University of Cape Town, South Africa, and promotes occupation as part of human rights (Mthembu, 2021). The focus on community-centered practice is aimed at social transformation in communities that have experienced collective trauma. Health care practitioners have an obligation to explore the broader scope and breadth of health care practice to include the impact of social policy and governance on the ability to provide equitable and inclusive care. Advocacy is defined as the act of speaking up or working on behalf of the interest of another person, group, or cause (Jacobs & McCormack, 2019). Health care professionals desires to make a difference and serve their client, community, and population include the need for professional advocacy, client advocacy, and advocacy relating to issues at a systems level, all of which are essential to balance disparities.

Relationship Between Health and Wellness Within Communities

The World Health Organization (2021) defines health as a state of complete physical, mental, and social well-being and not merely the absence of disease or infirmity. Wellness is defined as "the sense that one is living in a manner that permits the experience of consistent, balanced growth in the physical, spiritual, emotional, intellectual, social, and psychological dimensions of human existence" (Bezner, 2015).

Both in the United States and around the world, there has been a reported rise in people with chronic diseases related to lifestyles, for example, heart disease, cancer, chronic lung disease, hypertension, stroke, type 2 diabetes mellitus, and obesity (Rees & Williams, 2009; Dean et al., 2016). These and other chronic diseases are the leading causes of death and disability in the United States, and they are also a leading driver of health care costs (CDC, 2021). There are numerous modifiable risk factors associated with chronic disease hardship, such as tobacco use, poor dietary choices and physical inactivity (both strongly associated with obesity), excessive alcohol consumption, uncontrolled high blood pressure, and hyperlipidemia, that can be successfully addressed for individuals and populations (Bauer et al., 2014).

Physical and occupational therapists encounter clients daily in their practices who have unhealthy behaviors such as lack of physical activity, smoking, poor nutrition, inadequate sleep, and stress. Bezner (2015) recommends a move to transform the current medical system from one of treating illness to one of providing health and wellness in communities. Management of chronic lifestyle-related illnesses requires holistic, team-based care with collaborative and respectful interdisciplinary practitioners. Most practitioners advocate an interprofessional approach that emphasizes prevention of lifestyle-related chronic diseases through population and community promotion of health (Goodman et al., 2014). The health care systems focus on new health care delivery models for people with chronic diseases (Parra et al., 2017). A key element of these new models is the active involvement and partnership of health care practitioners with the person in the management of chronic conditions. The ideal partnership involves an integrated approach to patient care and self-management education (Reeves et al., 2017). Achieving optimal mental and physical health, in addition to addressing healthy nutrition, smoking cessation, healthy body composition, optimal sleep, and physical activity/exercise recommendations, improves the QOL for people living with chronic diseases in the community (Dean et al., 2016).

We believe that physical and occupational therapists have the opportunity to shift the way they view themselves relative to health promotion and wellness. The role of physical and occupational therapists in primary prevention is to assess, discuss, and educate clients on healthy behaviors and explain the connection between behavior and health. As part of their professional development, they should look for opportunities to fill gaps in their knowledge and skills regarding health and wellness by engaging in continuing education aimed at improving competency in health behavior change. Bezner (2015) emphasizes that all health care practitioners collaborate so that health-promoting interventions are coordinated and reinforced across all health care encounters and the patient or client feels supported and care is coordinated instead of disjointed and contradictory.

By connecting people who have chronic diseases or chronic disease risk factors to community resources, we can prevent or slow down the disease process, avoid complications, and reduce the need for additional health care when disease complications occur. Improved relationships between the non–health care community and clinicians result in participation of clients with proven programs. These programs are ideally with community organizations resulting in health care providers being eligible for reimbursement from health insurance payers (CDC, 2015). Improving availability and access to quality preventive services can help reduce disparities in health care. Health care programs at the community level provide people with chronic diseases an opportunity to prevent and reverse most chronic diseases, which improves a person's health outcome, **health promotion**, well-being, and QOL and downstream costs.

Barriers/Disparities in the Health Promotion in the Communities

Health inequities are defined as differences in the likelihood of achieving optimal health between different communities or within communities. Disparities in health opportunities may lead to unfair and avoidable differences in health outcomes for the individuals with chronic diseases, disability, and disenfranchised groups within various communities. Increased health care accessibility does not necessarily mean that health disparities will be reduced (Baciu et al., 2017). The burdens of disease and poor health, as well as the benefits of wellness and good health, continue to be inequitably distributed especially for individuals with chronic diseases and disabilities in communities.

Physical and occupational therapists should work collaboratively with the other stakeholders and focus to reduce health disparities in the communities to reduce differences in health outcomes. Bezner (2015) emphasizes that all health care practitioners collaborate so that health-promoting interventions are coordinated and reinforced across all health care encounters and the patient or client feel supported and care is coordinated instead of disjointed or worse, contradictory. Eliminating the root causes of health inequity will require considerable effort from all stakeholders in the communities; residents, businesses, religious leaders, community centers, government, health care practitioners, and academia, all of whom are in a position to promote health equity (Baciu et al., 2017). Nonetheless, health care practitioners, even in isolation, still have the opportunity to contribute to health equity and justice when they expand health care opportunities for the clients and in their community.

Community-Oriented Health Outcomes and Interprofessional Approach

Communities include diverse groups of people, as well as the locus (place, venue, or other unit) of programs, interventions, and other actions. There are various types of communities, including physical, work, social, and spiritual communities, each with distinctive priorities, needs, and cultures (Goodman et al., 2014). Community engagement is defined as the process of working collaboratively with and through groups of people affiliated by geographic proximity, special interest, or similar situations to address issues affecting the well-being of those people (National Institutes of Health, 2011). Partners in community engagement can include organized groups, agencies, institutions, or individuals. These partners may be engaged in health promotion, research, or policy making. Collaborative practice happens when multiple health workers from different professional backgrounds work together with clients, families, caregivers, and communities to deliver the highest quality of care across settings (WHO, 2010).

Partnerships are typically successful when members of the interprofessional team understand their roles and the roles of others. Relationships between partners need to be mutually beneficial, and any boundaries between partners need to be respected. These partnerships may be directed towards interprofessional education where team members are "engaged in learning with, from and about each other" (Purden, 2005, p. 226). When delivering patient care, an interprofessional approach can be affected by issues related to imbalances of authority, limited understanding of roles and responsibilities, and professional boundary friction (Reeves et al., 2017).

The CDC (2015) outlined seven core roles of community health practitioners in prevention and control of chronic disease, including mediating culturally between communities and health care systems, providing culturally appropriate and accessible health education and information, ensuring that people get the services they need, providing informal counseling and social support, advocating for individuals and communities, providing direct services and administering health screening tests, building individual and community capacity. The Interprofessional Education Collaborative (2016) updated their core competencies for interprofessional collaborative practice in 2016. One of the Values/Ethics (VE3) sub-competencies recognizes and embraces the cultural diversity and individual differences that characterize patients, populations, and the health team.

The development of a community-based interprofessional health care system that is efficient, equitable, and inclusive is essential to achieve healthier communities that lead to better health outcomes and QOL for all community members. Achieving social **justice** and equity are critical for health care to ensure that all individuals can maintain their highest level of health and wellness.

Case Studies

These two case studies provide real-life examples of culturally diverse groups and emphasize the importance of equity and justice in improving QOL and health promotion (Tables 2-2 and 2-3). The case studies are presented in a similar format, highlighting an interprofessional approach in community-based practice with a focus on cultural humility in the diverse communities.

Table 2-2

Case Study: Young Child, Interprofessional Evaluation

Joshua is a 10-month-old baby boy. He is the first child to his parents Alyssa and Johan. The family lives in a shared apartment with the child's paternal grandparents in the Bronx, New York. The family is originally from El Salvador and they have refugee status. The family members communicate with each other in Spanish. Joshua's parents completed high school at Bronx Central High and are currently employed. Alyssa missed many prenatal visits due to her work schedule. Joshua has been diagnosed with Down syndrome and there is concern of hearing loss. Joshua's pediatrician has recommended an Early Intervention (EI) evaluation. At the time of the evaluation, Alyssa confirmed that she has had a conversation with her EI Service Coordinator/Case Manager and has consented to the evaluations. The service coordinator recommended comprehensive multidisciplinary assessments to find the best support and intervention for the family.

EVALUATION PROCESS

Joshua's mother and paternal grandparents were present for the initial EI evaluations. The evaluations were scheduled for a Monday afternoon, as Alyssa starts work later this day. The EI team asked to schedule a home visit, which made Alyssa slightly uncomfortable. However, she eventually agreed to the visit. Alyssa was expecting two people and was surprised when a team of four arrived—a physical therapist, an occupational therapist, a speech therapist, and a social worker. Alyssa provided all medical and family history and indicated she has returned to work full time and that Joshua is cared for by his paternal grandparents. Johan works long hours and attends community college in the evenings; he is available to help with the baby on weekends.

The team asked questions to acquire more information about Alyssa's concerns and what baby Joshua is and is not yet able to do. The questions were in English and directed to Alyssa and she occasionally sought clarification about Joshua's development or routines in Spanish from her in-laws. Joshua became upset and cried midway through the interview and Alyssa became anxious as she was unable to calm him. Joshua's grandmother appeared upset and uncomfortable and verbalized that it was Joshua's mealtime and the child was hungry. The grandmother left to the kitchen to feed Joshua. The speech and occupational therapists stood at the kitchen door observing Joshua being fed. The evaluation team had questions regarding the food Joshua ate as well as the techniques used to feed him. These questions appeared to upset the family and Alyssa indicated it was time for her to leave for work and ended the evaluation session.

Define the Problems

1. What should be considered by health care practitioners prior to going into a community setting (e.g., home or school)?

Health care practitioners should be mindful and respectful when going into a home environment and understand that every family has its unique cultural beliefs, routines, and practices. They should understand health-related beliefs and spiritual influences. Health care practitioners should reflect on their own cultural heritage and possible biases and assumptions they might bring with them. Consider using an interpreter if needed, letting the family know the purpose of the visit prior to arrival, and reassure family members—this is especially important where they have sensitive refugee status. Schedule the visit when the primary caregivers are present, anticipate obstacles and resistance from family members, and explore how cultural humility could be applied during the initial visit maximizing use of time efficiently as a team. In preparation for the home visit the team should do their research to ensure a successful visit and establish an initial positive encounter with the family. The team should understand the implications of the family having refugee status, if applicable, as it relates to employment and health-related issues such as health insurance. Refugees are entitled to almost all assistance that any U.S. citizen can receive. The Office of Refugee Resettlement and New American Hotline are federal and New York state resources for the team to explore. It is important to be culturally responsive and recognize a few customs typically practiced and be prepared to use a translator if needed. The visit should be scheduled in advance with a clear understanding of the reason for the visit.

2. Define benefits of community-based intervention programs for this case.

Adopting a community-based design, in this case a home setting, allows the providers to work in the natural setting and understand the social context of the family. This allows for collaborative work between family members and health care practitioners. As a team the family and practitioners can explore the challenges and possibilities/solutions. The family members can have an active role in addressing issues that are of priority to them. A community-based program provides education, which promotes health, wellness, and prevention. This program will support the parents and caregivers, which increases their ability and capacity to support their child.

3. Describe potential barriers (e.g., gaps in the health care practitioner's knowledge of health beliefs and customs, community disparities and discrimination, biases, stereotypes, risk factors, minority status, social attitude, health-related beliefs, and spiritual influence).

Barriers in this case include gaps in the health care practitioner's knowledge of health beliefs and customs of the family. This is a family with refugee status. Therefore, mental health and post-traumatic stress must be considered. There

Table 2-3

Case Study: Older Adult, Community-Based Evaluation and Intervention

Nancy is a 73-year-old Caucasian female with a history of left cerebrovascular accident (CVA). During the COVID-19 pandemic of 2020 she relocated from central Illinois to Los Angeles to be closer to her children. Nancy lived her entire life in a small rural midwestern town. Nancy's stroke occurred 5 years ago and though she is independent with activities of daily living, she is having trouble negotiating her new environment and routine. She is cautious and lacks confidence in her abilities as she loses her balance frequently and relies on her cane more during ambulation. Nancy has had a few falls in recent months. Nancy's children are encouraging her to attend the daily exercise program at the recreation center, which she is hesitant to do. However, she agreed to a trial of the daily afternoon class at a senior citizen's community center.

Nancy has minimal experience with racial, ethnic, and language diversity including health care providers. Since attending the community program, she has expressed feeling uncomfortable and nervous. Despite these concerns, her family encouraged her to attend the fall prevention program. Her family also believes that this is an opportunity for her to be more involved within her new environment and community, make new friends, and learn about different cultures.

David is the director of the senior citizen center and is a registered nurse. The fall prevention program is run by Aisha, a physical therapist with 8 years of clinical experience. Aisha is an African American Muslim and a part-time employee of the center; she informs Nancy that it is necessary to complete a Timed Up and Go (TUG) test to determine her fall risk level and category. Aisha explained the importance of the test as well as the steps involved in the task. Nancy ignored Aisha's instructions and efforts and mostly communicated with David.

During her fall risk assessment check in, while David took Nancy's blood pressure, she asked if she could get a different physical therapist. When probed further by David, she expressed that Aisha has limited knowledge about her condition, she covers her head with a scarf, and is not trustworthy. David politely explained that it is not possible at this time to work with any other therapist and Aisha is a licensed physical therapist and has been working at the center for 2 years. He went on to explain that Aisha is an expert on fall prevention and runs similar programs at other centers. After Nancy's vitals were taken by David, Aisha approached Nancy and asked if she would be willing to start the TUG test with her. Nancy remained neutral, while Aisha explained that this is the best assessment for her situation. Aisha recognized some discomfort with Nancy and asked if anything was bothering her. Nancy revealed she had a negative experience with an African American woman years ago. Aisha, sensitive to the client's history, explained the test further, that she would take things slowly, and if, at any time, Nancy continued to feel uncomfortable, she would have someone else administer the test at a later time. Nancy agreed to have Aisha continue and completed the test. Afterward, Nancy told Aisha that her sensitivity and kindness made all the difference.

are also potential language barriers, financial barriers, and possible lack of knowledge on how to access health services. Other issues to consider include community disparities and discrimination, biases, stereotypes, and immigration/refugee status.

4. Describe the current problems/situation from a client, their family and friends, and interprofessional team's perspectives.

   Problems from the client's and family's perspective:

- Health care practitioners are intimidating and there is fear and anxiety related to family members' immigration status
- Lack of understanding of their family issues, beliefs, and customs
- Family feels judged
- Communication barriers
- Family health beliefs and customs are not understood
- Financial concerns
- Problems from the interprofessional team's perspective
- How to provide culturally responsive support
- Emotional support to parents and other family members
- How to provide services to and communicate with a culturally and linguistically diverse family
- Poor understanding of available social services
- Conflicting views and beliefs
- Coordination and efficient collaboration among team members

Develop the Solutions and Approaches

5. What cultural considerations should be thought of during interaction with the client and/or client's family members?

It is important to start off the relationship with the family members in a respectful manner to gain trust and build an alliance. This includes understanding the relationship between family members and family beliefs and the type of family structure. Effective communication, which includes being able to listen, is critical in establishing trust, as is consistency. Acceptance of diverse religious or spiritual beliefs and being sensitive to family members' customs, values, and practices are also important. Paying attention to nonverbal cues can help determine whether a differential power relationship is hindering communication.

6. How do you incorporate cultural humility into your decision-making process? Explore gaps in the health care practitioner's knowledge of health beliefs and customs as well as community disparities and discrimination.

It is important to explore and understand the beliefs of the client/family. Maintain a nonjudgmental outlook and focus on client-centered care with culturally appropriate approaches. Reflect on your own biases and be aware of potential historic biases against certain groups of people. Developing a tailored treatment plan for the client is possible with an egoless and humble approach. Openness and flexibility are key elements for the cultural humility.

7. What client outcomes and QOL factors should be considered (e.g., support wellness and QOL, mental health, social connections, physical health—well-being) in a community-based approach by an interprofessional team?

The focus should be on experiencing positive life encounters/events across settings and contexts, such as home, religious centers, recreation venues, or any community experience.

Client-centered outcomes support the holistic development of the child and the wellness of the caregivers. Educate, empower, and support the family in child development. QOL for the parents and family caregivers is critical for the well-being of the child. Consider associated stigma and the child's emotional and behavioral development. Social networks and resources that promote inclusion must be considered. Explore access to resources and support within the community and facilitate the ability to build or establish partnerships.

8. How can health care practitioners promote health equity through community practice and engagement? Explore community resources and partnerships, education, inclusion, awareness, support, and empowerment opportunities.

Recognize and acknowledge any disparities in the health care system. As a provider you need to understand and assess the resources available. Explore biases, stereotyping, and prejudice as these contribute to disparities. Be open to training and gaining knowledge regarding culture, which goes beyond knowledge, awareness, and sensitivity. When interacting with the different family members it is important to understand their perceptions of health service delivery. Examine the social context in which the family lives and collaboratively design interventions to address the family priority and needs and include a method to evaluate the success of these interventions. Issues that arise due to mistrust or communication should be addressed immediately. Share health information in an understandable way. Allow families to take charge of their own health decisions and respect the families' decisions. Understand the communities' capacities and resources to support this family within the community. Be aware that equality and equity are the main issues when **community resources** are not available and accessible for all individuals in the community.

9. Explore the benefits of a diverse workforce team.

A diverse workforce is represented by employees who are all different (age, gender, religion, sexual orientation, socioeconomic status). This brings varied views and opportunities and benefit both the health care teams and their clients.

A diverse workforce could also support removing barriers, increase access, and improve social justice in health care. A variety of viewpoints, expertise, and opportunities result in innovations. Within diverse employee groups, there is a benefit to include health care practitioners who grew up in the communities they serve as they will have a greater understanding of the community, its resources, and potential inequities. A diverse workforce builds respect and understanding of other cultures.

Reflective Questions

- Consider the different roles (therapist, educator/coach, counselor, provider of technical assistance) you have in a community setting.
- How do you educate yourself on your roles?
- What fears and possible stigmas are faced by families during the initial phases of diagnosis and developmental evaluations?
- Explore disparities in health care among two to three diverse populations.

Define the Problems

10. What should be considered in this community recreation setting?

The health care professionals should have a comprehensive profile and understanding of their clients prior to commencing an intervention. This should be obtained during the initial evaluation when consideration should be given to beliefs along with the medical and social history. Understanding Nancy's history of leaving an environment where she has lived her entire life will provide insight into her views, perceptions, and attitudes. Community services can help people navigate difficult life situations. The providers need to be familiar with the demographics of the population and the resources available in their community. Community health practitioners should also have the knowledge and skills to address a diverse array of daily living concerns and promote health and wellness. Since community service providers work directly with clients on preventative programs, they should comprehensively understand their clients' context. This includes environmental and personal factors such as physical, social, and attitudinal surroundings, in which a client lives (AOTA, 2020). Clinicians should understand the limitations and opportunities within their communities (Bezner, 2015).

11. Define benefits of this community-based intervention program.

The community-based program that Nancy attends focuses on prevention, health, and wellness. In Nancy's situation, the concern is with safety and falls. This type of program has a relapse prevention focus with chronic issues such as falls. Working in a recreation center provides opportunity for a more relaxed educational and wellness-focused environment with the opportunity for inclusion of family and friends. This community program will also provide Nancy with the chance to meet other people expanding her opportunity for socialization and friendships as well as increasing her exposure to the diverse population she now lives in. A community-based program could offer multiple other resources including leisure opportunities, counseling, and support for mental health.

12. Describe a few potential barriers (explore gaps in the health care practitioner's knowledge of health beliefs and customs, community disparities and discrimination, biases, stereotypes, risk factors, minorities, social attitude, health-related beliefs, and spiritual influence).

A few potential barriers could relate to the health care practitioner's difficulty understanding Nancy's beliefs and customs. The providers should have a thorough understanding of Nancy's health-related beliefs. An example would be understanding if Nancy believes it is too late to start with physical movement and if she is afraid of hurting herself. Community practitioners should explore their clients' beliefs about community services. Does Nancy believe rehabilitation is for serious illness and injury? Community practitioners should be able to explain and advocate the need for and understanding of preventative services.

The community's ethnic, racial, and religious diversity could impact Nancy's engagement and participation in, comfort with, as well as the outcome of therapy. It is important for these issues to be addressed through client education in a sensitive manner. Barriers to the therapeutic relationship in the form of biases and stereotypes on the part of the client and health care practitioners should be explored and addressed. An example would be stereotypes based on appearance such as a woman who wears a head covering.

13. Define the current problems/situation from the perspectives of the client, her family, her friends, and the interprofessional team.

Client: Nancy has relocated and is in an unfamiliar environment. She is dealing with loss—moving away from a home as well as a decline in physical health. She does not understand the culture of her environment and is fearful. She is in a new environment and is being exposed to unfamiliar and new experiences with people from different backgrounds. She has only immediate family as her social support network.

Family: Nancy's family is concerned about her physical health and safety. They are also looking to provide emotional support to their parent and opportunities to socialize in her new environment.

Interprofessional Team: The interprofessional team faces the challenge of a lack of trust from the client regarding their skills and knowledge. They are also experiencing racial profiling and explicit biases and stereotyping by their client. This type of situation could cause emotional distress to the practitioners and the client. There is a risk to forming a therapeutic relationship. The client's denial regarding the need for preventative community health interventions would impact outcomes of therapy. Health care professionals have a responsibility to provide services to the best of their ability and according to the needs of the client (Mroz et al., 2015). It could be a challenge for the practitioner to facilitate the client's care and keep the client and family well informed on their treatment when there is a lack of trust and respect on the part of the client. The interprofessional team should be proficient on collaborative goal setting as well as understand how to support of the client's participation and be considerate of the contexts that affect the client (Mroz et al., 2015).

Define the Solutions and Approaches

14. What cultural considerations should be thought of during interactions with the client or client's family members?

Nancy has recently moved from the Midwest. Through discussion it would be beneficial to understand Nancy's past and current context. Consider her age, upbringing, and prior experiences and determine how this influences her current beliefs. Consideration must be given to the influence of media, such as newspapers and television exposure. Apart from "on television" and a distant past experience, Nancy has had minimal interaction with a person using a scarf to cover her hair. It is also important to know that diversity exists within ethnic and cultural groups more so than between them.

15. How do you incorporate cultural humility into your decision-making process? Explore gaps in the health care practitioner's knowledge of health beliefs and customs, community including disparities and discrimination.

The situation between Nancy and Aisha could be contentious and requires Aisha to demonstrate professionalism. Incorporating humility into decision-making will promote leadership that considers the challenges and shows objective knowledge of the situation. This approach will serve the good of both the client and the clinician with a commitment to growth. Incorporating a cross-cultural communication model such as L.E.A.R.N. (Listen, Explain, Acknowledge,

Recommend, Negotiate) will provide the practitioner with a tool in building a therapeutic alliance (Ladha et al., 2018). Listen to the client's perception and understanding of the problem. Explain your perceptions of the problem. Acknowledge and discuss the differences and similarities. Recommend an intervention. Negotiate an agreement. The LEARN model is a cross-cultural tool that helps build mutual understanding and enhance client care (Berlin & Fowkes, 1983).

16. What interprofessional approach/collaboration should be considered to improve client's outcomes and QOL?

The interprofessional team can focus on the fall prevention program that has an impact on QOL. Since Nancy is new to the community, opportunities for socialization and involvement in community projects should be considered. Health and wellness education programs for aging would also be appropriate as well as social/emotional mental health services for coping with change, loss, and decline in ability. Clear and consistent communication between the interprofessional team and the client builds trust. A holistic approach with understanding and respect of other professionals along with inclusion of the client's and family's needs and beliefs leads to client-centered practice. Abiding to a client-centered approach supports the individual's engagement and functional performance while considering their ability to integrate with a group and their community. Core components of client-centered care are focused on the individual, this focus also needs to be on a population level to successfully enhance and implement health, wellness, and QOL programs (Mroz et al., 2015). Being client-centered in approach has practitioners explore possible barriers to access and integration from a perspective of health disparities and social disparities.

17. How can health care practitioners promote health equality through community partnerships and engagement? Define resources, education, inclusion, awareness, support, and empowerment opportunities.

The U.S. Census Bureau predicts that older Americans will make up more than 20% of the U.S. population starting in 2030 (Census Bureau, 2020). The older adult population experiences more chronic conditions such as degenerative diseases, physical disabilities, and mental illness. Community health services can provide enhanced client/patient safety through quality health service provision to the older adults within their communities. The role of a health care practitioner in primary prevention is to assess, discuss, and educate clients on healthy behaviors and explain the connection between behavior and health. Building interprofessional collaboration in the community setting requires effective communication and effective leadership of the health professionals and community members to effectively problem solve the concerns of the community members. Through partnerships with private institutions and local government and representatives there is a possibility to influence and improve client care and promote policy/legislation development.

18. How will this case in the community setting support wellness and QOL?

According to Rondón García and Ramírez Navarro (2018) health, leisure, environmental quality, functional capacity, level of satisfaction, social support, social networks, and positive social interactions are identified as determinants of well-being in an elderly population. These variables can be related to improvement of health and well-being. A senior community recreation center may be a part of supporting these health determinants. The degree of self-care capacity of an individual has an impact on the individual's mental health and wellness. A fall prevention program supports not only the physical aspects of health but also the mental aspects. Another factor for the elderly is isolation and loneliness. Community engagement and involvement provide a social network of support and structure.

19. Explore the benefits of a diverse workforce team.

A diverse work team can broaden the perspective and promote innovations and collaboration. Health care practitioners of varied academic and cultural backgrounds bring a wealth of knowledge and leadership to the community with increased problem-solving abilities and a comprehensive understanding of different belief systems, cultural biases, ethnic origins, and family structures that have an influence on the clients. A diverse work force will stand for and serve the nation's diverse population and could be involved in addressing health disparities related to chronic illness and conditions. Employing a diverse work force reduces perceptions of racism, ageism, sexism, and classism in institutions and practice.

Reflective Questions

- How would you recommend that cultural humility be included in pedagogy?
- What role do community health care practitioners play in reducing health disparities and increasing QOL in marginalized and underserved communities?

Conclusion

Health care practitioners working in communities collaborate and work in partnership with their clients and communities, sharing expertise and knowledge to make a difference in well-being. There are opportunities to integrate rehabilitation, health promotion, and prevention services into daily living through therapeutically intentional approaches and interactions that are respectful and supportive. Within the community context, health care professionals working in partnership with clients and communities can empower health decisions, advocate for inclusion, and design services that demonstrate a regard of culture and diversity. There should be a clearly focused awareness of disadvantaged communities with poor health outcomes such as communities of higher unemployment, underrepresented minorities, and low-income groups with a plan to provide support for better health outcomes. Health care education accrediting associations, educational institutes, and faculty must also endorse and authorize that the future practitioners have knowledge of social determinants of health, health disparities, and health inequities. Diversity, equity, inclusion, and justice principles must be integrated into our educational curricula to be conveyed, delivered, and implemented in community practice. Diversity of the health care workforce and leadership should be pursued with purposeful intent affirming the consequential trust and meaningful relationships within communities.

Community practitioners have an obligation to advocate for policies that will end health-related injustices, promote QOL, health, and wellness for all of their clients and for communities. Health care practitioners have a duty to attain inclusive knowledge on culture and humility and build these core concepts into their education and ultimately community clinical practice.

References

2018 Accreditation Council for Occupational Therapy Education Standards and Interpretive Guide (effective July 31, 2020). *Am J Occup Ther*, 72(Suppl._2), 7212410005p1–7212410005p83. doi: https://doi.org/10.5014/ajot.2018.72S217

American Council of Academic Physical Therapy (2020). Diversity, equity, inclusion. https://acapt.org/resources/diversity-equity-inclusion

American Occupational Therapy Association. (2015). Occupational therapy code of ethics (2015). *American Journal of Occupational Therapy, 69*(Suppl. 3), 6913410030. https://doi.org/10.5014/ajot.2015.696S03

American Occupational Therapy Association. (2017). Vision 2025. *American Journal of Occupational Therapy, 71*, 7103420010. https://doi.org/10.5014/ajot.2017.713002

American Occupational Therapy Association. (2020). Occupational therapy practice framework: Domain and process (4th ed.). *American Journal of Occupational Therapy, 74*(Suppl. 2), 7412410010. https://doi.org/10.5014/ajot.2020.74S2001

American Physical Therapy Association (2020). Diversity, equity and inclusion. https://www.apta.org/siteassets/pdfs/policies/codeofethicshods06-20-28-25.pdf

Baciu, A., Negussie, Y., & Geller, A. (2017). Communities in action: Pathways to health equity. National Academies Press. The Need to Promote Health Equity. https://www.ncbi.nlm.nih.gov/books/NBK425853/

Bartlett, T. (2017). Can we really measure implicit bias? Maybe not. *The Chronicle of Higher Education, 63*(21), B6-B7.

Bauer, U. E., Briss, P. A., Goodman, R. A., & Bowman, B. A. (2014). Prevention of chronic disease in the 21st century: Elimination of the leading preventable causes of premature death and disability in the USA. *Lancet (London, England), 384*(9937), 45-52. https://doi.org/10.1016/S0140-6736(14)60648-6

Berlin, E. A., & Fowkes, W. C., Jr. (1983). A teaching framework for cross-cultural health care. Application in family practice. *The Western Journal of Medicine, 139*(6), 934-938.

Bezner, J. R. (2015). Promoting health and wellness: Implications for physical therapist practice. *Physical Therapy, 95*(10), 1433-1444. https://doi.org/10.2522/ptj.20140271

Bjarnason, D., Mick, J., Thompson, J. A., & Cloyd, E. (2009). Perspectives on transcultural care. *The Nursing Clinics of North America, 44*(4), 495-503. https://doi.org/10.1016/j.cnur.2009.07.009

Braveman, B., & Suarez-Balcazar, Y. (2009). Social justice and resource utilization in a community-based organization: A case illustration of the role of the occupational therapist. *American Journal of Occupational Therapy, 63*, 13-23.

Braveman, P., Arkin, E., Orleans, T., Proctor, D., & Plough, A. (2017). *What is health equity? And what difference does a definition make?* Robert Wood Johnson Foundation.

Campinha-Bacote, J. (2003). Many faces: addressing diversity in health care. *Online Journal of Issues in Nursing, 8*(1), 3.

Census Bureau. (2020). Demographic turning points for the United States: Population projections for 2020 to 2060. https://www.census.gov/content/dam/Census/library/publications/2020/demo/p25-1144.pdf

Centers for Disease Control and Prevention. (2015). Addressing chronic disease through community health workers: A policy and systems-level approach. (Second Edition). Available at: https://www.cdc.gov/dhdsp/docs/chw_brief.pdf

Centers for Disease Control and Prevention. (2021). Health equity. https://www.cdc.gov/healthequity/index.html and https://www.cdc.gov/dhdsp/docs/chw_brief.pdf

Chang, M. C. & Richardson P. K. (2020). Use of standardized tests in pediatric practice. In J. Clifford-O'Brien & H. Kuhaneck (Eds.), *Case-Smith's occupational therapy for children and adolescents* (8th ed., pp.158-179).

Cross-Cultural Adaptability Inventory. (2007-2021). http://ccaiassess.com/

Dean, E., Greig, A., Murphy, S., Roots, R., Nembhard, N., Rankin, A., Bainbridge, L., Anthony, J., Hoens, A. M., & Garland, S. J. (2016). Raising the priority of lifestyle-related noncommunicable diseases in physical therapy curricula. *Physical Therapy, 96*(7), 940-948. https://doi.org/10.2522/ptj.20150141

Ekelman, B., Bello-Haas, V. D., Bazyk, J., & Bazyk, S. (2003). Developing cultural competence in occupational therapy and physical therapy education: A field immersion approach. *Journal of Allied Health, 32*(2), 131-137.

Erlen, J. A. (1998). Culture, ethics, and respect: The bottom line is understanding. *Orthopedic Nursing, 17*(6), 79-82.

Farrer, L., Marinetti, C., Cavaco, Y. K., & Costongs, C. (2015). Advocacy for health equity: A synthesis review. *The Milbank Quarterly, 93*(2), 392-437. https://doi.org/10.1111/1468-0009.12112

Foronda, C., Baptiste, D. L., Reinholdt, M. M., & Ousman, K. (2016). Cultural humility: A concept analysis. *Journal of Transcultural Nursing: Official Journal of the Transcultural Nursing Society, 27*(3), 210-217. https://doi.org/10.1177/1043659615592677

Foronda, C. L. (2008). A concept analysis of cultural sensitivity. *Journal of Transcultural Nursing: Official Journal of the Transcultural Nursing Society, 19*(3), 207-212. https://doi.org/10.1177/1043659608317093

Georgetown University. (2009). National Center for Cultural Competence. https://nccc.georgetown.edu/documents/ChecklistCSHN.pdf

Goodman, R. A., Bunnell, R., & Posner, S. F. (2014). What is "community health"? Examining the meaning of an evolving field in public health. *Preventive Medicine, 67*(Suppl 1), S58-S61. https://doi.org/10.1016/j.ypmed.2014.07.028

Greene-Moton, E. & Minkler, M. (2020). Cultural Competence or Cultural Humility? Moving Beyond the Debate. *Health Promotion Practice, 21*(1), 142-145. https://doi.org/10.1177/1524839919884912

GW Online Public Health (2020). Equity vs. equality: What is the difference? https://onlinepublichealth.gwu.edu/resources/equity-vs-equality/

Henderson, S., Horne, M., Hills, R., & Kendall, E. (2018). Cultural competence in healthcare in the community: A concept analysis. *Health & Social Care in the Community, 26*(4), 590-603. https://doi.org/10.1111/hsc.12556

Hook, J. N., Davis, D. E., Owen, J., Worthington, E. L., & Utsey, S. O. (2013). Cultural humility: Measuring openness to culturally diverse clients. *Journal of Counseling Psychology, 60*(3), 353-366. https://doi.org/10.1037/a0032595

Interprofessional Education Collaborative. (2016). Core competencies for interprofessional collaborative practice: 2016 update. Interprofessional Education Collaborative.

Isaacson M. (2014). Clarifying concepts: Cultural humility or competency. *Journal of Professional Nursing: Official Journal of the American Association of Colleges of Nursing, 30*(3), 251-258. https://doi.org/10.1016/j.profnurs.2013.09.011

Jacobs, K., & McCormack, G. L. (2019). *The occupational therapy manager*. AOTA Press.

Jongen, C., McCalman, J., & Bainbridge, R. (2018). Health workforce cultural competency interventions: a systematic scoping review. *BMC Health Services Research, 18*(1), 232. https://doi.org/10.1186/s12913-018-3001-5

Khan, S. (2021). Cultural humility vs. cultural competence and why providers need both. https://www.bmc.org/healthcity/policy-and-industry/cultural-humility-vs-cultural-competence-providers-need-both

Ladha, T., Zubairi, M., Hunter, A., Audcent, T., & Johnstone, J. (2018). Cross-cultural communication: Tools for working with families and children. *Paediatrics & Child Health, 23*(1), 66-69. https://doi.org/10.1093/pch/pxx126

Mroz, T. M., Pitonyak, J. S., Fogelberg, D., & Leland, N. E. (2015). Health policy perspectives—Client centeredness and health reform: Key issues for occupational therapy. *American Journal of Occupational Therapy, 69*(5). https://doi.org/10.5014/ajot.2015.695001

Mthembu, T. G. (2021). A commentary of occupational justice and occupation-based community development frameworks for social transformation: The Marikana Event. *South African Journal of Occupational Therapy, 51*(1), 72-75. https://doi.org/10.17159/2310-3833/2021a10

National Institutes of Health. (2011). *Principles of community engagement* (2nd ed). NIH Publication No. 11-7782. https://www.atsdr.cdc.gov/communityengagement/pdf/PCE_Report_508_FINAL.pdf

Nilsson, I. & Townsend, E. (2014). Occupational justice—Bridging theory and practice. Previously published in Scandinavian Journal of Occupational Therapy 2010; 17: 57-63. *Scandinavian Journal of Occupational Therapy, 21* Suppl 1, 64-70. https://doi.org/10.3109/11038128.2014.952906

Oliver, A. & Mossialos, E. (2004). Equity of access to health care: Outlining the foundations for action. *Journal of Epidemiology & Community Health, 58*, 655-658, https://jech.bmj.com/content/58/8/655#ref-8

Parra, D. C., Bradford, E., Clark, B. R., Racette, S. B., & Deusinger, S. S. (2017). Population and community-based promotion of physical activity: A priority for physical therapy. *Physical Therapy, 97*(2), 159-160. https://doi.org/10.1093/ptj/pzw006

Project Implicit. (2011). Implicit Association Test. https://implicit/education.html

Purden, M. (2005). Cultural considerations in interprofessional education and practice. *Journal of Interprofessional Care, 19*(Suppl 1), 224-234. https://doi.org/10.1080/13561820500083238

Rees, S., & Williams, A. (2009). Promoting and supporting self-management for adults living in the community with physical chronic illness: A systematic review of the effectiveness and meaningfulness of the patient-practitioner encounter. *JBI Library of Systematic Reviews, 7*(13), 492-582. https://doi.org/10.11124/01938924-200907130-00001

Reeves, S., Pelone, F., Harrison, R., Goldman, J., & Zwarenstein, M. (2017). Interprofessional collaboration to improve professional practice and healthcare outcomes. *The Cochrane Database of Systematic Reviews, 6*(6), CD000072. https://doi.org/10.1002/14651858.CD000072.pub3

Refugee Assistance Program Workers. Cultural Competence. (2017). http://rapworkers.com/wp-content/uploads/2017/08/cultural-competence-selfassessment-checklist-1.pdf

Rondón García, L. M., & Ramírez Navarrro, J. M. (2018). The Impact of quality of life on the health of older people from a multidimensional perspective. *Journal of Aging Research*, 2018, 4086294. https://doi.org/10.1155/2018/4086294

Stanford, F. C. (2020). The importance of diversity and inclusion in the healthcare workforce. *Journal of the National Medical Association, 112*(3), 247-249. https://doi.org/10.1016/j.jnma.2020.03.014

Stoto, M. A., Institute of Medicine (U.S.), Abel, C. H., & Dievler, A. (1996). *Healthy communities: New partnerships for the future of public health*. National Academies Press.

Stubbe, D. E. (2020). Practicing cultural competence and cultural humility in the care of diverse patients. *Focus (American Psychiatric Publishing), 18*(1), 49-51. https://doi.org/10.1176/appi.focus.20190041

Subica, A. M., & Brown, B. J. (2020). Addressing health disparities through deliberative methods: Citizens' panels for health equity. *American Journal of Public Health, 110*(2), 166-173. https://doi.org/10.2105/AJPH.2019.305450

Swihart, D. L., Yarrarapu, S., & Martin, R. L. (2021). *Cultural religious competence in clinical practice*. StatPearls Publishing.

Tervalon, M. & Murray-García, J. (1998). Cultural humility versus cultural competence: A critical distinction in defining physician training outcomes in multicultural education. *Journal of Health Care for the Poor and Underserved, 9*(2), 117-125. https://doi.org/10.1353/hpu.2010.0233

Townsend, E. & Wilcock, A. A. (2004). Occupational justice and client–centered practice: A dialogue in progress. *Canadian Journal of Occupational Therapy, 71*, 75-872.

Transcultural C.A.R.E Associates. (2020). Cultural assessment tools. http://transculturalcare.net/

U.S. Department of Health and Human Services. (2005). The Patient Safety and Quality Improvement Act of 2005. https://www.hhs.gov/hipaa/for-professionals/patient-safety/patient-safety-quality-improvement-act-2005/index.html

WestED. (2021). Improving learning healthy development and equality in schools and communities. https://www.wested.org/

World Health Organization. (2010). Framework for action on interprofessional education and collaborative practice. Geneva, Switzerland: WHO

World Health Organization. (2021). Constitution. Retrieved from https://www.who.int/about/who-we-are/constitution and https://www.who.int/healthsystems/topics/equity/en/

Yurt, C. (2021). Diversity, inclusion and equity visuals. Industrial Designer, MSc, PhD candidate.

Appendix A: Useful Resources for the Students and Faculty

Cross-Cultural Tools and Skills

- Cultural competence self-assessment checklist (Refugee Assistance Program Workers Cultural Competence, 2017) https://www.samdia.com/wp-content/uploads/2020/10/SELF-ASSESSMENT-of-Culture-Competence.pdf
- Inventory for Assessing the Process of Cultural Competence Among Healthcare Professionals-Revised (IAPCC-R; Transcultural C.A.R.E Associates, 2020) http://transculturalcare.net/
- Cross-Cultural Adaptability Inventory (CCAI; 2007-2021) http://ccaiassess.com/
- Implicit Association Test (Project Implicit, 2011) https://implicit.harvard.edu/implicit/selectatest.html
- Promoting Cultural Diversity and Cultural Competency: The Self-Assessment Checklist for Personnel Providing Services and Supports to Children with Disabilities & Special Health Needs and their Families (Georgetown University, 2009) https://nccc.georgetown.edu/documents/ChecklistCSHN.pdf
- Association of American Medical Colleges (AAMC). Tool for assessing cultural competence training. https://www.aamc.org/what-we-do/equity-diversity-inclusion/tool-for-assessing-cultural-competence-training
- U.S. Department of Health and Human Services (U.S. DHHS). Think cultural health. https://thinkculturalhealth.hhs.gov/
- U.S. Department of Health and Human Services (U.S. DHHS). Health Resources and Services Administration (HRSA). Culture, language and health literacy. https://www.hrsa.gov/about/organization/bureaus/ohe/health-literacy/culture-language-and-health-literacy
- U.S. Department of Health and Human Services (U.S. DHHS), Office of Minority Health (OMH). National standards for culturally and linguistically appropriate services (CLAS) in health and health care: Compendium of state-sponsored national CLAS Standards implementation activities. (2016). https://thinkculturalhealth.hhs.gov/assets/pdfs/CLASCompendium.pdf

Community Partnership

- Explore within the communities
- Recreation centers
- Local governmental facilities
- Adult care centers
- CDC's Healthy Communities Program (Steps, REACH, ACHIVE, CPPW, etc.)
- Special community support organizations MS, CP, Autism, etc., LGBTQIA organization
- Other non-governmental, community-based organizations and programs (https://acl.gov/programs/health-wellness)

Client Safety and Quality of Live: Social Services and Organizations, Parks, Recreations, Mental Health

- The Patient Safety and Quality Improvement Act of 2005 (U.S. Department of Health and Human Services, 2005) https://www.hhs.gov/hipaa/for-professionals/patient-safety/statute-and-rule/index.html
- WestED Improving Learning healthy development and equality in schools and communities, https://www.wested.org
- Parents, Families and Friends of Lesbians and Gays (PFLAG), https://www.pflag.org
- Gay & Lesbian Alliance Against Defamation, https://www.glaad.org
- Safe Schools Coalition, http://www.safeschoolscoalition.org/index.html
- The National Coalition for LGBT Health, https://healthlgbtq.org/

Appendix B: Professional Values and Standards

The APTA mission (The American Council of Academic Physical Therapy, 2020) focuses on improving Justice, Diversity, Equity and Inclusion (JDEI) in the profession and association and is one of APTA's strategic priorities. APTA's strategic plan includes an objective to foster the long-term sustainability of the physical therapy profession by making APTA an inclusive organization that reflects the ***diversity*** of the society the profession serves.

APTA—Code of Ethics for the Physical Therapists (American Physical Therapy Association, 2020)

Principle 1A. Physical therapists shall act in a respectful manner toward each person regardless of age, gender, race, nationality, religion, ethnicity, social or economic status, sexual orientation, health condition, or disability.

Principle 1B. Physical therapists shall recognize their personal biases and shall not discriminate against others in physical therapist practice, consultation, education, research, and administration.

Principle 8B. Physical therapists shall advocate to reduce health disparities and health care inequities, improve ***access*** to health care services, and address the health, wellness, and preventive health care needs of people.

AOTA mission (Statement and Vision 2025) (AOTA, 2017)

The position paper Occupational Therapy's Commitment to ***Diversity***, Equity, and Inclusion "affirms the right of every individual to ***access*** and fully participate in society," and was developed collaboratively by the Commission on Practice (COP), the Commission on Education (COE), the Coalition of Occupational Therapy Advocates for ***Diversity*** (COTAD), and the Multicultural, ***Diversity***, and Inclusion (MDI) Network.

AOTA—Code of Ethics for the Occupational Therapists (American Occupational Therapy Association, 2015)

Principle 3-Autonomy: Occupational therapy personnel shall respect the right of the individual to self-determination, privacy, confidentiality, and consent.

Principle 4-Justice: Occupational therapy personnel shall promote fairness and objectivity in the provision of occupational therapy services—fair and equitable treatment of persons. Individuals must have an equitable opportunity to achieve occupational engagement.

Principle 5-Veracity: Provide comprehensive, accurate, and objective information when representing profession—must be carefully balanced with cultural beliefs. Veracity is based on respect owed to others. Be honest, fair, accurate and respectful.

Principle 6-Fidelity: Occupational therapy personnel shall treat clients, colleagues, and other professionals with respect, fairness, discretion, and integrity (AOTA, 2015).

2018 Accreditation Council for Occupational Therapy Education (ACOTE®) Standards and Interpretive Guide (ACOTE®, 2018)

B.1.2. Sociocultural, Socioeconomic, *Diversity* Factors, and Lifestyle Choices: Apply, analyze, and evaluate the role of sociocultural, socioeconomic, and diversity factors, as well as lifestyle choices in contemporary society to meet the needs of persons, groups, and populations. Course content must include, but is not limited to, introductory psychology, abnormal psychology, and introductory sociology or introductory anthropology.

B.1.3. Social Determinants of Health: Demonstrate knowledge of the social determinants of health for persons, groups, and populations with or at risk for disabilities and chronic health conditions. This must include an analysis of the epidemiological factors that impact the public health and welfare of populations.

B.4.27. Community and Primary Care Programs: Evaluate access to community resources, and design community or primary care programs to support occupational performance for persons, groups, and populations.

B.5.2. Context of Service Delivery, Leadership, and Management of Occupational Therapy Services: Identify, analyze, and advocate for existing and future service delivery models and policies, and their potential effect on the practice of occupational therapy and opportunities to address societal needs.

B.7.1. Professional Ethics, Values, and Responsibilities: Demonstrate knowledge of the AOTA *Occupational Therapy Code of Ethics* and AOTA *Standards of Practice* and use them as a guide for ethical decision making in professional interactions, client interventions, employment settings, and when confronted with personal and organizational ethical conflicts.

Interprofessional Education Collaborative. (2016). Core Competencies for Interprofessional Collaborative Practice: 2016 Update. Washington, DC: Interprofessional Education Collaborative.

Competency 1. Work with individuals of other professions to maintain a climate of mutual respect and shared values. (Values/Ethics for Interprofessional Practice)

Competency 2. Use the knowledge of one's own role and those of other professions to appropriately assess and address the health care needs of patients and to promote and advance the health of populations. (Roles/Responsibilities)

Competency 3. Communicate with patients, families, communities, and professionals in health and other fields in a responsive and responsible manner that supports a team approach to the promotion and maintenance of health and the prevention and treatment of disease. (Interprofessional Communication)

Competency 4. Apply relationship-building values and the principles of team dynamics to perform effectively in different team roles to plan, deliver, and evaluate patient/population centered care and population health programs and policies that are safe, timely, efficient, effective, and equitable. (Teams and Teamwork)

Appendix C: Professional Reasoning Box

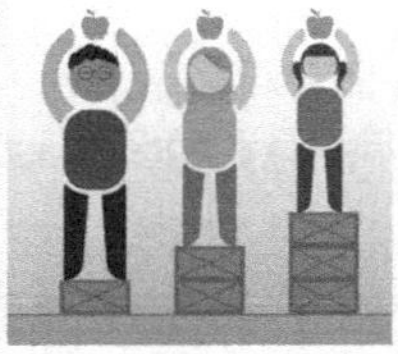	To be client-centered, inclusive, and provide the highest level of care a practitioner must have awareness and knowledge of population **diversity** and **health care disparities** in the communities they work in. Health care practitioners have the opportunity to be active participants in addressing **health care equity and justice** in their work in **community** settings as they plan, direct, perform, and reflect on client care.
While we continue to grow and increase our knowledge regarding appropriate therapeutic evaluation, intervention, and outcome tools we should enter the relationships with our clients with **cultural humility** honoring their beliefs and values, combined with our own willingness to learn from others and ongoing self-exploration (Stubbe, 2020).	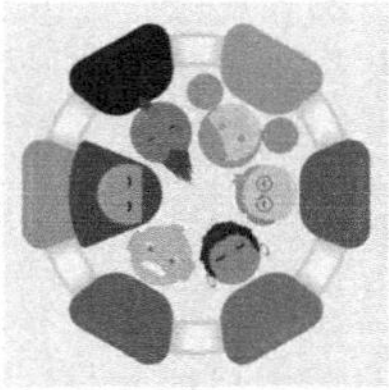
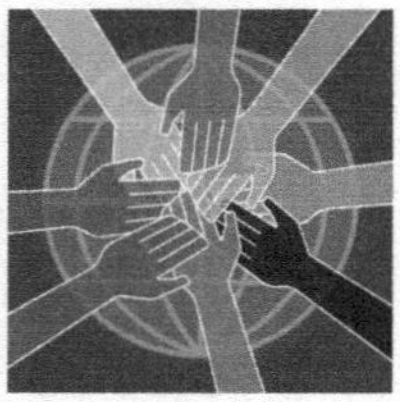	**Health care practitioners** create partnerships with communities and take their lead from community members. Be open to learning with, from, and about each member of the interprofessional team, client, and community members to enhance client's/communities'/populations' **health, wellness, and quality of life.**
A **client-centered approach** fosters a partnership between practitioners and the client with consideration given to the client's needs, wants, and desires while respecting beliefs, values and priorities. To be client centered is to provide the best care including advocating for inclusion and equity in the face of discrimination and disparity (AOTA, 2020; Mroz et al., 2015).	An **occupational justice** lens should be considered to maximize an individual client's as well communities' occupational potential and when working in communities promote occupations aimed at social transformation (Mthembu, 2021). prompting health care practitioners to be cognizant of social determinants of health and disparities.

CHAPTER 3

Theoretical Perspectives for Interprofessional Community-Oriented Practice

Nerida Hyett, PhD, MHSc, BOT, Grad Cert Higher Ed;
Brad Hodge, PhD, B. Psychological Science (with Hons);
Lisa Hanson, PhD, MBA, B. Physio (Hons), Grad Cert Higher Ed; and
Kerryn Bagley, PhD, B. Social Work (Hons)

Learning Objectives

At the end of this chapter, the reader will:

1. Describe the rationale for using theoretical perspectives in interprofessional community-oriented practice in relation to policy, research, and interprofessional frameworks (ACOTE B.2.1, B.2.2)
2. Explain and compare theoretical perspectives for practice with individuals and families in community-oriented settings to enhance health, well-being, and quality of life (ACOTE B.1.1.1, B.1.2)
3. Explain and compare theoretical perspectives for practice with communities and populations in community-oriented settings to enhance health, well-being, and quality of life (ACOTE B.1.3, B.4.27)
4. Apply theoretical perspectives for interprofessional community-oriented practice to a case study (ACOTE B.2.1, B.2.2)

The ACOTE Standards used are those from 2018.

Pizzi, M. A., & Amir, M. (Eds.). *Interprofessional Perspectives for Community Practice: Promoting Health, Well-Being, and Quality of Life* (pp. 37-52).

Key Words

Community-Based Health Service, Community Capacity Building, Community-Centered practice, Community-Centered Practice Framework, Community Development, Community-Oriented, Disease and Illness Prevention, Environment–Health–Occupation–Well-Being Model, Health Belief Model, Health Promotion, Primary Care, Social Determinants of Health, Theoretical Perspectives, Theory, Transtheoretical Model, United Nations Declaration of the Rights of Indigenous Peoples, United Nations Universal Declaration of Human Rights

Introduction

Health professionals in community-oriented health care settings need the ability to understand and apply theory to practice. Learning how to apply theory to practice begins with defining what is meant by theory and a theoretical perspective and exploring how this can inform and strengthen practice with a range of client groups. Health professionals working in community-oriented settings work with individuals as well as whole communities or populations. A community-oriented health professional will often manage a caseload of individual clients, while also working at the community level; designing and facilitating community groups, providing community health promotion, prevention, and education programs, and advocating and lobbying for population health issues. Working in a community-oriented health care setting requires specialist skills, including the ability to determine the social determinants of an individual's presenting issues, and to design group programs informed by community needs, key theories, and evidence. This ability to apply theory to practice also ensures practice is informed by policy, research, and interprofessional frameworks and will achieve optimal health and well-being outcomes.

What Is a Theoretical Perspective?

A **theory** describes relationships between different ideas, which are used to understand social phenomena and human behavior (Reitz et al., 2013). **Theoretical perspectives** are insights gleaned from theories that have been applied, tested, and validated for use in practice with different populations and environments. They provide a way of thinking about and unpacking a professional practice scenario, used by health professionals to form understandings and to make decisions regarding interventions. Health professionals, for example, refer to theoretical perspectives when selecting an assessment with a client. Theories inform how clinical observations and findings are interpreted and the construction of clinical reasoning, which ensures that health care is evidence-informed (Hoffmann et al., 2017). For purposes of this chapter, theoretical perspectives refer to the utilization of theories, frames of reference, and models of practice for use by all health professionals working in community-oriented practice and interprofessional teams.

The theoretical perspectives detailed here were selected because they are effective for informing community-oriented practice and enhancing community health, well-being, and quality of life (QOL) outcomes.

Key Theoretical Perspectives for Community-Oriented Health Care

Community-Oriented Versus Community-Based Health Care

The term **community-oriented** describes health care that is tailored to community issues, needs, and priorities. Community-oriented health care is often situated within a **community-based health service**, which is a health care organization that is located outside of institutions like hospitals or government health departments. However, just because a service is based or located in the community does not necessarily mean it is community oriented. A community-based health service might be limited to service provision with individuals and families and might not provide services at the community level. Therefore, the term community-oriented is used to encompass the approach to service provision within community-based health services or other settings, which is tailored to the community and includes whole-of-community programs and health interventions, in addition to services for individuals and families.

Primary Versus Tertiary Care

Health services are situated in communities to provide **primary care**, which includes a diverse range of health and medical services focused on prevention, education, and early intervention. Primary means first level of care that precedes secondary and tertiary care, which is increasingly more specialized and intensive. Secondary care includes those who are at risk for illness or disability. Tertiary care is often equated with need for specialized intervention, such as rehabilitation. In the context of cancer care, for example, primary care includes cancer screening and prevention strategies, whereas secondary could include targeted information sessions and strategies to prevent spread, while tertiary care involves treatments after a diagnosis, which can further extend to recovery after successful interventions or palliative services for deteriorating conditions.

The Declaration of Alma Ata is an international framework used to guide the implementation of primary health care (World Health Organization [WHO] and UNICEF, 1978). Primary care is most effective when it is community-oriented, and the Declaration advocates for primary care to be "the first level of contact of individuals, the family and community [with the health system] … bringing health care as close as possible to where people live and work … the first element of a continuing health care process" (WHO and UNICEF, 1978, p. 2).

The aim of primary care is to intervene early and prevent the development or progression of potentially unnecessary illness, injury, or disease. The Quadruple Aim framework defines the key components of effective primary care: to improve individual outcomes and experience, improve population health, reduce per capita health care costs, and improve the experience of providing care (Sikka et al., 2015). Primary care services are provided for all age groups including children, adolescents, adults, and older adults. All health professionals should work in primary care.

Disease and Illness Prevention

Health professionals deliver **disease and illness prevention** along the same spectrum of primary to tertiary health care intervention. In community-oriented health care, a major focus is on primary prevention that aims to prevent ill health for whole populations, by applying interventions in a wide range of settings, tailored to community contexts, but suitable for a wide range of community members (e.g., vaccination programs). Secondary or indicated prevention is increasingly more focused on community sub-groups and settings known to have a higher level of risk, such as substance use education for adolescents. The application of tertiary prevention is within individuals and groups who have diagnosed and established health conditions and aims to increase health-related QOL and reduce burden through prevention of exacerbation and the progression of the condition, reduction in disability and prevention of co-morbidities, for example, nutrition and exercise programs for people who have experienced their first heart attack (Centers for Disease Control and Prevention [CDC], 2017).

Health Promotion

One of the major focuses of community-oriented health care and primary care intervention is **health promotion**, which is defined by the Ottawa Charter as "the process of enabling people to increase control over, and to improve, their health" (WHO, 1986, para. 3). Community-oriented health professionals deliver health promotion through enabling, mediating, and advocating for resources that improve health of individuals and communities. Core objectives of health promotion interventions include 1) develop personal skills for health and well-being; 2) create supportive environments; 3) re-orient health services; and 4) strengthen community action and partnerships (WHO, 1986). Community-oriented health professionals utilize health promotion strategies with individuals, families, communities, and populations to improve health, well-being, and QOL outcomes. Health promotion informed by theoretical perspectives and health behavior frameworks is critical for community-oriented practice with individuals and whole communities, as theoretical perspectives lend support for assessment and interventions.

Case Study: Community-Oriented Health Care for Rural Youth

Kim is a community-oriented health professional working with individuals, families, and communities in a rural community-based health care setting. She manages a case load providing person-centered care with adolescents at risk for poor health outcomes, providing health assessment and screening, health promotion, prevention, and education interventions, social care assistance and advocacy to enable access to housing, employment support services, or welfare payments, and supported referral to other health and medical professionals. Kim also designs and facilitates community groups and programs focused on primary and secondary prevention, including health and well-being promotion and health education, social connection, and independent living skill development.

The community-based health service where Kim works is located in a town with a population size of 25,000 people. The nearest metropolitan city is located 155 miles or approximately 250 kilometers away. Kim is currently managing a case load of 30 young people aged between 12 to 25 years who have a wide range of presenting issues, for example, mental and emotional health, family and social issues including homelessness, substance misuse, gender, sexuality and reproductive health, and difficulties remaining engaged with school or work. Interprofessional services include a family physician, pediatrician, physical therapist, speech-language pathologist, occupational therapist, social worker, and psychologist, and Kim is able to work interprofessionally with her colleagues to achieve the best outcomes for her clients and the community.

Kim receives a referral from the physical therapist within her service for Jacob, a 15-year-old male. Jacob is a talented athlete and has been participating in a youth talent development program for football as well as playing competitively. Jacob's family is supportive of his commitment to the required training and skill development, so much so that he never missed a session. Jacob's father and grandfather played competitive organized football on representative teams and are model inspirations for Jacob to be accepted to a state or national team. Jacob had a good pre-season start and set high expectations for the official launch of competition. In the third round, Jacob sustained an unstable ankle fracture that required surgery for internal fixation of the fracture and his lower leg was immobilized in a cast for 6 weeks. On the seventh week, the cast was removed, and Jacob participated in rehabilitation with a physical therapist for 4 weeks. After conclusion of this stage of rehabilitation, Jacob was able to fully weight bear on the previously injured leg and was progressing as expected.

The physical therapist explained to Jacob that he is progressing well; however, Jacob is concerned by his loss of conditioning and very disappointed at how the season is ending without his participation. At this point in time, the physical therapist notices recent changes in Jacob's mood; he appears quiet and withdrawn and less motivated during the rehabilitation sessions. Conversations of his future aspiration to play football stops and he has lost interest in watching his previously favorite sport. This also caused him to limit contact with friends who are themselves still active in the sport. Jacob typically makes comments that "he can't see the point anymore" and that he cannot find an enjoyable activity to replace what he lost; without sport he feels like an "outsider" with his friends and community. The physical therapist, recognizing signs of mood changes, an overall loss of joy and declining motivation in Jacob, requests a health assessment for Jacob, with his parent's informed consent. Jacob agrees to see Kim for the assessment and while he expresses some reluctance is not confident that Kim can help him with his situation, he would like support to explore options for emotional coping strategies, for improving his sleep and diet, and making new friendships that do not involve sport.

Reflective Questions

1. What factors are influencing Jacob's engagement with community-based health services?
2. What theoretical perspectives could inform the physical therapist's decision to refer Jacob to adolescent health services?
3. What theoretical perspectives could inform Kim's approach to engaging Jacob in intervention, which includes optimizing his participation and achieving optimal health, well-being, and QOL outcomes?

Theoretical Perspectives for Working With Jacob

A number of theoretical perspectives exist that provide insights into how people access health services and what factors influence people's decisions to seek out and engage with health care. Two key theoretical perspectives are the Transtheoretical Model and Health Belief Model. Both can be applied to the case study to understand the factors that would influence Jacob's engagement with services and what factors Kim can prioritize to achieve optimal engagement and health behavior change. Summaries of the models are provided, followed by explanations of how they can be applied to practice with Jacob.

Transtheoretical Model

The Transtheoretical Model was originally developed to better understand the process of behavior change in tobacco smoking (DiClemente & Prochaska, 1982), but since then, the model has been used to understand behavior change in a range of areas (Bridle et al., 2005; Kleis et al., 2021). Traditionally the model was applied to behavior change for reducing unhealthy behaviors (Grant & Franklin, 2007); however, it is now applied to behavior changes to understand processes for adopting new healthy behaviors such as physical activity (Kleis et al., 2021).

The Transtheoretical Model is based on the assumption that behavior change is largely driven by changes to a person's beliefs about a behavior. Driving this change are a combination or balance of both positive and negative beliefs, or pros and cons, referred to as decisional balance (Figure 3-1). A person's positive and negative beliefs about a behavior can be formed by past experiences and preferences of the individual, opinions or preferences of the family or community, and policies and environmental characteristics. The Transtheoretical Model proposes that over the course of the change in behavior, decisional balance shifts so that the positive beliefs strengthen and the negative beliefs weaken, which increases the likelihood that one will maintain the target behavior. For example, if Jacob was to consider trying a different exercise and joining a gym, he would probably understand that exercise is good for him and he would feel physically better afterward (positive). But these positive beliefs conflict with negative beliefs; for example, Jacob might feel anxious about going to the gym for the first time (negative), or anticipate pain, fatigue, or discomfort (negative).

This combination of beliefs about the positive and negative implications of action or inaction influences the likelihood that people will undertake a behavior. To be successful in adopting and maintaining new health behaviors, higher positive and lower negative beliefs in regard to undertaking the behavior must be present. Additionally, a belief of being

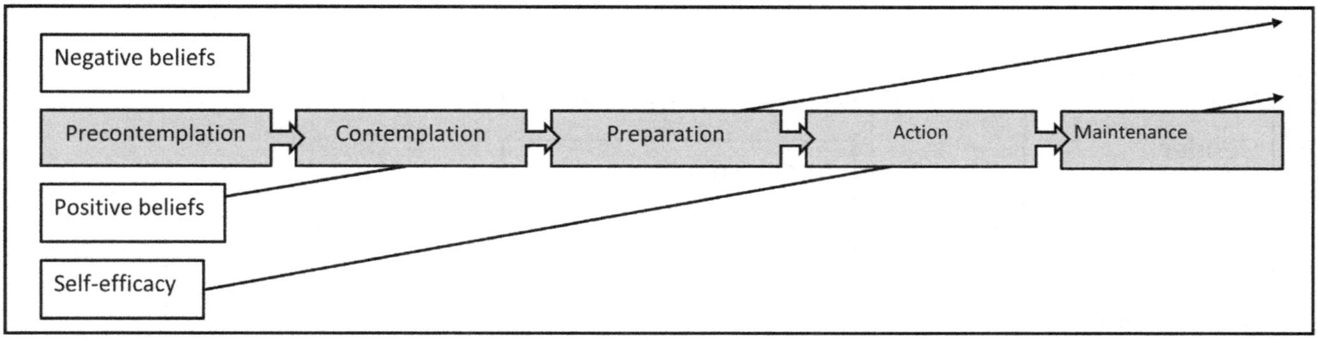

Figure 3-1. Components of Transtheoretical Model. (Adapted from DiClemente, C. C., & Prochaska, J. O. [1982]. Self-change and therapy change of smoking behavior: A comparison of processes of change in cessation and maintenance. *Addictive Behaviors, 7*[2], 133-142. https://doi.org/10.1016/0306-4603(82)90038-7)

capable of enacting that behavior should also exist, this is known as self-efficacy (Bandura, 1977; Bridle et al., 2005).

There are five stages of change described in the Transtheoretical Model (Figure 3-1): precontemplation, contemplation, preparation, action, and maintenance. While each stage is often described as distinct and linear in progression, the application of the model is fluid and the stages may overlap and become indistinct because of the nature of human behavior (Sutton, 2005). Community-oriented health professionals such as Kim and the physical therapist need to assess which stage a person is up to in their process of change by exploring their decisional balance (positive and negative beliefs), and tailor the intervention to the person's stage of change and level of self-efficacy to best support them through a process of reducing unhealthy behaviors and/or adopting positive health behaviors.

In the *precontemplation* stage, it is expected that positive beliefs about undertaking the behavior are low while negative beliefs are high, and as a result the individual has no recognition of a need to change behavior. It is also likely that self-efficacy is relatively low. If Jacob was in the precontemplation stage of change in regard to his mental and emotional health issues he is likely to have limited awareness of the issues and lack insight into the impact this is having on his well-being and QOL.

For a person to move from the precontemplation to *contemplation*, there needs to be an increase in positive beliefs and decrease in negative beliefs. The individual starts to realize a need for change and that their current action or inaction is not as beneficial as previously thought. In this contemplation stage the individual has not yet decided to change; however, they are beginning to become aware of a problem or need and are open to the possibility of change. Jacob is likely to be in the contemplative stage of change for his mental and emotional health issues because he is accepting of the referral to Kim and is open to exploring possibilities for making behavior change.

Kim will support Jacob through the *preparation* stage, which is characterized by a decision to change and planning ahead to begin a change process; this needs to precede active change behavior. During the *action* stage Jacob will undertake the necessary action to change his behavior, his positive beliefs will continue to rise, and self-efficacy will increase. There might still be struggle between positive and negative beliefs causing the new behavior to decline or pause, but there is progress.

In the final stage, the *maintenance* stage, the new behavior or cessation of behavior is somewhat fixed. During this stage, Jacob will feel capable because he has successfully changed his behavior and is experiencing the benefits of new behaviors. Kim and Jacob's family, however, will remain cognizant of the risk of relapse, which should reduce over time.

The Transtheoretical Model adds further context to the stages of change by detailing 10 processes that characterize the behaviors that people undertake to overcome the barriers encountered at different stages (Bridle et al., 2005), for example, consciousness raising (seeking out information or feedback), counter-conditioning (trying out alternative behaviors), forming helping relationships, applying reward and reinforcement, and stimulus control (e.g., using strategies for reducing exposure to triggers).

The Transtheoretical Model supports health professionals to understand the underlying drivers and processes of change and how these can be utilized to enable people to make changes to their behavior that improve health, well-being, and QOL. Understanding an individual's complex positive and negative beliefs about undertaking and not undertaking behaviors, clarifies some of the complexity in behavioral decision making. Understanding the role of self-efficacy as a driver of behavior provides an effective avenue for intervention for individuals like Jacob, in that he needs to believe he is capable of undertaking new behaviors, otherwise the likelihood of him doing so is very low. This theoretical perspective outlines the role of health professionals at each stage of change, demonstrating how to support people to adopt health-promoting behaviors and reduce behaviors that have negative impacts or risks, promoting early intervention.

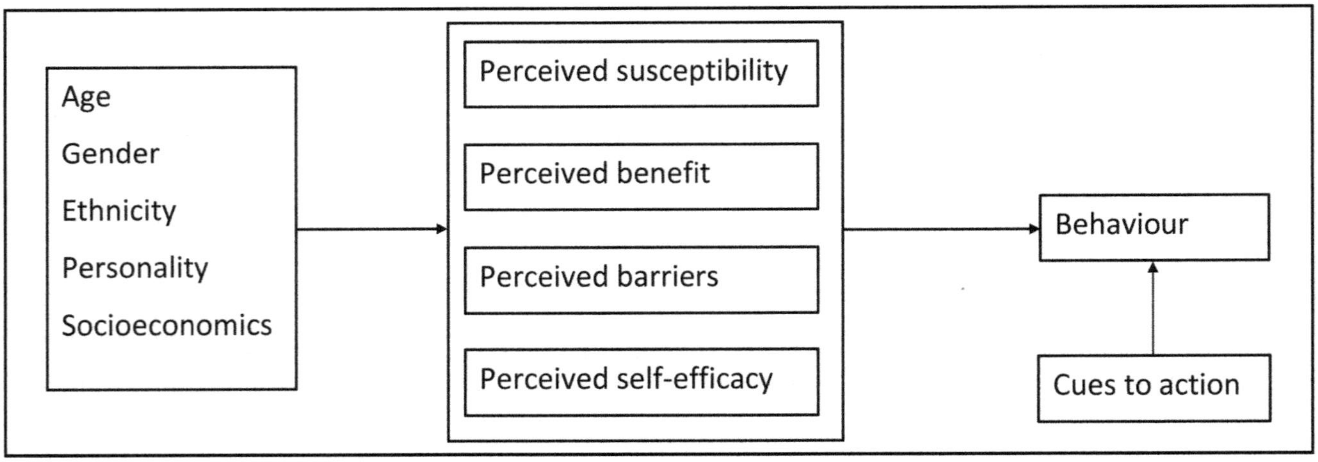

Figure 3-2. Health Belief Model. (Adapted from Rosenstock, I. M. [1974]. Historical origins of the Health Belief Model. *Health Education Monographs, 2*[4], 328-335. https://doi.org/10.1177/109019817400200403)

Health Belief Model

The Health Belief Model was created in an attempt to understand a person's reasoning process regarding participation in illness and disease screening and prevention programs when it is readily available through free access government-funded programs (Rosenstock, 1974). Unlike the Transtheoretical Model it is not focused on the change process but rather on the factors that predict whether or not a person will undertake a particular healthy behavior. Often, behaviors are perceived to have a singular cause, but more likely include multiple causes.

The Health Belief Model suggests that beliefs about the health outcomes and health behavior are the primary drivers of action or inaction (Rosenstock et al., 1988). Five core beliefs are described relating to people's understandings of their perceived susceptibility to and severity of illness, perceived barriers and benefits, and self-efficacy (Figure 3-2). Kim and the physical therapist can utilize this model in their practice with Jacob to construct holistic intervention plans for health promotion, early intervention, and education that will increase his likelihood of engaging positive health behaviors and achieving optimal health, well-being, and QOL.

Perceived susceptibility is an individual's beliefs about whether or not they are likely to experience a particular negative health outcome. *Perceived severity* is the individual's beliefs about how serious the implications of that health outcome might be. For example, in the case of Jacob's fractured ankle, he is more likely to perceive the outcomes of inaction as being very serious but neglects to see the significance of his mental and emotional health symptoms.

Perceived benefit and barriers refers to the beliefs about the health behavior that are needed to obtain a benefit and the barriers to engaging in the health behavior. If Jacob has the belief that undertaking a health behavior will lead to high beneficial outcomes, and perceives few barriers, he will be more likely to engage in the behavior. An opposite scenario could occur, where Jacob might recognize fewer benefits along with high barriers, such as discomfort or stigma, which would prevent initiation of a behavior.

Self-efficacy is the individual's beliefs about whether or not they can successfully undertake the behavior (Bandura, 1977). Enabling and engaging in health behaviors requires skills and expertise, therefore a person needs to hold the belief that they are capable of the behavior. For example, if the physical therapist has asked Jacob to complete a home exercise program to ensure Jacob understands the instructions and is able to implement this independently. If Jacob is unsure of the instructions when he is alone at home, thus low in self-efficacy, he will be less likely to attempt the program.

Additionally, these five health beliefs are influenced by a range of demographic variables including race, ethnicity, education, gender, and age (Champion & Skinner, 2008). In addition to the five beliefs, the Health Belief Model includes *cue to action* as a driver of behavior (Rosenstock, 1974). The cue to action captures the role that internal and external cues play in triggering action. Cues can be external, such as peers, the media or health promotion materials, or internal such as pain, fatigue, or tension (Rosenstock, 1974). Health professionals may also be the cue to action, for example, the physical therapist referral is likely to act as a trigger to action for Jacob by prompting him to undertake a particular behavior, booking a time with the physical therapist (Professional Reasoning Box A).

Application of the Theoretical Perspectives to the Case Study

Using the Transtheoretical Model, Kim can see Jacob is in the action stage of change for his ankle injury, but he is more contemplative about addressing his mental and emotional health issues. Jacob has accepted the referral and is open to exploring ideas for improving his physical and mental health and well-being, but she will need to spend time

Professional Reasoning Box A

CULTURALLY RESPONSIVE HEALTH CARE

Culturally responsive health care is a critical approach to practice that centers a person's culture at the forefront of their health care and is increasingly a requirement of professional practice standards. Culturally responsive health care is an extension of client-centered health care, which ensures that services are tailored to the person's cultural identity. Cultural identity includes a range of human diversity factors including race and ethnicity, religion, gender and sexuality, age and developmental stage, ability and disability, language, geographic location, education and employment status, family of origin and marital status, citizenship and immigration status.

Cultural responsiveness refers to how the health professional identifies, validates, and incorporates information about a person's cultural identity into their health care. Effective culturally responsive practice should include listening to the person and learning about their cultural identity, and recognition, validation, and affirmation of the person's cultural identity through selection of assessments and interventions and professional communications. Culturally responsive health care requires the establishment of a therapeutic relationship that demonstrates empathy and respect for the client's cultural identity, knowledge, and expertise. Culturally responsive health care practices should be incorporated into work within community-oriented settings to ensure health care settings are culturally safe for all people, families, and communities (Indigenous Allied Health Australia, 2019).

Culturally responsive health care with Jacob requires the health professionals to gain in-depth understandings of his cultural identity and to use these understandings to inform their intervention—for instance, Jacob is an adolescent male with a rural upbringing and close family relationships, with sporting values. Gaps in understanding would need to be addressed through Kim's assessment process, finding out more about Jacob's race and ethnicity, socioeconomic status, and values and interests beyond sport, which will reveal his strengths, but also barriers that might need to be addressed through her interventions.

exploring his positive and negative beliefs about change and his self-efficacy to ensure he is ready to prepare and plan for new behaviors. This will ensure that Jacob feels ready and has sufficient confidence and self-belief to engage in action and maintain changed behaviors over the longer term.

Using the Health Belief Model to understand Jacob's beliefs about susceptibility and severity, as well as benefits and barriers, will give Kim important information to predict Jacob's likelihood of change. Jacob might recognize but not fully understand how his ankle injury has led to social isolation impacting his mood, and how ongoing isolation and disengagement can be a risk for developing depression (Office of Disease Prevention and Health Promotion, U.S. Department of Health and Human Services, 2020). Health promotion can be used to increase his likelihood of engaging with the service and adopting new health behaviors by creating clear cues to action. A health promotion intervention, for example, could include assisting Jacob to identify symptoms of depression and highlighting the benefits of engaging in mindfulness relaxation and cognitive behavioral exercises, and of re-engaging in social activities. Kim can also provide education and support to Jacob's family, providing another effective external cue to action that will support Jacob to engage with the service and Kim's interventions.

Summary

Community-oriented health professionals work with individuals and families providing health promotion, education, prevention, and early intervention. Community-oriented health professionals working in community-based health services are often focused on primary care, which aims to reduce the need for the more specialized and intensive secondary and tertiary care interventions, which can be more difficult to access in rural locations.

Two key theoretical perspectives that were introduced and applied to Jacob were the Transtheoretical Model and the Health Belief Model. Both models are effective for identifying key factors that influence a person's engagement with community-based health services, particularly with primary care services focused on education, prevention, and early intervention. The Transtheoretical Model helps the community-oriented health professional to understand a person's readiness for change, their decisional balance (positive and negative beliefs about change) and perceptions of self-efficacy in order for that individual to participate more fully in their neighborhood and community. The Health Belief Model outlines ones' beliefs about susceptibility, severity, barriers and benefits, and self-efficacy that influence a person's likelihood for engaging in positive health behaviors. It is recommended that community-oriented health professionals utilize one or both of these theoretical perspectives in order to better understand individual and family presentations and for developing strategies to increase engagement in primary care services and positive health behaviors. This will ultimately help health professionals optimize one's health, well-being, and QOL outcomes.

Key Points

- Community-oriented health professionals work with individuals and families as well as at the community level with communities and populations.
- Community-oriented health professionals can work in community-based health services that are focused on primary care service provision including education, prevention, early intervention, and health promotion, which aims to reduce the need for secondary and tertiary care, which is more specialized and intensive, and can be more difficult to access in rural locations.
- The Transtheoretical Model and the Health Belief Model are two key theoretical perspectives recommended to inform practice with individuals and families which can increase engagement and improve health, well-being, and quality of life outcomes

Community-Oriented Practice With Communities and Populations

Case Study Continued "Connecting Rural Youth Through the Arts"

When Kim discusses Jacob's case with her interprofessional team, they reflect on the key presenting issues and realize there are a significant number of young people who are accessing the health service with similar challenges of mental and emotional health, social isolation, and loneliness. The rural community where the service is located has a strong sporting culture that is centered around the football club. There are limited community programs or groups available for young people that do not play sports, which is a key factor in making Jacob feel disconnected and like an outsider to his friends and community. Kim's role as a community-oriented health professional is to work with a health promotion network of community stakeholders, including representatives from local organizations, businesses, schools, and government, with a purpose of addressing community issues, needs, and priorities.

Kim presents the issue of youth social isolation to the health promotion network, and they decide to co-design, implement, and evaluate a community arts program with young people aged 12 to 17 years. The aim of the program is to foster social connections and friendships and reduce loneliness and social isolation, which are key social determinants of health, well-being, and QOL. Kim will work with young people and community leaders to design and host a photography-based arts exhibition, enabling young people to share their experiences of social isolation and connection through visual images and written or audio captions—a creative arts technique known as Photovoice. Jacob's football club has agreed to sponsor the initiative, and Jacob has planned to exhibit photos portraying his experiences of connection when playing sport, in addition to photos of his sense of isolation due to his injury.

The group experience improves Jacob's well-being and QOL by strengthening friendships with peers from his school who do not play football. He has decided to continue sharing photographs and captions on his social media page as a coping strategy and to raise awareness about mental health in his community. Kim's involvement in the development of the community arts initiative is informed by a range of theoretical perspectives, which ensures she is able to work effectively with the community stakeholders and achieve optimal health, well-being, and QOL outcomes with the community (Professional Reasoning Box B and C).

Reflective Questions

1. Why is a community-oriented approach important to address the issue of social isolation in rural youth?
2. What theoretical perspectives could have informed Kim's contributions to this initiative?
3. How can community-oriented practice draw from interprofessional collaboration?

Application of the Health Belief Model and the Transtheoretical Model at the Community Level

Many of the theoretical perspectives utilized in health care are drawn from western contexts and paradigms, which have a strong focus on individualism and person-centered health care. This creates a challenge for community-oriented health professionals designing and delivering programs at the community and population levels. Individually focused theoretical perspectives can offer valuable insights for community-level work; however, the limitations of this need to be considered; that theories have been designed and tested for use with individuals and the utility for community-level work has not yet been evaluated and published in peer reviewed research. The two theoretical perspectives described earlier in this chapter for working with Jacob (the Transtheoretical Model and the Health Belief Model) can be applied for working with the community to design the arts initiative. This provides a way of understanding factors that might influence or predict the likelihood of community participation.

Professional Reasoning Box B

NOTHING ABOUT US WITHOUT US

The active engagement of consumers and communities in the development and design of services and programs has gained increasing importance among health professionals in recent years and has become a focus in health policy agendas internationally.

This emphasis on engagement and inclusion of consumers, however, is not new, it reflects a decades-old history of advocacy and activism in the disability community, particularly associated with the Disability Rights Movement, from which the philosophy "Nothing about us without us" emerged (Charlton, 1998). "Nothing about us without us" reflects the idea that the people who are the end users of a service or are affected by a policy, should have a right to influence and contribute to its development.

Since the 1990s, the "nothing about us without us" mandate has been taken up outside the Disability Rights Movement and applied in other domains, including, for example, adolescent health (McDonagh & Bateman, 2012) and dementia advocacy (Bryden, 2015). The philosophy is reflected in the evolution of consumer-engaged practices and approaches such as co-design and co-production. These approaches to developing programs and services recognize that consumers and communities are experts in their own lives and emphasizes the need to work *with* rather than *for* consumers and communities to ensure that the outcomes meet the identified needs of the end users.

Professional Reasoning Box C

THE DOMINANCE OF INDIVIDUALISM IN HEALTH CARE

The majority of health care settings are positioned to provide individual focused health care because of the ways in which services are planned, funded, and delivered. This focus on individual service provision, however, ignores or fails to address the social and environmental determinants of ill health, which causes and maintains high levels of burden of disease. Similarly, health care professionals and researchers have largely focused on establishing theoretical perspectives and practices for individual or person-centered care (Gerlach et al., 2017).

More recently, there have been calls for developing and expanding community-based health care services and systems that extend current programs to include whole-of-community health and well-being interventions. This requires service planning and delivery that identifies the community as client and service partner, and the co-design of health and well-being programs that address social and environmental determinants of ill health (Hyett et al., 2016; South et al., 2017). This shift or expansion in thinking will take time to adapt and test and trial approaches for working with communities and building an evidence base for this work. In the meantime, individual focused models can be adapted and used where relevant, however, limitations need to be considered.

The Transtheoretical Model could be used to understand community members' readiness for participating in the arts initiative based on motivation and self-efficacy factors. It could be used to determine stages of change for community members and community sub-groups and advise what types of interventions might be helpful to increase participation based on their stages of change. If it was determined, for example, that some community members were in an action stage of change, this sub-group could be given leadership positions to model and support participation of community members in more contemplative or pre-contemplative stages.

The Health Belief Model can provide insight into how community members make decisions about participating in the initiative and what factors might support their engagement. Using this model, Kim can design promotional materials targeting self-efficacy, increasing community confidence in their ability to participate. This could be done by sharing stories about positive experiences of participation via social media and providing information on how to be involved.

Community-Oriented Theoretical Perspectives

The use of community-oriented theoretical perspectives shifts the focus from individual to community and recognizes that many determinants of ill health stem from social and environmental determinants that are beyond individual control. Community-oriented approaches to health care target the root cause of health issues and factors that perpetuate illness and disease that originate in the environments and contexts in which people live.

A wide range of theoretical perspectives exist that can be used by community-oriented health professionals like Kim to guide their practice with communities. Several theoretical perspectives are described below (in the form of models, frameworks, and theories) that could be used by Kim to inform her work with the health promotion network and community stakeholders to co-design the arts initiative.

Social Determinants of Health

When using any theoretical perspectives health and human service providers must look beyond their clinical silo and discipline-specific understanding of an illness or injury and consider how social factors such as living arrangements, education, or working conditions as well as the socioeconomic, environmental, and political landscape affects the health and well-being of individuals and families, communities, and populations. The WHO (2008) defines these social determinants of health as "the circumstances in which people grow, live, work, and age, and the systems put in place to deal with illness. These conditions in which people live and die are, in turn shaped by political, social and economic forces" (WHO, 2008, p. iii). For example, Jacob's presenting issues will be influenced by his family and community context, which could include social determinants of low health literacy, low household income or socioeconomic status, underemployment or unemployment, food and housing insecurity, higher prevalence of substance dependence, rural isolation, and/or poor access to health care services. Providing education and coping strategies on the management of Jacob's mental and emotional health issues will only address part of the problem and if social determinants remain as problems for the family, Jacob's recovery and goal attainment will be restricted. Evidence-informed practice requires interventions to address the social determinants impacting an individual and family. Addressing social determinants also has positive effects for the broader community who are also restricted by these living conditions.

Kim can develop interventions that address social determinants of poor mental and emotional health and social disconnection for the rural youth by working with the health promotion network and community stakeholders to build supportive infrastructure and a community context that enables connection and participation. For example, Kim will need to secure a safe and accessible meeting space for the group of rural youth, which could involve applying for funding, finding and booking a suitable location, reimbursing travel costs, and providing information resources for families. Kim would need to identify which social determinants are having a major influence and develop solutions to address these. For example, there might be a lack of arts initiatives in the rural community because of a historical lack of funding, Kim might need to advocate and apply for funding then establish the initiative and ensure it is sustainable over the long term. Another example might be that young people do not attend programs after school because a lack of safe public transport, Kim might need to establish transportation to allow youth participation.

Social Justice, Inclusion, and Human Rights–Based Approaches

Working with the community to address social and environmental determinants of ill health recognizes that many of the factors that impact community health, well-being, and QOL originate in the societal systems and structures in which we live, including governments, policies, laws, and institutions. The use of social justice, equity, and human rights–based theoretical perspectives can support community-oriented health professionals to identify determinants of ill health caused by injustice and violations of human rights, and how across communities, experiences of ill health might be different and inequitable for different sub-groups. A human rights–based approach is about designing and facilitating programs that improve community awareness of and ability to self-advocate for their rights, and plan and implement actions to change systems and structures that perpetuate inequities and injustice. Two key frameworks for rights-based approaches include the **United Nations Universal Declaration of Human Rights**, which states 30 universal human rights that are required for equity, justice, dignity, and freedom of all peoples (1948). Released in 1948, it was a shared commitment of global leaders at the time protect fundamental human rights and never allow the human suffering and loss experienced during and after World War II. Released in 2007, the **United Nations Declaration on the Rights of Indigenous Peoples** is an extension of the Universal Declaration of Human Rights, and details 46 unique rights of Indigenous peoples for survival, dignity, and well-being (2007). Both frameworks have been developed by the United Nations to recognize the importance of specific rights for humans to live healthy, free, and just lives, and for there to be equality among people and groups. Using a rights-based framework, health professions may have responsibilities to develop health care policies that uphold human rights, justice, and equity, and prevent violation.

Using the Declarations, Kim could work with the rural youth by providing education on human rights and rights of Indigenous peoples, to enable the youth to learn and grow confidence with self-advocacy. Kim could leverage support from the community stakeholders for this education and advocacy, to address barriers to community participation, for example, stigma or discrimination based on race, ethnicity, disability, or age.

Community Development

Community development or community organizing is an orientation toward the practice of working with communities that encompasses a range of approaches and strategies enabling partnership and increased community-led decision making and self-determination (Minkler, 2012). The process is characterized by collective action, toward an identified shared issue or need, and enactment of strategies that increase and develop the community's ability to address and overcome the issue (Labonte, 2012; Lauckner et al., 2011).

Authors have described community development as a multilayered process that requires different steps, processes, and actions, to achieve the desired goal. Relationship building, partnership development, and capacity building are core processes (Lauckner et al., 2007; Lauckner et al., 2011). Community development requires strategies and actions to change power structures and relations within communities, or a redistribution of power from institutions to the community, such as power over decision making in health planning and programs (Labonte, 2012). Processes must incorporate strategies for enhancing people's abilities to influence decision making about issues that impact on their livelihoods and support the development of reciprocal and equal partnerships between communities and organizations to ensure processes do not have unintended negative consequences for communities that can result from paternalistic and top-down ways of working (Labonte, 2012).

A useful taxonomy developed by Rothman and Tropman (1987, in Lauckner et al., 2011) describes three approaches to community development, including:

1. Social planning: a top-down, data-driven approach of technical problem solving used by health professionals to identify community issues and determine actions.
2. Social action: a bottom-up, community-driven approach to identify, advocate, and address oppression, exclusion and resulting disadvantage by power and resource redistribution.
3. Locality development: a top-down and bottom-up, partnership approach, where health professionals engage with community members in identifying goals and actions to enable and catalyze actions and change (Lauckner et al., 2011).

Kim's involvement with the health promotion network and partnerships with the community stakeholders best aligns with a locality development approach to community development. Kim can further utilize this approach by working with the rural young people to identify their goals for the arts initiative and creating a plan for presenting the exhibition that is driven by the young people's ideas, aspirations, and interests, and creates opportunities for participation and belonging. A community development way of working would enable long-term partnerships with the community, extending beyond the arts initiative, ensuring the community maintains an ability to initiate and sustain infrastructure and programs that address inequities in participation and improve community health.

Community-Centered Practice Framework

The Community-Centered Practice Framework supports health professionals to shift from a person-centered to a community-centered care approach (Hyett et al., 2017, 2018). When the physical therapist began working with Jacob, for example, they used a person-centered care approach that is best practice for working with individuals—maintaining the person at the center of their care. Similarly, when Kim's focus shifts from Jacob to the community, the same key principles of equal partnership and collaboration need to be maintained and applied. A community-centered approach enables a clinician to conceptualize the community as the client and maintain the community at the center of care, ensuring an equal partnership is developed for service provision and services are directed toward community-driven goals, needs, and health challenges.

The Community-Centered Practice Framework was developed through research of exemplar models of community participation in Australia and Canada and is informed by social sciences and critical theories (Hyett et al., 2017, 2018). The Framework provides guidance for applying theory to practice with communities, to increase health professionals' understanding of the different components of community work. There are four components included in the Framework that can be applied concurrently or nonsequentially are outlined in Figure 3-3 (Hyett et al., 2018).

The first components of community-centered practice described in this Framework require health professionals to build an understanding of community identity including the peoples, leaders, groups, networks, organizations, institutions, and businesses (Hyett et al., 2018). The aim is to look beyond who is immediately visible in the community to explore and develop understandings of community diversity.

The next component is about exploring the health-promoting activities that are meaningful for the community. Health professionals are encouraged to explore how community members engage in different activities that promote health and well-being. This information gathering assists in the development of community-driven goals that enhance health, well-being, and QOL. Exploring community participation in shared or joint activities also reveals diverse expertise in communities that can contribute to health promotion initiatives including community roles, skills, values, experiences, assets, and capital (Hyett et al., 2018).

The third component involves identifying community resources and barriers that can be used to support participation or are challenges to participation. Resources can be identified within social and cultural capital, for example, relationships with people within a cultural group can be drawn

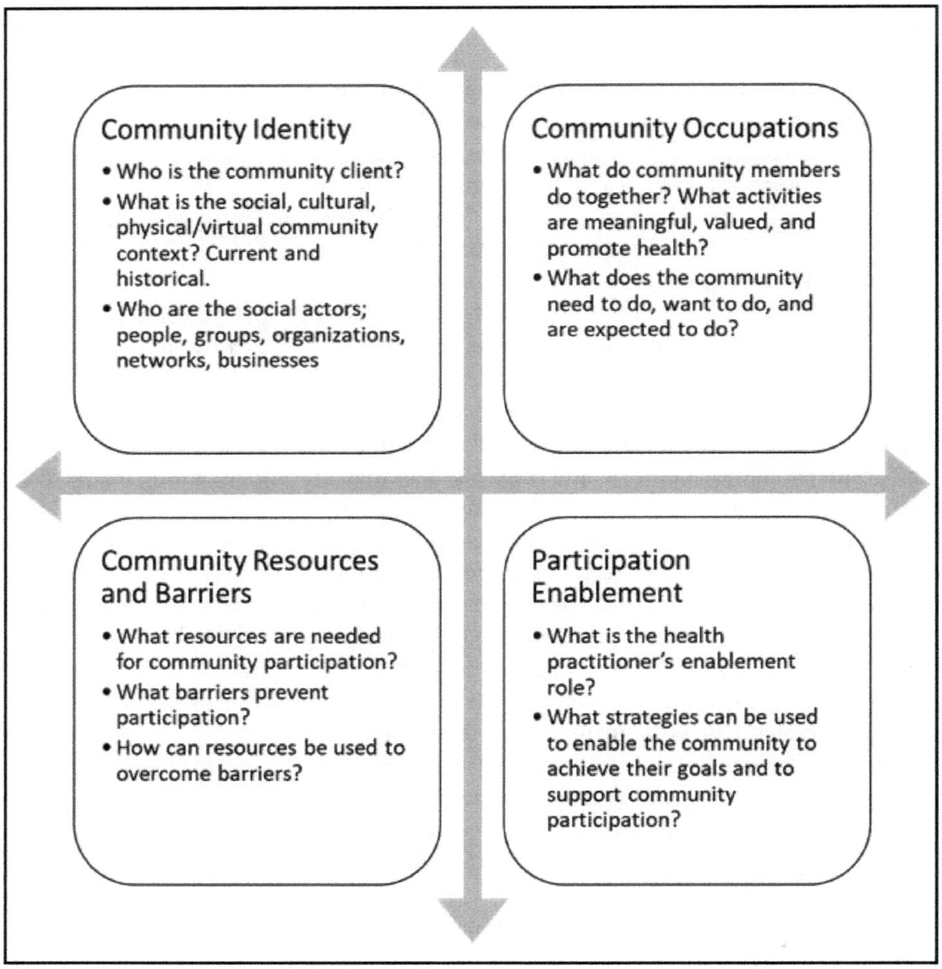

Figure 3-3. Community-Centered Practice Framework. (Adapted from Hyett, N., Kenny, A., & Dickson-Swift, V. [2018]. Re-imagining occupational therapy clients as communities: Presenting the community-centred practice framework. *Scandinavian Journal of Occupational Therapy, 26*[4], 246-260. https://doi.org/10.1080/11038128.2017.1423374)

upon to establish support networks, understandings of the community culture and history can inform health promotion strategies. Resources can also be economic (e.g., community-based business support and fundraising initiatives; Hyett et al., 2017, 2018). Many participation barriers within communities are attributed to social and environmental determinants of health. Changing and removing barriers to community participation that are caused by social and environmental determinants requires a process of power redistribution, to enable community members to influence and change the circumstances in which they live which are having a negative impact on their health. This requires critical analysis and interventions that target leaders and decision makers.

The final component is focused on developing strategies for community participation using information gathered from the previous phases to co-design strategies in partnership with the community. Strategies must be community-centered and utilize previous successful mechanisms of community participation. The health professional offers their expertise and specialist knowledge to inform the design and facilitation of strategies (e.g., expertise in health promotion and education). Evidence-informed strategies could include (but are not limited to) relationship building and partnership development, resource mobilization and leveraging, community building using social media and typical face-to-face methods, leadership development and community capacity building, community health promotion and education, and advocacy, protest and political lobbying (Hyett et al., 2017, 2018; Townsend et al., 2013; Whiteford & Townsend, 2011).

Kim could utilize the Community-Centered Practice Framework to guide her work with the community in co-designing the arts initiative by working through all four components in partnership with the community stakeholders. This would enable Kim to gain an in-depth understanding of the rural youth and their identity as a community group, and to work in partnership to identify strengths and resources and reduce barriers to social connection and participation. Kim would draw on her specialist expertise to add value (e.g., providing education on mental and emotional health, and coping skills for managing stress and anxiety).

Environment–Health–Occupation–Well-Being Model

The Environment–Health–Occupation–Well-Being (E-HOW) Model, developed by Dr. Michael Pizzi, an occupational therapist, provides health professionals with an approach to working with communities to enhance well-being and QOL (Pizzi & Richards, 2017). The model can be used by all professionals. Similar to other practice models, Pizzi and Richards (2017) argue the E-HOW Model is informed by core assumptions or concepts, which provide a set of theoretical perspectives to guide practice. The core assumption of this model is that well-being and QOL can be achieved through community work that is focused on creating supportive environments and opportunities for health promoting and meaningful community participation (Pizzi & Richards, 2017). The E-HOW Model is grounded in a dynamic systems perspective meaning that change in one aspect of the model (i.e., system) will influence another (therefore, making it dynamic; Figure 3-4).

The core assumptions and principles of the E-HOW Model include: 1) communities strive to and want to improve their health, well-being, and QOL; 2) there is a dynamic relationship between health, environments, and people's capacity for participating in health promoting and meaningful activities that can be utilized to improve well-being and QOL; 3) health behavior change can occur when people are conscious of the need for change; 4) effective community initiatives should incorporate strategies to improve people's control over decisions that impact their health, provide opportunities for participation in socially and culturally meaningful activities, and be underpinned by interprofessional collaboration (Pizzi & Richards, 2017). Importantly, this model fills the gap in community-level theoretical perspectives by providing a way of working with communities on well-being and QOL, which is different to many other theoretical perspectives that often specifically target health or disease outcomes.

Kim could apply the E-HOW Model to practice by including QOL as a goal and outcome indicator, and consulting with the team and drawing from interprofessional collaboration to achieve this goal with the rural youth. A relevant QOL outcome indicator could be enhanced friendships and social connection. Working as an interprofessional team, Kim could draw on strengths from the distinct disciplinary knowledge, as well as the team's shared understandings of health, illness, and recovery for interprofessional collaborative practice that achieves the highest standard of care for the community (Interprofessional Education Collaborative, 2016). All team members share abilities in supporting safe, equitable, accessible, and meaningful community participation (Interprofessional Education Collaborative, 2016). The physiotherapist can provide insights into physical activity requirements and mobility and body mechanics, increasing accessibility of the community program for people with injury or disability. The occupational therapist could inform the arts activity design and facilitation making sure the activity is meaningful for all community participants and supports social connections. The social worker could advocate for stakeholder support and funding, making sure the program was accessible for people who do not have access to transport or resources needed to attend the group. A psychologist can help to design supports for people with mental health barriers, supporting their coping abilities during group sessions especially if sensitive topics are raised. Finally, the speech therapist would develop and embed communication supports for youth that need them.

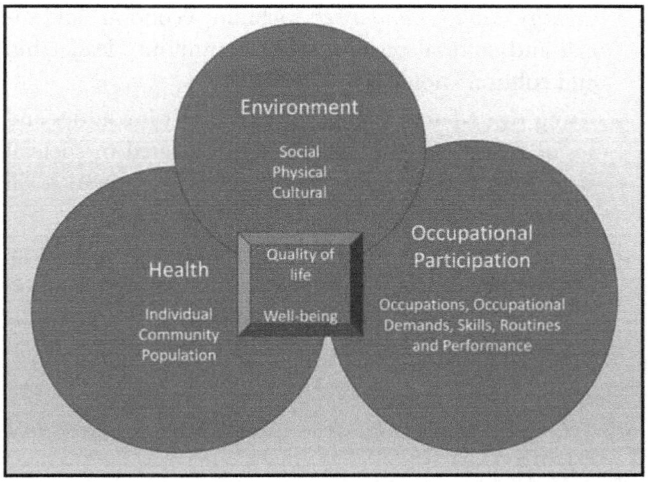

Figure 3-4. E-HOW Model. (Reproduced with permission from Michael A. Pizzi.)

Key Principles for Community-Oriented Practice

There are a number of commonalities between the different approaches that reflect best practice principles for working with communities to improve health, well-being, and QOL. Key overarching principles that are common across theoretical perspectives, which should inform Kim's work with the community in the case study include:

1. Taking time to *understand the community* context and community member's perspectives on the issue.
2. *Build relationships, partnerships and trust* with community members, local leaders, networks, groups, organizations, and businesses.

3. *Identify resources and assets* including economic and social and cultural resources like community leadership and cultural knowledge.
4. Using *rights-based approaches* that target inequities and *social determinants of health*; issues located in societal structures and systems that cause and perpetuate ill health.
5. Using *strengths-based approaches* that focus on building community capacity and mobilizing existing resources to improve health, well-being, and QOL *with* communities and not *for* them.

Summary

Community-oriented health professionals work with individuals, families, communities, and populations to improve health, well-being, and QOL. Theoretical perspectives provide community-oriented health professionals with evidence-informed approaches and specialist skills for making decisions about and implementing effective practice strategies and interventions. Health professionals working with communities are guided by international policy frameworks, for example, the Declaration of Alma Ata and the Ottawa Charter of Health Promotion, in addition to professional competency standards. The theoretical perspectives outlined in this chapter are based on current research, which ensures that theories are robust and suitable for applying to practice. Community-oriented health professionals must draw from theoretical perspectives to underpin and guide their practice to ensure optimal outcomes are achieved with clients.

The Transtheoretical Model and the Health Belief Model were introduced and applied to the case study, demonstrating effective theoretical perspectives for practice with individuals and families in community-oriented settings that enhance health, well-being, and QOL. The Transtheoretical Model assists health professionals to guide clients through a process of behavior change and to uptake positive behaviors or reduce negative behaviors, supporting goal attainment; while also providing guidance on how to approach working with people who are ambivalent or lack self-efficacy. The Health Belief Model is used by health professionals to predict a person's likelihood for engaging in positive health behaviors using five beliefs or factors. The Model is used for education and awareness raising interventions to increase a person's insight into their susceptibility to illness and the possible severity or risks of not engaging in health interventions. Both models provide important perspectives for health promotion and primary care services, for example, interventions that increase self-efficacy are supported by both models.

When working at the community-level, several theoretical perspectives for community-oriented care can be applied to enhance health, well-being, and QOL with communities and populations, including social justice, inclusion, and human rights-based approaches, community development, community capacity building, social determinants of health, Community-Centered Practice Framework, and the E-HOW Model. These theoretical approaches are critical for addressing social and environmental determinants of ill health, which are beyond individual control. These theoretical perspectives can be applied to practice by health professionals and interprofessional teams in partnership with communities to co-design initiatives that will have positive outcomes for the whole community. Teams can draw on disciplinary strengths and interprofessional capabilities to provide valuable input into the design and delivery of initiatives, optimizing community health, well-being, and QOL.

Key Points

- Community-oriented health professionals work at the community level with communities and populations, as well as with individuals and families.
- Community-oriented health professionals work with communities to improve whole-of-community health, well-being, and quality of life, and can develop and co-design initiatives with communities that address specific concerns of communities and sub-groups.
- Several theoretical perspectives are recommended to inform practice with communities and populations that can leverage community strengths and improve health, well-being, and quality of life outcomes, which are social justice, inclusion, and human rights-based approaches, community development, community capacity building, social determinants of health, Community-Centered Practice Framework, and the E-HOW Model.

References

Bandura, A. (1977). Self-efficacy: Toward a unifying theory of behavioral change. *Psychological Review, 84*(2), 191. https://doi.org/10.1037/0033-295X.84.2.191

Bridle, C., Riemsma, R. P., Pattenden, J., Sowden, A. J., Mather, L., Watt, I. S., & Walker, A. (2005). Systematic review of the effectiveness of health behavior interventions based on the transtheoretical model. *Psychology & Health, 20*(3), 283-301. https://doi.org/10.1080/08870440512331333997

Bryden, C. (2015). *Nothing about us, without us!: 20 years of dementia advocacy*. Jessica Kingsley.

Centers for Disease Control and Prevention. (2017). *Picture of America: Prevention*. https://www.cdc.gov/pictureofamerica/index.html

Champion, V. L., & Skinner, C. S. (2008). The Health Belief Model. In K. Glanz, B. K. Rimer, & K. Viswanath (Eds.), *Health behavior and health education: Theory, research, and practice* (Vol. 4, pp. 45-65). Jossey-Bass.

Charlton, J. I. (1998). *Nothing about us without us: Disability oppression and empowerment*. University of California.

DiClemente, C. C., & Prochaska, J. O. (1982). Self-change and therapy change of smoking behavior: A comparison of processes of change in cessation and maintenance. *Addictive Behaviors, 7*(2), 133-142. https://doi.org/10.1016/0306-4603(82)90038-7

Gerlach, A. J., Teachman, G., Laliberte-Rudman, D., Aldrich, R. M., & Huot, S. (2017). Expanding beyond individualism: Engaging critical perspectives on occupation. *Scandinavian Journal of Occupational Therapy, 25*(1), 1-9. https://doi.org/10.1080/11038128.2017.1327616

Grant, A. M., & Franklin, J. (2007). The transtheoretical model and study skills. *Behaviour Change, 24*(2), 99-113. https://doi.org/10.1375/bech.24.2.99

Hoffmann, T., Bennett, S., & Del Mar, C. (2017). *Evidence-based practice across the health professions* (3rd ed.). Elsevier Health Sciences.

Hyett, N., Kenny, A., & Dickson-Swift, V. (2017). Approaches for building community participation: A qualitative case study of Canadian food security programs. *OTJR: Occupation, Participation and Health, 37*(4), 199-209. https://doi.org/10.1177/1539449217727117

Hyett, N., Kenny, A., & Dickson-Swift, V. (2018). Re-imagining occupational therapy clients as communities: Presenting the community-centred practice framework. *Scandinavian Journal of Occupational Therapy, 26*(4), 246-260. https://doi.org/10.1080/11038128.2017.1423374

Hyett, N., McKinstry, C., Kenny, A., & Dickson-Swift, V. (2016). Community-centred practice: Occupational therapists improving the health and wellbeing of populations. *Australian Occupational Therapy Journal, 63*(1), 5-8. https://doi.org/10.1111/1440-1630.12222

Indigenous Allied Health Australia. (2019). Cultural safety through responsive health practice. https://iaha.com.au/wp-content/uploads/2020/02/Cultural-Safety-Through-Responsive-Health-Practice-Position-Statement.pdf

Interprofessional Education Collaborative. (2016). Core competencies for interprofessional collaborative practice: 2016 update.

Kleis, R. R., Hoch, M. C., Hogg-Graham, R., & Hoch, J. M. (2021). The effectiveness of the Transtheoretical Model to improve physical activity in healthy adults: A systematic review. *Journal of Physical Activity & Health, 18*(1), 94-108. https://doi.org/10.1123/jpah.2020-0334

Labonte, R. (2012). Community, community development, and the forming of authentic partnerships. Some critical reflections. In M. Minkler (Ed.), *Community organizing and community building for health and welfare* (pp. 95-108). Rutgers University Press. http://ebookcentral.proquest.com/lib/latrobe/detail.action?docID=988156

Lauckner, H., Krupa, T. M., & Paterson, M. L. (2011). Conceptualizing community development: Occupational therapy practice at the intersection of health services and community. *Canadian Journal of Occupational Therapy, 78*(4), 260-268. https://doi.org/10.2182/cjot.2011.78.4.8

Lauckner, H., Pentland, W., & Paterson, M. (2007). Exploring Canadian occupational therapists' understanding of and experiences in community development. *Canadian Journal of Occupational Therapy, 74*(4), 314-325. https://doi.org/10.2182/cjot.07.005

McDonagh, J. E., & Bateman, B. (2012). 'Nothing about us without us': Considerations for research involving young people. *Archives of Disease in Childhood - Education and Practice, 97*(2), 55-60. https://doi.org/10.1136/adc.2010.197947

Minkler, M. (2012). Part one: Introduction. In M. Minkler (Ed.), *Community organizing and community building for health and welfare* (3rd ed., pp. 1-26). Rutgers University Press.

Office of Disease Prevention and Health Promotion, U.S. Department of Health and Human Services. (2020). Healthy People 2030: Mental health and mental disorders. https://health.gov/healthypeople/objectives-and-data/browse-objectives/mental-health-and-mental-disorders

Pizzi, M. A., & Richards, L. G. (2017). Promoting health, well-being, and quality of life in occupational therapy: A commitment to a paradigm shift for the next 100 years. *American Journal of Occupational Therapy, 71*(4), 7104170010p7104170011-7104170010p7104170015. https://doi.org/10.5014/ajot.2017.028456

Reitz, S. M., Scaffa, M. E., & Merryman, M. B. (2013). Theoretical frameworks for community-based practice. In M. E. Scaffa & S. M. Reitz (Eds.), *Occupational therapy in community-based practice settings* (2nd ed., pp. 31-50). F.A. Davis Company. http://ebookcentral.proquest.com

Rosenstock, I. M. (1974). Historical origins of the Health Belief Model. *Health Education Monographs, 2*(4), 328-335. https://doi.org/10.1177/109019817400200403

Rosenstock, I. M., Strecher, V. J., & Becker, M. H. (1988). Social learning theory and the health belief model. *Health Education Quarterly, 15*(2), 175-183. https://doi.org/10.1177/109019818801500203

Sikka, R., Morath, J. M., & Leape, L. (2015). The Quadruple Aim: care, health, cost and meaning in work. *BMJ Quality & Safety, 24*(10), 608. https://doi.org/10.1136/bmjqs-2015-004160

South, J., Bagnall, A.-M., Stansfield, J. A., Southby, K. J., & Mehta, P. (2017). An evidence-based framework on community-centred approaches for health: England, UK. *Health Promotion International*, dax083-dax083. https://doi.org/10.1093/heapro/dax083

Sutton, S. (2005). Another nail in the coffin of the Transtheoretical Model? A comment on West (2005). *Addiction, 100*(8), 1043-1046. https://doi.org/https://doi.org/10.1111/j.1360-0443.2005.01172.x

Townsend, E. A., Beagan, B., Kumas-Tan, Z., Versnel, J., Iwama, M., Landry, J., Stewart, D., & Brown, J. (2013). Enabling: Occupational therapy's core competency. In E. A. Townsend & H. J. Polatajko (Eds.), *Enabling occupation II: Advancing an occupational therapy vision for health, well-being, and justice through occupation* (pp. 87-133). Canadian Association of Occupational Therapists.

United Nations. (1948). United Nations Universal Declaration of Human Rights. https://www.un.org/en/about-us/universal-declaration-of-human-rights

United Nations. (2007). United Nations Declaration on the Rights of Indigenous Peoples. https://www.un.org/development/desa/indigenouspeoples/declaration-on-the-rights-of-indigenous-peoples.html

Whiteford, G. E., & Townsend, E. A. (2011). Participatory Occupational Justice Framework (POJF 2010); enabling occupational participation and inclusion. In F. Kronenberg, N. Pollard, & D. Sakellariou (Eds.), *Occupational therapies without borders: Towards an ecology of occupation-based practices* (Vol. 2, pp. 65-84). Elsevier.

World Health Organization. (1986). Ottawa Charter for Health Promotion. http://www.who.int/healthpromotion/conferences/previous/ottawa/en/

World Health Organization. (2008). Closing the gap in a generation. Health equity through action on social determinants. Commission on social determinants of health. Final report. http://whqlibdoc.who.int/hq/2008/WHO_IER_CSDH_08.1_eng.pdf

World Health Organization and UNICEF. (1978). Primary Health Care: Report of the International Conference of Primary Health Care. The International Conference on Primary Health Care, Alma Ata.

Part II

PROMOTING PHYSICAL HEALTH

4

CHAPTER

Promoting Physical Health

Infants, Children, and Youth

Cheryl A. Hall, PT, DHSc, MBA; Alexander Lopez, JD, OT/L, FAOTA; and Sandra M. Ribeiro, PT, DPT, MSEd

Learning Objectives

At the end of this chapter, the reader will:

1. Explain the benefits and goals of physical activity on overall development in childhood and the effects throughout the life span (CAPTE 2J; ACOTE B.1.1)
2. Describe effective interventions to caregivers designed to increase physical activity for health and well-being of children (CAPTE 3E; ACOTE B.1.3., B.4.10).
3. Develop interprofessional, culturally sensitive plans of care designed to increase physical activity throughout childhood by implementing parent-guided strategies (CAPTE 3F; ACOTE B.1.2)
4. Implement the principles of the teaching–learning process using educational methods and health literacy education approaches through activity design, clinical training, and instruction to all stakeholders (ACOTE B.4.21)
5. Be able to coordinate a community-based interdisciplinary group focused on providing physical activity opportunities for children before, during and after school, based on the needs of the child and family (CAPTE 2J; ACOTE B.4.25)
6. Be able to identify key community-based resources for family members and caregivers to access with their children of all ages and developmental skill levels (CAPTE 3F; ACOTE B.5.2)
7. Be able to develop a community-based program to encourage, engage, and provide instruction to parents and caregivers in promoting health and well-being through physical activities in their children (CAPTE 3E; ACOTE B.3.4)

The ACOTE Standards used are those from 2018.

Pizzi, M. A., & Amir, M. (Eds.). *Interprofessional Perspectives for Community Practice: Promoting Health, Well-Being, and Quality of Life* (pp. 55-75).

Key Words

Community Engagement, Container Baby Syndrome, Health Promotion, Interprofessional, Motor Development, Physical Activity, Play, Quality of Life, Well-Being

Introduction

Promoting Health, Well-Being, and Quality of Life in Children Through Physical Activity

As per the Centers for Disease Control and Prevention (CDC), family and **community engagement** in **physical activity** incorporates an **interprofessional** team approach, which is described as a means of integrating parents and professionals into the various venues where children work and **play** (CDC, 2020a,b,c). Physical activity is defined as movement of the body produced by energy expenditure by skeletal muscles and is categorized into levels of activity, such as moderate to vigorous (World Health Organization [WHO], 2020). Although sometimes used synonymously when referring to children, play, although complex in its scope, is defined as "The work of children. It consists of those activities performed for self-amusement that have behavioral, social, and psychomotor rewards. It is child-directed, and the rewards come from within the individual child; it is enjoyable and spontaneous" (Encyclopedia of Children's Health, n.d.). Parent engagement in school requires that parents work with school staff to improve the quality of a child's health and education. Where there is parent involvement, there are children who are doing better in school, are engaged in their school communities, and making better choices about their health and behaviors. When parents are engaged, they can learn from those in the school environment and integrate that information into their families' lives as a result. For example, parents who are educated in school nutrition, physical education, and physical activity and are given ways to promote healthy programs in their schools are more likely to use that information and strategies at home to promote wellness activities at home (CDC, 2020a,b,c).

In-school physical activity does need not only take place on the playground or in physical education class. The CDC encourages the engagement of all school personnel, children, administrators, parents, and others to help promote physical activity in the school environment and proposes the use of activity breaks, using equipment such as balls, mats, and music to engage children in movement. These breaks from sitting are easy to implement and have a host of benefits to children such as: improving concentration and on-task activities, reducing fidgety behaviors, improving motivation, engagement and learning, and increasing the amount of a child's daily physical activity (CDC, 2018a,b,c). At-school activity is not the only time children can be engaged in physical activities. Before and after school also provide opportunities for the development of healthy habits and an improvement in **quality of life** (QOL) and well-being throughout the life span. QOL is an individual's perception of the positive and negative aspects of one's own life and varies based on many factors, including but not limited to health, socioeconomic status, culture, values, family structure, and family and community support (CDC, 2018a,b,c). **Well-being** is "a positive outcome that is meaningful for people and for many sectors of society because it tells us that people perceive that their lives are going well," which is closely related to QOL (CDC, 2018a,b,c).

Community-based programs, such as Out of School Time (OST) is an after-school program that is designed to take place in any safe community setting, schools, and Boys and Girls Clubs. This type of program can be staffed with members of the school, health care providers, and parents, if properly qualified, to supervise and participate in such a program (CDC, 2021). An important benefit of programs like this is that they can be developed according to age and can include infants and young toddlers, young children, youth, and adolescents. In addition, with the proper professional participation and supervision (school-based personnel, nursing and rehabilitation professionals), these programs can be inclusive for all children including those with chronic illness and those with unique needs. This type of inclusive program can not only foster a sense of acceptance to others, but can enhance the QOL for all children and their families by fostering peer interactions and friendships (CDC, 2020a,b,c).

In this chapter, we will discuss the evolution of movement and the application of age-appropriate activities in children to encourage lifelong health, fitness, improved QOL, and well-being across the life span using an interprofessional approach. We will also discuss the importance of identifying and participating in community-based resources and the impact of those resources on overall community health.

Movement in Infancy and Early Toddlerhood

What Prompts Early Motor Activity?

Well-known 1970s children's television host Fred Rogers famously known as Mr. Rogers, said, "Play is often talked about as if it were a relief from serious learning; but for children, play is serious learning. Play is really the work of childhood" (Moore, 2020). Studies show that early play experiences are necessary and important to social-emotional development in early childhood (Nandy, 2020). In addition, gross motor and cognitive development have a strong association in early childhood as children learn to explore their environment and learn about their surroundings through movement and interaction with objects in their surroundings (Veldman, 2019).

As infants grow and develop, the systems responsible for movement are changing as well. Physiologically, bone and soft tissue develop because of hormonal messengers to direct bone growth and the mechanical forces applied to each, and this occurs, in infants and young children, as a direct relationship of typical **motor development** (LoRang, 2019). Motor development is defined as "the continuous, age-related process of change in movement as well as interacting constraints (or factors) in the individual, environment, and task that drive these changes" (Haywood & Getchell, 2019, p. 5). This is a continuation of what occurs in utero, but the forces exerted on the musculoskeletal structures are coming from gravity and limb movement, either in its entirety or segmentally. It is during this time that infants and young toddlers begin to experience the multisensory, multisystem effects of movement, such as those associated with postural control and stability, vestibular input, voluntary control and purposeful movement, the integration of eye-hand coordination and processing input to the visual-perceptual systems and the neuromotor and musculoskeletal systems. This is a vital period between birth and 3 years old during which infants begin to roll, creep on all fours, sit, walk independently, run, kick a ball, and hop. This development is based on the interaction of numerous factors such as maturation of the neuromuscular system, the child's physical growth and behavior, the pace of maturation of these two domains and biological maturity, the remaining effects of prior movement experiences, and the novel movement experiences (Malina, 2004). At the crux of motor development is how "environmental experiences interact with growth and maturity to influence motor development and proficiency" (Malina, 2004, p. 50).

A variety of environmental stimuli is essential for growth and development. Based on the fact that the earliest myelination of the brain begins in the areas responsible for motor and sensory function, Tierney (2009) reported sensory experiences influence gross motor skill development and cited an important physiological relationship between music and movement in the developing brain. Music is also associated with development in many areas such as communication and language, social development and conceptual development in math, reading, technology, culture, and art and design, positively affecting all developmental domains and contributing to overall well-being and QOL (Battelley, 2020).

Early exposure to music is a cross-cultural phenomenon in societies worldwide and occurs in the earliest days of the infant's life. In many cultures, infants are carried and sung to by their mothers or are lulled to sleep with gentle lullabies. Early exposure to music during routine parent-child interactions pairs music to movement carried throughout infancy and early childhood. Young infants stop and observe their mother's "performance," and older infants will engage in rhythmic movement of their own making. As they get older, children use this early association to develop their own motor patterns, preferences for movement, and motor experiences (Trehub, 2018).

The infant is a complex organism that receives sensory input, oftentimes without the caretaker realizing it. Touch is one of the essential and most-often experienced type of sensory input received by an infant and very young child as a result of routing care. Based on numerous infant massage studies, Field et al. (1986) found that tactile input has been shown to have many positive effects on growing premature infants, including higher motor scores on the Brazelton scale compared to those infants who did not receive massage. Visual input is essential for postural development and "even while lying down, the body is still in motion" (Adolph & Franchak, 2017, p. 4), and if we consider the infant's early days, they are often positioning on their back. Even though they appear stationary, their vestibular, tactile, visual, auditory, and motor systems are receiving multiple sensory inputs and responding to those various stimuli with movement. For example, notice a newborn infant resting on his back. A sudden loud sound will provoke a startle response, with all extremities responding with random movement; the infant's eyes widen as a primitive response to fight or flight, even though we know that this is not possible, and this loud sound often provokes the infant to begin crying. Most often, in infants, crying is appreciated as a whole-body experience, complete with flailing extremities and other random body movements. Therefore, although we addressed music as a specific source of sensory input as it relates to brain development and movement, research has shown the importance of many types of sensory experiences that facilitate motor development in infants and young toddlers. As children get older, their motor experiences become more complex. As they are exposed to and are able to seek out their own novel interactions with the environment, they learn to respond to multiple sensory inputs at once. This early exposure to sensory input through parent/caregiver–guided opportunities continues to forge the development of the young brain and the ability to fine-tune complex motor skills.

> **Key Point**
>
> **CONTAINER BABY SYNDROME**
>
> According to the American Academy of Pediatrics (AAP), the effects of keeping infants in carriers with less "tummy time" have yielded findings as follows: abnormal head shape (plagiocephaly), lower locomotor scores on the Alberta Infant Motor Scales (Piper et al., 2000), an inverse relationship to time spent in prone and BMI and delays in social communication up to 12 months of age and in cognition up to 2 years of age.

Container Baby Syndrome

Container baby syndrome is defined as "a collection of movement, behavior and other problems caused by a baby or infant spending too much time in a container—any commonly-used piece of baby equipment that resembles a container" (*What is Container Baby Syndrome?* Physical Therapy Guide to Container Baby Syndrome, 2020). These items include, but are not limited to car seats, nursing pillows, jumpers, strollers, and vibrating chairs (Physical Therapy Guide to Container Baby Syndrome, 2020). There is no evidence of delayed development in infants and children prior to the availability of baby containers compared to today's children who spend an average of 5.7 hours per day ± 3.5 hours, ranging from 0 to 16 hours per day, in infant seating devices (Callahan, 1997). In fact, research supports the opposite. There is a positive association between tummy time and age-appropriate gross motor and overall development, increased mobility in prone, supine, crawling, and walking, the prevention of brachycephaly, and a lower body mass index (BMI) in children ages 0 to 12 months (Hewitt, 2020; Malina, 2004).

In addition, as previously discussed, a variety of sensory experiences contributes to all areas of development and improved health indicators in infants and children. Studies show that infants who spend more time on their tummies, have a lower BMI score and higher scores on motor development assessments at 2 months and then again at 4 months, as tummy time increases (Koren et al., 2019). A systematic review by Carson et al. (2017, p. 59) compiled 96 studies, which concluded "physical activity, especially prone for infants... were consistently found to be favorable with a number of health indicators" and emphasized the importance of consistent physical activity in children of all ages. Placing infants in these devices reduces tummy time and limits their ability to interact with their environment in a way that reduces the type sensory input, motor experiences, and achievement of developmental milestones throughout childhood. Collectively, these findings support the importance of environmental interactions and the development of proficient motor skills in infants and children.

In conjunction with the consideration of proper positioning of infants for developmental purposes, Healthy People 2030 cites one of the goals for healthy infants is to "Improve the health and safety of infants" (U.S. Department of Health and Human Services [USDHHS], n.d.). One of the developmental objectives is MICH-14, which states, "Increase the proportion of infants who are put to sleep on their backs" (USDHHS, n.d.). This objective, when measured, showed that 78.7% of infants born in 2016 were placed on their backs to sleep. The target goal for 2030 is 88.9%, with the purpose being the prevention of sudden infant death syndrome and sleep-related deaths (USDHHS, n.d.). However, as with infants being placed in "containers," with limited opportunities for "tummy time," data shows associations between increased incidence of plagiocephaly and craniosynostosis and the Back to Sleep initiative and plagiocephaly, craniosynostosis, and motor delays (Andrews, 2017; Branch, 2015).

Engagement and Collaboration: Caregiver and Professionals as Partners

The importance of physical activity should not be underestimated, even in the youngest populations. It is vital to encourage movement in young children through play and age-appropriate motor skills, by providing novel movement experiences necessary to require adaptation and refinement of higher-level skills. Children who participate in physical activity early on have a wider variety of movement experiences, which, in turn influences continued engagement in physical activity and proficiency in motor skills. As children mature cognitively, they improve in self-assessment of their physical abilities, and those who see themselves as more skillful will continue to participate in physical activity (Stodden et al., 2008). Herein lies the foundation where early physical activity and development of proficient motor skills exist. This can determine if a child will integrate regular physical activity as a lifestyle behavior or not, whether through structured or unstructured activities throughout the life span.

Contemporary research shows that structured physical activity is more beneficial than unstructured physical activity, where kindergarten children who engaged in a combination of structured and unstructured activities or structured activities only, had superior gross motor skills 2 years later when compared to their same-age peers who engaged in only unstructured activities (Dapp, 2021). Similar findings were present in the development of fine motor skills (Dapp, 2021). However, unstructured physical activity has its benefits as well, and while structured physical activity leads to skillfulness and neurocognitive benefits in adolescents, unstructured outdoor physical activity has a greater positive effect on moderate to vigorous physical activity in younger children and preschoolers (Subramanian et al., 2015; Gordon et al., 2013).

For interprofessional team members providing care to infants and young toddlers, the goal should be promotion of good health and the development of healthy habits that continue throughout the life span; however, incorporating too many providers at one time can be overwhelming to family members and have a negative impact on outcomes and increase cost of care (Schuetz et al., 2021). Well-defined roles of each team member are essential in carrying out effective interventions with families and these roles require time to learn about each member's goals of intervention, develop effective communication between team members, and to have consistent leadership and support (Schuetz et al., 2021). Only then, can the team work collaboratively to achieve the desired outcomes. An example of this model is found in the Transition to Home (TtH) model that found families with limited resources (socially disadvantaged, lacking in family support) were those most in need of support from an interprofessional team. Although the population studied were parents of preterm infant, many caregivers find themselves alone and unsure of what are appropriate resources to help encourage motor development in their children, do those resources exist in their communities for their children, and if they do, how can they and their children have to access them.

Pediatricians are becoming aware of the services provided through Early Intervention programs and are adept as screening children for developmental delays. Therefore, these formal points of entry into an organized system make it easier to address the needs of these infants and children in a system that is continually trying to implement a collaborative model (Bruder et al., 2019). The goal of typical development is found in the International Classification of Functioning, Disability and Function (ICF-CY), the child and youth version (Adolfsson et al., 2018). Traditionally, this model is used as a model of disability assessment; however, the ICF-CY version focuses on participation and engagement, important factors for the assessment of health and well-being of children (Adolfsson et al., 2018).

Hwang et al. (2012) used the ICF-CY framework as a model to investigate biopsychosocial factors that affect development, specifically, what influenced activity and participation. In this study, the home environment was found to be "very influential...based on the bioecological model, family system perspective and empirical evidence" (Hwang et al., 2012, p. 305). In addition, the home environment has a greater effect on early development, and is associated with similar outcomes, as the child gets older. Thus, supporting the need for creating a home environment that incorporates opportunities for physical activity and other healthy behaviors throughout infancy and early childhood. What better way to incorporate the skills of the interprofessional team. With the support of the child's primary care provider, physical therapists, and occupational therapists and other health professionals can develop activity programs by teaching parents how to set up play areas to encourage tummy time and exploration of their play areas. Speech-language pathologists can provide information about the importance of modeling language and speaking to infants and children. Music therapists can provide fun ways to use music to encourage movement, language, and sensory integration. Nutritionists can offer insight and strategies on how to prepare fun, healthy foods and snacks. Teachers, nurses, psychologists, and community partners can also work together to offer families an array of community-based resources, and experiences designed to educate and promote health and well-being throughout the life span. Such resources can be found in public libraries and can include infant/toddler reading groups, music, and movement activities. Community-based programs that offer parent-child play groups, such as local YMCAs, houses of worship, and other community-based organizations that support children and families. The ability to provide families with a collection of rich resources is essential and interprofessional team collaboration is one way to help promote and encourage healthy development for everyone.

Case Study 4-1 addresses an infant with issues related to common movement concerns. These issues leave parents feeling frightened and unsure of what to do and how to proceed. Do the issues of concern warrant a full evaluation by an Early Intervention team or something less formal, community-based? If community-based resources are indicated, what resources are available in the community? Which are appropriate for Sammy and his family? How can Sammy's parent access these resources? What is the cost? How can Sammy's parent find out more about which resources are right for Sammy? Whom can she contact to find out all of these things? Sammy's pediatrician? A pediatric therapy office? The local public library? A community-based nursery or preschool? Consider the previous information and the following content to answer these questions and those at the end of the first part of the case study.

Since infants and very young children cannot engage in the structured activities enjoyed by older children, activity can be encouraged in other ways. Play offers children the benefits of stimulating cognitive, social, physical, and emotional development (Ginsburg, 2007). Free play, to the degree that it can exist in infants and young toddlers, provides opportunities for learning whereby they can create and explore their environment in a meaningful way. Infants can engage in mouthing toys to help learn about their environment and play with their hands and feed to learn about their bodies in relation to space. Toddlers also use their newfound mobility to explore their surroundings, climbing and running, negotiating uneven surfaces, challenging their balance and postural control in an upright position, and begin to increase their movement repertoire. As they do, they refine their skills and continue to challenge themselves with jumping, stair-climbing, and negotiating playground equipment. It is important to recognize that not all children have the same opportunity for the same type of play experiences in early childhood.

Socioeconomic disparities can affect the ability and quality of play in children and families living in poverty, and

Case Study 4-1

Sammy is an 8-month-old-year-old boy. Sammy has a history of premature birth. He was born at 35 weeks' gestation and weighed 4 lbs., 8 oz. APGARS were 5,1 7,5 and 8.10 He was transferred to the Neonatal Intensive Care Unit (NICU) due to mild respiratory distress for which he received oxygen via nasal cannula for 5 days and was then stable on room air. His postnatal course was also remarkable for jaundice, for which he was treated with phototherapy. Sammy remained in the NICU for 3 weeks and was discharged to home with his mother.

Sammy is an only child and lives in a private two-story home with his mother. Extended family live nearby, but Sammy's mother is the primary caretaker. Sammy is seen regularly by his pediatrician for well visits. His mother brought him to the emergency department of the local hospital 3 weeks ago when Sammy demonstrated difficulty breathing and a cough that sounded like "a seal barking." He was diagnosed with reactive airway disease and was prescribed an Albuterol nebulizer mist to be administered as needed.

Developmental milestones: Sammy rolled belly to back at 4 months, tripod sitting when placed at 5 months, rolled back to belly at 6 months, and sat alone at 7 months. Sammy does not like to be on his belly to play and rolls to his back immediately. He demonstrates a mild flattening to the right parietal-occipital area, but no limitations were noted with active neck rotation to either side and head righting reactions were consistent and age-appropriate.

1. What might be a possible concern that can develop with lack of "tummy time"?
2. What type of physical activities can be used to help Sammy's mother encourage tummy time?
3. What strategies can Sammy's mother use to encourage the next phase of age-appropriate motor skills?
4. What are the implications for future development if Sammy does not develop mastery of these earlier skills?
5. What community resources would you recommend for Sammy and his mother to take part in to help create a healthy and stimulating home environment?

this is especially true in older children, as well as infants and toddlers. Parents in families living in poverty have less time to invest in playing with their children due to multiple jobs and other responsibilities interfering with opportunities for age-appropriate play with their children. In addition, economic hardship, a higher likelihood of parental substance abuse in the home, fewer opportunities for safe outdoor play, and lack of financial resources to purchase toys, blocks, books, and other developmentally suitable learning items, also impact play experiences and opportunities for these children (Milteer, 2021).

The American Academy of Pediatrics (AAP), offers parents and caregivers tips for keeping young children active and healthy (Milteer, 2021). Some of them are as follows:

1. Teach parents about the importance of free, unstructured play in the normal development of children. Especially in younger children, free play allows for higher levels of physical activity, especially outdoor play. Encouraging children to run, roll, reach for their feet, bring climb, crawl, creep, push or throw a ball, kick a ball, climb over objects, jump in place or over obstacles, or anything that gets children moving, is beneficial to their physical health and well-being and their overall motor development. Assisting their movement by bringing their hands to their feed, moving them from side to side or through developmental transition, modeling activities for older children and parent participation is motivational for children, and children will model behaviors that they see in their parents, including healthy behaviors.
2. Simple, inexpensive toys (e.g., dolls, jump ropes, blocks, balls, buckets) allow children to be creative, more physically involved, and more imaginative than expensive toys. Setting up these toys to encourage movement in infants by putting toys out of their reach can encourage movement and exploration of their environment. Older children have wonderful imaginations, so a bucket and a beanbag or a ball can become a tossing game. Blocks can be set up to be kicked down or knocked over, not only for physical activity, but for cognitive and visual motor development as well.
3. Playtime is an opportunity to engage fully with their children, to bond and promote social-emotional health. Anytime talking or singing can be incorporated into playtime, an opportunity for development of communication, language, and social skills presents itself. During these experiences, infants will imitate facial expressions and mouth movements, and they will learn about emotion and social connections; all-important skills in all domains of development.
4. Use positive reinforcement and encouragement to help children try things that may be difficult at first. Encouraging children to continue to be active and playful by cheering and clapping for their best efforts enhances confidence and self-esteem. Children who are more confident in their motor skills tend to participate in sports and physical activity as teens and adults.
5. Discuss the importance of physical activity to help prevent obesity in children and explain how habits in childhood will continue into adulthood. Therefore, encourage parents and caregivers to encourage and engage in healthy behaviors (more physical activity and less screen time) with their children. Parents are primary models of

behaviors for their children; this includes bad behaviors too, so ensure that parents are modeling positive behaviors that encourage healthy eating, regular physical activity, and other healthy habits.

6. Provide parents and caregivers with resources that can help provide resources to help with familial financial, education, and mental health issues. Making oneself familiar with available resources for families is very important, and being knowledgeable about community groups, activities, and interprofessional team members and their roles is essential to carrying out a successful plan designed to serve families and their children in local communities. As health care team members, we need to establish relationships with local pediatricians. These partnerships are vital to help us assist families to find resources outside of the medical model right in their own communities. It is in their neighborhoods, towns, and villages that families will find long-term support, friendship, and vital connections with others.

Integrating healthy physical activity habits early on can help prevent obesity and obesity-related problems later in life and these healthy habits can lead to an integration of physical activity into a healthy lifestyle across the life span.

As we recognize and appreciate the benefits of mostly unstructured, self-driven play in the infant and young toddler, the importance of environmental exploration in the development of motor skills and acknowledge the adverse implications of limited physical activity on motor development, let us examine the motor experience in late toddlerhood and in the preschool-aged child.

Movement in Early Childhood

The Importance of Physical Activity in Early Childhood

According to the WHO, physical activity during early childhood is defined as "any bodily movements produced by skeletal muscle that result in a substantial increase over the resting energy expenditure" (WHO, 2022).

Early childhood is divided into two categories: toddlerhood, between 2 to 3 years of age and preschool age, from 3 to 5 years of age (Stanborough, 2019). During this stage, physical development in children increases steadily in height, weight, and muscle mass. Early childhood is a dynamic developmental period with evolving movements for greater participation, social development, and independence (Gerber et al., 2010). A significant time for a dramatic change in mobility for toddlers is from 18 months. It is during this time when proficiency in standing mobility begins. An increase in frequency of upright mobility in walking, running, and stair climbing is evident. This change in independent mobility in standing provides a natural challenge for joint positioning and core muscle development necessary in the development of postural stability. Postural alignment during this early stage develops to support the achievement of higher-level gross motor function and the maintenance of a healthy body though participation in physical activities. The toddler enjoys walking around the house, the playground, or preschool, and experiences changes in physical, mental, and social abilities. This freedom of movement allows for increased speed, negotiation of obstacles, and exploration through sensory-motor activities. Exploration of the world in an upright position offers opportunities for problem solving and developing confidence in earlier and newly developing skills. Zeng et al. (2017) reports that physical activity in early childhood positively affects motor and cognitive skills, and it is easy to surmise that skillful motor and cognitive abilities have a positive effect on an individual's confidence, overall health and well-being, and QOL.

Engaging Caretakers in Supporting Health and Well-Being

Primary caretakers are integral in supporting development, especially mobility skills, which have benefits beyond walking. When a child is confined or mobility is restricted, the child has a limited repertoire in which to explore and learn. Opportunities for a variety of movement experiences allows for an expansion of the child's social, cognitive, and physical world through exposure to new environments. Trial and error, innate in the development of locomotor skills stimulates the brain to interpret and respond to the environment. This type of response occurs progressively throughout life when learning new motor skills and facilitates neuroplasticity in the brain to occur (Scott et al., 2020). Opportunities for free play and physical activity are vital components that should be promoted throughout childhood. When parents can share in this experience, a mutual mindset of health and well-being and patterns of enjoyment can develop between the caregiver and child.

Since parents play an important role in promoting habits essential to a child's well-being and health, the interdisciplinary team can offer benefits to any potential barriers to participating in encouraging their child's motor skill and physical health. Parents cite their own fears that limit their child's physical activity in early childhood in order to protect them from injuries and falls. Although this age group has a higher risk of nonfatal falls and drowning, caregivers can be directed to educational resources in the National Action Plan for Child Injury Prevention (CDC, 2012), and with proper guidance, they can be partners in promoting a better QOL for their children in the short and long term. In addition, Healthy People 2030 also provide helpful resources for parents and caregivers, including guidelines of limiting screen time to less than 1 hour to discourage sedentary behaviors and promote physical activity (USDHHS, n.d.).

Studies show that the quality of interactions between children and adults paired adequate levels of engagement and opportunities to explore are essential to a young child's development (Slot & Beses, 2018). Since adults supervise young children, it is important that adults create programs that incorporate safe and risk-taking play activities. It is in this age group where being exposed to exciting and challenging tasks foster a child's self-esteem (Little, 2016). At this young age, parents are responsible for creating opportunities for activity and modeling the lifestyle they want to impart on their children. In playing together, young children learn the value of the activity and integrate habits of healthy behaviors and participation well beyond the early childhood years. As the toddler learns to communicate, share ideas, set boundaries, and partake in activities that are fun, they develop preferences toward types of physical activity. The child can request opportunities to participate in specific activities in which they feel comfortable, such as Pee-Wee sports leagues, karate classes, dance classes, and other programs designed for young children. As the child participates, they become more adept in their skills, and with skill comes confidence, which enables them to seek out, engage, and participate in other challenging activities in the community, school, and home environments.

Developmental Milestones for the Foundation of Health and Well-Being

As the child moves beyond 3 years of age, their motor skills progress rapidly, yielding an advanced repertoire of play. The steady progression of physical activity, which refers to the amount of exercise completed, is an initiative of the Department of Health and Human Services with national objectives to promote health, prevent disease, and improve QOL (USDHHS, n.d.). During the toddler years, the child shows a determination to develop skills, such as jumping, that produce power in muscles of the lower legs required for future success in physical activity such as sports. The child develops coordination and visual motor control through ball playing. Motor skills expand through practice in ability to kick, throw, and catch a ball. Developmental delay in early childhood have been linked to decreased participation in organized sports and psychosocial development (Neville et al., 2021). Starting around the preschool age, a child develops motor skills such as hopping on one leg, walking on a taped line, and skipping. Difficulty in these skills and activities may hinder the development of postural control and balance reactions that influence higher-level physical activities. These higher-level skills encourage confident participation in present and future activities responsible in the promotion of health and well-being throughout the life span (Robinson et al., 2020). Activities to enhance these motor skills can be easily incorporated during age-appropriate play activities. Any member or members of the interdisciplinary team can provide knowledge and resources to families and share helpful, parent-friendly websites such as Healthy Kids, Healthy Future from Nemours Children's Health. This website lists a guide on best practices for physical activity (Nemours' Integrated Approach to Child Health and Obesity Prevention in Delaware, 2014). A study by Wang et al. (2020) investigating possible variables affecting the rate of motor skills between family income, parents' education level, and family activity found no correlation between any of variable and the rate of motor skill development. However, providing more opportunities for children to play with friends and participate in sports activities were found to support motor skills and correlate positively with motor skill acquisition (Wang et al., 2020).

Strategies for Promoting Physical Activity in the Young Child

The ability to imitate motor skills increases a child's repertoire of movement by visually observing and learning from other children or adults in structured activities such as dance class, karate, sports, or in unstructured, natural activities (Scott et al., 2020). Some children who have difficulty with motor imitation may need support from interdisciplinary team members, including health care providers such as physical therapists, occupational therapists, and speech-language professionals. The inability to imitate others impedes full participation in simple games or makes it difficult for the child to learn on their own from watching others move (Scott et al., 2020). Decreased participation in physical activity can be compounded in families who discourage children from these activities because of noise production and/or limited space such as apartments (Rahman, 2012).

Health professionals can educate/teach parents and adults to increase physical participation through a variety of modalities, such as music and videos that incorporate yoga, dance, and simple exercise routines. QOL and overall well-being of children improves with physical activity. In safe community spaces, such as playgrounds, parks, beaches, and other open areas, children will more readily engage in activities with adults and will improve the physical activity level in both the children and their adult caregivers. In providing these bouts of physical activity, the young child can meet specified guidelines of 15 minutes of physical activity per hour for 12 hours; this level of activity leads to 3 hours per day, which is the amount recommended by the U.S. Institute of Medicine National Center on Health, Physical Activity and Disability (USDHHS, 2018). Health professionals can educate parents using websites, helping to organize activities, prepare schedules, explore community resources, or facilitate referrals to other members of the interprofessional team (e.g., social workers, dieticians, and nutritionists). The consensus is to provide a variety of free, creative play options, which can occur indoors and outdoors, while trying to monitor and minimize time spent sitting time spent throughout the day (Chow et al., 2015). Adults should consider the complexity of the games and the child's ability to understand instruction while being able to provide adequate strategies for enjoyable experiences. Families who understand the richness and benefits of these activities and practice together, will foster the child's self-awareness, game rules, and task-specific learning. The development of motor skills allows for greater engagement in recreation, group activities with peers, and school participation.

Health Benefits of Physical Activity in Early Childhood

As a child matures, an increase in endurance develops with greater mastery of running, galloping, skipping, and bike riding. The standards of physical activity for children younger than 6 years have been reported by the Physical Activity Guidelines Advisory Committee in a 2008 report (USDHHS, n.d) showing a positive association in outdoor games, jumping, scooter riding, bike riding, and swimming with overall Gross Motor Quotients on motor skills tests (O'Neil et al., 2014). These unstructured activities contribute to the development of motor skills. When performed in a safe environment with proper supervision, these activities can promote healthy habits throughout childhood and into adolescence and adulthood.

Many children may also attend structured activities that further increase the benefits of physical activity. The most common for children are aquatic programs, T-ball, and community-based dance classes. In providing structured and unstructured play, children can accrue at least 3 hours of physical activity or exercise every day with benefits to bone health and healthy weight status (USDHHS, 2020). An increase in physical activity promotes bone ossification during early childhood, counteracting the effects of vulnerability to nutritional deficiency, fatigue, illness, or excessive weight or pressure. Weight-bearing through the extremities adds pressure and force for bone development but should not be excessive (Smith et al., 2015). Although it is difficult to measure the amount of physical activity in this age group, frequent bouts of activity are typical, and toddlers appear to be achieving their recommended 180 minutes per day of physical activity (Bruijns et al., 2020). However, almost 50% of the children tested in a two independent sample study did not meet the guidelines of achieving at least 15 minutes of physical activity per hour per day. In both samples, more boys (53.5% and 57.6%) than girls (33.5% and 45.9%) met the physical activity guidelines. There were no noted differences across racial/ethnic and parent education groups (Pate et al., 2015).

Typically, a child should grow incrementally within standards of length and height for a given age on standardized growth charts. If the child is gaining weight at an average beyond a normal target of 5 pounds per year for their height, a referral to a registered dietitian or physician may be warranted (Whitlock, 2005). Currently, 22.8% of U.S. children ages 2 to 5 years are overweight or obese (≥85th percentile) in conjunction with a trend of declining physical activity (Ogden et al., 2014). Another report indicates that 26.7% of American children ages 2 to 5 years are obese or overweight (Ogden et al., 2014). Since exercise requires energy expenditure to fuel the skeletal muscles and reduces the amount of insulin required to metabolize glucose, understanding the benefits of physical activity early in life is important. Essentially, prevention of a disease is preferred over having to manage and treat the long-term consequences of disease (Romanelli et al., 2020). To manage body weight and prevent an unhealthy BMI, the U.S. Department of Health and Human Services recommends that children engage in at least 60 minutes of moderate to vigorous intense activities while not exceeding caloric intake (USDHHS, n.d). Children predisposed to obesity or engage in sedentary play should be monitored closely and guided to engage in physical activity. The role of the interdisciplinary team is essential in helping to coordinate these efforts. According to research-based evidence, the ecological environment of the family or school, within the larger social context of the community and society, is an area to address strategies to manage childhood obesity (Smith et al., 2020). Physical activity in late infancy and throughout childhood has been linked to lower BMI and less body fat (Datar & Sturm, 2004). Physical activity participation also provides an alternative to the sedentary past time of watching television and playing video games. A National Longitudinal Study of Youth indicates that 17% of infants and 48% of toddlers watch about 1 hour of television and 25% of the toddlers watched over 3 hours of television daily, indicating long periods of sedentary behavior (Certain et al., 2002).

Caregiver knowledge of nutritional standards also helps children grow strong while maintaining a healthy weight and activity level. The interdisciplinary team can collaborate to provide caregivers with information, referral sources, counseling, and strategies for developing awareness of healthy behaviors. The team of professionals can include mental health professionals, physicians, dietitians, and they can work together within the contextual environment of the family and/or school. Community resources and personnel such as athletic trainers in gyms, group exercise programs at local community centers, support groups through local clinics, churches, or community centers can be utilized as well. Each member has a role in supporting the 2010 Dietary Guidelines for Americans, which recommends a balance between energy consumption and utilization to maintain a healthy weight with the emphasis on the consumption of nutrient dense foods and reducing added sugars and sold fats (U.S. Department of Agriculture and USDHHS, 2020).

Dietary guidelines include:

- Increase vegetables and fruit intake, especially dark green and orange vegetables, and beans and peas.
- Consume at least half of all grans as whole grains, replacing refined grains.
- Increase intake of fat-free or low-fat milk and milk products, such as milk, yogurt, cheese, or fortified soy beverages.
- Choose a variety of protein foods, which include seafood, lean meat and poultry, eggs, beans and peas, soy products, and unsalted nuts and seeds.
- Choose foods that provide more potassium, dietary fiber, calcium, and vitamin D.
- Use oils to replace solid fats.

Strategies for Promoting Physical Activity in the Preschool Child

The development of healthy habits and routines starts early in life. Childhood development is linked to school readiness and physical abilities for future childhood success (Sabol et al., 2018). In early childhood, starting at 3 to 4 years old, development of the ability to dress and undress, engage in creative play, and complete obstacles at the playground begins. Caregivers and adults promote independence and skill development for participation in daily activities in order for the child to learn to dress himself, develop hygiene skills, and share in the chores and tasks within the home and preschool environments. Parents' viewpoints on fostering independence may vary. Some families prefer to assist the child immediately, not allowing a waiting time for the child to complete the task. This is true especially if the child takes longer when learning a new skill, and even more the case for busy families who are on rigid schedules, which do not allow for adequate practice time of the skill needed for integration into motor plan necessary for skill mastery (Ayllón et al., 2019). Aside from learning daily skills, the ability to care for oneself develops self-determination and has positive mental health and well-being outcomes, as well as being a key to future goal-directed planning and independence (McMahon et al., 2019). Another aspect of self-determination is the ability to learn to advocate for oneself in requesting, responding, and expressing preferences with adults (Hui & Tsang, 2012).

One of the items on the list of Physical Determinants in *Healthy People 2030* is to support a child's healthy behaviors and address barriers (Office of Disease Prevention and Health Promotion [ODPHP], n.d.). Adults who are involved with the child daily are responsible to shape and guide the child's early behaviors in physical play, sedentary behaviors, food choices, and healthy routines. As a young child attends preschool or day care, this new environment and the adults present continue to influence the child's health and well-being. All educators have a role. Administrators provide the funding for special activities, equipment and space for recreation, and community relationships. Teachers create the classroom learning experience and opportunities to develop physical skills, leadership, and resilience; all components necessary to healthy growth and well-being (Slot & Beses, 2018). Parents are also encouraged to work with school professionals to support them in promoting healthy habits at school. In order to maximize a child's ability to take part in activities with his peers, teachers can work with families and other health professionals to identify any developmental delays that interfere with a child's functional ability by completing a comprehensive, school-based evaluation. Although there are tests that measure motor skill development, there is scant research or testing tools available that quantify the level of a young child's physical activity. Available tools, although based on subjective observation, include the Observational System for Recording Physical activity in Children-Preschool Version and Children's Activity Rating Scale, and both offer information about **health promotion** programs (Burdette et al., 2004). Such programs are designed to enable people to improve their health through involvement in social and environmental interventions, and do so with the help of public policies, community support, and environments that support, educate, and strengthen communities to help people address their own health challenges (WHO, 2021).

To promote physical activity, preschools offer a type of movement education program that generally use rhythmic activities like music or dancing, to reinforce and encourage physical play or games (McMahon et al., 2019). Others encourage activities by utilizing toys, materials, or sensory-driven experiences in sight, sound, or touch, or solve simple problems with a toy or puzzle. At times, simple games of "duck, duck, goose," "freeze tag," or "hopscotch" can be introduced during the school day (Allvin, 2019). Guidelines from a U.S.-based organization, the Institute of Medicine (IOM), recommends that childcare centers provide preschoolers with a combination of light, moderate, and vigorous physical activity for at least 15 minutes per hour (Cheadle et al., 2014). It is important to consider that there are differences in childcare programs in the types of programs and geographical location. The interprofessional team can be helpful in guiding families in making choices and providing insight into what to look for when exploring these early childhood programs. In one study conducted in the state of Nebraska, the quality of physical activity programs was compared between childcare centers and family childcare homes in rural versus urban communities. Findings favored the urban programs in that they provided portable play equipment, provided families with information on children's physical activity and outdoor play, and completed professional development training on topics such as outdoor play and learning (Dinkel et al., 2020).

In order to guide movement programs offered at preschools, the National Association for Sport and Physical

Education has developed the Active Start physical activity guidelines for children younger than 5 years of age, which included a recommendation of 60 minutes of structured and unstructured of physical activity daily (Society of Health and Physical Educators; Advanced Solutions International, n.d.). The specific, fundamental movement skills that should be incorporated into a school movement program are unclear and lack sufficient conclusive evidence. This is an area where high-quality research is needed in early childhood (Wick et al., 2017). To reduce the risk of obesity or sedentary behaviors, regardless of skill level, a young child should have frequent movement experiences throughout the day and participate in play activities for short periods several times per day (Patrick et al., 2001). Adults who are involved in the young child's life, both at home and school, should monitor children for any signs of motor problems, such as lack of fundamental movements, difficulty with age-appropriate motor skills, or difficulty in keeping up with same-age peers. The lack of ability to keep up with peers, with simultaneous lack of skill, may interfere with advanced motor skills and a reluctance to participate in physical and play activities (Advanced Solutions International, n.d.). The interprofessional team, including physical educators, are integral in identifying children who are falling behind in their abilities in comparison to peers. Evaluations and services such as physical therapy, occupational therapy, and adaptive physical education can offer support and remediation of motor skills or modifications to adjust to a child's physical abilities. The lack of physical activity in schools continues to be an area of concern. A study completed in schools found that children spent more time sitting (76%), standing (13%), and only engaged in low to moderate intensity physical activity 11% of the time while in school (Chow et al., 2015).

The consensus is that it is best for a child to have regular movement experiences and active play to promote movement skills, develop standards of health, and promote well-being for an improved QOL. In providing large muscle activities like running, jumping, hopping, and stair climbing, children in preschool can accumulate the 60 minutes of structured physical activity per day. The provision of indoor and outdoor play areas and opportunities for play and physical activity are the building blocks for the adoption of a healthy lifestyle and behaviors in a child's early years. Ultimately, healthy habits begin with the adults in the child's life helping to create relationships that encourage and model healthy behaviors and build a physical environment that promotes the development of a healthy mindset of interests and actions.

Case Study 4-2 addresses a young child who is showing issues of decreased engagement with others with others and moving into a new school environment. The school staff are often the first ones to notice developmental delays that relate to the child's well-being. Multiple factors are examined: the family environment, the child, and any barriers. The decision-making process involves the decision to wait or initiate an interdisciplinary team evaluation. Should the child be referred to a physician? When is the right time to discuss these findings with the parent? Will the parent be open to the information or leave the preschool? Is this parent aware of the milestones? Will the educational environment foster sufficient opportunities to develop and make gains or will this child need professional support? Did this child receive any prior services? Did mother receive any information on social services support or community support? How will the educational environment and family system work together? Consider the previous information and the following content to answer these questions and those at the end of the first part of the case study.

Assessments

The use of assessments can provide insight to caregivers or children in determining their current level and optimize their level of health and wellness in the areas of daily activities, habits, social situation, physical activity, and environment health and wellness. The selection of the assessment should depend on the specific area of interest to the individual and supported by the interdisciplinary team. Table 4-1 provides suggested tools and parameters for selection based on desired area functional assessment.

Physical Activity in Older Children and Adolescence

Physical Play and Motor Skills Development in Preadolescence and Adolescence

Late childhood and adolescence represent a period of rapid growth and development and the formation of habits and routines that can have a lasting effect on health and well-being (Rodriguez-Ayllon et al., 2019). Children advance their personal capacities by engaging and participating in activities that foster performance skills such as social interaction, emotional regulation, and executive functioning. Physical activities provide a medium for exercising performance skills in various contexts (social, cultural, and physical). The extent of participation is dependent on the acquisition and degree of proficiency of age-appropriate milestones needed to meaningfully activities. For example, a 6-year-old immigrant child, Luis, enjoyed playing soccer with his friends and family in his native country. However, the extent of his ball control skills is limited to pushing the ball forward with limited activation of other body parts. Luis recently moved into a neighborhood where no one speaks

Case Study 4-2

Sammy is a 3.5-year-old boy who started preschool after his single mother returned to full time work about 1 hour away. This is Sammy's first time attending preschool since he had been cared at home with either his mother or grandmother, while his mother worked part-time. During the preschool intake, mother indicates that Sammy is a shy child, born prematurely, and does not have any siblings. In completing the information regarding developmental abilities, mother states that Sammy prefers sitting and playing with his Legos, understands and talks in sentences, and enjoys drawing. Sammy is toilet trained, eats independently, but needs helps in dressing. Sammy will be attending preschool daily from 8 am to 5 pm.

After the first 3 months at preschool, his teachers have been watching Sammy. They are sharing concerns with his mother about his clumsiness and frequent falling. The teachers further add that Sammy fatigues easily during dance class and refuses to participate in the preschool gym class. Teachers inquire about Sammy's past early development. Mother reports that Sammy sat alone at 7 months and moved into walking without ever crawling, since he did not like being on his belly. Since he was born prematurely at 35 months, mother has been careful in keeping him healthy and safe. He has been diagnosed with reactive airway disease and starts to cough when he runs. The teachers explained that Sammy is not able to walk up and down the stairs, the jungle gym outside, and prefers to sit and play with his toys rather than his classmates. Teachers recommended that Sammy should be evaluated to determine any delays and ways to support his ability to play.

1. What ecological factors may have contributed to a delay in motor abilities?
2. What are personal factors possibly contributing to his decreased physical activity?
3. Were the teachers appropriate in raising concerns?
4. How can Sammy's physical participation be improved?
5. Would early parental guidance, prior to entering preschool, have helped Sammy's participation level?
6. If Sammy is not encouraged to physical participate or provided with support, what type of future physical activity level is expected? Will he join sports? Can his health become more of a concern?

his native language. Luis is shy and reluctant to engage with others because he cannot communicate with his neighborhood peers. His parents are concerned that he feels unwelcomed and discriminated against by his peers. Luis' feelings of alienation or marginalization by his peers may discourage participation in valued activities and lead to a plateau in development. The social context (peers) denies Luis opportunities to develop advanced gross motor skills such as kicking, striking, punting, and dribbling skills. A child who does not have the affordances or opportunities to engage in physical play will have limited opportunities to expand foundational skills to more complex and dynamic motors skills needed in organized sports. The importance of mastering and advancing foundational motor skills in middle childhood and adolescence cannot be underestimated.

As children interact with their social and physical contexts, the demands and expectations of performance become increasingly challenging. As children transition from middle childhood into adolescence, demands and expectations necessitate greater motor skills proficiency. Acquisition of age-appropriate physical milestones occurs when a child can explore external contexts through physical activities (Sigmundsson et al., 2017). The ability to stay on an age-appropriate motor developmental trajectory consistent with peers depends on the environmental demands, constraints, and resources made available to the child. As play becomes more organized and complex and children gain motor competence, they explore alternative or novel ways to perform, strengthening and expanding existing neurological pathways and advancing their motor repertoire of skills (Sigmundsson et al., 2017). Considering Luis' motor performance, Luis may perform a kick with little coordination of movement between the upper and lower body. The lack of coordination leads to a coupling of body structures to ensure accuracy. However, as the child continues to engage in physical soccer play, the child will begin to demonstrate more significant synergies complicated movements. Thus, these movements appear purposeful, smooth, and accurate. Luis will begin to kick with greater speed, rhythm, and timing, demonstrating synchronize, coordinated movements of the upper and lower body. As improved motor capacities and physical prowess improve, so do the range of opportunities for children to engage in mainstream recreational and organized play. Moreover, as Luis becomes more aware and confident of his capacities to perform physical activities, his motivation to participate would increase. Gu and Solmon (2016) found a strong correlation between a positive self-appraisal of physical skills, engagement in physical activities, and overall QOL.

Table 4-1

Assessment Tools and Resources

ASSESSMENT	AREA OF ASSESSMENT	PRODUCT LOCATION
The Assessment of Life Habits or Life-H: Assesses daily activities to social participation and self-perception	Performance measurement to determine a child's participation, QOL, and well-being. Three applications based on ages: 1. Children from birth to 4 years of age 2. Children from 5 to 13 years of age 3. General (teenagers, adults, and seniors) Life habit categories that are comprised in "daily activities" or "social roles."	International Network on the Disability Creation Process (INDCP) Address: 525 Boulevard Wilfrid-Hamel Est, Local F-117.4 Quebec, Qc, G1M2S8 Telephone: 418-529-9141, ext. 6202 Fax: 418-780-8765 Email: ripph@irdpq.qc.ca
Children's Assessment of Participation and Enjoyment and Preferences for Activities of Children or CAPE	Examines child's participation in activities outside of school by looking at the diversity, intensity, and location of the child's activities and enjoyment of these activities.	Pearson Address: 330 Hudson in New York City, New York Telephone: 800-627-7271 Fax: 800-232-1223 Web: https://www.pearson.com/
Child and Adolescent Scale of Participation or CASP	A brief, caregiver completed questionnaire measuring participation at home, school, and community.	CanChild Institute for Applied of Health Sciences, McMaster University 1400 Main Street West, Room 408 Hamilton, Ontario Canada, L85 1C7 Telephone: 905-525-9140, ext. 27850 Fax: 905-529-7687 Email: canchild@mcmaster.ca
Measurement of Quality of the Environment or MQE	Assesses the role of the environmental factors in maintaining life habits.	INDCP Address: 525 Boulevard Wilfrid-Hamel Est, Local F-117.4 Quebec, Qc, G1M2S8 Telephone: 418-529-9141, ext. 6202 Fax: 418-780-8765 Email: ripph@irdpq.qc.ca
Pediatric QOL Inventory or PedsQL	Measures the core dimensions of health following the World Health Organization and the role of the school functioning. The scales are physical functioning, emotional functioning, social functioning, and school functioning.	Mapi Research Trust ePROVIDE Address: 27 rue de la Villette 69003 Lyon France Telephone: +33 4 72 13 65 75 Web: eprovide.mapi-trust.org/

(continued)

Table 4-1 (continued)

Assessment Tools and Resources

ASSESSMENT	AREA OF ASSESSMENT	PRODUCT LOCATION
Child Engagement in Daily Life Measure	A parent or caregiver questionnaire to identify child's participation in activities and enjoyment of the activities.	CanChild Institute for Applied of Health Sciences, McMaster University Address: 1400 Main Street West, Room 408 Hamilton, Ontario Canada, L85 1C7 Telephone: 905-525-9140, ext. 27850 Fax: 905-529-7687 Email: canchild@mcmaster.ca
Ages and Stages Questionnaire or ASQ	A reliable developmental and social-emotional screening for children.	Brookes Publishing Co. Address: P.O. Box 10624 Baltimore, MD 21285-0624 Telephone: 1-800-638-3775 Fax: 410-337-8539 Web: agesandstages.com
Lifestyle and Health Risk Questionnaire	A checklist of levels of physical activity, nutrition, sleep, mental health, social support, weight, other lifestyle risk factors and conditions.	Web: https://intermountainhealthcare.org

Key Point

The CDC recommends children and adolescents (ages 6 through 17 years) engage in 60 minutes of moderate-to-vigorous physical activity daily. In addition to the cardiopulmonary and musculoskeletal benefits of physical activities, children who engage in physical activities also demonstrate improved performance skills (social, emotional, and cognition).

Children who exhibit minor delays in motor performance but have the potential to develop skills are often alienated, marginalized, or deprived of opportunities to engage in organized or recreational play (Townsend & Wilcock, 2004). They may appear awkward or clumsy. They may not perform physical tasks with the smoothness and automaticity of their peers. The ungainliness in motor performance leads to a cascading effect of exclusion. They often have fewer opportunities to exercise skills that can promote engagement in meaningful activities. Recreational activities such as recess play, after-school programs, and organized sports provide opportunities for children to engage in physical play. Failure to provide opportunities to expand on basic foundational motor skills can lead to an interruption in play, social, and emotional performance skills in children (Hulteen et al., 2018). Motor skills and physical activity are universal elements in developing all performance skills. In early development, children rely on rudimentary, poorly coordinated movement skills to perform simple play. However, as children move into late childhood and adolescence, they broaden and refine fundamental skills that allow them to use their bodies and minds with proficiency in various activities. For example, Dorsey et al. (2011) found that overweight and obese children demonstrate less proficiency in physical activities then nonoverweight counterparts. They found that children with obesity demonstrated impairments in locomotion skills such as running. Children demonstrated inefficiencies in posture and limb control. This is consistent with Han et al. (2018) who found that overweight children have impairments in fundamental movement skills compared to their healthy weight peers. They found that children were less likely to engage in physical activities. However, they posited that the lack of skill could be addressed by skilled interventions. One such example would be a program developed by an interdisciplinary team led by a pediatric cardiologist and physical therapist known as Fit Families for Life (https://you.stonybrook.edu/fitfamilies). Fit Kids for life is a comprehensive lifestyle wellness program designed to reduce risk factors associated with childhood obesity. Fit Kids for Life provides a forum to learn and acquire the fundamental skills needed to break the vicious cycle of childhood obesity. Children develop fundamental skills and confidence to engage in physical activities and improve their QOL.

Addressing the alienation, marginalization, and eventually disengagement of physical activities in children requires a dynamic interprofessional approach (Lopez & Block, 2011; Nilsson, & Townsend, 2010). A concerted effort between school and health professionals can be effective in advancing motor performance. One such program, PAR FORE (Perseverance, Accountability, Resilience, Fellowship, Opportunity, Respect, Empowerment), an after-school golf program for at-risk youth designed to address the detrimental effects of sedentary and health-compromising (gang participation) activities in under-served communities (https://www.parfore.org). An interprofessional team consisting of an occupational therapist, a physical therapist, a school educator, and a golf professional designed a program incorporating golf fitness and mentoring for middle school children. The program was designed to advance health-promoting behaviors such as active play and golf fitness. As a result, adolescents engage in productive activity (golf) that advanced physical and social health. The physical and occupational therapist collaborated on designing health promotion activities related to physical and mental health while the golf professional provided skilled golf instruction on golf fitness and performance. As a result, adolescents learned valuable life skills inherent in the sport and met physical activity requirements set by the CDC (USDHHS, 2018). The program successfully provided opportunities to engage in structured physical fitness activities for children in dangerous, underserved communities (Lopez & Block, 2011).

Contextual Demands and Constraints on Physical Health Promotion

Several factors facilitate or hinder engagement and participation in physical play among children and adolescents. This, in turn, can lead to maladaptive patterns of activity, which can lead to poorer health and well-being among children and adolescents. Cultural, social, and familial expectations can influence a child's motivation to engage in physical activities. Socioeconomic status and physical environments can also promote or hinder physical play (Lopez & Block, 2011).

Children who live in poverty are often deprived of physical and social environments that provide safe outlets for outdoor physical play. They lack the affordances such as safe playgrounds and parks necessary for play to advance motor skill competence. Barriers included perceived crime-related safety concerns, inconvenient park locations, and poorly managed recreational spaces that affected park use by children in low-income areas. The emergence of exclusive travel team culture has led to a shift in focus in access to organized sports. Families from low-income areas do not have the resources to commit to travel sports (Huang et al., 2020). Thompson (2018) reported that only 34% of children from families earning less than $25,000 played a team sport in 2017, vs. 69% from homes earning more than $100,000. The surge in the team sports culture has affected sports play that was otherwise accessible to low-income areas. Organized sports such as soccer, basketball, cross country, and baseball have all been affected by an elitist sports organization (Thompson, 2018). Children living in poverty are deprived of such opportunities in a competitive youth sports market where families can spend from $700 to $35,000 a year for private lessons, camps, and travel teams (Picchi, 2019). The consequences to children living in poverty are devastating. Children who lack alternatives ways to occupy their time succumb to health-compromising activities such as passive (social isolation and inactivity) or self-destructive activities (gang participation; Lopez & Block, 2011).

Coakley (2011) identified the myriad of benefits associated with participation in organized youth sports. Youth sports are essential in developing motor skills that contribute to physical proficiency and social networks among their peers. It facilitates health and a sense of overall well-being and builds character. Lastly, it provides a purposeful and healthy means for occupying a child's time. Schools can counteract the inequities of an unsafe environment with high-quality physical education. The mental and physical health benefits of participation in physical education classes are unequivocal (Park et al., 2017). Nevertheless, schools have reduced resources for physical education (Society of Health and Physical Educators [SHAPE], 2016). It is estimated that only 29.9% of high school students attend physical education classes (CDC, n.d.). Public school programs have shifted resources and reduced opportunities for children to participate in physical activities (SHAPE America, 2016). As a result, physical education is often underappreciated and underutilized. School physical education curriculum may be the primary source of physical activity and fitness for adolescents (USDHHS, 2001). This is particularly concerning for children who live in under-represented and impoverished communities where access to play environments is limited. It has been reported that city schools have the lowest average minutes per day of recess (Ramstetter & Murray, 2017). It has been well-documented that the quantity and quality of school physical education play a significant role in adolescents' health-related fitness (McKenzie et al., 1996). Moreover, it is essential for brain function. Movement activates the brain creating a state of arousal and a readiness to learn (Ratey & Hagerman, 2008). Children who engage in physical activity throughout the school day have demonstrated improved academic performance. Unfortunately, schools fail to recognize the relationship between movement and thinking (Archer & Garcia, 2014; CDC, 2010).

Teachers and health professions can collaborate to identify optimal individual and classroom learning opportunities and environments. Occupational, physical, and speech therapists as interprofessional teams can provide motor-based multisensory experiences that can facilitate learning. Teachers can incorporate learning activities that engage both the mind and the body. Role-play, walking and learning groups, and game play increase participation and creates lasting memories of the activity and the content covered.

One method of incorporating movement in the classroom is utilizing the Total Physical Response (TPR) developed by James Asher (1981). Teachers and students use their bodies to act out or gesture the meaning of words or concepts. Another method of encouraging movement and learning is the use of acute walking and learning groups. The movement provides sensorimotor feedback (kinesthetic, proprioceptive, auditory, and visual) and can support episodic memory and long-term memory (Sng et al., 2018).

Often referred to as "the latchkey generation," the Generation X child had little supervision (Swanzen, 2018). Generation X children preceded the technological advances in gaming and social media. Generation Xers engaged in exploratory and creative play. Child's play was sparked by curiosity and spontaneity—children engaged in unplanned, imaginative outdoor play. The outdoor physical and imaginative play was the predominant mode of play. Today, the U.S. society views play in a more measured and controlled fashion (McQuade et al., 2019). Play is organized and scheduled. Parents plan "play dates" and select the environments in which children play. Parents strive to provide the best play experiences to encourage development. As children enter middle and high school years, parents continue to control their access to play (McQuade et al., 2019). Whether it is music, dance, or sports, parents will plan their course. The parents push a single-sport or art agenda, limiting the scope of a child's play to a single concentrated activity (Hereth, 2019). This parenting mindset reduces opportunities for the child to advance performance skills. Moreover, children who engage in single-sport activities are prone to loss of motivation, overscheduling, and anxiety from unrealistic expectations from parents (Myer et al., 2015). However, in their attempt to provide a dynamic play experience, they constrain the child's ability to explore and engage in imaginative physical play. They manage learning experiences without giving them the opportunity to experience adversity and learn from failing experiences. Children benefit from variety in play. Variety provides opportunities to use their body and minds in different ways. It encourages problem solving and increases self-awareness. For example, participation in dance can foster advanced development of rhythm and timing skills that may carry over on the football field. Dance can also help improve flexibility and muscle balance reducing an athlete's propensity for injury (Quick Quick Slow Ballroom Dance Studio, 2018). Independent exploration and imagination allow a child to challenge their minds and bodies in novel ways and increase their repertoire of skills (Myer et al., 2016). Children who engage in heterogenous activities are more likely to achieve mastery in a range of activities than mastery in a single activity (Myer et al., 2016). Engaging in a variety of physical activities benefits brain development and prevents injuries. Variability in play encourages adaptability in function. Novel tasks require adaptative responses to unexpected situations and advancing motor learning and executive functioning (DiCesare et al., 2019). For example, skill-building programs that promote both mental and physical health can be effective in addressing the whole child's QOL. Individuals from different health and education professions can provide a unique perspective in addressing these concerns. Educators, occupational therapists, psychologists, and social workers can offer a unique perspective in what motivates engagement in play while physical education educators, physical therapists, and coaches can advise on methods for improving a child's gross motor skills. Moreover, nongovernmental civic groups and local governmental agencies can form partnerships in developing after-school programming to promote physical play and fitness among children. Camhi et al. (2021) found that interprofessional collaborations supported learning outcomes among children in an after-school gardening program. The comprehensive nature of collaboration breadth and weight of the content and delivery of community-based programs. Interprofessional teams can use this information in a variety of ways to promote physical health and well-being for older youth and adolescence.

Technology and virtual environments have also had some implications for reducing physical activities and motor performance in late childhood and adolescence. Excessive use of mobile devices, internet media, the proliferation of streaming services, and gaming has been implicated in reducing physical activity levels among children and adolescents (Domoff et al., 2019).

In a study conducted by Cadoret et al. (2018), subjects demonstrated reduced gross motor proficiency (postural control, locomotion, and object manipulation). The study reported the concern for the spiraling effects of disengagement associated with delayed motor performance. They report a lack of competence and confidence to engage in physical activities (Cadoret et al., 2018; Robinson et al., 2015). On the other hand, there has also been an explosion of exergaming platforms (McConnon, 2020) that can provide encouraging opportunities to provide meaningful opportunities for gamers to engage in physical activities. Case Study 4-3 explores some of the barriers to participation in physical activity in older children and adolescents.

Our society has seen a significant shift in the way children engage and participate in physical activities. The changing dynamics of structured and unstructured play, organized sports, physical education, and emergence of technology have changed the way children develop motor competence and engage in physical activities. Although the way in which children play has changed, so has the science and evidence that supports physical activity (McQuade et al., 2019). McQuade et al. (2019, p. 93) reported a consensus that "modern play is more sedentary, passive, solitary and indoor, and less likely to be active, creative, and outdoor." The explosion of technology platforms (e.g., application, web, nedia, gaming, mobile) has increased screen time and reduced active play significantly today. Concurrently, there is a proliferation of research supporting the need for physical activity among children. Moreover, the research in neuroplasticity suggests that children can develop skills needed to develop motor proficiency at any age (Dorn et al., 2019). The degree of

Case Study 4-3

Sam is a 13-year-old boy who is graduating from his eighth-grade middle school class and will be transitioning into high school in the fall. Sam is mildly obese. He presents with low muscle tone and thoracic kyphosis and forward head posture on the cervical range. Sam is independent with all his ADLs and is doing exceptionally well in school. Sam is more comfortable around adults than his peers. He has a great sense of humor that is highlighted by sarcasm when communicating with adults. Sam does not participate in organized sports or extracurricular activities. Sam enjoys gaming and binge-watching shows on a streaming service. Sam does not have any interest in playing sports or joining clubs. He can spend up to 5 to 8 hours a day watching TV and playing video games. Because his mother is the sole provider, she is unable to monitor his online activity. Sam describes himself as a gamer who does not like sports. However, he does enjoy playing sports-themed video games. He has learned a great deal about sports playing video games. Sam continues to demonstrate difficulties with gross motor skills. In his physical education class, he displays avoidant behaviors because children tease him. He self-reports that he is not good at throwing, kicking, and running and does not like when the other children make fun of him. Sam was seen by a physical and occupational therapist when he was in third grade but was discharged from services after 1 year.

1. What ecological factors may have contributed to a delay in motor abilities?
2. What are personal factors possibly contributing to his decreased physical activity?
3. What can be done to improve his motor performance?
4. What can be done to improve Sam's physical participation?
5. If you were charged with putting an interprofessional team together to address Sam's concerns, which professionals would you include?

proficiency may not meet competitional standards but may be sufficient to support development of other performance skills. Motor proficiency and interest can improve given opportunity and guidance.

Conclusion

Interprofessional teams of educators and health professions are poised for addressing issues related to engagement and participation in physical activities among children. However, many educators and practitioners often work within the bounds of their clinics and schools. Practitioners need to advocate and network with community stakeholders (e.g., educators, community youth groups, faith-based groups) to address the health, well-being, and QOL of children who might be marginalized, alienated, and deprived of opportunities to engage in physical play. They must take a proactive stand in not only educating community members but also take action-oriented approaches, such as public advocacy, to meet the needs of children. Children who engage in physical play activities are likely to develop lifelong health-promoting lifestyles. Therefore, educating stakeholders (parents, health professionals, and educators) on the need for active engagement and participation in physical activities can be the first step in promoting health and wellness in children (Burner et al., 2019). If children are discouraged by their motor competencies and contexts that do not support their need or desire for physical activity, it could result in dire health-related consequences.

References

Adolfsson, M., Sjöman, M., & Björck-Åkesson, E. (2018). ICF-CY as a framework for understanding child engagement in preschool. *Frontiers in Education, 3.* https://doi.org/10.3389/feduc.2018.00036

Adolph, K. E., & Franchak, J. M. (2017). The development of motor behavior. Wiley interdisciplinary reviews. *Cognitive Science, 8*(1-2), 10.1002/wcs.1430. https://doi.org/10.1002/wcs.1430

Advanced Solutions International, I. (n.d.). National PE standards: Shape America sets the standard. National Physical Education Standards-SHAPE America Sets the Standards. https://www.shapeamerica.org/standards/pe/.

Allvin, R. E. (2019). MAKING CONNECTIONS - FORMAR CONEXIONES: Radical transformation in higher education is required to achieve real equity. *YC Young Children, 74*(5), 60–66. https://www.jstor.org/stable/26842307

Andrews, B. T. (2017). Correlative vs. causative relationship between neonatal cranial head shape anomalies and early developmental delays. *Frontiers in Neuroscience, 11*(708), 1-4. https://doi.org/10.3389/fnins.2017.00708.

Archer, T. & Garcia, D. (2014). EDITORIAL: Physical exercise influences academic performance and well-being in children and adolescents. *International Journal of School and Cognitive Psychology, 1.* doi:10.4172/1234-3425.1000e102.

Asher, J. J. (1981). The total physical response: Theory and practice. *Annals of the New York Academy of Sciences, 379*, 324-331. https://doi.org/10.1111/j.1749-6632.1981.tb42019.x

Ayllón, E., Moyano, N., Lozano, A., & Cava, M. J. (2019). Parents' willingness and perception of children's autonomy as predictors of greater independent mobility to school. *International Journal of Environmental Research and Public Health, 16*(5), 732. https://doi.org/10.3390/ijerph16050732

Battelley, H. (2020). Play, music and movement. International *Journal of Birth & Parent Education, 7*(4), 17.

Branch, L. G. (2015). Deformational plagiocephaly and craniosynostosis: trends in diagnosis and treatment after the "back to sleep" campaign. *The Journal of Craniofacial Surgery, 26*(1), 147-150. https://doi.org/10.1097/SCS.0000000000001401.

Bruder, M. B., Catalino, T., Chiarello, L. A., Mitchell, M. C., Deppe, J., Gundler, D., Kemp, P., LeMoine, S., Long, T., Muhlenhaupt, M., Prelock, P., Schefkind, S., Stayton, V., & Ziegler, D. (2019). Finding a common lens. *Infants & Young Children, 32*(4), 280-293 https://doi.org/10.1097/IYC.0000000000000153

Bruijns, B. A., Truelove, S., & Johnson, A. M. (2020). Infants' and toddlers' physical activity and sedentary time as measured by accelerometry: A systematic review and meta-analysis. International *Journal Behavioral Nutrition Physicial Activity, 17*(14). https://doi.org/10.1186/s12966-020-0912-4.

Burdette, H. L., Whitaker, R. C., & Daniels, S. R. (2004). Parental report of outdoor playtime as a measure of physical activity in preschool-aged children. *Archives of Pediatrics & Adolescent Medicine, 158*(4), 353. https://doi.org/10.1001/archpedi.158.4.353

Burner, A., Bopp, M., Papalia, Z., Weimer, A., & Bopp, C. M. (2019). Examining the relationship between high school physical education and fitness outcomes in college students. *Physical Educator, 76*(1), 285-300.

Cadoret, G., Bigras, N., Lemay, L., Lehrer, J., & Lemire, J. (2018). Relationship between screen-time and motor proficiency in children: a longitudinal study. *Early Child Development and Care, 188*(2), 231-239.

Callahan, C. W. (1997). Use of seating devices in infants too young to sit. *Archives of Pediatrics & Adolescent Medicine, 151*(3), 233-235. https://doi.org/10.1001/archpedi.1997.02170400019004.

Camhi, S., Richman, L., & Cory, N. (2021). An inter-professional framework for quality improvement of school gardening programming. *International Journal of School Health, 8*(3).

Carson, V., Lee, E. Y., Hewitt, L. et al. (2017). Systematic review of the relationships between physical activity and health indicators in the early years (0-4 years). *BMC Public Health, 17*, 854. https://doi.org/10.1186/s12889-017-4860-0

Centers for Disease Control and Prevention. (n.d.) Physical activity facts. https://www.cdc.gov/healthyschools/physicalactivity/facts.htm

Centers for Disease Control and Prevention. (2010). The association between school based physical activity, including physical education, and academic performance. Atlanta, GA: Centers for Disease Control and Prevention, US Dept of Health and Human Services. https://www.cdc.gov/healthyyouth/health_and_academics/pdf/pa-pe_paper.pdf

Centers for Disease Control and Prevention. (2012). National action plan for child injury prevention. Atlanta, GA: Centers for Disease Control and Prevention. https://www.cdc.gov/safechild/publications.html.

Centers for Disease Control and Prevention. (2018a). Strategies for classroom physical activity in schools. Atlanta, GA: Centers for Disease Control and Prevention, U.S. Department of Health and Human Services. https://www.cdc.gov/healthyschools/physicalactivity/pdf/2019_04_25_Strategies-for-CPA_508tagged.pdf

Centers for Disease Control and Prevention. (2018b). Health-related quality of life (HRQOL): HRQoL concepts: What is quality of life? Atlanta, GA: Centers for Disease Control and Prevention, U.S. Department of Health and Human Services. https://www.cdc.gov/hrqol/concept.htm

Centers for Disease Control and Prevention. (2018c). Health-related quality of life (HRQOL): Well-Being concepts. Atlanta, GA: Centers for Disease Control and Prevention, U.S. Department of Health and Human Services. https://www.cdc.gov/hrqol/wellbeing.htm

Centers for Disease Control and Prevention. (2020a). CDC Healthy Schools: Parents for Healthy Schools. Atlanta, GA: Centers for Disease Control and Prevention, U.S. Department of Health and Human Services. https://www.cdc.gov/healthyschools/parentsforhealthyschools/p4hs.htm?CDC_AA_refVal=https%3A%2F%2Fwww.cdc.gov%2Fhealthyschools%2Fparentengagement%2Fparentsforhealthyschools.htm

Centers for Disease Control and Prevention. (2020b). CDC Healthy Schools: Parents for Healthy Schools. Atlanta, GA: Centers for Disease Control and Prevention, U.S. Department of Health and Human Services. https://www.cdc.gov/healthyschools/parentsforhealthyschools/resources.htm

Centers for Disease Control and Prevention. (2020c). The association between school based physical activity, including physical education, and academic performance. Atlanta, GA: Centers for Disease Control and Prevention, U.S, Department of Health and Human Services. https://www.cdc.gov/healthyyouth/health_and_academics/pdf/pa-pe_paper.pdf

Centers for Disease Control and Prevention. (2021). Out of school time. Atlanta, GA: Centers for Disease Control and Prevention, U.S. Department of Health and Human Services. https://www.cdc.gov/healthyschools/ost.htm

Certain L. K., et al (2002). Prevalence, correlates, and trajectory of television viewing among infants and toddlers. *Pediatrics, 109*(4), 634-642.

Cheadle, A., Rauzon, S., & Schwartz, P. M. (2014). Community-level obesity prevention initiatives. *National Civic Review, 103*(1), 35-39. https://doi.org/10.1002/ncr.21172

Chow, B. C., McKenzie, T. L., & Louie, L. (2015). Physical activity and its contexts during preschool classroom sessions. *Advances in Physical Education, 05*(03), 194-203. https://doi.org/10.4236/ape.2015.53024

Coakley, J. (2011). Youth sports: What counts as "positive development?" *Journal of Sport and Social Issues, 35*(3), 306-324.

Dapp, L. G. (2021). Physical activity and motor skills in children: A differentiated approach. *Psychology of Sport and Exercise, 54*, 1-8. https://doi.org/10.1016/j.psychsport.2021.101916.

Datar, A., & Sturm, R. (2004). Physical education in elementary school and body mass index: Evidence from the early childhood longitudinal study. *American Journal of Public Health, 94*(9), 1501-1506. https://doi.org/10.2105/ajph.94.9.1501

DiCesare, C. A., Montalvo, A., Foss, K. D. B., Thomas, S. M., Hewett, T. E., Jayanthi, N. A., & Myer, G. D. (2019). Sport specialization and coordination differences in multisport adolescent female basketball, soccer, and volleyball athletes. *Journal of Athletic Training, 54*(10), 1105-1114.

Dinkel, D., Dev, D., Guo, Y., Sedani, A., Hulse, E., Rida, Z., & Abel, K. (2020). Comparison of urban and rural physical activity and outdoor play environments of childcare centers and family childcare homes. *Family & Community Health, 43*(4), 264-275. https://doi.org/10.1097/fch.0000000000000267

Domoff, S. E., Borgen, A. L., Foley, R. P., & Maffett, A. (2019). Excessive use of mobile devices and children's physical health. *Human Behavior and Emerging Technologies, 1*(2), 169-175.

Dorn, L. D., Hostinar, C. E., Susman, E. J., & Pervanidou, P. (2019). Conceptualizing puberty as a window of opportunity for impacting health and well-being across the life span. *Journal of Research on Adolescence, 29*(1), 155-176.

Dorsey, K. B., Herrin, J., Krumholz, H. M. (2011). Patterns of moderate and vigorous physical activity in obese and overweight compared with non-overweight children. *Int J Pediatr Obes*, 6(2-2), e547-555. doi: 10.3109/17477166.2010.490586

Encyclopedia of Children's Health. (n.d.). Play. http://www.healthofchildren.com/P/Play.html

Field, T. M., Schanberg, S. M., Scafidi, F., Bauer, C. R., Vega-Lahr, N., Garcia, R., Nystrom, J., & Kuhn, C. M. (1986). Tactile/kinesthetic stimulation effects on preterm neonates. *Pediatrics, 77*(5), 654–658.

Gerber, R. J., Wilks, T., & Erdie-Lalena, C. (2010). Developmental milestones: Motor development. *Pediatrics in Review, 31*(7), 267-277. https://doi.org/10.1542/pir.31-7-267

Ginsburg, K. (2007). The Importance of play in promoting healthy child development and maintaining strong parent-child bonds. *Pediatrics, 119*(1). https://doi.org/10.1542/peds.2006-2697

Gordon, E. S., Tucker, P., Burke, S. M., & Carron, A. V. (2013). Effectiveness of physical activity interventions for preschoolers: A meta-analysis. *Research Quarterly for Exercise and Sport, 84*(3), 287-294. https://doi.org/10.1080/02701367.2013.813894

Gu, X., & Solmon, M. A. (2016). Motivational processes in children's physical activity and health-related quality of life. *Physical Education and Sport Pedagogy, 21*(4), 407-424.

Han, A., Fu, A., Cobley, S., & Sanders, R. H. (2018). Effectiveness of exercise intervention on improving fundamental movement skills and motor coordination in overweight/obese children and adolescents: A systematic review. *Journal of Science and Medicine in Sport, 21*(1), 89-102. https://doi.org/10.1016/j.jsams.2017.07.001

Haywood, K. M., & Getchell, N. (2019). *Life span motor development* (7th ed.). Human Kinetics.

Hereth, H. (2019). Why are high school sports participation numbers flat? HeraldNet. https://www.heraldnet.com/sports/participation-in-local-high-school-sports-holding-steady/

Hewitt, L. K. (2020, May). Tummy time and infant health outcomes: A systematic review. *Pediatrics, 145*(6), e20192168. https://doi.org/10.1542/peds.2019-2168

Huang, J.-H., Hipp, J. A., Marquet, O., Alberico, C., Fry, D., Mazak, E., Lovasi, G. S., Robinson, W. R., & Floyd, M. F. (2020). Neighborhood characteristics associated with park use and park-based physical activity among children in low-income diverse neighborhoods in New York City. *Preventive Medicine, 131*, 105948. https://doi.org/10.1016/j.ypmed.2019.105948

Hui, E. K., & Tsang, S. K. (2012). Self-determination as a psychological and positive youth development construct. *The Scientific World Journal, 2012*, 1–7. https://doi.org/10.1100/2012/759358

Hulteen, R. M., Morgan, P. J., Barnett, L. M., Stodden, D. F., & Lubans, D. R. (2018). Development of foundational movement skills: A conceptual model for physical activity across the lifespan. *Sports Medicine*, 48(7), 1533–1540. https://doi.org/10.1007/s40279-018-0892-6

Hwang, A.-W., Liao, H.-F., Chen, P. C., Hsieh, W. S., Simeonsson, R. J., Weng, L. J., & Su, Y. N. (2012, May 16). Applying the ICF-CY framework to examine biological and environmental factors in early childhood development. *Journal of the Formosan Medical Association, 113*(5). https://www.sciencedirect.com/science/article/pii/S0929664612000915

Koren, A., Kahn-D'angelo, L., Reece, S. M., & Gore, R. (2019). Examining childhood obesity from infancy: The relationship between tummy time, infant BMI-z, weight gain, and motor development—An exploratory study. *Journal of Pediatric Health Care, 33*(1), 80-91. https://doi-org.arktos.nyit.edu/10.1016/j.pedhc.2018.06.006

Little, H. (2016). Promoting risk-taking and physically challenging play in Australian early childhood settings in a changing regulatory environment. *Journal of Early Childhood Research, 15*(1), 83-98. https://doi.org/10.1177/1476718x15579743

Lopez, A., & Block, P. (2011). PAR FORE: A community-based occupational therapy program. In: F. Kronenberg, S. Algado, & N. Pollard (eds.), *Occupational therapy without borders* (2nd ed., pp. 285-292). Churchill Livingstone.

LoRang, C. R. (2019). Building your baby from the ground up: In defense of free-range and baby-led movement. *Journal of Evolution and Health: A Joint Publication of the Ancestral Health Society and the Society for Evolutionary Medicine and Health, 4*(1). https://doi.org/10.15310/J34145988

Malina, R. (2004). Motor development during infancy and early childhood: overview and suggested direction for research. *International Journal of Sports and Health Science,* (2), 50-66. https://doi.org/10.5432/ijshs.2.50

McConnon, A. (2020, February 17). Video game makers want to get players off the couch. *The New York Times*. https://www.nytimes.com/2020/02/17/business/video-games-exercise-fitness.html

McKenzie, T. L., Nader, P. R., Strikmiller, P. K., Yang, M., Stone, E. J., Perry, C. L., Taylor, W. C., Epping, J. N., Feldman, H. A., Luepker, R. V., & Kelder, S. H. (1996). School physical education: effect of the Child and Adolescent Trial for Cardiovascular Health. *Preventive Medicine, 25*(4), 423–431. https://doi.org/10.1006/pmed.1996.0074

McMahon, J., Emerson, R. S., Ponchillia, P., & Curtis, A. (2019). Measures of self-perception, level of physical activity, and body mass index of participants of sports education camps for youths with visual impairments. *Journal of Visual Impairment & Blindness, 113*(1), 43-56. https://doi.org/10.1177/0145482x18818611.

McQuade, L., McLaughlin, M., Giles, M., & Cassidy, T. (2019). Play across the generations: Perceptions of changed play patterns in childhood: Play across the generations. *Journal of Social Sciences and Humanities, 5*(2), 90-96.

Milteer, R. G. (2021). The importance of play in promoting healthy child development and maintaining strong parent-child bond: Focus on children in poverty. *Pediatrics*, e204-e213. https://doi.org/10.1542/peds.2011-2953

Moore, H. (2020, August 15). Why play is the work of childhood. Fred Rogers Center for Early Learning and Children's Media. https://www.fredrogerscenter.org/2014/09/why-play-is-the-work-of-childhood/

Myer, G. D., Jayanthi, N., Difiori, J. P., Faigenbaum, A. D., Kiefer, A. W., Logerstedt, D., & Micheli, L. J. (2015). Sport specialization, part I: Does early sports specialization increase negative outcomes and reduce the opportunity for success in young athletes? *Sports Health, 7*(5), 437-442.

Myer, G. D., Jayanthi, N., DiFiori, J. P., Faigenbaum, A. D., Kiefer, A. W., Logerstedt, D., & Micheli, L. J. (2016). Sports specialization, part II: Alternative solutions to early sport specialization in youth athletes. *Sports Health, 8*(1), 65-73.

Nandy, A. N. (2020, August). Parental toy play and toddlers' socio-emotional development: The moderating role of coparenting dynamics. *Infant Behavior & Development*, 60. https://doi.org/10.1016/j.infbeh.2020.101465

Nemours: Health & Prevention Services. Health Kids, Healthy Future. Healthy Kids, Healthy Future (2021). https://healthykidshealthyfuture.org/

Nemours' Integrated Approach to Child Health and Obesity Prevention in Delaware. SlideServe. (2014). https://www.slideserve.com/demont/nemours-integrated-approach-to-child-health-and-obesity-prevention-in-delaware

Neville, R. D., Guo, Y., Boreham, C. A., & Lakes, K. D. (2021). Longitudinal association between participation in organized sport and psychosocial development in early childhood. *The Journal of Pediatrics*, 230. https://doi.org/10.1016/j.jpeds.2020.10.077.

Nilsson, I., & Townsend, E. (2010). Occupational justice—Bridging theory and practice. *Scandinavian Journal of Occupational Therapy, 17*(1), 57-63.

Office of Disease Prevention and Health Promotion (n.d.). Healthy People 2030. U.S. Department of Health and Human Services. https://health.gov/healthypeople

Ogden, C. L., Carroll, M. D., Kit, B. K., & Flegal, K. M. (2014). Prevalence of childhood and adult obesity in the United States, 2011-2012. *Journal of the American Medical Association, 311*(8), 806. https://doi.org/10.1001/jama.2014.732.

O'Neill, J. R., Williams, H. G., Pfeiffer, K. A., Dowda, M., McIver, K. L., Brown, W. H., & Pate, R. R. (2014). Young children's motor skill performance: Relationships with activity types and parent perception of athletic competence. *Journal of Science and Medicine in Sport, 17*(6), 607-610. https://doi.org/10.1016/j.jsams.2013.10.253

Park, J. W., Park, S. H., Koo, C. M., Eun, D., Kim, K. H., Lee, C. B., ... & Jee, Y. S. (2017). Regular physical education class enhances sociality and physical fitness while reducing psychological problems in children of multicultural families. *Journal of Exercise Rehabilitation, 13*(2), 168.

Pate, R. R., O'Neill, J. R., Brown, W. H., Pfeiffer, K. A., Dowda, M., & Addy, C. L. (2015). Prevalence of compliance with a new physical activity guideline for preschool-age children. *Childhood Obesity, 11*(4), 415-420. https://doi.org/10.1089/chi.2014.0143

Patrick, K.S., et al (2001). Bright Futures in Practice: Physical activity. National Center for Education in Maternal and Child Health.

Physical Therapy Guide to Container Baby Syndrome. American Physical Therapy Association. (2020). https://www.Physical Therapy Guide to Container Baby Syndrome, 2020)/symptomsconditionsdetail/physical-therapy-guide-to-container-baby-syndrome

Picchi, A. (2019) Game over: Middle-class and poor kids are ditching youth sports. CBS News. https://www.cbsnews.com/news/uneven-playing-field-middle-class-and-poor-kids-are-ditching-youth-sports/

Piper, M. C., Darrah, J., Boyce, N., Maguire, T. O., & Redfern, L. (2000). *Motor assessment of the developing infant*. Saunders.

Quick Quick Slow Ballroom Dance Studio. (May 18, 2018). https://www.quickquickslow.com/blog/why-every-football-player-should-take-ballroom-dance-lessons.

Rahman, S. (2012). A study on the opportunity and type of play of the children living in the apartments in Dhaka City. Master of Early Childhood Development. BRAC University and Columbia University.

Ramstetter, C. & Murray, R. (2017). Time to play: Recognizing the benefits of recess. *American Educator, 41*(1), 17-23. https://www.aft.org/sites/default/files/ae_spring2017ramstetter_and_murray.pdf

Ratey, J. J., & Hagerman, E. (2008). *Spark: The revolutionary new science of exercise and the brain*. Little, Brown.

Robinson, L. E., Stodden, D. F., Barnett, L. M., Lopes, V. P., Logan, S. W., Rodrigues, L. P., & D'Hondt, E. (2015). Motor competence and its effect on positive developmental trajectories of health. *Sports Medicine, 45*(9), 1273-1284.

Robinson, L. E., Wang, L., Colabianchi, N., Stodden, D. F., & Ulrich, D. (2020). Protocol for a two-cohort randomized cluster clinical trial of a motor skills intervention: The promoting activity and trajectories of Health (PATH) study. *BMJ Open, 10*(6). https://doi.org/10.1136/bmjopen-2020-037497.

Rodriguez-Ayllon, M., Cadenas-Sánchez, C., Estévez-López, F., Muñoz, N. E., Mora-Gonzalez, J., Migueles, J. H., ... & Esteban-Cornejo, I. (2019). Role of physical activity and sedentary behavior in the mental health of preschoolers, children and adolescents: a systematic review and meta-analysis. *Sports Medicine, 49*(9), 1383-1410.

Romanelli, R., Cecchi, N., Carbone, M. G., Dinardo, M., Gaudino, G., Miraglia del Giudice, E., & Umano, G. R. (2020). Pediatric obesity: Prevention is better than care. *Italian Journal of Pediatrics, 46*(1). https://doi.org/10.1186/s13052-020-00868-7.

Sabol, T. J., Bohlmann, N. L., & Downer, J. T. (2017). Low-income ethnically diverse children's engagement as a predictor of school readiness above preschool classroom quality. *Child Development, 89*(2), 556–576. https://doi.org/10.1111/cdev.12832

Schuetz Haemmerli, N., von Gunten, G., Khan, J., Stoffel, L., Humpl, T., & Cignacco, E. (2021). Interprofessional collaboration in a new model of transitional care for families with preterm infants—The health care professional's perspective. *Journal of Multidisciplinary Healthcare, 14*, 897-908. https://doi.org/10.2147/JMDH.S303988

Scott, M. W., Emerson, J. R., Dixon, J., Tayler, M. A., & Eaves, D. L. (2020). Motor imagery during action observation enhances imitation of everyday rhythmical actions in children with and without developmental coordination disorder. *Human Movement Science, 71*, 102620. https://doi.org/10.1016/j.humov.2020.102620

SHAPE America – Society of Health and Physical Educators. (2016). Shape of the nation: Status of physical education in the USA. https://www.shapeamerica.org/Common/Uploaded%20files/uploads/pdfs/son/Shape-of-the-Nation-2016_web.pdf

Sigmundsson, H., Trana, L., Polman, R., & Haga, M. (2017). What is trained develops! theoretical perspective on skill learning. *Sports, 5*(2), 38.

Slot, P. L., & Bleses, D. (2018). Individual children's interactions with teachers, peers, and tasks: The applicability of the inclass pre-K in Danish preschools. *Learning and Individual Differences, 61*, 68-76. https://doi.org/10.1016/j.lindif.2017.11.003

Smith, B., Trujillo-Priego, I., Lane, C., Finley, J., & Horak, F. (2015). Daily quantity of infant leg movement: Wearable Sensor algorithm and relationship to walking onset. *Sensors, 15*(8), 19006-19020. https://doi.org/10.3390/s150819006

Smith, J. D., Fu, E., & Kobayashi, M. A. (2020). Prevention and management of childhood obesity and its psychological and health comorbidities. *Annual Review of Clinical Psychology, 16*(1), 351-378. https://doi.org/10.1146/annurev-clinpsy-100219-060201

Sng, E., Frith, E., & Loprinzi, P. D. (2018). Temporal effects of acute walking exercise on learning and memory function. *American Journal of Health Promotion, 32*(7), 1518-1525.

Stanborough, R. J. (2019, December 9). *Ages and stages: How to monitor child development*. Healthline. https://www.healthline.com/health/childrens-health/stages-of-child-development

Stodden, D., Goodway, J., Langendorfer, S., Roberton, M., Rudisill, M., Garcia, C., & Garcia, L. (2008, May). A developmental perspective on the role of motor skill competence in physical activity: An emergent relationship. *Quest, 60*(2), 290-306. https://doi.org/10.1080/00336297.2008.10483582

Subramanian, S. K., Sharma, V. K., Arunachalam, V., Radhakrishnan, K., & Ramamurthy, S. (2015). Effect of structured and unstructured physical activity training on cognitive functions in adolescents—A randomized control trial. *Journal of Clinical and Diagnostic Research, 9*(11), CC04-CC9. https://doi.org/10.7860/JCDR/2015/14881.6818

Swanzen, R. (2018). Facing the generation chasm: The parenting and teaching of generations Y and Z. *International Journal of Child, Youth and Family Studies, 9*(2), 125-150.

Thompson, D. (2018). American meritocracy is killing youth sports. *The Atlantic*.

Tierney, A. L. (2009). Brain development and the role of experience in the early years. *Zero to Three, 30*(2), 9-13.

Townsend, E., Wilcock, A. A. (2004). Occupational justice and client-centred practice: A dialogue in progress. *Canadian Journal of Occupational Therapy, 71*(2), 75-87. doi:10.1177/000841740407100203

Trehub, S. E. (2018). Multimodal music in infancy and early childhood. In Y. R. Kim (Ed.), *The Oxford Handbook of Music and the Body* (pp. 383-386). Oxford University Press. https://doi.org/10.1093/oxfordhb/9780190636234.013.7

U.S. Department of Agriculture & U.S. Department of Health and Human Services. (2020). *Dietary Guidelines for Americans, 2020-2025*. (9th ed.). DietaryGuidelines.gov

U.S. Department of Health and Human Services, (n.d.). Infants: Overview and objectives. Healthy People 2030. https://health.gov/healthypeople/objectives-and-data/browse-objectives/infants

U.S. Department of Health and Human Services (2008). Physical activity. Guidelines Advisory Committee Report, 2008. Washington, DC: U.S. Department of Health and Human Services.

U.S. Department of Health and Human Services (2018). Physical activity guidelines for Americans (2nd ed.). https://health.gov/paguidelines/second-edition

Veldman, S. L.-S. (2019). Associations between gross motor skills and cognitive development in toddlers. *Early Human Development, 132*, 39-44. https://doi.org/10.1016/j.earlhumdev

Wang, H., Chen, Y., Liu, J., Sun, H., & Gao, W. (2020). A follow-up study of Motor Skill Development and its determinants in preschool children from middle-income family. *BioMed Research International, 2020*, 1-13. https://doi.org/10.1155/2020/6639341

Whitlock, E. P. (2005). Screening and interventions for childhood overweight: A summary of evidence for the U.S. Preventive Services Task Force. *Pediatrics, 116*(1). https://doi.org/10.1542/peds.2005-0242

Wick, K., Leeger-Aschmann, C. S., Monn, N. D., et al. (2017). Interventions to promote fundamental movement skills in childcare and kindergarten: A systematic review and meta-analysis. *Sports Medicine, 47*, 2045-2068. https://doi.org/10.1007/s40279-017-0723-1

World Health Organization. (2020). Physical activity: What is physical activity? https://www.who.int/news-room/fact-sheets/detail/physical-activity

World Health Organization. (2021). Health Promotion. https://www.who.int/westernpacific/about/how-we-work/programmes/health-promotion

World Health Organization: WHO. (2022, October 5). Physical activity. https://www.who.int/news-room/fact-sheets/detail/physical-activity

Zeng, N., Ayyub, M., Sun, H., Wen, X., Xiang, P., & Gao, Z. (2017). Effects of physical activity on motor skills and cognitive development in early childhood: A systematic review. *BioMed Research International, 2017*, 1-13. https://doi.org/10.1155/2017/2760716

5

CHAPTER

Promoting Physical Health
Adults

Mark Amir, PT, DPT, MPH, DipMDT; Michael A. Pizzi, PhD, OTR/L, FAOTA; Katie J. Galezniak, MS, OTR/L; Avi Friedman, DPT; Ashleigh Augello, MOT, OTR/L; and Melissa Neagles, OTR/L

Learning Objectives

At the end of this chapter, the reader will:

1. Identify social and cultural barriers to physical health and wellness for adults (ACOTE B.1.2, B.1.3; CAPTE 7D8, 7D37)
2. Describe practice strategies to address health and wellness in the adult population (ACOTE B.4.10; CAPTE 7D11, 7D16)
3. Understand social determinants of health and their impact on physical health (ACOTE, B.1.3, B.7.0; CAPTE 7D10)
4. Be able to demonstrate use of health promotion models in practice (ACOTE B.2.1, B.3.4, B.4.23; CAPTE 7D13, 7D34)
5. Recognize the risk and protective factors related to physical health and adults (ACOTE B.1.2, B.1.3; CAPTE 7D16)
6. Promote physical health for individuals, communities and populations as part of the interprofessional team (ACOTE B.4.23, B.4.25; CAPTE 7D7, 7D39, 7D13, 7D24)

The ACOTE Standards used are those from 2018.

Pizzi, M. A., & Amir, M. (Eds.). *Interprofessional Perspectives for Community Practice: Promoting Health, Well-Being, and Quality of Life* (pp. 77-96).

Key Words

Economic Stability, Education Access and Quality, Health Belief Model, Health Care Access and Quality, Micro-Breaks, Neighborhood and Built Environment, Ottawa Charter for Health Promotion, Physical Activity, Population-Based Framework, Protective Factors, Risk Factors, Secondary Conditions, Social and Community Context, Social Determinants of Health, Stages of Change Model

Introduction

This chapter addresses physical health in adults through an interprofessional lens, with a focus on wellness and prevention. Physical health refers to the level of functioning of the body's musculoskeletal, cardiovascular, and neurological systems working together to be able to participate in all forms of physical activity throughout the individual's life span (World Health Organization [WHO], 2018b). The WHO adds that "health is state of complete physical, mental and social well-being and not merely the absence of disease or infirmity" (WHO, 2021c). In promoting physical health, an interprofessional team perspective is crucial. Although many health care professionals engage with clients for the first time only after a health episode presents itself, there is a growing opportunity to improve the client, community, and population health through physical activity, which will minimize health-related risks in the adult and aging population.

In this chapter, adult physical health assessment, intervention, and program design are highlighted. The potential to influence well-being through interprofessional initiatives, at the individual and societal level, for communities and populations, is investigated. Health promotion and preventative interventions that target lifestyle choices and habits, wellness screens, sleep, ergonomics, and environment are examined. Additionally, chronic illness and prevention of further disease processes and disability will also be explored. Discussions include a look into the roles and potential roles of health professionals and barriers to implementation.

Case Study

Angie is a 42-year-old single mother of three children ages 2, 5, and 10 years old. She recently moved from a city apartment to a suburban house to be closer to her parents who are helping with caring for her children. Angie works full-time for a marketing company and spends half the workweek working from the office and the other half from home. Although her work hours are Monday through Friday 8 am to 4:30 pm, she often works later into the evening and occasionally on weekends. Her work tasks require extensive computer use and she recently developed wrist and hand pain, which her physician diagnosed as carpal tunnel syndrome. On occasion, Angie works while sitting on her couch, which she states produces neck and low back pain. The pain has become significant enough to interfere with Angie's everyday physical and social activities as well as house chores and child caring. Daily activities (e.g., household management, meal preparation, folding laundry) that were once done with ease are now taking an increased amount of time to complete due to her pain, as well as decreased endurance and generalized weakness from her sedentary lifestyle of having a desk job with little physical activity. Before having her kids, Angie participated in outdoor activities of walking and biking but with her aches and pains, workload, and family demands, finds little time for personal care. Additionally, she has been consuming alcohol more frequently and reports having interrupted sleep. Due to her physical situation, Angie experiences increased anxiety about her current life situation and ability to engage in daily activities, including work.

Reflective Questions

1. Describe the impact of Angie's life situation in relation to her overall quality of life (QOL).
2. How specifically does her physical health impact her QOL, as well as impact her social, mental/emotional, and family health?
3. What are some health promotion strategies that can be implemented to interrupt a downward spiral of physical health?

Defining and Promoting Physical Health for Adults

According to the WHO, "Regular physical activity is proven to help prevent and manage noncommunicable diseases (NCDs) such as heart disease, stroke, diabetes and several cancers. It also helps prevent hypertension, maintain healthy body weight and can improve mental health, quality of life and well-being" (2021a, para. 1). Physical activity, more than just exercise, is any activity that includes moving the body. To maximize participation in physical activity, movement should be meaningful and important for the person, community, or population. Popular forms of physical activity include formal and structured exercise, biking, walking/running/jogging, and sports activities. Advancing into middle age and later into older adulthood, physical activity may take the form of lighter forms of these activities. Health professionals should bear in mind that it is the individuals value placed on the activity that will help sustain and maintain engagement in any physical activity.

Physically engaging in activities can also be described as muscular wellness, the relationship between one's muscles and bones, to support dynamic movement and stability. When there is a breakdown of muscular wellness, pain can develop, such as complaints of low back pain, which are the most commonly presented (Ferrari et al., 2015). Movement is a critical factor in mitigating musculoskeletal risks for disease and injury. Having a regular movement regimen that incorporates regular exercise decreases obesity and improves wellness. For example, for those suffering from osteoporosis, body weight exercises have been shown to improve bone density and decrease the risk for fractures (Rizzoli et al., 2010). Health professionals (e.g., rehabilitation professionals coordinating with exercise physiologists, athletic trainers, personal trainers, physicians) can create activity-specific programs to mitigate physical deterioration from ailments such as osteoporosis. Proper posture can also be key for the myriad individuals who maintain static positions, either standing or sitting, for extended periods of time, be it at work or at home. Proper posture and movement patterns can also be addressed in situations where repetitive movements are required, such as excessive typing or lifting items in a warehouse. These excessive movement patterns, similar to sports injuries, as well as postural abnormalities often result in stresses to the musculoskeletal system and can result in arthritis and even further complications such as ligament or tendon sprains and strains (Wilder & Sethi, 2004). They can be alleviated with restorative movements that reduce chronic stress with short duration breaks called a **micro-break** or by countermovements creating homeostatic muscular balance. Micro-breaks can be any form of a short burst of stretch, lasting up to 30 seconds, that target a specific area of the body to be considered at risk of injury. Rehabilitation professionals can coordinate work site programs with employers so that chronic postures leading to musculoskeletal impairments can be avoided using a daily stretching and micro-break program (da Costa & Vieira, 2008; Haines et el., 2002). The physical well-being is codependent on mental, social, and environmental factors addressed in part throughout this chapter and the book. Each can have an influence on overall physical health and the interprofessional team should continue to seek and eliminate barriers to physical health.

Guiding Principles for a Globally Healthy Active World

The Global Action Plan on Physical Activity 2018–2030 (WHO, 2018b), calls for promotion of healthier and more active lives across the world. The mission is:

> to ensure that all people have access to safe and enabling environments and to diverse opportunities to be physically active in their daily lives, as a means of improving individual and community health and contributing to the social, cultural, and economic development of all nations (p. 20).

This mission considers the importance of creating opportunities and environments in which physical activity can occur, and not simply provide the physical activity in isolation of other factors that influence health, well-being, and QOL. It is a proactive call to action for all health professionals to engage individuals, communities, and populations in physical activity to promote health and well-being. This important document also provides guiding principles (Table 5-1) for promoting physical health that support the mission.

The population-based framework in which to enact these guiding principles is made up of four objectives, which include the creation of 1) active societies; 2) active environments; 3) active people; and 4) active systems. This framework considers dynamic systems thinking, whereby one action (or inaction) impacts others in various ways toward an outcome. In this instance, the framework is implying the dynamic between societies, the environments that make up societies, the people that make up the environments and society, and the systems that influence all of them. Earlier, the authors spoke about health professionals' creating opportunities within environments in which meaningful physical activity can be implemented. This framework supports that concept.

Considering Angie's case:

1. What criteria or changes are required for Angie to meet related to the objectives of the Global Action Plan of Physical Activity?
2. Name two professionals you would consider adding to your team to make sure Angie meets each of the objective goals?

Table 5-1

Key Terms and Definitions

PRINCIPLE	DEFINITION
Human rights approach	The WHO Constitution enshrines that the highest attainable standard of health is a fundamental right of every human being. As an essential resource for everyday living, health is a shared social and political priority for all countries. In the 2030 Agenda, countries committed to invest in health, achieve universal health coverage, and reduce health inequalities for people of all ages and abilities. Implementation of this action plan should employ a rights-based approach and incorporate a commitment to engaging and empowering individuals and communities to actively participate in the development of solutions.
Equity across the life course	Disparities in physical activity participation by age, gender, disability, pregnancy, socioeconomic status, and geography reflect limitations and inequities in the socioeconomic determinants and opportunities for physical activity for different groups and different abilities. Implementation of this action plan should explicitly consider the needs at different stages of the life course (including childhood, adolescence, adulthood, and older age), different levels of current activity and ability with a priority towards addressing disparities and reducing inequalities.
Evidence-based practice	The recommended policy actions are informed by a robust scientific evidence base, as well as practice-based evidence from active evaluation and demonstration of impact. The cost-effectiveness for many interventions is already established; implementation of the plan should continue to build and develop this evidence base.
Proportional universality	Proportional universality describes an approach to the resourcing and delivery of services at a scale and intensity proportionate to the degree of need. At a global, national, and subnational level, there is a need to focus efforts on reducing inequity in the opportunities for physical activity. Therefore, proportional allocation of the resources to the actions needed to engage the least active and those who face the greatest barriers to increasing participation should be a priority.
Policy coherence and health in all policies	Physical activity can deliver benefits for individuals, communities, and Member States across a range of SDGs, and therefore action is required across and between a wide range of policies and partners to achieve sustained change and impact. The SDGs recognize that people's health and the health of the planet are not mutually exclusive, and that environmental sustainability is critical to health improvement.
Engagement and empowerment of policymakers, people, families, and communities	People and communities should be empowered to take control of the determinants of their health through active participation in the development of policies and interventions that affect them in order to reduce barriers and to provide motivation. Active engagement to mobilize communities is one of the most powerful ways to change behavior and change social norms.
Multisectoral partnerships	A comprehensive, integrated and intersectoral approach consistent with SDG17 is essential to increase population levels of physical activity and reduce sedentary behavior. Implementation of this action plan should foster collaboration across and between all stakeholders at all levels, guided by a shared vision to realize the multiplicative benefits of a more active world (WHO, 2018b, pp. 22-23).

Social Determinants of Health and Physical Activity for Adults

While it is important to acknowledge the importance of engaging in meaningful physical health-related activities, it is equally important to understand how inactivity and sedentary behaviors impact health, well-being, and QOL. There are many factors related to engaging in physical activity to develop and maintain physical health. Social Determinants of Health (SDOH) "are the conditions in the environments where people are born, live, learn, work, play, worship, and age that affect a wide range of health, functioning, and quality-of-life outcomes and risks" (U.S. Department of Health and Human Services, 2020b, p. 1). Primary SDOH that impact physical health and participation in activity that promotes physical health include:

1. Economic Stability
2. Education Access and Quality
3. Health Care Access and Quality
4. Neighborhood and Built Environment
5. Social and Community Context

Economic Stability

People who do not have any meaningful financial means tend to live in poverty, and thus do not have the means to purchase proper food to maintain a nutritional status for physical health, for housing, or to meet other needs to maintain physical health, let alone participate in health-related physical activity. People living in poverty are also more likely to die from preventable disease and more likely to have a disability. Disability also is correlated with having more potential to live in poverty, especially when the disability occurs earlier in the adult life and more so in low- and middle-income countries or regions (Lena et al., 2017). Having employment is important to sustain economic stability; however, finding and maintaining employment can often be a difficult task. All these factors also impact one's mental health, which has a direct impact on participation in physical activities (Williams & Do, 2021).

Education Access and Quality

There are many studies that correlate levels of education with health status, noting that more educated young people (who become adults) are more likely to be healthier and live longer (U.S. Department of Health and Human Services, 2020a), health inequities in general are impacted (Marmot & Bell, 2009), and longevity decreases among those with less education (Shiels et al., 2017). According to Zajacova and Lawrence (2018), "less educated adults report worse general health, more chronic conditions, and more functional limitations and disability" (p. 3). When working with individuals and populations, health professionals' general knowledge of educational levels can inform them about health literacy issues, as well as adapting traditional health education and physical activity recommendations.

Health Care Access and Quality

HP2030 objectives for health care access and quality include the following: 1) Increase the proportion of people with a usual primary care provider; 2) Reduce the proportion of people who can't get medical care when they need it; 3) Reduce the proportion of people who can't get prescription medicines when they need them; and 4) Increase the number of community organizations that provide prevention services (U.S. Department of Health and Human Services, 2020a). Other objectives include access to and affordability of dental care and health professionals of all disciplines having knowledge of evidence-based preventive services. Access to health care makes a life and death difference, as does the quality of that health care. Working with an interprofessional team perspective can lead to increased individual member's knowledge of other member's roles so that collectively they can meet the needs of a client and community. If access to any individual is difficult, each member can provide health education, (e.g., physical activity recommendations and strategies) which can be effective in improving physical health. If access is limited, there is a risk of a lower overall quality of care, which interprofessional teams should be aware of and compensate for.

Neighborhood and Built Environment

The WHO statement about health and well-being includes environmental. The Ottawa Charter for Health Promotion (WHO, 1986) states:

> Health is created and lived by people within the **settings** of their everyday life; where they learn, work, play, and love. Health is created by caring for oneself and others, by being able to make decisions and have control over one's life circumstances and by

ensuring that the society one lives in creates conditions that allow the attainment of health by all its members. Caring, holism, and ecology are essential issues in developing strategies for health promotion and wellness. (p. 1)

The Ottawa Charter statement reflects the need to explore the environments where people engage as influences on their health and well-being. From a community and population perspective, it speaks clearly to health professionals to take a clear look at environmental barriers and supports during any intake or needs assessment to optimize health, well-being, and QOL. Some environmental considerations include: cultural biases, clean air or water, walkable spaces, community levels of violence and drug use, accessible community centers, and availability of preventive services. All these factors, taken together or separately, will impact one's physical and mental health and well-being.

Social and Community Context

Relationships are an essential determinant of health, no matter the context in which they occur. Families, schools, workplaces, and communities are such contexts; social ties influence health, well-being, and QOL (Umberson et al., 2010a). "Social ties can instill a sense of responsibility and concern for others that then lead individuals to engage in behaviors that protect the health of others, as well as their own health. Social ties provide information and create norms that further influence health habits. Thus, in a variety of ways, social ties may influence health habits that in turn affect physical health and mortality" (Umberson & Montez, 2010b, p. S56). Well-being in one's own family and community is affected by socioeconomic status, cultural or racial discrimination, and sense of safety in the community or residence, even within a family unit. It is crucial that health professionals explore social connectedness as it impacts and helps determine one's health status, physical health and sense of well-being, and QOL. One way to support increased physical health accessibility is by increasing access to health services at the **community** level. Relying on client motivation and support for long term changes from occasional visits to a health care professional is not likely to be sufficient at community level physical health (Krist et al., 2013). Offering **secondary prevention** services in nontraditional settings (churches, recreational, and community centers, home-based, or internet programs) may increase participation (Lawlor et al., 2018). Multicomponent individually tailored secondary preventative services outside of the traditional clinical setting, for cardiovascular disease, for example, have positive effects on physical activity, diastolic blood pressure, cholesterol, and mental health (Lawlor et al., 2018). Optimal individual health benefits from access and support at the community level.

Health care professionals can prioritize preventative care, as well as address nonmedical factors of health with clients. For better health outcomes, delivery at the medical and community levels should be integrated. Ideally, clinicians initiate preventive services by bringing in a medical framework, and the community assists to reinforce and provide motivation for lifestyle changes that reduce risk (Krist et al., 2013). One way of achieving this goal is by utilizing Community Health Centers (CHC). One in three Americans with low-income use CHCs to access primary health care (Manning, 2015). Under a CHC model, primary care providers interact with multiple medical disciplines as well as social support systems and community service organizations (Manning, 2015). Additionally, stakeholders include board members and patients that helps to address the specific needs of a community and supports cultural competency. Rehabilitation professionals are ideal collaborators in developing community-based integrated prevention services.

1. What types of CHCs are available in your neighborhood that would be helpful for Angie's case?
2. What resources can you provide as a health care professional that would add value to a CHC and Angie?
3. What other disciplines are available at a CHC that could assist your goal of creating community-based programs of prevention related to Angie's case?

Risk and Protective Factors Related to Physical Health

The Centers for Disease Control and Prevention (CDC) has established that lack of physical activity (or sedentary behaviors) is a high-risk factor for development of chronic disease such as obesity, some cancers, cardiovascular disease, and diabetes 2 (CDC, 2019). Sedentary behaviors are one category of behaviors that impact health and well-being. Lacking motivation to engage in activity, not having safe and supportive environments and communities, working too many hours and not engaging in self-care, diet and nutrition, smoking, lack of sleep, and engaging in risky behaviors (e.g., unsafe sexual encounters) are but a few of the other risk factors for ill health and the possibility of contributing to chronic illness.

Concomitantly, there are many physical health benefits for engaging in activity and protecting and maintaining physical health. Daily exercise and physical activity increase one's flexibility, mobility, joint strength, and cardiovascular status. Engaging in something every day, even if for 10 minutes, can be beneficial (U.S. Department of Health and Human Services, 2018). Having a motivation to engage daily promotes positive mental as well as physical health. Maintaining a work-life balance, being aware of one's own needs for self-care, and having a healthy diet are all protective factors for one's physical health. Engaging in physical activity has also shown cognitive benefits that helps to improve overall health as people age (U.S. Department of Health and Human Services, 2020b).

Interprofessional teams that address both risk and protective factors, as well as the barriers to physical activity engagement, can establish realistic goals and intervention plans. For example, employers can be encouraged to offer workplace wellness programs, as working adults with access to health care are more likely to receive preventative care services like blood pressure checks, cholesterol screens, mammograms, and vaccinations. This is a ripe opportunity for collaboration with various stakeholders since less than half of all working adults reported having access to such programs (Isehunwa et al., 2017). Furthermore, employees with a lower socioeconomic status who participate in workplace wellness programs may have moderate positive effects on health behaviors (van Heijster et al., 2021). Wellness initiatives in the workplace can be as simple as offering gym membership reimbursement or time off from work for preventative well visits with a primary care physician.

Understanding Health Behaviors for Physical Health Promotion

Health behaviors are defined as behaviors enacted and implemented that impact once's health, well-being, and QOL (Short & Molborn, 2015). These behaviors can result in outcomes that are positive for physical health (e.g., structured exercise program engagement, healthy diets, positive mindset, sufficient sleep) or one's that can lead to ill health (e.g., excessive alcohol, excessive eating, not wearing seatbelts, not having proper vaccinations to ward off disease, being sedentary, smoking). Health behaviors are influenced by SDOH.

> "While these nonmedical factors include individual characteristics, such as level of education, health literacy, income, and health beliefs, many others derive from an individual's social and physical contexts – families, schools, workplaces, neighborhoods, and the larger political economic organization of society – "upstream" factors that further enable or constrain health." (McKinlay, 1979, as cited in Short & Molborn, 2015, p. 78)

Health behaviors are influenced by a dynamic interplay of many factors, especially the context in which people live, work, play and love. Thus, it is imperative health professionals understand not just behaviors that impact engagement in physical health–related activity, but the contexts in which they occur to enable positive health lifestyles. It is also crucial that there is at least a basic understanding of some models for health behavior change. Below the authors use alcohol use and sleep as two health behaviors that illustrate these points and that are a potential contributor to physical health decline. Both sleep and alcohol, both of which are human health behaviors, can influence work, social, and personal environments and can be difficult to identify as contributors to other complaints in a clinical setting.

Alcohol and Health

The National Institute on Alcohol Abuse and Alcoholism (NIAAA) provides clear and alarming facts and statistics regarding the impact of alcohol consumption on human health and well-being. Excessive alcohol hinders brain communication pathways, which can alter coordination, mood, behavior, and functional performance (WHO, 2018b). Diagnoses as a result of excessive alcohol consumption include, but are not limited to, cardiomyopathy, arrhythmias, cerebrovascular accident, hypertension, steatosis, alcoholic hepatitis, fibrosis, and cirrhosis. In addition, alcohol consumption can weaken the immune system, increase risk of cancer diagnoses, and directly impact overall health and wellness in the adult population (U.S. Department of Health and Human Services, n.d.). As stated by WHO in a 2016 review, "3 million deaths, or 5.3 percent of all global deaths (7.7% for men and 2.6% for women), were attributable to alcohol consumption" (2018a). Health care professionals should be alert to potential alcohol use among their clients and maintain an open and safe environment for dialogue. While alcohol abuse can risk an individual's social, family, and work life, it should not be perceived as a risk to discussing such behaviors in the clinical environment. Lastly, resources such as a Twelve Step program (Parker & Guest, 1999) and collaboration with experts in the field of substance abuse can be one of the interprofessionals on a behavioral change team.

Sleep Hygiene

Sleep is a vital function that permits the body and mind to rejuvenate and prepare for future activity (Uehli et el., 2014; Vgontzas et al., 2010). With proper sleep, one can feel refreshed and more alert while completing daily tasks. The *Occupational Therapy Practice Framework: Domain and Process, Fourth Edition* (AOTA, 2020) defines *rest and sleep* as "activities related to obtaining restorative rest and sleep to support healthy, active engagement in other occupations" (p. 32), with occupation defined as activities engaged in throughout life that are meaningful and important to an individual. Adequate sleep assists the body to maintain overall health and wellness, therefore reducing the risk of acquired health diseases and musculoskeletal injuries (Uehli et el., 2014). Lack of sleep negatively effects clear thinking, recall, and concentration on tasks (Shoen, 2021a; Uehli et el., 2014; Vgontzas et al., 2010). It is recommended young adults have a minimum of 7 hours of sleep every night to have proper cognitive and behavioral functions (Vgontzas et al., 2010).

However, despite this recommendation, high-quality sleep is not always prioritized, and many adults may not be aware of the benefits of sleep as medically beneficial.

Sleep quantity and quality directly impact physical performance. Inconsistent sleep and wake cycles add to the stress of the universal strains on sleep in the adult population (Vgontzas et al., 2010). The relationship between sleep and other areas of life is cyclical. Sleep affects social relationships, employment, substance use choice, and mental health. These negative effects then have a downward spiral that further deteriorates the quality and sometimes the quantity of sleep. Several studies of college students found poor sleep quality "can lead to significant emotional imbalance, fatigue, poor concentration, impaired memory, and generally lower life satisfaction" (Vgontzas et al., 2010; Ye et al., 2015, p. 88). These impacts may cause the individual to seek substances (e.g., caffeine, alcohol) or become irritable thus deteriorating social networks. There is also a noticeable connection between decreased sleep performance and adopting additional unhealthy habits. This is evident through the marketing and implementation of medication, controlled substances, and a variety of beverages and foods that maximize sleep performance or enhance wakefulness and productivity (Pacheco & Rehman, 2021; Shoen, 2021b; Suni & Truong, 2020).

For individuals without a medical or chronic condition, it is important to follow sleep guidelines developed by the CDC. These sleep habits, also referred to as "sleep hygiene," include the following:

- Be consistent. Go to bed at the same time each night and get up at the same time each morning, including on the weekends.
- Make sure your bedroom is quiet, dark, relaxing, and at a comfortable temperature.
- Remove electronic devices, such as TVs, computers, and smartphones, from the bedroom.
- Avoid large meals, caffeine, and alcohol before bedtime.
- Get some exercise. Being physically active during the day can help you fall asleep more easily at night (CDC, 2016).

The CDC also recognizes that lack of sleep is directly and indirectly linked to chronic disease such as obesity, depression, cardiovascular disease, and type 2 diabetes (2016). Smallfield et al. (2021), through a systematic review, found there is moderate evidence supporting mind-body self-care education to promote sleep and support sleep hygiene for people with chronic conditions. They also discussed the importance for interprofessional teams and health professionals to provide education around topics of nutrition, physical activity, sleep hygiene, and relaxation to promote healthier sleeping habits and routines.

When not addressed effectively, poor sleep can result in severe consequences. Inadequate sleep can result in considerable emotional discrepancy, lethargy, difficulty with attentiveness, and impaired problem solving. Sleep disturbances have been linked to impaired function of immune systems, anabolic and regenerative processes, neurophysiologic organization, consolidation of the memory, and cognitive function (Uehli et el., 2014; Vgontzas et al., 2010). In extreme cases sleep disturbances may lead to development of delirium and increased mortality (Boyko et al., 2012). Education about proper sleep as a physical and mental health–promoting intervention can be an effective tool to support daily activity engagement, improve overall well-being, increase concentration, alertness, and attention and improve general QOL.

1. How would you as part of the interprofessional team begin a conversation with Angie to maximize health behaviors?
2. What other risk factors can you identify in Angie and within your community that will require interprofessional collaboration?
3. What would a sleep hygiene intervention look like for Angie?

Promoting physical activity, modifying sleep, or eliminating drinking habits requires actionable change from the participant. The Stages of Change Theory and Health Belief Model are two of many that are highlighted here. The next two sections expand on the Stages of Change and Health Belief Model's to help the reader gain an in depth perspective.

Stages of Change Model

The Stages of Change Model, also known as the Transtheoretical Model (TTM), was developed by DiClemente and Prochaska (1982) and consists of several stages: precontemplation (not aware of the need for health behavior change and/or no intention to change), contemplation (now aware of a health problem and thinking about making a change), preparation (creates a plan for a change), action (implementing the plan for a change), maintenance (maintaining a commitment to the changes made that result in improved health), and the termination stage whereby there is full integration and ongoing engagement in the new health behavior that intervention is no longer needed.

In a systematic review of the use of the TTM related to health behavior change and physical activity, the authors concluded that the best time for enabling health behavior change is during the precontemplation and contemplation stages. They also stated that behavior change is more readily made and integrated when interventions for exercise and physical health activity are made face to face (Kleis et al., 2021). The implication for health professionals is that all individuals may not have any idea, despite overwhelming health education messages via social media and television, that exercise and physical activity can mitigate health issues (precontemplation). It also implies that, when made aware, people are more likely to make a health behavior change in

Table 5-2

Construct Definition

HEALTH BELIEF	DEFINITION	EXAMPLE RELATED TO PHYSICAL HEALTH
Perceived susceptibility	One's belief about how susceptible one is to contract an illness or develop a health condition	"I will never have a heart condition because no one in my family has heart disease."
Perceived severity	Perceived seriousness of an illness or severity of symptoms if contracted	"I don't need a COVID vaccine because I am healthy, and I won't end up in the hospital."
Perceived benefits	The positive things that can happen if enacting a health behavior	"If I do get a COVID vaccine, I am more protected from the virus and symptoms will be much less if I do contract the virus."
Perceived barriers	How difficult or costly it is to adopt a new behavior	"I need a lot of equipment or join a gym to exercise, and I can't afford it, so I won't exercise."
Self-efficacy	Having the motivation, determination, and willingness to achieve goals and take actions	"I can get out of bed and take a daily walk and need to for better physical health."

physical activity to improve health and well-being. The important factor is how it is communicated and the timing of that health communication.

Health Belief Model

Rosenstock (1974) created the Health Belief Model (HBM) that explores a person's beliefs about health and well-being and how those beliefs influence one's health behaviors (Table 5-2). The HBM is composed of constructs that focus on those beliefs and influences on those beliefs.

Another concept that influences health behaviors, according to the HBM, are cues to action. These are internal or external cues (e.g., pain, having a near accident while not wearing a seatbelt, seeing billboards about healthy diets to decrease obesity).

While one possesses health beliefs based on past experiences and knowledge acquired over time, the HBM is used most often after a health condition has emerged. It can also be used in prevention. Reitz et al. (2010), who cite Rosenstock (1974) discuss that, to prevent illness, positive beliefs must outweigh the negative and the "individual believes that:

1. He or she is personally susceptible to the disease or illness,
2. The occurrence of the health problem is severe enough to negatively impact his or her life,
3. Taking specific actions would have beneficial effects,
4. The barriers to such actions do not overwhelm the benefits, and
5. The individual is exposed to cues for action, then it is likely the health behavior will occur" (p. 53).

Having knowledge about one's ability or perceptions for change, as well as their beliefs about health and behavior change is essential for interprofessional teams. The same concepts can be used when creating community programs focused on health behavior changes.

Physical Health and Prevention

Preventing disease and disability is key for a healthier global community. What follows are five areas of health in which interprofessional teams can work together from a public health perspective to enable change in individuals, communities, and populations.

Chronic Disease and Obesity Management

Achieving and maintaining a healthy weight in adulthood can be a difficult journey for many. This is evidenced by the fact that three chronic diseases—heart disease, cancer, and type 2 diabetes—are the leading causes of death and disability in the United States and the leading drivers of health care costs (CDC, 2019). One in three deaths in the United States each year is due to cardiovascular disease (CDC, 2021). The presence of a chronic disease can lead to complications that affect overall health and QOL. Chronic diseases negatively impact pain levels, functional abilities, employment, finances, mental health, and relationships (Levine et al., 2019). There is a sequelae of health issues that can accompany chronic disease. For example, uncontrolled diabetes can lead to damage to the eyes, skin, nerves, heart, blood vessels, and kidneys, seizures, coma, and premature death (The Healthline Editorial Team, 2018, August 20).

Table 5-3

Construct Definition

HEALTHY LIVING STRATEGY	WHAT IT IS	WHERE TO FIND IT
Assessing your weight	Body mass index and waist circumference	https://www.cdc.gov/healthyweight/assessing/index.html
Healthy weight	To learn about weight loss, caloric intake and weight management/maintenance	https://www.cdc.gov/healthyweight/index.html
ChooseMyPlate	For managing healthy eating and habits for eating	https://www.myplate.gov
Physical activity basics	Learn about different types of physical activities and amount of activity needed	https://www.cdc.gov/physicalactivity/basics/index.htm

Adapted from Centers for Disease Control and Prevention. (2019). *Lack of physical activity.* National Center for Chronic Disease Prevention and Health Promotion (NCCDPHP). https://www.cdc.gov/chronicdisease/resources/publications/factsheets/physical-activity.htm

These chronic diseases are linked to being overweight or obese (U.S. Department of Health and Human Services, 2020a) and may be preventable. Obesity is directly linked to diet and lack of physical activity, which translates into poorer physical health. Lack of activity is a leading indicator for developing chronic diseases, so it is evident there is a dynamic interplay between physical activity, weight management, and chronic disease.

Current global statistics show that obesity and being overweight has risen to epidemic proportions. The following are key facts (WHO, 2021b):

- Worldwide obesity has nearly tripled since 1975.
- In 2016, more than 1.9 billion adults, 18 years and older, were overweight. Of these over 650 million were obese.
- Thirty-nine percent of adults aged 18 years and over were overweight in 2016, and 13% were obese.
- Most of the world's population live in countries where overweight and obesity kills more people than underweight.
- Thirty-nine million children under the age of 5 years were overweight or obese in 2020.
- Over 340 million children and adolescents aged 5 to 19 years were overweight or obese in 2016.
- Obesity is preventable.

There are many reasons people become overweight or obese from poor diets and lack of or low physical activity. Many of the factors are also related to the SDOH, such as poverty, community factors, health care access, and health food availability.

Changes in dietary and physical activity patterns are often the result of environmental and societal changes associated with development and lack of supportive policies in sectors such as health, agriculture, transport, urban planning, environment, food processing, distribution, marketing, and education (WHO, 2021a, p. 1).

While much more attention needs to be paid to the social determinants of physical health, especially related to healthy weight management, people of any weight for whom there is opportunity can begin to transform their physical health. Healthy People 2030 lists several objectives related to obesity and overweight and possible interventions (Table 5-3). The CDC also lists several strategies for assessment and management of being overweight or obese to live a healthier life and enable a healthy lifestyle.

Increasing one's physical activity levels and decreasing caloric intake are common and well-known strategies for weight reduction. However, health professionals and interprofessional teams must also pay attention to the person and community needs and intervene holistically. This means to also consider factors that impact caloric intake and physical activity: stress and mental health, motivation and readiness to change, current levels of activity and reasons for such, food availability (and other SDOH), as well as the current level of physical health. One assessment captures many of these factors and is focused on current activity levels of individuals as well as readiness to change.

The Pizzi Healthy Weight Management Assessment (PHWMA) was designed to capture the above factors and is focused on one's perceived levels of activity and current health behaviors, one's readiness to change maladaptive behaviors, and the stress related to making changes. While it is an individual client assessment, it can be used with populations and community programs by assessing individuals and examining the common threads of responses to effectively, with the client, community, or population, successfully intervene to promote healthier living. What follows is an example of some questions on the assessment:

Please use the following numbers to tell me if you want to make changes in that area.

1. I do not want to change this area
2. I am thinking about making a change in this area
3. I have decided to make a change in this area
4. I already started making changes in this area
5. I need to maintain or keep my behavior/changes I have made in this area

CATEGORY	WANT TO CHANGE? Circle your answer				
Doing play, fun or leisure activities	1	2	3	4	5
Keeping a schedule for things I do in my day	1	2	3	4	5
My physical health	1	2	3	4	5
Eating habits and routines (e.g., in front of the TV, eating too late at night)	1	2	3	4	5
Time I spend in front of the TV or on a computer	1	2	3	4	5

Reproduced with permission from Michael A. Pizzi.

A well-researched strategy for healthy weight management is high-intensity interval training (HIIT). It has been shown that moderate to vigorous intensity exercise or activity is most beneficial for weight management and can help prevent development of chronic disease (U.S. Department of Health and Human Services, 2018). Other health weight management assessments are detailed in Table 5-3.

Cardiovascular Prevention

Cardiovascular health involves the health of the heart and blood vessels, which can be affected by health behaviors and other factors including genetics (CDC, 2020b). "Regular physical activity is proven to help prevent and manage noncommunicable diseases such as heart disease, stroke, diabetes and several cancers. It also helps prevent hypertension, maintain healthy body weight and can improve mental health, quality of life and well-being" (WHO, 2022, para. 3). The federal physical activity guidelines recommend at least 150 to 300 minutes of moderate-intensity, or 75 to 150 minutes of vigorous-intensity aerobic physical activity per week to obtain the optimal level of health (Whitfield et al., 2019). In addition, muscle-strengthening exercises are recommended more than twice every week for each of the major muscle groups (Whitfield et al., 2019; Garber et al., 2011). Yet only one in four U.S. adults is getting the recommended level of physical activity (CDC, 2019). Rehabilitation professionals are best suited in leading an interprofessional team in cardiovascular prevention strategies because of their ability to assess the client's health status, physical function, response to the exercise prescription, and overall goals (Garber et al., 2011). When initiating an exercise for a sedentary individual, short bouts of even 10 minutes a day can be a good starting point with a goal of increasing both the volume and intensity of the exercise over time (Garber et al., 2011). A general daily walking program and counting steps (volume) as well as measuring heart rate (intensity) can be used as educational and motivational tools. These recommendations apply to both adult male and female across all communities.

Mental Health

There is considerable research on the relationship between physical activity, physical health, and improved or sustained mental health and brain health (maintaining active neural connections through physical activity; Ohrnberger et al., 2017; U.S. Department of Health and Human Services, 2018). For positive relationships between these areas of health to occur, one needs to move regularly and not always at a high intensity and consistently (every couple of hours if sitting) for positive health outcomes to be achieved. There are numerous opportunities for movement every day (e.g., stretching and walking around during TV commercials) that can improve mental and emotional health, overall life satisfaction, happiness, and QOL. As mentioned previously, engaging in physical activity of one's interest and choice is the most beneficial. For example, if someone is in their early 60s and never exercised in a structured way, but enjoyed dancing, then dancing and musical activities would be most beneficial for cardiovascular, muscular strengthening, and mental/emotional health. Sustainability of that activity would also be more likely, which is the ultimate goal of physical activity related to physical health.

Engaging in physical activity can be a preventive strategy for mental health conditions, and aid in optimizing cognition, QOL, mood, and sleep, while also acting to minimize anxiety. Table 5-4 presents common benefits of physical activity on various mental health constructs that can be used as general guidelines for clients with any level of ability.

An excellent assessment of physical and mental health, and one's life satisfaction, is the Short Form-36 (SF-36; Ware & Sherbourne, 1992). The SF-36 assesses eight health-related concepts that explore mental and physical health within a previous 4-week time frame. Likert scales and yes/no questions are asked throughout. This helps health professionals gather preliminary information about the impact of physical and mental health on one's activity and role performance.

1. What chronic disease is Angie most at risk of developing? How would you address that within your professional scope of practice? What resources would you need to add to your team to maximize the physical health requirements that minimize the chronic disease you identified?

Table 5-4

Physical Activity Benefits on Mental Health

AREA OF MENTAL HEALTH	BENEFIT OF PHYSICAL ACTIVITY
Cognition	Reduced risk of dementia (including Alzheimer's disease) Improved cognition (executive function, attention, memory, crystallized intelligence, processing speed)
Quality of life	Improved life satisfaction and happiness
Mood and depression	Reduced risk of depression Reduced depressed mood
Anxiety	Reduced short-term feelings of anxiety (state anxiety) Reduced long-term feelings and signs of anxiety (trait anxiety) for people with and without anxiety disorders
Sleep	Improved sleep outcomes (increased sleep efficiency, sleep quality, deep sleep; reduced daytime sleepiness, frequency of use of medication to aid sleep) Improved sleep outcomes that increase with duration of acute episode

Adapted from U.S. Department of Health and Human Services. (2018). ***Physical activity guidelines for Americans*** (2nd ed.). https://health.gov/sites/default/files/2019-09/Physical_Activity_Guidelines_2nd_edition.pdf

Preventing Secondary Conditions for People With Physical Disabilities

People with physical disabilities, given their limited mobility status, are prone to what is termed "secondary conditions" or those that result from limited participation in physical activity and mobility. **Secondary conditions** can be defined as those physical, medical, cognitive, emotional, or psychosocial consequences to which persons with disabilities are more susceptible by virtue of an underlying impairment, including adverse outcomes in health, wellness, participation, and QOL (Hough, 1999, p. 162). These can include pain, bowel and bladder complications, bed sores (decubiti), fatigue, depression, and being overweight or obese.

People with disabilities often are treated primarily for their existing disability, with little concern or thought regarding the prevention of secondary conditions. However, using more of a public health and prevention model, interprofessional teams have opportunities to "diminish the possibilities of secondary conditions associated with the lifestyle of the disabled (e.g., inactivity secondary to a disability)" (Pizzi, 2010, p. 379). The public health perspective has been noted in the need for a paradigm shift to incorporate more health promotion for developing and maintain functional independence for people with developmental disabilities, who are prone to the secondary conditions noted earlier (Frey et al., 2001):

> ... having a disability is viewed as increasing one's risk for a variety of preventable problems that can limit health, functional capacity, participation in life activities and independence. A prevention framework that incorporates rehabilitation interventions and themes of consumer empowerment can be offered using a public health orientation. (p. 362)

Preventing secondary conditions improves the health, well-being, and QOL of people with disabilities. All health professionals can utilize a prevention and public health approach during all interventions, which begins during assessment. Examples of preventing secondary conditions can include development of health education materials on self-management of decubiti, positioning strategies, or a physical activity program for wheelchair users to maintain aerobic capacity and strength. The CDC provides a list of resources (Table 5-5) all health professionals can use.

Additional Interventions for All Health Professionals

Healthy People 2030 (HP2030) describes various health objectives (Table 5-6) related to physical activity and promoting physical health. Also provided are evidence-based resources for interventions. These include:

In the HP2030, there is also evidence-based information for promoting physical health using social support interventions in community settings and family-based interventions. These apply to all the above objectives.

Table 5-5

Resources for Secondary Health Prevention

RESOURCE	WHAT IT IS	WHERE TO FIND IT
2018 Physical Activity Guidelines for Adults with Disabilities	Guidelines and intervention ideas for physical activity.	https://health.gov/sites/default/files/2019-09/Physical_Activity_Guidelines_2nd_edition.pdf
Inclusive Fitness Trainers	Have specialized training on understanding exercise precautions for people with disabilities, and utilizing safe, effective, and adapted methods of exercise training to provide exercise.	https://www.acsm.org/get-stay-certified/get-certified/specialization/cift
Move Your Way	Interactive. How to get started and physical activity needs.	https://health.gov/moveyourway
Healthy Weight & Obesity Briefs	Considerations for people and organizations to help prevent obesity.	https://www.cdc.gov/ncbddd/disabilityandhealth/materials/factsheets.html
Exercise Is Medicine	Resources and tools for reviewing activity each visit.	https://www.exerciseismedicine.org
National Center on Health, Physical Activity and Disability	Focuses on improving the health, wellness, and quality of life of people with disabilities. The Center promotes and facilitates increased participation in all types of physical activity including exercise, recreation, leisure, and sport.	https://www.nchpad.org
I Can Do It, You Can Do It	Encourages physical activity for people with disabilities.	http://committoinclusion.org/i-can-do-it-you-can-do-it/

Adapted from Centers for Disease Control and Prevention. (2021). *Promoting health for adults*. National Center for Chronic Disease Prevention and Health Promotion (NCCDPHP). https://www.cdc.gov/chronicdisease/resources/publications/factsheets/promoting-health-for-adults.htm

Orthopedic Health

There are many musculoskeletal injuries that can occur throughout life, whether through sport, work activities, or declining physical health, that medical professionals try and minimize with various movement strategies. Orthopedically, medical professionals most commonly manage arthritis issues and their sequela. Rheumatoid arthritis (RA) is an autoimmune disease, causing joint breakdown of most commonly the hands, wrists, and knees and producing symptoms of pain, swelling, and deformity (CDC, 2020a). Other areas of the body can also be affected, such as the lungs, heart and eyes (CDC, 2020a). Much of the known cause of RA is from a genetic predisposition but the likelihood of RA increases with age, smoking, and obesity (CDC, 2020a). It is most often treated with prescription medications, which can be more effective when self-care strategies, such as physical activity and weight loss are also implemented (CDC, 2020a). A more common movement related problem is found with osteoarthritis (OA), which is a joint condition that is caused by a breakdown of cartilage, usually in the hands, hips, and knees (CDC, 2020a). As the cartilage in the joint wears down, from excessive repetitive movement or from prolonged sedentary lifestyle, the underling bone is negatively impacted. Symptoms can include pain, loss of movement and swelling, and creates further risk of joint injury from improper joint function. These two arthritic conditions demonstrate that whether disease is primarily genetically predisposed or are developed due to lifestyle and behaviors, there are interventions that can be used to minimize their impact and improve QOL.

One of the best mechanisms to reduce OA symptoms and decrease further joint deterioration is through physical activity of strengthening exercises, weight loss, and pain-relieving medications (CDC, 2020a). While activity modification is not as immediately helpful for people with OA, it is still a supplement to use with other treatment options. Surgery is a last option alternative if other interventions failed or were insufficient with improving the individuals QOL. Teaching prevention strategies, such as reducing weight, maintaining an active lifestyle, and reducing chronic load on joints are interventions that are commonly used by health care providers. To enhance the effectiveness of these interventions, an interprofessional team should consider coordinating strategies that include social and emotional support as well as identifying community resources such as fitness centers or community activity centers, where individuals can socialize as they can safely participate in an active program. Arthritic conditions are a major cause for loss of work in the working population and reducing one's QOL at any age (Theis et al., 2018). In the older population, these joint conditions can lead to a high risk of falls that further increases disability and reduces health, increases cost, and impacts QOL (Barbour et al., 2012).

Table 5-6

Healthy People 2030 Objectives and Interventions

OBJECTIVES	INTERVENTIONS
Increase the proportion of adults who do enough aerobic physical activity for substantial health benefits.	Physical Activity: Individually Adapted Health Behavior Change Programs Physical Activity: Community-Wide Campaigns
Increase the proportion of adults who do enough aerobic physical activity for extensive health benefits.	Physical Activity: Individually Adapted Health Behavior Change Programs Physical Activity: Community-Wide Campaigns
Reduce the proportion of adults who do no physical activity in their free time.	Physical Activity: Individually Adapted Health Behavior Change Programs Physical Activity: Community-Wide Campaigns
Increase the proportion of health care visits by adults with obesity that include counseling on weight loss, nutrition, or physical activity.	Physical Activity: Interventions Including Activity Monitors for Adults with Overweight or Obesity
Increase the proportion of adults with arthritis who get counseling for physical activity.	Physical Activity: Interventions to Increase Physical Activity, Reduce Pain and Address Disability
Increase the proportion of adults who do enough aerobic and muscle-strengthening activity.	Physical Activity: Individually Adapted Health Behavior Change Programs
Reduce the proportion of adults with obesity.	Physical Activity: Interventions Including Activity Monitors for Adults with Overweight or Obesity
Reduce cholesterol in adults.	https://health.gov/healthypeople/objectives-and-data/browse-objectives/heart-disease-and-stroke/reduce-cholesterol-adults-hds-06
Increase the proportion of adults who walk or bike to get places.	https://health.gov/healthypeople/objectives-and-data/browse-objectives/physical-activity/increase-proportion-adults-who-walk-or-bike-get-places-pa-10
Improve cardiovascular health in adults.	Healthful Diet and Physical Activity for Cardiovascular Disease Prevention in Adults Without Known Risk Factors: Behavioral Counseling

Adapted from U.S. Department of Health and Human Services. (2020a). *Healthy People 2030*. Office of Disease Prevention and Health Promotion. https://health.gov/healthypeople

Nutritional Support

In addition to teaching about movement and active lifestyle strategies, nutrition can have a dramatic impact on our community members. Nutrients from food provide the body what it needs to function and can influence overall health. Nutrients, along with body hormones, environmental factors, physical activity level, and genetics create a synergistic effect on our performance and growth (Nayak et al., 2021). Depending on the exercise level and activity goals, nutritional supplements can further enhance health and activity performance, but care should be taken with supplements since when they are combined, they can vary in efficacy and effect (U.S. Department of Health and Human Services, 2021, March 29). Some foods can have an inflammatory effect on our body while others are anti-inflammatory. Foods that include excessive sugar can cause and exacerbate diabetes, heart disease, and arthritic pain and can lead to obesity even in young children (Della Corte et el., 2018; López-Alarcón et al., 2014). Simply educating the community on reducing overall sugar consumption can have dramatic benefits in reducing downstream medical issues throughout life. Adding fruits and vegetables, fatty fish, and adding spices, for example, can help mitigate inflammation (Islam et al., 2016) and targeting specific conditions, such as OA, with supplements of glucosamine and chondroitin adds additional health benefits (Jüni, 2016; McAlindon et al., 2000; Nayak et al., 2021).

Holistic management of the individual and a community can get complex when a health care professional attempts to make changes on their own. It is necessary to create a well-informed and well-rounded interprofessional group of health care stakeholders such as rehabilitation professionals, nutritionists, psychologists, and other medical experts that address the many issues influencing physical health, beyond movement and activity.

Physical Activity and Health Recommendations

There are two major types of physical activity recommendations that promote health and well-being for adults:

aerobic activity and muscle strengthening. The newest recommendations come from an abundance of evidence that any amount of moderate-to-vigorous activity can offer health benefits (U.S. Department of Health and Human Services, 2018). The benefits of activity, proper exercise, along with nutrition, are not new and have been known to benefit individual's health for over 2000 years (Keadle et al., 2021). For the past several decades, major organizations interested in exercise and public health, such as the CDC and American College of Sports Medicine (ACSM) offered guidelines related to dosing the amount of exercise for the general adult population (Haskell et al., 2007). Too much activity can cause stress and breakdown of body structures as does lack of proper intake of nutrients (Keadle et al., 2021). ACSM's guidelines include "moderate-intensity aerobic (endurance) physical activity for a minimum of 30 minutes on five days each week or vigorous-intensity aerobic physical activity for a minimum of 20 minutes on three days each week" and "activities that maintain or increase muscular strength and endurance a minimum of two days each week" (Haskell et al., 2007, p. 1). Activities and exercises that are over 5 hours per week offer even more health benefits (U.S. Department of Health and Human Services, 2018). When advising sedentary individuals, or those with chronic conditions that limit physical ability, a slow and steady start is advisable, such as starting with a daily walking routine at a comfortable pace on level ground for at least 10 minutes and increasing the duration to the recommended 30-minute time frame. As individuals gain endurance, confidence, and the habit of exercising, an increase of intensity such as higher walking speed or climbing hills can add to the challenge and health benefit. One motivational tool that can be used, especially when health care professionals promote physical activities is sharing the evidence that greater activities reduce the risk of common ailments such as cardiovascular disease (CVD), stroke, diabetes, cancer, as well as anxiety and depression (Haskell et al., 2007). This is especially powerful when working with individuals that have an early mild diagnosis that is still manageable without surgery or intense medical needs. Learning about the individual's life goals and values can help health care teams identify what motivates their clients and can be used to maintain the interest in activity modification. Encouraging clients to participate in group activities available in the community will add to their compliance of staying active.

When dosing the quantity of aerobic activities, a simple tool that can be used to educate first-time exercisers who do not have cardiovascular disease is to teach them how to measure their heart rate as a measure of exercise intensity. ACSM recommends an exercise intensity where the heart rate reaches at least 60% of the individual's maximum level. A rough guideline to assess the maximum heart rate is to use the following formula: 220 – age = maximum heart rate. As an example, a 45-year-old person would have a maximum heart rate of 175 beats per minute (220 - 45 = 175). An exercise level of at least 60% of the 175 maximum heart rate would require the individual to remain active at a pace that maintains their heart rate at about 105 beats per minute (175 x 60% = 105). An even simpler recommendation could be to instruct clients to walk at the fastest pace they can tolerate while still maintaining a conversation, referred to as the "talk Test" (Foster et al., 2008). For example, if while walking, the exerciser cannot finish a sentence without losing their breath, they are above the 60% exercise recommendation. This is not to indicate they shouldn't push to maintain the highest level of activity but simply to use it as a guide to learn when they should try and push their tolerance and when it is better to slow down and let the body recover from the activity. At the other end of the exercise tolerance, when the heart rate reaches 90% of maximum, the exercise intensity is very high and should not be maintained for more than a few short minutes. This is similar to running a sprint such as trying to catch a bus or a train that is a few hundred feet away and is about to leave the station. That level of exercise is excellent for cardiovascular health but cannot be sustained over a long duration. Both recommendations, slow and steady activity intertwined with short bursts of high intensity, can be recommended when a more comprehensive assessment of the client is utilized. Teaming up with exercise physiologists or certified athletic trainers can be helpful in fine tuning an activity plan for individual clients.

Learning Activities

1. Create a physical activity action plan for Angie that will reduce her chronic disease risk factors.
2. Create three measurable goals for Angie to improve her physical health.

Community Programs

Maintaining an interest in activity participation should include community resources and events such as school fundraisers where groups meet to walk together to raise money or awareness for a specific cause. Medical organizations, schools, and community groups such as a local fire department often have such events that individuals can participate in and train for. Participating in these events offers the benefits of exercise, social interaction, and emotional increase of doing good in one's community. Health care professionals can motivate their clients to attend and even coordinate such events if they do not yet exist. Organizing with public regulators to issue permits for such events may be a challenge so addressing all stakeholders impacted by these events should be assessed and discussed among the interprofessional team. In many communities, local nonprofit organizations, such as the YMCA provide affordable programs for all age groups that include physical activities and community

Table 5-7

Programming Resources for Health Promotion

PROGRAM	DESCRIPTION	WEBSITE
What Works: Strategies to Increase Physical Activity	Evidence-based strategies to increase physical activity across sectors and settings.	https://www.cdc.gov/physicalactivity/activepeoplehealthynation/strategies-to-increase-physical-activity/index.html
What's Your Role? Strategies by Sector	Evidence-based strategies to increase physical activity for individual community sectors, including real-world examples and resources for government, education, health care, and faith-based settings.	https://www.cdc.gov/physicalactivity/activepeoplehealthynation/everyone-can-be-involved/index.html
Active People, Healthy Nation	An initiative to help people become more physically active by 2027 to improve their overall health and quality of life and to reduce healthcare costs.	https://www.cdc.gov/physicalactivity/activepeoplehealthynation/index.html
The CDC Guide to Strategies to Increase Physical Activity in the Community	This document provides guidance for program managers, policy makers, and others on how to select strategies to increase physical activity in the community.	https://www.cdc.gov/obesity/downloads/PA_2011_WEB.pdf
Physical Activity Guidelines for Americans	Describes the amounts and types of physical activity needed to maintain or improve overall health and reduce the risk of chronic disease.	https://health.gov/sites/default/files/2019-09/Physical_Activity_Guidelines_2nd_edition.pdf
State and Local Examples	Examples of promoting physical activity on state and local levels.	https://www.cdc.gov/nccdphp/dnpao/state-local-programs/physicalactivity.html
CDC Workplace Health Promotion	Resources for workplace health promotion.	https://www.cdc.gov/workplacehealthpromotion/index.html
The Built Environment Assessment Tool (BEAT)	This tool helps assess core features and qualities of the built environment that affect health, especially walking, biking, and other types of physical activity.	https://www.cdc.gov/nccdphp/dnpao/state-local-programs/built-environment-assessment/index.htm
CDC's Designing and Building Healthy Places	This website offers tools and evidence-based health strategies for community planning, transportation, and land-use decisions.	https://www.cdc.gov/healthyplaces/default.htm
Increasing Access to Safer and Healthier Modes of Transportation	Strategies to increase physical activity levels while also using other modes of transportation. Also addresses social determinants of health.	https://www.cdc.gov/policy/hi5/publichealthinnovators/
Evidence-based Strategies and Community Examples	Examples for increasing physical activity and health that are community-based.	https://www.cdc.gov/policy/hi5/publichealthinnovators/

Adapted from Centers for Disease Control and Prevention. (2021). Promoting health for adults. National Center for Chronic Disease Prevention and Health Promotion (NCCDPHP). https://www.cdc.gov/chronicdisease/resources/publications/factsheets/promoting-health-for-adults.htm.

events that help motivate participants throughout their life cycle (YMCA of the USA, 2021). Some commercial health insurance companies may cover gym membership fees or may have prenegotiated discount rates for their enrollees. Health care professionals who are more skilled at navigating the complexity of private health insurance coverage should assist their clients in receiving these benefits (Blue Cross Blue Shield Association, 2021).

The CDC describes many types of programming that can promote physical health for adults. Table 5-7 describes several of those programs and resources.

1. Identify three community-sponsored physical events that Angie can train and participate in over the next 6 months. How would you encourage her to get involved?
2. Consider your own health insurance. If that was the same as Angie's, would it provide gym membership reimbursement? If not, what is the cost of your local gym membership, YMCA or similar community center that your clients can become active with?
3. What barriers can you perceive Angie will have in YOUR community with participation in physical activity events?

Interprofessional Collaboration to Promote Physical Health for Adults

The current model of health care in the United States lacks coordination among professionals and their common clients resulting in overutilization of resources and administering unnecessary or misapplying care (Donaldson et al., 2000). Health care delivery is reactive in nature in the sense that interventions occur after an illness or an injury is already present, rather than as a preventive measure. Once a health issue arises, patients and health care professionals find navigating through the maze of regulations and processes confusing and a waste of resources (Wolfe, 2001). Physicians will normally recommend increasing physical activity as part of a treatment plan after a diagnosis of cardiac condition, stroke, or after performing a joint replacement surgery but rarely is physical health promoted as critical to well-being during routine annual physicals or when treating patients for common conditions. The 2010 passage of the Patient Protection and Affordable Care Act was an attempt to first and foremost "increase the number of people with health insurance by expanding government programs and subsidizing private insurance premiums" (Atlas, 2017, para. 1). The proposition was that lack of health insurance coverage was a barrier to accessing health care, especially for low income, underinsured, and uninsured individuals. A second major goal was to improve quality of care by expanding prevention services of individuals with the purpose of improving population health. Unfortunately, achieving part of the first goal, providing health insurance to the uninsured, did not improve population health or impact prevention services since the focus remained on interventions after an episode of illness, which has been the current model used for several decades. Health professions did not expand on the opportunity to educate their patients on prevention care, such as exercise, nutrition, sleep, and related behaviors of health as the access to health care professionals increased with fewer uninsured in the population. This was not necessarily the fault of health care providers individually but may reflect the current system of heath delivery. While most physicians self-report to practicing population health along with primary care, few of them acknowledge the ability to integrate their activities within their practice or system (Jamison et al., 2021). The Interprofessional Education Collaborative (2016) recommend four core competencies to help professionals maximize integration of services:

1. Values/Ethics for Interprofessional Practice—Work with individuals of other professions to maintain a climate of mutual respect and shared values.
2. Roles/Responsibilities—Use the knowledge of one's own role and those of other professions to appropriately assess and address the health care needs of patients and to promote and advance the health of populations.
3. Interprofessional Communication—Communicate with patients, families, communities, and professionals in health and other fields in a responsive and responsible manner that supports a team approach to the promotion and maintenance of health and the prevention and treatment of disease.
4. Teams and Teamwork—Apply relationship-building values and the principles of team dynamics to perform effectively in different team roles to plan, deliver, and evaluate patient/care and population health programs and policies that are safe, timely, efficient, effective, and equitable.

Health care students and professionals can self-administer the Interprofessional Professionalism Assessment Instrument (Frost et al., 2019) to evaluate their personal level of demonstrating interprofessionalism behaviors when working within a team. Once personal weaknesses are examined, resources from professional organizations and the Interprofessional Education Collaborative can be used to improve behaviors and expand a personal knowledge base. Improving one's own behaviors can begin the journey toward improving interprofessional collaboration that would hopefully translate to better community and population physical health.

Knowing that health care is currently focused on treating those that are already impaired, and professionals lack the opportunity to coordinate care should encourage emerging health care students and professionals to begin a shift toward interprofessionalism and prevention of physical health deterioration in their clients. Using the concepts outlined in this chapter, such as focusing on health behaviors of increasing activities, exercise, and nutrition simultaneously with decreasing negative behaviors such as being sedentary, overeating, and poor sleep can begin the shift toward preventive care and population health. Recognizing that each professional is an expert in their discipline should encourage collaboration with a team of resources in the community. This team approach of utilizing community resources, beyond simply making a referral, would help the individual and would also begin a broader community and population level health care improvement.

Conclusion

The promotion of physical health is an opportunity for health care professionals to optimize an individual, a community, and a population's well-being. As the focus in health care changes to prevention and health promotion, interprofessional teams of health professionals can decrease potential physical impairments and hospitalizations, and increase abilities needed to sustain daily living. Increasing basic everyday activity levels, such as walking or re-engaging people or communities in favored daily physical activities, can be a first step toward personal physical health improvement. Utilizing resources highlighted in this chapter that provide parameters for physical health intervention and guidance can assist any health care professional in directing a client, community, or population toward removing barriers and maximizing the benefits of physical health.

References

American Occupational Therapy Association. (2020). Occupational therapy practice framework: Domain and Process—Fourth Edition. *American Journal of Occupational Therapy, 74*(2), 7412410010p1-7412410010p87. https://doi.org/10.5014/ajot.2020.74S2001

Atlas, S. W. (2017). *The path to affordable health care.* Hoover Institution. https://www.hoover.org/research/path-affordable-health-care

Barbour K. E., Stevens, J. A., Helmick, C.G., Luo, Y. H., Murphy, L. B., Hootman, J. M., Theis, K. A., Anderson, L. A., Baker, N. A., & Sugerman, D. E. (2012). Falls and fall injuries among adults with arthritis—United States. *Morbidity and Mortality Weekly Report, 63*(17), 379-383.

Blue Cross Blue Shield Association. (2021). Fitness your way discounts. https://www.fepblue.org/manage-your-health/incentives-discounts/gym-discounts

Boyko, Y., Ørding, H., & Jennum, P. (2012). Sleep disturbances in critically ill patients in ICU: how much do we know? *Acta anaesthesiologica scandinavica, 56*(8), 950-958.

Centers for Disease Control and Prevention. (2016). Tips for sleep hygiene. Sleep and Sleep Disorders. https://www.cdc.gov/sleep/about_sleep/sleep_hygiene.html

Centers for Disease Control and Prevention. (2019). Lack of physical activity. National Center for Chronic Disease Prevention and Health Promotion (NCCDPHP). https://www.cdc.gov/chronicdisease/resources/publications/factsheets/physical-activity.htm

Centers for Disease Control and Prevention. (2020a). Disability and health related conditions. Disability and Health Promotion. https://www.cdc.gov/ncbddd/disabilityandhealth/relatedconditions.html

Centers for Disease Control and Prevention. (2020b). *Prevent Heart Disease.* Centers for Disease Control and Prevention. https://www.cdc.gov/heartdisease/prevention.htm#print

Centers for Disease Control and Prevention. (2021). Promoting health for adults. National Center for Chronic Disease Prevention and Health Promotion (NCCDPHP). https://www.cdc.gov/chronicdisease/resources/publications/factsheets/promoting-health-for-adults.htm

da Costa, B. R., & Vieira, E. R. (2008). Stretching to reduce work-related musculoskeletal disorders: a systematic review. *Journal of Rehabilitation Medicine, 40*(5), 321-328.

Della Corte, K. W., Perrar, I., Penczynski, K. J., Schwingshackl, L., Herder, C., & Buyken, A. E. (2018). Effect of dietary sugar intake on biomarkers of subclinical inflammation: A systematic review and meta-analysis of intervention studies. *Nutrients, 10*(5), 606.

DiClemente, C. C. & Prochaska, J. O. (1982). Self-change and therapy change of smoking behavior: A comparison of processes of change in cessation and maintenance. *Addictive Behaviors, 7*(2), 133-142. https://doi.org/10.1016/0306-4603(82)90038-7

Donaldson, M. S., Corrigan, J. M., & Kohn, L. T. (Eds.). (2000). *To err is human: Building a safer health system.*

Ferrari, S., Manni, T., Bonetti, F., Villafañe, J. H., & Vanti, C. (2015). A literature review of clinical tests for lumbar instability in low back pain: Validity and applicability in clinical practice. *Chiropractic & Manual Therapies, 23*(1), 1-12.

Foster, C., Porcari, J. P., Anderson, J., Paulson, M., Smaczny, D., Webber, H., ... & Udermann, B. (2008). The talk test as a marker of exercise training intensity. *Journal of Cardiopulmonary Rehabilitation and Prevention, 28*(1), 24-30.

Frey, L., Szalda-Petree, A., Traci, M., & Seekins, T. (2001) Prevention of secondary health conditions in adults with developmental disabilities: A review of the literature. *Disability and Rehabilitation, 23*(9), 361-369. https://doi.org/10.1080/096380010006674

Frost, J. S., Hammer, D. P., Nunez, L. M., Adams, J. L., Chesluk, B., Grus, C., ... & Bentley, J. P. (2019). The intersection of professionalism and interprofessional care: Development and initial testing of the Interprofessional Professionalism Assessment (IPA). *Journal of Interprofessional Care*, 33(1), 102-115.

Garber, C. E., Blissmer, B., Deschenes, M. R., Franklin, B. A., Lamonte, M. J., Lee, I. M., ... & Swain, D. P. (2011). Quantity and quality of exercise for developing and maintaining cardiorespiratory, musculoskeletal, and neuromotor fitness in apparently healthy adults: guidance for prescribing exercise.

Haines, H., Wilson, J. R., Vink, P., & Koningsveld, E. (2002). Validating a framework for participatory ergonomics (the PEF). *Ergonomics, 45*(4), 309-327.

Haskell, W. L., Lee, I. M., Pate, R. R., Powell, K. E., Blair, S. N., Franklin, B. A., ... & Bauman, A. (2007). Physical activity and public health: updated recommendation for adults from the American College of Sports Medicine and the American Heart Association. *Circulation, 116*(9), 1081.

Hough J. (1999). Disability and health: A national public health agenda. In R. J. Simeonsson & D. B. Bailey (Eds.), *Issues in disability and health: The role of secondary conditions and quality of life* (pp. 161-203). North Carolina Office on Disability and Health.

Interprofessional Education Collaborative. (2016). Core competencies for interprofessional collaborative practice: 2016 update. Interprofessional Education Collaborative. https://hsc.unm.edu/ipe/resources/ipec-2016-core-competencies.pdf

Isehunwa, O. O., Carlton, E. L., Wang, Y., Jiang, Y., Kedia, S., Chang, C. F., Fijabi, D., & Bhuyan, S. S. (2017). Access to Employee wellness programs and use of preventive care services among U.S. adults. *American Journal of Preventive Medicine, 53*(6), 854-865. https://doi.org/10.1016/j.amepre.2017.08.001

Islam, M., Alam, F., Solayman, M., Khalil, M., Kamal, M. A., & Gan, S. H. (2016). *Dietary phytochemicals: Natural swords combating inflammation and oxidation-mediated degenerative diseases.* Oxidative Medicine and Cellular Longevity.

Jamison, S. D., Higginbotham, L. B., Chambard, M. L., White, D. P., Porterfield, D. S., & Flower, K. B. (2021). Preventive medicine physicians' role in health care organizations' pursuit of the triple aim. *Journal of Public Health Management and Practice, 27*(1), S133-S138.

Jüni, P. (2016). *Alternative treatment options for osteoarthritis: Facts and evidence on glucosamines and chondroitin.* International Association for the Study of Pain.

Keadle, S. K., Bustamante, E. E., & Buman, M. P. (2021). Physical activity and public health: Four decades of progress. *Kinesiology Review, 10*(3), 319-330.

Kleis, R. R., Hoch, M. C., Hogg-Graham, R., & Hoch, J. M. (2021). The effectiveness of the Transtheoretical Model to improve physical activity in healthy adults: A systematic review. *Journal of Physical Activity & Health, 18*(1), 94-108. https://doi.org/10.1123/jpah.2020-0334

Krist, A. H., Shenson, D., Woolf, S. H., Bradley, C., Liaw, W. R., Rothemich, S. F., Slonim, A., Benson, W., & Anderson, L. A. (2013). Clinical and community delivery systems for preventive care: An integration framework. *American Journal of Preventive Medicine, 45*(4), 508-516. https://doi.org/10.1016/j.amepre.2013.06.008

Kuo F., Pizzi M., Chang W., Fredrick, A., & Koning, L. (2016b). An exploratory study on the clinical utility of the Pizzi Healthy Weight Management Assessment (PHWMA) among Burmese high school students. *American Journal of Occupational Therapy, 70*, 7005180040p1-7005180040p9. https://doi.org/10.5014/ajot.2016.021659, 2016

Lawlor, E. R., Bradley, D. T., Cupples, M. E., & Tully, M. A. (2018). The effect of community-based interventions for cardiovascular disease secondary prevention on behavioural risk factors. *Preventive Medicine, 114*, 24-38. https://doi-org.ezproxy.lib.usf.edu/10.1016/j.ypmed.2018.05.019

Lena, M. B., Kuper, H., & Polack, S. (2017). Poverty and disability in low- and middle-income countries: A systematic review. *PLoS One, 12*(12). http://dx.doi.org/10.1371/journal.pone.0189996

Levine, S., Malone, E., Lekiachvili, A., & Briss, P. (2019). Health care industry insights: why the use of preventive services is still low. *Preventing chronic disease, 16*.

López-Alarcón, M., Perichart-Perera, O., Flores-Huerta, S., Inda-Icaza, P., Rodríguez-Cruz, M., Armenta-Álvarez, A., ... & Mayorga-Ochoa, M. (2014). Excessive refined carbohydrates and scarce micronutrients intakes increase inflammatory mediators and insulin resistance in prepubertal and pubertal obese children independently of obesity. Mediators of Inflammation.

Manning, T. (2015). Community health centers in low-income areas. *Communities & Banking*, 29.

Marmot, M. G., & Bell, R. (2009). Action on health disparities in the United States: Commission on social determinants of health. *Journal of the American Medical Association, 301*(11), 1169-1171.

McAlindon, T. E., LaValley, M. P., Gulin, J. P., & Felson, D. T. (2000). Glucosamine and chondroitin for treatment of osteoarthritis: a systematic quality assessment and meta-analysis. *Journal of the American Medical Association, 283*(11), 1469-1475.

McKinlay, J. B. (1979). A case for refocusing upstream: The political economy of illness. Patients, Physicians and Illness: A Sourcebook in Behavioral Science and Health (pp. 9-25).

Nayak, S. K., Jena, S., Sahu, P. K., Tiwari, P., & Chaudhury, H. C. (2021). Nutraceuticals as supplements in the management of arthritis: A review. *International Journal of Pharmaceutical Research, 13*(1).

Ohrnberger, J., Fichera, E., & Sutton, M. (2017). The relationship between physical and mental health: A mediation analysis. *Social Science & Medicine, 195*, 42-49. https://doi.org/10.1016/j.socscimed.2017.11.008

Pacheco, D., & Rehman, A. (2021, September 15). Using marijuana as a sleep aid. Sleep Foundation. https://www.sleepfoundation.org/natural-sleep-aids/marijuana-for-sleep

Parker, J., & Guest, D. L. (1999). *The clinician's guide to 12-step programs: How, when, and why to refer a client*. Taylor & Francis.

Pizzi, M. (2010). Health promotion for people with disabilities. In M. E. Scaffa, S. M. Reitz, & M. A. Pizzi (Eds.), *Occupational therapy in the promotion of health and wellness* (pp. 376-396). F.A. Davis.

Pizzi, M. (2016). *Pizzi Healthy Weight Management Assessment* [PHWMA]. Unpublished assessment.

Reitz, S. M., Scaffa, M. E., Campbell, R. M., & Rhynders, P. A. (2010). Health behavior frameworks for health promotion practice. In M. E. Scaffa, S. M. Reitz, & M. A. Pizzi (Eds.), *Occupational therapy in the promotion of health and wellness* (pp. 46-69). F.A. Davis.

Rizzoli, R., Bianchi, M. L., Garabédian, M., McKay, H. A., & Moreno, L. A. (2010). Maximizing bone mineral mass gain during growth for the prevention of fractures in the adolescents and the elderly. *Bone, 46*(2), 294-305.

Rosenstock, I. M. (1974). Historical origins of the Health Belief Model. *Health Education Monographs, 2*(4), 328-335. https://doi.org/10.1177/109019817400200403

Shiels, M. S., Chernyavskiy, P., Anderson, W. F., Best, A. F., & Haozous, E. A. (2017). Diverging trends in premature mortality in the US by sex, race, and ethnicity in the 21st century. *Lancet, 389*(10073), 1043-1054.

Shoen, S. (2021, September 10, a). Night owls experienced more sleep problems than other chronotypes during pandemic. Sleep Foundation. https://www.sleepfoundation.org/

Shoen, S. (2021, September 10, b). Sleep benefits of tart cherry juice. Sleep Foundation. https://www.sleepfoundation.org/nutrition/tart-cherry-juice

Short, S. E., & Mollborn, S. (2015). Social determinants and health behaviors: Conceptual frames and empirical advances. *Current Opinions in Psychology, 5*, 78-84. https://doi.org/10.1016/j.copsyc.2015.05.002

Smallfield, S., Fang, L., & Kyler, D. (2021). Self-management interventions to improve activities of daily living and rest and sleep for adults with chronic conditions: A systematic review. *American Journal of Occupational Therapy, 75*(4).

Suni, E., & Truong, K. (2020, November 6). Nutrition and sleep. Sleep Foundation. https://www.sleepfoundation.org/nutrition

The Healthline Editorial Team. (2018, August 20). Diabetes complications. Type 2 Diabetes. https://www.healthline.com/health/diabetes-complications

Theis, K. A., Roblin, D. W., Helmick, C. G., & Luo, R. (2018). Prevalence and causes of work disability among working-age US adults, 2011–2013, NHIS. *Disability and Health Journal, 11*(1), 108-115.

Uehli, K., Mehta, A. J., Miedinger, D., Hug, K., Schindler, C., Holsboer-Trachsler, E., ... & Künzli, N. (2014). Sleep problems and work injuries: A systematic review and meta-analysis. *Sleep Medicine Reviews, 18*(1), 61-73.

Umberson, D., Crosnoe, R., & Reczek, C. (2010a). Social relationships and health behavior across the life course. *Annual Review of Sociology, 36*, 139-157.

Umberson, D., & Montez, J. K. (2010b). Social relationships and health: A flashpoint for health policy. *Journal of Health and Social Behavior, 51*(Suppl), S54-S66. https://doi.org/10.1177/0022146510383501

U.S. Department of Health and Human Services. (n.d.). Alcohol's effects on the body. National Institute on Alcohol Abuse and Alcoholism. https://www.niaaa.nih.gov/alcohols-effects-health/alcohols-effects-body

U.S. Department of Health and Human Services. (2018). Physical activity guidelines for Americans (2nd ed.).https://health.gov/sites/default/files/2019-09/Physical_Activity_Guidelines_2nd_edition.pdf

U.S. Department of Health and Human Services. (2020a). Healthy People 2030. Office of Disease Prevention and Health Promotion. https://health.gov/healthypeople

U.S. Department of Health and Human Services, (2020b). Social determinates of health. Office of Disease Prevention and Health Promotion. https://health.gov/healthypeople/objectives-and-data/social-determinants-health

U.S. Department of Health and Human Services. (2021, March 29). Office of dietary supplements - dietary supplements for exercise and athletic performance. NIH Office of Dietary Supplements. https://ods.od.nih.gov/factsheets/ExerciseAndAthleticPerformance-HealthProfessional/

van Heijster, H., Boot, C. R., Robroek, S. J., Hengel, K. O., van Berkel, J., de Vet, E., & Coenen, P. (2021). The effectiveness of workplace health promotion programs on self-perceived health of employees with a low socioeconomic position: An individual participant data meta-analysis. SSM-Population Health, 100743.

Vgontzas, A. N., Liao, D., Pejovic, S., Calhoun, S., Karataraki, M., Basta, M., ... & Bixler, E. O. (2010). Insomnia with short sleep duration and mortality: The Penn State cohort. *Sleep, 33*(9), 1159-1164.

Ware, J. E., & Sherbourne, C. D. (1992). The MOS 36-item Short-Form Health Survey (SF-36): I. Conceptual framework and item selection. *Medical Care, 30*, 473-483.

Whitfield, G. P., Carlson, S. A., Ussery, E. N., Fulton, J. E., Galuska, D. A., & Petersen, R. (2019). Trends in meeting physical activity guidelines among urban and rural dwelling adults—United States, 2008–2017. *Morbidity and Mortality Weekly Report, 68*(23), 513.

Wilder, R. P., & Sethi, S. (2004). Overuse injuries: Tendinopathies, stress fractures, compartment syndrome, and shin splints. *Clinics in Sports Medicine, 23*(1), 55-81.

Williams, M. R., & Do, D. P. (2021). The compounded burden of poverty on mental health for people with disabilities. *Social Work in Public Health, 36*(4), 419-431.

Wolfe, A. (2001). Institute of Medicine report: crossing the quality chasm: a new health care system for the 21st century. *Policy, Politics, & Nursing Practice, 2*(3), 233-235.

World Health Organization. (1986). Ottawa Charter for Health Promotion. https://www.euro.who.int/__data/assets/pdf_file/0004/129532/Ottawa_Charter.pdf

World Health Organization. (2018a). Alcohol. World Health Organization. https://www.who.int/en/news-room/fact-sheets/detail/alcohol

World Health Organization. (2018b). More active people for a healthier world. Global action plan on physical activity 2018-2030. https://apps.who.int/iris/bitstream/handle/10665/272722/9789241514187-eng.pdf?sequence=1&isAllowed=y

World Health Organization. (2021a). Physical activity. https://www.who.int/health-topics/physical-activity#tab=tab_1

World Health Organization. (2021b). Obesity and overweight. https://www.who.int/news-room/fact-sheets/detail/obesity-and-overweight, License: CC BY-NC-SA 3.0 IGO.

World Health Organization. (2021c). Constitution. https://www.who.int/about/governance/constitution

World Health Organization. (2022). *Physical Activity*. World Health Organization; World Health Organization. https://www.who.int/news-room/fact-sheets/detail/physical-activity

Ye, L., Hutton Johnson, S., Keane, K., Manasia, M., & Gregas, M. (2015). Napping in college students and its relationship with nighttime sleep. *Journal of American College Health, 63*(2), 88-97.

YMCA of the USA. (2021). Who we are. What We Do. https://www.ymca.org/what-we-do

Zajacova, A., & Lawrence, E. M. (2018). The relationship between education and health: reducing disparities through a contextual approach. *Annual Review of Public Health, 39*, 273-289.

6

CHAPTER

Promoting Physical Health

Older Adults

Pamela Bartlo, PT, DPT, CCS and Michele Karnes, EdD, OTR

Learning Objectives

At the end of this chapter, the reader will:

1. Describe age-related changes that can impact health and safety for older adults. (ACOTE St. B.1.1, B.1.3, B.3.6, B.4.1, B.4.2; CAPTE 7C)
2. Explain various assessments or tests that can be used to determine fitness level, safety for exercise, and methods to determine the appropriate activity parameters for that individual (ACOTE St. B.1.3, B.1.4, B.3.2, B.4.4, B.4.5, B.4.6, B.4.7, B.4.8, B.4.9; CAPTE 7D19a, 7D19d, 7D19f, 7D19i, and 7D19m)
3. Describe factors related to parameters for exercise or activity for the older adult and how to determine appropriate parameters for each person (ACOTE St. B.3.4, B.3.5, B.3.6, B.3.7, B.4.2, B.4.3, B.4.7, CAPTE 7D20 and 7D27i)
4. Describe relationships of rehab professionals and how they can all impact promotion of physical activity for the older adult (ACOTE St. B.4.21, B.4.22, B.4.23, B.4.24, B.4.25, B.4.26; CAPTE 7D 24, 7D28, 7D34, 7D37, and 7D39)
5. Apply information to case study for activity for an older adult

The ACOTE Standards used are those from 2018.

Key Words

Aerobic Exercise, Aging, Falls Prevention, Older Adult, Physical Activity, Pizzi Health and Wellness Assessment, Prevention, Resistance Exercise, Wellness

Pizzi, M. A., & Amir, M. (Eds.). *Interprofessional Perspectives for Community Practice: Promoting Health, Well-Being, and Quality of Life* (pp. 97-120).

Case Study

A 67-year-old adult comes to a wellness program inside a local community center. The wellness program incorporates physical therapy, occupational therapy, nutrition, and social work. The person is seeking out the wellness center to improve their overall health and activity. They would like to start exercising again as they are afraid to get less mobile as they get older, and they would like to stop some of their joint aches and pains. They would like to maintain their independence as they age and are looking to improve their diet too although they want to still eat "bad foods once in a while."

The person has a history of:

- Coronary artery disease with a heart attack 4 years ago (currently takes a beta blocker)
- High blood pressure (currently takes an ace inhibitor)
- High cholesterol (currently takes a statin)
- Gastric acid reflux disorder (currently takes a proton-pump inhibitor)
- Mild osteoarthritis in both knees (currently takes naproxen)
- Takes a multi-vitamin, Vitamin D, and fish oil, all daily

Your systems evaluation showed:

- Vital signs within acceptable limits
- Range of motion and strength somewhat limited, but mostly intact for age
- Balance with mild impairments but the person denies any falls in the past 6 months
- ADLs, gait, and other mobility are all independent, but some with slower motions and some mild impairments noted

Each health care professional will want to work with the person within their discipline as well as part of a team to establish the appropriate dietary recommendations, physical activity program, adjustments and modifications to ADLs, safety in their environment, and independence and quality of life (QOL) issues.

Reflective Questions

1. What are two of the most important factors to consider when developing an initial wellness program for a person?
2. How may the person's cultural background impact your recommendations for physical activity and wellness?
3. How will you determine which specialized tests would be most beneficial for use with the individual?
4. What factors should you take into account when prescribing exercise frequency, duration, and intensity for physical activity and how will you monitor the person's response to the activity?
5. What findings will you use to determine appropriate modifications or equipment needs for use during mobility and ADLs?

Introduction

People need to be physically active throughout their life span. All individuals are recommended to perform physical activity for at least 150 minutes per week at a moderate intensity level (U.S. Department of Health and Human Services [USDHHS], 2018a). According to this report, performance of 150 minutes or more of weekly physical activity has been shown to reduce or prevent a myriad of physical and medical conditions. For a variety of reasons, many adults, especially **older adults**, do not achieve the minimum amount of recommended **physical activity**. Some of the reasons for this lack of activity can be related to anatomical, physiological, and other system changes that occur as a person ages and that can impact function. Loss of flexibility and bone density can lead to balance deficits and a possible risk of falls (Centers for Disease Control and Prevention [CDC], 2020a, 2020b). Visual and vestibular changes may also lead to safety risks as individuals age (Ehrlich et al., 2019; Liston et al., 2014; Pothula et al., 2004; Sousa et al., 2011). Physical activity can positively impact older adults, even into older adulthood (Mora & Valencia, 2018). Aerobic activity, resistance movements, flexibility and stretching, and balance training can help to maintain function and safety as a person ages. The American College of Cardiology (ACC) and the American Heart Association (AHA) found that physical activity can help protect against some health conditions including cognitive decline and mental health (Arnett et al., 2019). AOTA (2020c) also strongly promotes engagement in activities or occupations that enable individuals "to maximize their capacity to participate in life activities that are important and meaningful to them, to promote overall health and wellness" (para. 1), discovering the appropriate activity is essential. Therefore, maintaining or improving physical health is an important part of overall wellness and well-being.

Performing at least the minimum amount of recommended weekly physical activity can help prevent complications from hypertension, diabetes, cardiovascular disease, some forms of cancer, renal disease, and other conditions (Chodzko-Zajko et al., 2009; Powell et al., 2018). There is no particular mode of activity that is significantly more beneficial than any other. Therefore, it is more important to encourage any physical activity a person will consistently engage in instead of requiring a specific activity that the person may not like and will only perform once or twice. For example, activities could include walking, biking, tai chi, or gardening. Talking with the person about their likes and dislikes, motivations, and limitations will help the health professional work with the person in selecting the best physical activity(ies) for them. Health professionals need to assess the person's physical abilities and possibly their baseline fitness level and capabilities to make appropriate activity recommendations. The use of standardized outcome measures may assist with this. These will be discussed more later in this chapter.

Health professionals should assist the person with developing activity parameters to initiate a physical activity program and then safely advance the person's fitness or physical ability levels. Occupational therapists, as part of the health team, can conduct an analysis of occupational performance (AOTA, 2020a). This would entail not only assessing the physical capabilities of the older adult, but the environment and social connections associated with the physical activity. Determining the barriers to engagement in physical activity is an essential step in promoting engagement and follow-through until a health-promoting routine is developed.

It is also important for health professionals to help people find appropriate community programs or opportunities that will help them to engage in exercise or physical activities outside of a rehabilitation setting. This may help to engage the older adult in social connections, which are essential to promoting health, well-being, and QOL. These types of programs may help the older adult in adopting long-term lifestyle behavioral changes. The ultimate goal is for the health professional to work with the individual to establish a lifestyle of physical activity and engagement that will help them manage the **aging** process and maintain functional safety and independence into older adulthood.

This chapter will examine the assessment of physical capacity and functioning for older adults and the measures the health professional can utilize in their assessment. The focus will then shift to intervention parameters with attention paid to several aspects of promoting physical health. These will include movement and exercise, as well as a discussion of nutrition and psychosocial aspects on a smaller scale. Particular attention will be paid to the role of multiple health professionals and the benefits of interdisciplinary involvement. Lastly, the chapter will explore community programs and technology to assist with promoting physical health for the older adult. Specific programs will be mentioned, as well as some thoughts on components to include in new programs. Additionally, strategies for facilitating behavior change will be included as this should be part of building long-term, health-promoting actions that an older adult can engage in.

Gauging Intention for Action

When considering evaluating a person's ability for engaging in exercise or a physical activity that would benefit their health, wellness, and perhaps QOL, it is important to understand where the person is in terms of their interest in engaging in these activities. There are many theories and health models that help the health professionals understand this aspect. A few theories or models are presented in this section, along with examples of how they have been used in practice to promote health and wellness.

Health Belief Model

The Health Belief Model has been used in many individual, group, and even community health improvement programs. Janz and Becker (1984) describe the model as a framework for community-based practice and wellness promotion. They explain that using this model, the person examines their susceptibility or risk, as well as the severity of negative effects from disease, illness, or health conditions such as cardiovascular, respiratory, and other health aspects that will be covered in this chapter. The beliefs or perceived benefits of actions on these negative effects are also considered by the individual. Barriers that may prevent positive steps and facilitators that promote the positive actions are identified and weighed out. As the individual weighs out the perceived risk(s), benefits(s), barriers, and facilitators to the behavior change, they come to a decision as to whether they should change to the new healthier behavior. This can result in one large change or small changes that move toward the goal of full behavior change.

Transtheoretical Model of Health Behavior Change

In the model called *Transtheoretical Model of Health Behavior Change*, people go through health behavior change in stages (Prochaska & Velicer, 1997). The individual may begin at any point in the stages and hopefully move through the cycle of stages to arrive at an action toward health behavior change and then the maintenance period. Some people may begin at the **precontemplation** stage, where they have no thought that there may be a problem and have no intention to change behavior. The next phase, **contemplation**, finds the individual recognizing that there is an issue and realizing there needs to be an intervention of some sort. In the **preparation** stage, the individual is conducting the necessary tasks to begin changing behavior(s). For example buying loose-fitting clothing and sneakers to join a neighborhood walking group. When an individual engages in the actual activity, for example, meets the walking group on the appointed day and time, they enter the **action** stage. The next stage is the maintenance stage, where the person sustains the behavior for at least a period of several months. This could be a neighbor who routinely walks with the group. Unfortunately, there is another stage, that of **relapse**. This is either a temporary or permanent stop of the healthy behavior. Unfortunately, this may be a pattern for some individuals, for example, the occasional walker who quits the group entirely or will walk with the group occasionally.

Brief Motivational Interviewing

Motivational Interviewing (MI) is another suggested model that fits well within interprofessional practice, such as in the case of adopting health activity behaviors. According to Connors et al. (2019), MI can be used as "a directive, client-centered counseling style for eliciting behavior change by helping clients explore and resolve ambivalence" (para. 4). Through the use of short periods of MI, health professionals can explore the goals, roadblocks, and successes of physical activity recommendations that are based on the older adults' thought process, perceptions, and values regarding their health, wellness, and overall QOL. It is suggested that further investigation into the MI technique be conducted so as to use the model for effective behavior change and/or adoption.

There are many theories and models that health professionals may utilize when helping their older adult clients to engage in more physical activity or when developing health and wellness groups. The important takeaway, however, is to determine where the older adult is in recognizing the need for physical activity, helping them to choose activities or exercises they are interested in and enjoy, assessing their abilities and need for modification or adaptation, and to help them make a connection to the available activity of choice.

How to Gauge the Person's Readiness to Change

There are many screening tools that can be used to specifically measure a person's willingness to modify behavior. However, one the easiest and effective ways to do this, is to ask the person. Simply ask them if they've thought about changing the specific behavior (i.e., losing weight, starting to be more active, stopping smoking). The health professional can ask the person about any barriers they perceive to changing behavior and can help problem-solve ways to mitigate or eliminate those barriers. The health professional can then assist the person in developing their plan to change their behavior and be guided by one of the models noted above to provide structure and a foundation for intervention.

Assessment

Assessment of Health, Well-Being, and Activity Participation

It is important for the health professional to assess the general health and wellness of a person. This can include assessment of health status, activity performance, QOL, and overall wellness. The most basic, yet comprehensive assessment tool may be the Short Form 36 Health Survey (SF-36). This quick form assesses the person's perceptions of their health over a broad spectrum of categories. It has been shown to be effective when self-completed and when assisted by a health professional (Bito & Fukuhara, 1998).

Another reliable and valid assessment of one's perceived health and well-being is the Pizzi Health and Wellness Assessment (PHWA; Pizzi, 2001, in press; Serwe et al., 2019). The PHWA can be a self-assessment or administered by a health professional, whereby the client assesses one's own perceived level of health in six areas, then answers activity-based questions focused on each of those areas. The person also rates oneself in their readiness to change a health behavior for the better, and their interest level in changing that health behavior. The assessment has been used with all adult populations, as well as health professional students, and has been shown to have long lasting impact in helping one make necessary and sustained health behavior changes

The Wellness Evaluation of Lifestyle (WEL; Myers et al., 2000) looks at wellness across five areas of a person's life and includes psychosocial, as well as physical, domains. The Interest Checklist UK (Klyczek et al., 1997) assesses someone's interest in and ability to perform basic leisure activities, as well as some forms of exercise. The Physical Activity Scale for the Elderly (PASE; Washburn et al., 1993) is quick and asks the person how often they performed certain activities over the previous 7 days and how long each activity was performed. The scale includes both active and sedentary activities. There are many other tools to consider, and each health professional should assess the tools to find the best fit for their area of practice and the clients they work with. The tools above and a few others used to assess wellness and health can be found in Table 6-1.

Changes With Aging

As people age, there are often physical system changes that occur. People typically experience muscle, bone, and physiology changes due to the aging process. Without specific exercise or physical activity to combat these processes, muscle mass, strength, and endurance may decrease as one ages, which can result in reduced health and abilities to conduct daily activities (Charlier et al., 2016). Health professionals need to understand the natural changes with aging.

Table 6-1

Standardized Tools to Assess Wellness, Physical Activity, or Overall Health

WELLNESS TOOL	AREAS ASSESSED	CLINICAL IMPLICATIONS
Short Form 36 Health Survey-36 (SF-36; Ware & Sherbourne, 1992)	36 items related to health and overall body function. Self-reported scale.	Gives person's perception of their health in physical, emotional, and social domains, as well as pain and mental health, bodily pain, general and mental health.
Wellness Evaluation of Lifestyle (Meyers et al., 2000)	Five life tasks assessed: Spirituality, Self-Direction, Work and Leisure, Friendship, and Love.	Measurement of score in each section, but person also reflects on if they are content with that area.
Interest Checklist UK (Klyczek et al., 1997)	Person marks activities that interest them off a large checklist of sedentary and active items. The person also reports current participation and desire to participate in the activity in the future.	Can be used to examine what physical level the person is currently at, what they'd like to do, and whether they will need interventions to be able to perform that task in the future.
Physical Activity Scale for the Elderly (PASE; Washburn et al., 1993)	Self-reported physical activity over the previous 7 days.	Gives a clear picture of what the sedentary and physical activities in both frequency of days performed and duration performed on those days.
Pizzi Health and Wellness Assessment (PHWA; Pizzi, 2001)	Self-assessment of health in eight areas that may affect the person.	Used to communicate with person about health issues that may impact function and develop health promoting interventions as appropriate for those health issues.
International Physical Activity Questionnaire-S (IPAQ; Craig et al., 2003)	Self-reported levels of physical activity focusing on intensity of activity.	More geared toward physical activity or exercise, so used most often for exercise prescription or to modify activity intensity.
IPAQ-L (Craig et al., 2003)	Self-reported levels of physical activity focusing on leisure activity, home activities, and work tasks.	Geared toward leisure activities and daily tasks. Gives a more well-rounded view of physical activity when combined with IPAQ-S.

However, they also need to be able to assess what level of physical capacity a person may have, what their physical limitations or impairments may be, and the impact of body systems on their abilities. The physical activity program should be designed for overall health and **wellness** and **prevention** of further medical or physical impairments as the person ages. Traditional exercise programs may work for some older adults, but more likely, general activity that is meaningful to the individual will create long-term adherence.

Muscular Changes With Aging

Muscle changes can occur in all peripheral muscles as an individual ages. Muscle mass decreases naturally as people age. Both with use and disuse, as adults age, there is an intrinsic decrease in muscle mass. The loss is typically greater in those with disuse, but the exact proportion has not been established. Loss of muscle mass and strength can be of great concern for large lower extremity muscles and core, spine, and postural muscles. Weakness in these muscle groups can lead to gait disorders and other functional limitations (LaRoche et al., 2011; Seidel et al., 2011). A change in muscle fiber type, through disuse or as a natural aging process, also impacts muscle weakness. Muscle unit loss also contributes to loss of strength (Doherty et al., 1993; Kaya et al., 2013; McKinnon, 2015; Roos et al., 1997). The combination of muscle fiber type loss, muscle unit loss, and then personal disuse can create a large functional impact for a person.

Muscle mass decreases also occur in the respiratory system (Janssens et al., 1999). Skeletal muscle change and other anatomical changes in the pulmonary system contribute to a decreased endurance as a person ages. Aerobic exercises, as well as resistance exercises peripherally, can improve respiratory endurance (American College of Sports Medicine [ACSM], 2017). Physical activity and exercise are recommended to maintain respiratory capacity even as respiratory muscle changes occur during natural aging. One study did show that the decline in pulmonary function due to aging was not significantly improved through exercise training (Roman et al., 2016). However, preliminary evidence has shown there may be mild benefits to respiratory function for those who danced for at least 20 minutes (Philip et al., 2020). Though some exercise may not be appropriate, specific low-intensity activities and occupations may be beneficial to not only respiratory status but overall QOL. Thus, it is important for the health professional to assess the person's pulmonary capacity through outcome measures and develop interventional strategies to maintain respiratory function and capacity as the person ages. The use of daily activities, leisure activities or hobbies, or the person's job can also be used to promote respiratory endurance. The more active the person is for longer durations, the more the pulmonary and cardiovascular systems will be maintained. The health professional can work with the person to identify ways to use the activity in which they are already participating to maintain endurance. As people age, overall pulmonary endurance decline can affect exercise intensity and duration, which is why it is important for older adults to stay physically active and thus lessen this decline.

How to Assess Impact of Musculoskeletal Changes

The health professional should utilize standardized tests and measures, which could include traditional manual muscle testing techniques, or it could involve functional movement tests. Assisting the person in the community would involve different tests than seeing a person in a rehabilitation clinic. So, the tests should be appropriate to the person and environment. See Table 6-1.

Case Reflection

The person in this chapter's case study may experience strength and endurance impairments due to the aging process, as well as their medical history. Describe how the medical conditions the person in the case study has, along with their age, will impact muscle strength and how you would address that in your scope of practice. How might you prevent disability through exploring strength and endurance issues, and how might you improve abilities and well-being?

Visual Changes With Aging

Visual changes are also common as people age, and these can lead to a variety of functional impairments in mobility, safety, self-care, and independence. Visual acuity, contrast sensitivity, depth perception, and visual field disturbances can impact function and even present hazards for the older adult. Based on findings from multiple studies, health professionals should screen for vision-related limitations as part of typical patient assessment and to promote safe, physical activity. Recommendations for safe ways to be physically active in various environments, with visually safe protocols may be appropriate intervention goals.

An occupational therapist can assess the home and the older adults' abilities to perform daily tasks in order to develop strategies for increasing safety and engagement in daily activities (AOTA, 2017). Several home assessments are available, such as the Rebuilding Together Safe AT HOME Checklist (2012; www.rebuildingtogether.org) and the Home Safety Self-Assessment Tool (HSSAT; Tomita et al., 2014).

How to Address Visual Changes

Major roles of health professionals are to assess and then help modify or adapt the environment, to better enable the individual to participate in their desired activities while enhancing safety. Teaching safe practices is also recommended. For example, increasing lighting and contrast or adding raised bump dots can aid the person in engaging in their desired activity (Berger, 2013). AOTA also suggests organizing items by color or size, using large print and adaptive equipment, or removing obstacles in the room may increase both safety and abilities. By evaluating the individual, the environment, and identifying those activities that are most important to the older adult, the therapist can help to provide avenues for participation and physical activity.

Vestibular Changes With Aging

Vestibular system changes are also common and can compound safety issues for someone as they age with or without visual impairments. With aging comes decreased sensitivity to spatial changes in part due to the vestibular system changes. The changes to the components of the central nervous system, as well as the responses sent through the central nervous system all decline with age. These vestibular changes contribute to the dizziness and imbalances frequently seen in people over the age of 60 years (Brosel & Strupp, 2019; Zalewski, 2015). Approximately 30% of people over the age of 60 years experience dizziness and imbalance (Brosel & Strupp, 2019). The dizziness symptoms contribute to fall risk and possible injury. Understanding vestibular system changes and possible interventions to help maintain function as much as possible will have safety and functional benefits. A thorough assessment of the vestibular system includes positional testing, visual system assessment, balance tests, and specific tests for impairments specific to the vestibular system. In-depth discussion of these assessments is beyond the scope of this text, but the health professional should refer the person to a rehab professional that specializes in vestibular assessment and intervention if it is not a skill they possess.

How to Address Vestibular Changes With Aging

Physical therapists can perform vestibular testing to ascertain the location of the vestibular involvement and thus determine appropriate intervention strategies. These could include exercises for problems with vestibulo-ocular reflexes, benign paroxysmal positional vertigo (BPPV), or semi-circular canal hypofunction. Occupational therapists can also help address vestibular impact on ADLs based on positioning and head movements during ADL performance.

According to Cohen et al. (2006), occupational therapists are well-equipped to assist those with vestibular disorders. Therapists are able to identify desired physical activities, analyze performance, and possibly identify actions that may trigger symptoms. The therapist and older adult can work to add graded activity, modify the environment, provide modifications, or identify adaptive devices that may promote engagement in the activity. Occupational therapists can instruct the individual of safe ways to carry out their activities should vestibular symptoms be present. Referral to an occupational therapist with vestibular rehabilitation expertise should be considered.

Risk of Fall

Fall risks also become important threats to health in older people. The health professional is integrally involved in **falls prevention** and should determine which strategies are most appropriate for the individual. There are standardized tests and measures for detecting specific fall risks, endurance, and overall fitness level that can be valuable in this population. Health professionals should be competent in performing assessments related to functional safety, balance, endurance, overall fitness, health, and well-being. These may include but are not limited to the Timed Up and Go Test (TUG), Five times sit to stand test (FTSTS), 30-second chair rise test, 2-minute step test, Short Physical Performance Battery (SPPB), Berg Balance test, 2 or 6-minute walk test, and other tests (Table 6-2). The Functional Reach Test may help the health professional understand whether the older adult loses their balance as they engage in a functional task that can help fall risk assessment (de Waroquier-Leroy et al., 2014). Fear of falling, reduction in abilities due to physical factors, and environmental factors may emerge as limitations for the older adult. These factors can negatively impact physical health and activity choices within the home in addition to decreased independent functioning.

Fear of falling is a recognized fall risk factor and there are several assessments to evaluate an individual's fear of falling. Fear of falling can also significantly reduce activity engagement and physical activity. Deshpande et al. (2014) found that activity restriction due to fear of falling was an independent predictor of a decline in older adults' physical function. Determining the fear of falling through self-report measures and objective fall risk through performance-based measures, will assist the health professional in recommending appropriate physical activities to maximize the person's physical abilities while minimizing their safety risks. An overall assessment that can also help detect limitations in daily activity is the Katz Index of Independence in Activities of Daily Living (Shelkey & Wallace, 2001). The health professional can use findings from specific components of the Katz Index to identify fall risk and need for intervention. The CDC has an available toolkit for health professionals who are interested in establishing or enhancing falls prevention efforts. The Stopping Elderly Accidents, Deaths, and Injuries, or STEADI Initiative (CDC, 2020c) provides free online information, tools, and training for health professionals that seeks to establish an interprofessional approach to fall prevention assessment and intervention. An algorithm provides a step-by-step fall risk screening, assessment, and intervention process. The toolkit can be accessed at https://www.cdc.gov/steadi/index.html.

How to Assess Fall Risk

All health professionals should assess the fall risk of a person related to that health disciplines' scope of practice. The team should work together to assess the greatest areas of risk for that person and determine a plan of care to improve the physical factors contributing to that risk, as well as the environmental, supports, and emotional factors.

Case Reflection

Although the person in the chapter case study denies any incidence of falls, it is important to fully assess their balance and risk of falling. They have common risk factors related to falls, which are taking multiple medications, various medical and orthopedic conditions, and increasing in age. The health professional should assess the impact of these factors on balance and fall risk, which translates to potential health, well-being, and QOL issues. Further training and patient education may be needed to prevent falls in the future (see Professional Reasoning Box A).

Flexibility Assessment

Health professionals should also assess musculoskeletal flexibility as a factor of balance and safety. Therefore, assessing risk factors for falls and health and wellness factors is an important role for therapy practitioners. SilverSneakers, a health and fitness program designed for adults 65+ that is included with many Medicare Plans, recommends a self-test for determining fitness. The self-assessment includes the

Table 6-2

Standard Outcome Measures for Physical Capacity or Endurance for the Older Adult

OUTCOME MEASURE	EQUIPMENT NEEDED	OUTCOME	CLINICAL IMPLICATIONS
Duke Activity Status Index (Hlatky et al., 1989)	None, person self-reports on paper or computer survey	Asks questions about functional status and physical activities.	Gives health professionals an overall assessment of the person's self-reported activity level and functional mobility.
2 Minute Walk Test (Bohannon et al., 2015) 6 Minute Walk Test (Sanderson & Bittner, 2006)	30-meter (100-foot) walkway, stopwatch, chair, stethoscope, and sphygmomanometer	Distance ambulated in 2 or 6 minutes and vital sign response to activity.	Can be equated to VO_2 max, comparison with age-appropriate norms.
Five Times Sit to Stand Test (Bohannon, 2006)	Standard height chair (16 inches off floor) and stopwatch	Time needed to perform sit to stand 5 times.	Measure of basic function and physical capacity and can correlate with fall risk.
30 Second Chair Stand Test (Jones et al., 1999)	Standard height chair (16 inches off floor) and stopwatch	Count the number of times the person can perform sit to stand in 30 seconds.	Measure of basic function and physical capacity and can correlate with fall risk.
Timed Up and Go (Podsiadlo & Richardson, 1991)	Standard height chair, 3-meter (10 foot) walkway, stopwatch	Time it takes a person to stand, ambulate 10 feet, turn around, ambulate back, and sit down.	Measures functional mobility and is a good predictor of fall risk.
Seated Step Test (Simonsick et al., 2008)	Standard height chair, step 12 inches, 16 inches, 18 inches, stopwatch, metronome, stethoscope and sphygmomanometer	Person alternates stepping each foot on the step, keeping time with the metronome for 2 minutes. At the end of each stage if vital signs haven't changed significantly, the step height is raised, and the test continues.	Measure of lower extremity function and endurance.
Short Physical Performance Battery (National Institute on Aging, 2017)	Standard height chair, 3-meter (10-foot) walkway, stopwatch	Person completes three physical tests. Each is scored and then a composite score is calculated too.	Assesses lower extremity function, fall risk, balance, and overall mobility and safety.
Two Minute Step Test (Pedrosa, 2009)	12-inch step and a stopwatch	Measure a height on the wall between the person's iliac crest and patella. Person lifts the lower extremity in a stepping motion until the top of the thigh is even with the mark. Count how many times the person can do this in 2 minutes.	Shows dynamic balance, lower extremity function, and is a good predictor of fall risk.
Modified Shuttle Test (Singh et al., 1992)	20-meter (66 feet) walkway and a metronome	Person ambulates from one end of the 20-meter course to the other in a specific time. Time increments get faster as the test progresses.	Can correlate to VO_2 max rates, measures physical capacity, and overall functional endurance.

VO_2 max = maximal oxygen uptake.

following: Sit to Stand, Arm Curl, Chair Sit and Reach, Back Scratch, Stand up and Go, and March in Place for a determined number of repetitions or time intervals (https://www.silversneakers.com/blog/fitness-test/; Fetters, 2017). Health professionals can also test the older adult on a number of these items as part of their overall assessment. It is commonly understood that as people age, they have decreased muscle and joint flexibility. However, attempts to maintain or improve flexibility can be beneficial in overall function, injury prevention, and physical abilities (Stathokostas et al., 2013). See the intervention section of this chapter for discussion regarding parameters of flexibility interventions.

Professional Reasoning Box A: Fall Risk

Falls are a very complex and costly problem that increases as a person ages. There has been much research into fall risk and fall prevention over the last decade. That makes it difficult for the health professional to keep up with all the latest evidence-based recommendations. The CDC provides a guideline booklet to assist health professionals and community groups to develop evidence-based programs that aim to prevent falls (National Center for Injury Prevention and Control, 2015). This booklet along with other health discipline–specific texts and articles can guide the health professional to the best evaluation and intervention strategies to use with people at risk for falls. Addressing this risk can make a far-reaching impact into the person's function, independence, and QOL.

A PDF file of the Guideline Booklet can be found on the CDC's website at https://www.cdc.gov/falls/programs/community_prevention.html#:~:text=This%20guide%20is%20designed%20to%20be%20a%20practical,prevention%20programs%20by%20providing%20examples%2C%20resources%2C%20and%20tips.

How to Assess Flexibility

Physical therapy, occupational therapy, nursing, and other disciplines can measure flexibility through some of the standardized tests mentioned above. Health professionals can also get a general assessment through observation of functional movement, such as during performance of ADLs or other desired and necessary activities. If the person has joint, muscle, or limb deficiencies, they can be more acutely assessed and formalized rehabilitation interventions can be determined. If the loss of motion is generalized due to older age, physical activity may be enough intervention to limit the impact of loss of flexibility. The health professional can advise the person on physical activity movements that will maintain motion through aging.

Mental Health Assessment

Another key element that can negatively influence physical health and wellness is depression. Depression and anxiety are quite common as a person ages, especially in those that are more socially isolated. There are several assessment scales that health professionals can utilize to screen for issues with depression or anxiety. See Table 6-3 for a few such scales available to health professionals. If a potential risk of depression or anxiety is found through the assessment tool, the health professional should reach out to the person's primary care provider and seek further assistance and intervention from the interprofessional team. The intervention section below discusses a few benefits to mental health through physical activity.

How to Assess Mental Health Impact

Health professionals should use the screening tools in Table 6-3. If further assessment is necessary, the health professional should refer the person to the primary care provider or other mental health provider.

Case Reflection

It would be important to screen the person for any depression or anxiety. Cardiovascular issues are closely associated with increased rates of depression and anxiety. The person in this case study also has chronic reflux and orthopedic issues. As the person tries to cope with chronic pain from the orthopedic issues, they may begin to feel effects of depression. They may also feel some symptoms related to anxiety surrounding the impact of reflux on diet choices, interactions with family and friends around meals, or other discomfort associated with the symptoms from their reflux. Screening for these complications will allow the health professional to assist the person in finding the appropriate resources to address the depression or anxiety. At that point, it would be appropriate for the health professional to refer the person to another doctor or specialist to address those needs while the health professional addresses the wellness needs within their scope of practice.

Intervention

Physical activity has been shown to be beneficial as people age (ACSM, 2017; Galloza et al., 2017; USDHHS, 2018b). Sadly, according to a USDHHS (2018a), only 27% of older adults met the recommended physical activity guidelines. As people age, activity becomes more physiologically taxing, joint aches occur more regularly, and other physical and orthopedic impairments develop that may impact parameters of activity engagement. Therefore, many adults begin to become more sedentary and fail to engage in physical activity. Physical activity recommendations exist to help prevent cardiovascular and other health conditions as people age (ACSM, 2017; Whelton et al., 2018). Increasing physical activity was shown to decrease risk for falls by 32% to 40% in older adults (USDHHS, 2018a). That included severe falls that would require hospitalization. Aerobic and resistance types of physical activity provide many benefits and

Table 6-3

Standardized Scales for Depression/Anxiety Screening

SCALE NAME	COMPONENTS OF SCALE	OUTCOME OF SCALE
Patient Health Questionnaire-9 (PHQ-9; Spitzer et al., 1999)	9 items assessing how person has felt about certain activities over past 2 weeks	Designed to measure symptoms of depression in primary care settings.
Beck Depression Inventory-II (BDI-II; Beck, 1996)	21 questions asking about specific feelings over past 2 weeks	Designed to measure the severity of depression. Especially when used over multiple weeks and months.
Psychological Risk Factor Survey (PRFS; Feltz & Eichenauer, 2001)	5 sections assessing anger/hostility, emotional guardedness, social isolation, anxiety, and depression	Designed for specific use with cardiovascular patients to screen for psychosocial factors that impact the cardiovascular risk for that person.
Hospital Anxiety and Depression Scale (HADS; Zigmond & Snaith, 1983)	14 questions asking hospital patients how they felt over 1 week	Designed to assess anxiety and depression symptoms in hospital patients. Goal is then to reduce the impact of physical illness on the total score.

complication prevention for people as they age (Chodzko-Zajko et al., 2009, Galloza et al., 2017). Prolonging life expectancy, eliminating or delaying impairments from chronic medical conditions, improvement in balance and safety, and QOL have all been shown to occur due to physical activity (ACSM, 2017; Galloza et al., 2017; Whelton et al., 2018).

Parameters of Physical Activity

Parameters of physical activity programs can vary, and specific intricacies are beyond the scope of this text. However, the health professional can assist with the implementation of physical activity for an older adult. First, the desired mode of activity should be discussed. It is important that this mode of activity doesn't exacerbate other orthopedic or medical problems the person may have. Physical activity should also be accessible, easy for the person to manage independently, and provide a safe avenue for exercise or activities based on that person's capabilities and risk.

Both aerobic and resistance activities should be a part of the person's exercise program. Aerobic activity should follow the minimum guidelines of 150 minutes of moderate-intensity exercise per week (USDHHS, 2018a). Resistance activities should be performed minimally 2 to 3 days per week (ACSM, 2017). The physical activity intensity should start at a level appropriate for that person as assessed through individualized tests and measures, and the health professional should recognize that this level can vary greatly between individuals. Age is not always an indicator of a person's fitness abilities, so exercise testing should guide the initial intensity prescription. When the older adult begins to perform aerobic activity, the initial goal should skew toward longer duration and lower intensity. This will allow the body to adapt to the new movements and reduce musculoskeletal injury, yet still provide activity gains that can be measured to continue and motivate participation. As the person progresses their physical activity, the health professional can increase the intensity and strive for greater aerobic and resistance intensities (ACSM, 2017). Specific activity modes should be selected by the health professional and the individual. However, the AHA (2018) gives some suggestions of moderately intense physical activities. These could include brisk walking, water aerobics, forms of dancing, working in the garden, tennis, and biking. The AHA also provides examples of vigorous-intensity aerobic activities, which include activities such as running, lap swimming, aerobic dance, cycling, and rope jumping. Specific exercises can be beneficial to the individual as well. Resistance activities should begin with around 8 to 10 repetitions of each movement for 1 to 2 sets (ACSM, 2017). The weight, number of repetitions, and number of sets can be modified and increased/decreased as appropriate based on the person's responses. Similar to intensity, the initial duration of activity can vary greatly and may be regardless of age. The ideal goal is for the individual to achieve at least 30 minutes of physical activity at a moderate intensity, thus allowing them to achieve the minimum weekly activity recommendations (Powell et al., 2018).

If orthopedic or other medical conditions prevent longer duration activity, a person can break that effort into smaller time segments. Interval training involving moderate-intensity activity mixed with rest or lower intensity activity may allow the person to maintain physical activity longer (Keating et al., 2020). Breaking up the activity duration into smaller segments spaced throughout the day can also be beneficial. Performing three sessions of 10-minute bouts of physical activity can be beneficial physiologically and may be easier for the person to complete due to compounding factors impacting activity duration (ACSM, 2017). At a minimum, physical activity should be performed 3 days per week. If the person is performing moderate intensity activity, it is recommended

Professional Reasoning Box B: Parameters of Physical Activity

So many factors go into the decisions regarding mode, intensity, duration, and frequency of physical activity prescription. For many years the ACSM has aggregated resources from a multitude of health professional disciplines to establish activity parameters (2017). The health professional completes their discipline-specific systems examination and discusses the person's desires and goals. Many of these health professionals struggle with where to start the actual activity prescription. They ask what if I make it too tough? What if the person hates it and doesn't want to continue? How hard should I tell them to work out? These are common questions that come up across health disciplines. The ACSM guidelines are a good place to start for the health professional. Taking into account medical conditions, orthopedic or functional limitations, and then referencing the guidelines in the latest ACSM manual, the health professional should be able to establish some good starting parameters. The health professional should then use vital signs, subjective, and other measurable responses to activity to modify the parameters to fit that individual's needs.

they try to perform that for 5 to 6 days per week (ACSM 2017). The more active the person is, the less intense that activity needs to be for physiologic gains. As previously stated, resistance activity should be performed at least 2 days per week and complement the overall activity goals of the individual. Incorporating group activity may be beneficial to increase support and camaraderie, thus increasing adherence to the physical activity program. Adherence rates may be as high as 70% with group activity due to social connectedness and other important factors (Farrance et al., 2016).

The health professional should work and consider the interest of the individual person to develop a plan for activity that can be performed with relative ease. Plans that are too complicated, involve too much equipment, or take too much time may be difficult to adhere to, so the person will just stop being active altogether. An occupational therapist, through the occupational therapy process, can gain information about the person's health, the environment they engage in, factors related to their ability to engage in the desired activity, and their perceived QOL and well-being. The PHWA (Pizzi, 2001) facilitates this process and should be explored as a useful tool in the evaluation process. As a self-assessment, the individual can determine their own health and wellness goals and the impediment to carrying out what is most valued. Another program, the Lifestyle Redesign Program process (Mandel et al., 1999) can also aid occupational therapy practitioners and older adults evaluate how their occupations or activities, and their habits and daily choices influence their overall health and well-being. This can be an early step in identifying healthy activities to promote physical activity. Physical therapists can utilize various activity and endurance tests and measures, along with discussion with the person to develop a thorough plan that will meet the physical activity guidelines and be enjoyable to the person. Using assessment results, the health team can work toward helping the individual remove barriers, adopt adaptations, and improve their ability to pursue the desired activities. The goal is to increase/maintain physical activity as the person ages, so it's important to help the person establish a plan that will work for them and to develop adaptive modifications periodically as they age or if other medical or physical changes occur.

How to Determine Physical Activity Parameters

Physical therapists and occupational therapists can utilize ACSM guidelines, knowledge of exercise physiology, vital signs at rest and with movement, and other standardized endurance tests to determine appropriate parameters for the person to use when they initiate physical activity. The parameters should then be modified based on the person's responses during activity.

Speech-language pathologists will perform standardized tests to determine greatest system impairments such as cognitive, motor planning, soft palate issues, and so on. Parameters for interventions will be based on those tests and re-evaluated and modified periodically based on the person's response. In the case of wellness and not rehabilitation settings, the speech-language pathologist will determine cognitive activities for the person to do to minimize cognitive decline and maintain higher level functioning.

Case Reflection

Since the person in the case study of this chapter is relatively young and with stable medical and orthopedic issues, the health care professional would want to attempt moderate physical activity with the person first. If it is tolerated, the person could work up to vigorous activity bouts worked into the moderate activity program. If the person's medical or orthopedic issues make moderate intensity activity difficult, then the health care professional should help establish a lighter intensity program that will still yield physical benefits (Professional Reasoning Box B).

Lighter Intensity Physical Activity

At times, a person may not have the ability or desire to perform moderate intensity activity as recommended. This could be due to physical limitations or other factors. Although not as beneficial, there is some evidence that light intensity activity still has some health benefits, especially for sedentary individuals (Füzéki et al., 2017). Typical household tasks may provide benefits to the individual. A 2019 study by Rees-Punia et al. indicated that engaging in light physical activities, such as walking the dog, folding laundry, and taking the stairs may have health benefits. Thus, it seems that any movement, when compared to being sedentary, can positively influence health and wellness. The health professional should work with the person to determine which intensity levels are most appropriate for that person and for the specific activity(ies) they are performing. An individual may be able to perform moderate intensity for one mode of activity and light intensity for another. Using subjective feelings and vital signs, when able, the person can increase or decrease their intensity between light and moderate and still achieve benefits of activity.

How to Determine Light Intensity Activity

Health professionals can encourage the person to partake in household and functional tasks intermittently throughout the day, most days of the week. The person should be instructed that they should be able to carry on a conversation during the activity. Use of subjective exertion scales may be appropriate if the person can understand them. However, the health professional can just discuss with the person the symptoms or feelings they have with different types, durations, and intensities of activities. The health professional could use the information from that discussion to guide the person on the type and parameters of activity that will be light intensity for them.

Physical Activity Influence on Chronic Conditions

Health professionals can play an important role in helping older adults to promote their physical health. Since exercise and physical activity have been shown to reduce and prevent complications from certain medical conditions, finding the appropriate activities and intensity levels are important (Arnett et al., 2019; Whelton et al., 2018). For example, hypertension (HTN) is a common medical condition found in 49.6% of adults as young as 20 years old, and most were taking HTN medications (Arnett et al., 2019). HTN is a major contributor to cardiovascular disease leading to heart attacks, strokes, and death, frequently due in part to HTN. **Aerobic exercise** can reduce the elevated systolic and diastolic blood pressures (ACSM, 2017; Fagard, 2001), thus, in turn, reduce the risk of cardiovascular related medical events. Encouraging physical activity in people with HTN is an effective and valuable strategy of overall health. Cardiovascular disease and related conditions can also be positively impacted through physical activity. Coronary artery disease, congestive heart failure, peripheral vascular disease (arterial and venous), and stroke have all been shown to be able to be positively impacted by physical activity (ACSM, 2017). Physical activity will improve circulation, the muscle's ability to utilize delivered nutrients and oxygen, removal of waste products, and many other positive physical changes. Another common societal medical condition is diabetes mellitus, which negatively affects most body systems. Physical activity for people with diabetes is integral in minimizing the disease's impact on some of these systems. Physical activity has been shown to improve blood glucose utilization in muscle, hepatic, and adipose tissue (Duclos et al., 2011). Physical activity's influence on people with diabetes provide other benefits that include improved QOL, glycemic control, muscle strengthening, and decreased cardiovascular risk (Cauza et al., 2005; Ferrer-García et al., 2011) as well as weight management.

Cancer can occur in many varieties and at any age in life. However, the prevalence of cancer is higher in older adults. Some studies have shown cancer rates 10 to 11 times higher in older adults compared to younger adults (Ershler, 2003; Yancik & Ries, 2004). Many forms of cancer can affect the older person's muscle strength, physical endurance, and QOL. Pharmacologic, surgical, and radiation treatment interventions can also greatly impact a person's physical abilities. A full discussion of the effects of cancer on the body systems or an in-depth discussion of exercise for people with cancer are beyond the scope of this chapter. However, the health professional should be aware that aerobic and resistance activities can help counteract some of the negative effects on the body by cancer and/or the treatments used to combat the cancer (D'Ascenzi et al., 2019). The health professional should prescribe physical activity based on the individual's type of cancer, current and past interventions, and current fitness and functional abilities.

Osteoporosis is another condition that affects older adults at larger numbers. During the span between 2005 and 2010, it was found that 16.2% of older adults had osteoporosis at the lumbar spine or femur neck (Looker & Frenk, 2015). People with osteoporosis typically have lower independence and QOL (Bloomfield & Smith, 2003). The main complication with osteoporosis is a reduction in bone mineral density and bone quality. Therefore, a person with osteoporosis may benefit from physical activity involving weight-bearing activities (ACSM, 2017). Both aerobic and **resistance activities** may be beneficial. High-impact activities or high-intensity motions should be avoided to prevent possible bone fracture.

Other orthopedic conditions may be improved via aerobic and/or resistance activity too. Physical activity can keep joints mobile and maintain muscle mass and strength. Even if the orthopedic impairment cannot be corrected, keeping the joint and muscle healthy around it will minimize functional loss of the person. The health professional should tailor any physical activity recommendations based on the person's orthopedic issue and their current physical abilities. Parameters of the activity should create benefit without causing more pain, impacting other joints through poor motion, or increase the person's risk of injury or fall due to the underlying orthopedic issue.

Neurologic conditions such as Parkinson's disease, spinal cord injury, traumatic brain injury, cerebral palsy, and many others can be improved or at least positively impacted by physical activity. Examining each person's neurologic condition, their physical limitations, and their medical stability will guide the health professional in the appropriate activity prescription or functional activity at that time. Progression in physical activity levels should occur as tolerated by that person. The full benefits of activity for specific neurologic conditions can be found in other resources devoted to those particular conditions.

How to Encourage Activity for Those With Chronic Conditions

Physical therapists can work with the person to determine which activities would be safe for them and provide adequate physiologic impact. Modifications may need to be made to activities or equipment due to neurologic or orthopedic impairments.

Occupational therapists can help the individual to identify the activities that are most important to them. Based on this, the occupational therapist may consider discussing the ways the person can manage their symptoms while engaging in those activities requiring physical activity. By modifying the task or the environment, engaging in work simplification and energy conservation techniques, and recommending adaptive devices or technologies, the occupational therapist can encourage and support physical activity engagement (AOTA, 2020b). The occupational therapist should also provide patient education about the disease or condition, the effect that symptoms may have on activity engagement, and then discuss options. By encouraging the person to take one day at a time, perform the desired and necessary activities based on how they feel that day, and taking action to reduce symptoms or prevent further decline is an important element of the therapist-person relationship.

Case Reflection

The person in this chapter's case study does have some chronic medical and orthopedic conditions. The interprofessional team should work together, including collaboration with the person involved, to decide which interventions will be most helpful and most likely to maintain long term. These include physical activity, but also nutrition and diet, stress management, and other factors that impact QOL.

Muscle and Joint Flexibility Interventions

Maintenance or improvement of muscle and joint flexibility has been deemed important as people age (Li et al., 2019; Pollock et al., 1998) and allow greater endurance and independence. This is vital as a person ages to help prevent falls and avoid sedentary behavior. The systematic review by Stathokostas et al. (2013) concluded that flexibility exercises in older adults increased joint motion and some functional outcomes. They also showed no additional risk of including flexibility exercises in an overall physical activity program for older adults. Their systematic review highlighted that the present research on stretching for older adults varies greatly in parameters. Study protocols regarding body parts stretched, type of stretches performed, and times for stretch hold were different between every study analyzed. Therefore, there are no concrete parameter recommendations available at this time. Also, there has not been a direct link shown between stretching/maintaining flexibility and improving daily function (Stathokostas et al., 2013). However, although there is not a proven direct benefit of stretching to improving function, there is also no evidence of any health or functional risks associated with flexibility exercises or stretching. In light of a lack of risk from stretching and a possible improvement, the health professional can help the person initiate flexibility activities or stretching to see if that individual experiences any benefits. Parameters should be kept toward the lighter end of time of stretch hold and number of stretch repetitions until the person has seen their individual response.

Occupational therapists, as part of the interprofessional team, can work with the older adult on appropriate functional activities that provide range of motion movements to improve flexibility. Liu et al. (2018) suggest that occupational therapy practitioners use task-oriented exercises that encourage physical activity with their clients. Health professionals can consult CDC Guidelines (2003) to determine appropriate functional tasks based on the Metabolic Equivalent of Task (MET) level for varying abilities. For example, someone with moderate capabilities could engage in yard work or carrying groceries rather than carry out a formal exercise program. Even those with lower abilities can be encouraged to perform simple household tasks such as folding laundry or hanging clothing in a closet. Even this type of simple activity could work to slowly increase range of motion and flexibility, balance, and endurance. This is an important aspect for the older adult as flexibility, stamina, and other physical factors can typically also interfere with ADLs and those activities that lead to independence, engagement in desired and necessary activities, and help to fulfill QOL.

How to Impact Muscle and Joint Flexibility

Physical therapists, occupational therapists, chiropractors, and other health professionals can show the person basic flexibility motions for spine flexion and extension, shoulder motions, hip and knee motions, and some ankle motions. It is more important to have the person keep general mobility throughout the trunk and limbs than it is to have very specific stretches that they perform. The health professional can refer the person to community tai chi, yoga, or other stretching type classes in their area if they exist too.

Balance Interventions and Decreasing Risk of Fall

As previously discussed in this chapter, balance and fall risk are closely associated. Health professionals can assist the individual with activity interventions that will help improve or at least maintain balance as they age. Aerobic activity doesn't typically have a direct effect on balance and falls, but there is an indirect association. As someone improves the endurance of individual muscle groups, it allows them to use those muscles for longer periods of time before quality of movement suffers. Aerobic training also improves pulmonary endurance that will allow greater oxygen delivery to the tissues and thus allow longer periods of time of muscle use before quality of movement suffers. Strength or resistance training, with a focus on the lower extremities, can also help improve balance in older adults (Buchner et al., 1997; USDHHS, 2018b). The ACSM guidelines are a good place for health professionals to start when assessing an older individual in initiating aerobic and/or resistance training (ACSM, 2017). The minimum weekly recommendations of 150 minutes of moderate intensity activity is also a good guide for the health professional to use (ACSM, 2009; USDHHS, 2018a).

Tai chi is another intervention that has a long history of use with older adults for physical function and balance. There are multiple studies that show that the performance of tai chi postures or exercise routines can improve balance in older adults (Qi et al., 2020: Wang et al., 2021). This improvement in balance will improve functional abilities, as well as decrease fall risk in older adults (Gallant et al., 2019; Penn et al., 2019). The fluid movement, weight shifting, and intermittent single limb stance makes tai chi a way to improve balance throughout the body and not just one system. Tai chi postures and sequences can be adapted to sitting, supported standing, or assisted postures too that allows the person to perform the activity without being at increased risk of falling. When performed in a group setting, tai chi can increase socialization, more likely influencing participation in this activity.

Dance has also been shown to improve physical function and endurance in older adults (Joung & Lee, 2019; Liu et al., 2021; Rodrigues-Krause et al., 2019). The movements associated with dance help with motor planning and spatial relations. The person's sense of position in space can also be improved with dance. These benefits are found regardless of the type of dance and one study even found that dance was more beneficial to balance than stretching (Joung & Lee, 2019). The health professional should encourage the person to pick whatever music and movement they enjoy in order to increase participation enjoyment. Safety must be ensured if the person is at risk of falls, but even slight swaying to music can have benefits. Boxing is a slightly newer intervention with older adults, which may improve balance and decrease risk of falls. Programs have been finding that the repetitive motions of boxing can help with balance (Combs et al., 2013; Horbinski et al., 2021; Park et al., 2017). The evidence to support boxing training is not conclusive yet, but it is an intervention to explore with the older adult based on their interest, physical presentation, and availability of an established boxing program for older adults.

Other interventions, including traditional balance exercises, may also maintain balance for the older adult. Care should be taken to select the intervention that the person will enjoy the most and thus maintain long term. Safety, needed equipment, availability of a program, and other factors discussed so far in this chapter, will help the health professional decide which interventions are appropriate to offer the older adult.

How to Lessen Fall Risk

Physical therapists, occupational therapists, nursing, and other health professionals will address fall risk with a person. Primary care providers should be asking the person if they have fallen and referring them to rehabilitation professionals if needed. Physical therapists and occupational therapists can talk with the person about general techniques to prevent falls such as removing loose rugs or other items on the floor, not moving, or walking in the dark or low light, wearing proper footwear, and so on. Specific fall assessment tools may indicate if the person should do specific balance, strengthening, or endurance activities to lessen their risk of fall.

Case Reflection

It would be beneficial to do some basic to moderate balance training exercises and interventions for the person. They are aging and have some circulatory and orthopedic issues that impact lower extremity function. Those impairments could lead to safety and balance issues. Balance assessments should be performed including standardized tests, vestibular screening, and specific positional and ADL testing of balance. Then the health professionals should work together, and with the individual, to determine how to best improve balance and prevent falls. Since the person has not reported a fall yet, now is the time to work on balance with them to prevent future falls.

Impact of Physical Activity on Mental Health

There is more than lack of exercise that impacts health among older adults. Mental and emotional deficits can also be very debilitating. Based on depression and anxiety screening during the assessment, health professionals should refer the person to mental health care providers for intervention as needed. There are simple strategies that rehabilitation and other health professionals can employ as adjuncts to assist individuals with mental health, such as stress management and basic coping strategies. Even so, the act of engaging in physical activity has benefits on mental health (Reguera-García et al., 2020; van der Zwan et al., 2015). People can improve their ability to cope, decrease depression and anxiety levels, and improve overall QOL. There are numerous studies showing a direct improvement in depression or anxiety and QOL with regular physical activity. A dose-relationship between exercise and depression or anxiety has not been shown in research (ACSM, 2017). This means that the person doesn't need to perform high level or vigorous activity in order to see improvement in depression or anxiety. A study by Ku et al. (2018) found a positive association between light physical activity and a reduced risk of depressive symptoms. Kaya (2020) conducted a randomized control study with 40 women over the age of 55 years. Half of the participants engaged in a three times per week swimming program for 12 weeks, while the control group of 20 women had no prescribed program. Results revealed that those in the experimental group had a significant decrease in depression levels ($p < .01$), as measured by the Beck Depression Scale. Another study conducted by Fakhari in 2017 found a statistically significant difference in depression mean scores in the experimental group who participated in a Tai Chi program ($p < .01$), three times per week for 12 weeks, when compared to the control group who did not participate. Thus, finding the desired type of exercise or physical activity that an older adult adheres to can greatly contribute to overall positive mental health.

How to Address Mental Health

Health professionals should screen for mental health issues, especially depression and anxiety. If any screening tool indicates a possible issue, the occupational therapist, physical therapist, nurse, dietician, primary care provider, and so on, should refer the person to a specialized mental health provider. For general wellness, health professionals can talk to the person about the importance of maintaining social contact with others, strategies for stress management, relaxation techniques, and who/what agencies to contact if they need any help with emotional or psychosocial factors.

Impact of Nutrition With Aging

Nutrition is also important as people age. Referral to a nutritionist or registered dietician should occur for full dietary recommendations and development of a nutrition plan specific for an individual. However, any health professional should be able to discuss basic nutritional needs as people age, educate on healthy vs. unhealthy weight loss or gain, and provide general nutritional education. Maintenance of vitamins and minerals such as calcium and vitamin D can help the overall well-being during the aging life span. These measures can help prevent bone density loss thus decreasing a person's risk of osteoporosis. Dietary intake of calcium is one example of appropriate nutritional management that may be required with consultation of a dietician or the person's physician (Yao et al., 2021). Older adults should also be encouraged to consume lower levels of sodium, saturated fats, cholesterol, and simple sugars. They should be encouraged to eat unsaturated or "healthy" fats, complex carbohydrates, proteins, and foods high in antioxidants (e.g., blueberries, certain seeds, certain legumes). Antioxidants, for example, may help limit memory loss, vision loss, and some chronic diseases (Frei, 1995; Liu, 2003). There are specific foods that can interact with cardiac medications so a blanket one size fits all recommendation should not be the rule. Rather, health professionals should educate the person with specific medical conditions on typical risk factors for that condition and relate it to one's physical health and well-being. Dietary implications and modifications should be made and discussed after fully understanding how nutrition influences all body systems relevant to the individual.

Weight loss can assist with orthopedic and other medical issues as a person ages. However, weight loss should be done responsibly. The person should seek the assistance of a nutritionist or registered dietician to establish a safe plan for weight loss while also making sure they aren't limiting beneficial nutrients and minerals. The health professional should educate the person that weight loss without trying or without a known cause may be a concern and could indicate a deeper medical issue. The individual should seek further medical care if there is weight loss of greater than 5 to 10 pounds with no known cause.

Case Reflection

The individual in the chapter's case study has some unique nutritional needs. Between the reflux disease and cardiovascular history, it would be important for the health professionals to address general nutrition and dietary modifications related to those conditions. These include limitation of salts, simple sugars, and saturated fats due to his cardiac disease. Dietary modifications due to his reflux disease would include eating smaller meals more frequently throughout the day and limiting saturated fats, caffeine, foods that are spicy, or high in acids such as citrus fruits It is even more important to ensure that the person receives specific, individualized intervention from a registered dietician.

How to Manage Nutrition With Aging

The nutritionist or registered dietician should be contacted for specific dietary recommendations. For general wellness, the physical therapist, occupational therapist, nurse, chiropractor, physician assistant, or other health professional should discuss the factors above related to vitamins, minerals, fats, and so on. Discussion on how to read labels and what to look for and what to avoid in foods may also help the older adult manage their diet better.

Adherence to Physical Activity

Adherence, especially over the long term, is an important factor to consider when promoting healthy behaviors in any person. In 2010, it was found that 55% of adults over the age of 50 years did not meet the recommended physical activity guidelines (de Lacy-Vawdon et al., 2018). Many factors contribute to the likelihood of a person continuing with exercise or activity. Health professionals should look to bolster factors that will encourage adherence to physical activity as an individual ages. The professional should also seek to help remove or lessen the impact of barriers to physical activity such as the availability of equipment or expense of participation. Motivation, choice of activity modality, and social support contribute to a person adhering to an activity program. Also, physical limitations, competing priorities, and perceptions of benefits impact whether a person will continue with physical activity or not (Franco et al., 2015).

Group support, good instructors that are helpful and motivating, and classes two to three times per week led to greater adherence to physical activity in older adults (de Lacy-Vawdon et al., 2018). One study examined long-term adherence past the initial 6-month initiation of a physical activity program. The researchers found that environmental and social barriers were the most directly linked to long-term adherence (Brown et al., 2020). This reiterates the importance of the health professional working with the individual to find a routine or program that will be easiest for them to maintain. The health professional should work with the patient addressing the following factors that will contribute to adherence to physical activity:

- Easy access to and easy ability to perform the activity
- Assessing any possible limitations to certain activities
- Modifications may be needed due to musculoskeletal, neurologic, cardiovascular, or other system impairments
- Exercise tolerance, strength, flexibility, and endurance will also need to be assessed and then considered in the prescription of physical activity
- Addressing any psychological factors impacting activity and helping to establish social support (Allison & Keller, 1997)

The health professional should work with the person to determine the mode of physical activity they would be most willing to perform. The more amenable to the type of activity, the more likely the person is to perform it regularly. The person should be assisted to determine their own goals of any physical activity program. Whether to improve fitness, maintain safety, maintain endurance, and so on, the individual should determine what their primary goal(s) is/are and then the health professional can help design a program to fit those goals.

Involving a person's spouse has also been shown to improve exercise adherence especially long term (Greenberg et al., 2004; Osuka et al., 2017). If a person does not have a spouse, involving their significant other, partner, friend, or other social support may be as effective to encourage exercise adherence (Duncan & McAuley, 1993; Oka et al., 1995). It is almost irrelevant who the support is from. The fact that an individual has social support, and a feeling of connection will help them maintain adherence to physical activity. It is therefore important to try to involve family members or friends in the prescription of a physical activity program. Walking programs, group exercise classes, belonging to the same gym, or other activities that allow simultaneous exercise will make it easier for the person and their significant other to motivate each other to continue with activity. Group activity programs also show great benefit to adherence in older adults (Beauchamp et al., 2018). The feeling of connection and social participation helps the person stay motivated for exercise. Group motivation and a sense of team or camaraderie help encourage continuation of regular exercise. Knowing that others will still be there encourages the person not to miss the exercise session. When developing group

Professional Reasoning Box C: Adherence to Exercise

Many health professionals struggle to keep people adhering to a lifestyle behavior modification. Whether it be physical activity, diet modification, or using an assistive device for mobility safety, adherence is often difficult to maintain long term. The expert health professional looks for ways to bolster that adherence. They work with the person to identify barriers to adherence and then address those as best they can (Brown et al., 2020). This may be the most important factor in improving adherence rates to any behavior. Addressing or eliminating barriers allows the individual the ability to perform the behavior routinely. The more often the behavior is performed, the more routine it becomes. The more routine a behavior is, the more it is solidified as a habit and lifestyle and not just a short-term intervention. So, it is imperative that the health professionals work with the person right at the beginning of care to identify barriers or potential barriers and come up with ways to combat those.

activities, health professionals should try to make exercise programs fun, energetic, and variable. The program should have individualized parameters based on each person's abilities, while still allowing group motivation and support. The most important thing is that a person continues to adhere to a physical activity program as they age. Working with them to address the parameters and factors outlined above will help to bolster their adherence rate and therefore their health and physical abilities.

How to Encourage Adherence to Activity

As discussed earlier, the health professional must involve the individual with determining which activity they will be most willing to continue with on their own. Physical activity for lifelong behavior change occurs outside of a rehabilitation setting, so the health professional must assist the person in finding what activity they can and will continue without extraneous support needed (Professional Reasoning Box C).

The WHO (2020) also offers a booklet on physical activity and sedentary behaviors, which can be found at https://apps.who.int/iris/bitstream/handle/10665/336656/9789240015128-eng.pdf?sequence=1&isAllowed=y.

Interprofessional Perspectives

Almost as important as working with the individual to develop a physical activity plan, is the health professional working with other health care disciplines in the development and adherence to that plan. The WHO stated that interprofessional collaborative practice occurs when "multiple health workers from different professional backgrounds work together with patients, families, careers, and communities to deliver the highest quality of care" (WHO, 2010, p. 7). Thus, finding and establishing a team approach to the promotion of physical exercise and activities should be a priority. Research has shown that program management and sustainability is enhanced when a collaborative approach is used (El Ansari et al., 2001).

There are new and emerging roles for health professionals who work with older clients and community members. According to the National Council on Aging (NCOA), less than one-third of older adults meet the recommended 30 minutes of moderate exercise at least five times per week and muscle-strengthening activities for at least 2 days per week for major muscle groups (NCOA, 2021). Using evidence-based programs, therapists can guide older adults in specific exercises, programs, or functional activities that are best suited to their physical health and interests. It may be beneficial for people to participate in programs led by various rehab professionals. This will allow education and possible intervention for various physical limitations including, but not limited to gait speed, safety, ADLs, and self-care. When rehabilitation professionals work together as a team, the person is more likely to maintain functional independence in the community.

The Interprofessional Education Collaborative (IPEC) is an initiative that includes the major health professional national associations (2021). The collaborative was established in an effort to develop "a collaborative to promote and encourage constituent efforts that would advance substantive interprofessional learning experiences to help prepare future health professionals for enhanced team-based care of patients and improved population health outcomes" (IPEC, 2021, para. 2). IPEC Competency #4 seeks to prepare practitioners who can work together to "plan, deliver, and evaluate patient/population centered care and population health programs and policies that are safe, timely, efficient, effective, and equitable" (2016, p. 10). In line with this collaborative goal, professionals who seek to increase physical activity as a way of reducing negative health outcomes should create opportunities to develop an interprofessional approach. Currently, many examples of interprofessional team successes can be found in the literature for specific diagnoses and outcomes. For example, a collaborative health care team approach was found to facilitate more appropriate health care utilization by adults with type-2 diabetes (Janson et al., 2009), result in statistically significant weight loss and decreased body mass index in patients with obesity (Nagelkerk et al., 2018) and reduce mental health hospital admissions (Bauer et al., 2019).

Though more studies are needed that focus on patient outcomes and interprofessional practice, results are promising.

Strategies to increase physical activity as a way to reduce or prevent chronic conditions and illnesses are well documented. However, Warburton and Bredin (2016), stated that physical activity "promotion should not be done in isolation, but rather part of a larger promotion of the importance of engaging in healthy lifestyle behaviours" (p. 501) including increased physical activity, smoking cessation, healthy nutrition, stress control, adequate sleep, and reduced alcohol consumption. A multidisciplinary team can provide aspects of these healthier behaviors. Physical therapy, for example, can assess abilities and teach individuals about exercise that would be appropriate and achievable. Occupational therapy can work with the individual on stress reduction and how to incorporate health management tasks, such as walking or riding a bicycle, into existing habits so they become part of the daily routine. Dieticians and nutritionists can address healthy eating that results in weight loss and ability to be more physically active. Other members of an interprofessional health care team can identify other specific interventions that may be helpful. In addition, Schwarz et al. (2019) suggest that "in order to increase physical activity participation aiming at chronic disease prevention, the optimal strategy should make use of a number of proven approaches that are grounded in relevant theories and targeting the individual and their environment" (p. 4).

An example of a comprehensive multi-tiered interprofessional community-wide program focusing on falls prevention in older adults can be seen in the **Step Up to Stop Falls Collaborative Project** (Health Foundation of Western and Central New York [HFWCNY], 2021a). Team members included health professionals such as primary and specialty care physicians, nursing, occupational, speech, and physical therapy, pharmacy, emergency services, faith-based and community partners, students, older adults, and others. The overarching goals were to focus on balance and exercise, home safety, professional practice change, older adult education, and examination of older adult's medical history.

Specific to rehabilitation professionals, health professional education was provided so therapists were prepared to receive referrals for older adults who were identified to be at risk for falls. Further, therapists were assessed for competency in providing standardized fall risk assessment and screenings. Fall risk factor standardized assessments, such as one-legged stance and TUG, were taught or reviewed, so therapists could be evidence-based in their approach. Education emphasized the importance in determining if the older adult had a fear of falling, experienced falls or near falls, had difficulty in their daily tasks, and vision screening was included. Similarly, various interventions including occupational therapist- and physical therapist-specific treatment goals were included in the education.

Occupational therapists focused on balance, environmental risk factors, and home hazard assessment, teaching energy conservation and work simplification, and recommendations for adaptive devices to enable engagement in ADLs and IADLs in a safe manner. Physical therapy focused on vestibular and balance goals, strength and conditioning, footwear assessment, and other older adult–specific needs. Rehab professionals were also taught tai chi, an evidence-based activity for falls prevention (Hosseini et al., 2018). Therapists were encouraged to work with experts in tai chi to develop programs that were easily accessible to the older adults in facilities and the community. Pharmacists, physicians, nurses, and other health professionals helped with medication management. This included reviewing the older adult's medication list to detect falls risks due to inappropriate combinations of medications, obtaining appropriate prescriptions, and managing their medication schedules. Community members who frequently interacted with older adults, such as hairdressers, barbers, activities program staff, and ambulance staff, were taught to recognize falls risk factors and identify frequent fallers so they could refer to fall prevention professionals. A toolkit inclusive of education, assessment, videos, and other materials was produced from the collaborative partners and is available at https://hfwcny.org/resource/step-stop-falls-toolkit/.

Data collection and analysis determined that approximately 1200 older adults were engaged in falls prevention programs, 2000 older adult homes were assessed, 500 health care professionals were engaged in education (HFWCNY, 2014). Findings also revealed that those over 80 years of age were highly represented in falls prevention activities and programs. Overall findings indicate the collaborative efforts reduced falls in all counties in New York that were involved in the initiative while remaining counties in the state had no decrease in the number of falls (HFWCNY, 2021b).

Technology

The growing field of eHealth can also yield positive results for increasing physical activity as part of an approach to wellness and prevention of disease, illness, and disablement. Duan et al. (2021) conducted a recent meta-analysis that included 15 studies that evaluated the use of a multiple health behavior change (MHBC) eHealth interventions. Results indicated a significant increase in physical activity and adoption of a healthy diet. The authors also suggested that research is emerging on the use of eHealth tools for promoting a healthier lifestyle.

Mobile phone or tablet software apps, part of the eHealth umbrella, may provide an alternative approach to health behavior adoption. In a systematic review and meta-analysis, Yerrakalva et al. (2019) evaluated an initial 11,829 studies that contained elements of mHealth or eHealth technologies. A mere six studies met inclusion criteria and were included in the systematic review, with five of the studies being eligible for inclusion in the meta-analysis. The technologies included in the studies contained one or more of the following: pedometer, accelerometer, blood pressure and glucose monitoring, sleep, heart rate, group or individualized education, goal setting, virtual coaching, educational or exercise video, messaging and rewards, and/or prompts. Evaluation of the studies revealed that mHealth app interventions may have been associated with decreased sedentary time, increased physical activity, and increased fitness; however, the researchers warned that improved study rigor and long-term benefits are needed. Syncing to smart activity monitors, goal setting, self-monitoring, instructions and education, and reward seemed to be more effective, and the researchers suggested that future studies should assess the use of apps along with professional support. Thus, it seems there are opportunities for health care professionals to assess and adopt technologies that can complement their interventions aimed at improving physical activity and other health behaviors for adults with and without challenges. Since technology is constantly changing, the health professional should assess what is available to that person and the benefits and drawbacks of the technology aid prior to incorporating it into physical activity recommendations. The authors of this chapter chose not to list or recommend specific technology or eHealth devices as they are changing so rapidly and could be outdated quickly.

How to Incorporate Technology

Each health professional may be familiar with different technologies and their applications. However, the biggest factors to the use of technologies will be the availability of the technology and the ability of the person to use it.

Community Programs

There are existing programs that older adults can access, but the person may need guidance as to the right fit for them. The NCOA's Active Choices, Active Living Every Day, Enhance Fitness, Fit and Strong, Geri Fit, Healthy Moves for Aging Well, Walk with Ease (2021) are some such programs. Although each one is slightly different, the intention is to create a program that allows easy, affordable access to physical activity for older adults. Some incorporate formal health assessments while others just encourage physical activity that the person varies based on their responses.

Silver Sneakers is a national program offered through Medicare Advantage plans.* It allows older people to exercise at specific fitness/gym locations or take exercise classes online (Tivity Health, 2021). The classes are designed for specific types of activity. Some are geared more toward strength, some toward balance, and so on. The person can pick the classes that appeal to them. The programs are offered free or at very low cost to the person through their medical insurance. Significant others are encouraged to join too and most of the classes are offered in a group format, thus increasing socialization value.

In recent years, technology has increased the amount of remote or telehealth-type exercise programs (Jennings et al., 2020). Telehealth monitoring has been used in cardiac rehab programs, return to work programs, and other realms of health care. With the 2020 COVID-19 pandemic, most non-emergency health and medical programs had to close or shift to remote delivery. One study showed that remote delivery of an exercise program did still decrease negative health risks (Jennings et al., 2020). As technology improves and older adults become more adept at utilizing technology, more programs could look to expand into a remote delivery. This would expand the ability to offer exercise programs to even more people, especially when geographic barriers exist. If specific community activity programs do not exist in a person's area or aren't open access, the NCOA has resources which outline components that can aid to create an effective program for older adults (Belza, 2007). The health professional could assist the person in understanding and implementing these components for physical activity.

Why Promoting Physical Activity for the Older Adult Is Important

As discussed in this chapter, there are anatomical and physiological changes that negatively influence people as they age. These changes can contribute to impairments with muscle strength and mass, bone density, joint and ligament motion, balance and safety, endurance, independence levels, and overall QOL. Strategies and interventions that reduce the natural decline and increase levels of physical activity can positively impact and many times reduce impairments. Health professionals should work within their scope of practice and with other disciplines to help create a comprehensive plan for the older adult to continue with safe physical activity. Using each health professional's expertise, the individual can be guided toward safe and effective activity that they could continue on their own or with community support.

As discussed throughout this chapter, the most important factor in physical activity for the older adult is individualization. The health professional should work with the person to identify parameters that are appropriate for them, as well as potential barriers. Establishing a clear plan for physical activity and involving social support will help bolster the

*Medicare Advantage plans are offered by private insurance companies in conjunction with the government to replace the traditional part A and B plans. The extra fitness membership benefits associated with Medicare Advantage plans can vary based on the private insurance company.

adherence to the program. Adhering to physical activity can help mitigate chronic medical conditions, orthopedic complications, balance and risk of falls, and maintain functional strength and endurance. Maintenance of flexibility may also help decrease risk of falls and retain functional independence. Use of group classes or programs, often held within communities, whether in person or remote, may increase adherence to the physical activity program. The various disciplines of health professionals should work as an interprofessional team for assessment and interventions related to physical activity. As technology improves, there may be further methods to encourage adherence to an exercise routine. Taking all this into account allows the health professional to provide individual, community-oriented or population-based assistance in the establishment of a physical activity program. Initiating and maintaining physical activity is paramount for the older adult.

References

Allison, M., & Keller, C. (1997). Physical activity in the elderly: Benefits and intervention strategies. *The Nurse Practitioner, 22*(8), 53.

American College of Sports Medicine. (2017). *American College of Sports Medicine exercise testing and prescription* (10th ed.). Wolters Kluwer.

American Heart Association. (2018). American Heart Association recommendations for physical activity in adults and kids. https://www.heart.org/en/healthy-living/fitness/fitness-basics/aha-recs-for-physical-activity-in-adults

American Occupational Therapy Association. (2017). Occupational therapy's role with fall prevention. https://www.aota.org/-/media/Corporate/Files /AboutOT/Professionals/ WhatIsOT/PA/Falls.pdf

American Occupational Therapy Association. (2020a). Occupational therapy practice framework: Domain and process, 4th edition. *American Journal of Occupational Therapy, 74*(Suppl. 2), 7412410010. https://doi.org/10.5014/ajot.2020.74S2001

American Occupational Therapy Association. (2020b). Occupational therapy's role with chronic disease management. https://www.aota.org/-/media/Corporate/Files/AboutOT/Professionals/WhatIsOT/HW/Facts/FactSheet_ChronicDiseaseManagement.pdf

American Occupational Therapy Association. (2020c). Occupational therapy's role with health promotion. https://www.aota.org/-/media/Corporate/Files/AboutOT/ Professionals/ WhatIsOT/HW/Facts/FactSheet_HealthPromotion.pdf

Arnett, D. K., Blumenthal, R. S., Albert, M. A., Buroker, A. B., Goldberger, Z. D., Hahn, E. J., Himmelfarb, C. D., Khera, A., Lloyd-Jones, D., McEvoy, J. W., Michos, E. D., Miedema, M. D., Muñoz, D., Smith, S. C., Jr., Virani, S. S., Williams, K. A., Sr., Yeboah, J., & Ziaeian, B. (2019). 2019 ACC/AHA guideline on the primary prevention of cardiovascular disease: A report of the American College of Cardiology/American Heart Association Task Force on Clinical Practice Guidelines. *Circulation, 140*(11), e596-e646. https://doi.org/10.1161/CIR.0000000000000678

Bauer, M. S., Miller, C., J., Kim, B., Lew, R., Stolzmann, K., Sullivan, J., Riendeau, R., Pitcock, J., Williamson, A., Connolly, S., Rani Elwy, A., & Weaver, K. (2019). Effectiveness of implementing a collaborative chronic care model for clinician teams on patient outcomes and health status in mental health: A randomized clinical trial. *JAMA Network Open, 2*(3). doi:10.1001/jamanetworkopen.2019.0230

Beauchamp, M. R., Ruissen, G. R., Dunlop, W. L., Estabrooks, P. A., Harden, S. M., Wolf, S. A., Liu, Y., Schmader, T., Puterman, E., Sheel, A. W., & Rhodes, R. E. (2018). Group-based physical activity for older adults (GOAL) randomized controlled trial: Exercise adherence outcomes. *Health Psychology, 37*(5), 451-461. https://doi.org/10.1037/hea0000615

Beck, A. T. (1996). *Beck Depression Inventory II*. The Psychological Corporation. Harcourt Brace & Company. https://www.nctsn.org/measures/beck-depression-inventory-second-edition

Belza, B. (2007). *The PRC-HAN Physical Activity Conference Planning Workgroup. Moving ahead: Strategies and tools to plan, conduct, and maintain effective community-based physical activity Programs for older adults*. Centers for Disease Control and Prevention.

Berger, S. (2013). Effectiveness of occupational therapy interventions for older adults living with low vision. *The American Journal of Occupational Therapy, 67*(3), 263–265. https://doi-org.ezproxy.daemen.edu/10.5014/ajot.2013.007203

Bito, S., & Fukuhara, S. (1998). Validation of interviewer administration of the Short Form 36 Health Survey, and comparisons of health-related quality of life between community-dwelling and institutionalized elderly people. *Japanese Journal of Geriatrics, 35*(6), 458-463. https://doi-org.dyc.idm.oclc.org/10.3143/geriatrics.35.458

Bloomfield, S. A., & Smith, S. S. (2003) Osteoporosis. In: J. L. Durstine & G. E. Moore (Eds.), *ACSM's Exercise Management for Persons with Chronic Diseases and Disabilities* (2nd ed., pp. 222-229). Human Kinetics.

Bohannon, R. W. (2006). Reference values for the five-repetition sit-to-stand test: A descriptive meta-analysis of data from elders. *Perceptual and Motor Skills, 103*(1), 215-222.

Bohannon, R. W., Wang, Y. C., & Gershon, R. C. (2015). Two-minute walk test performance by adults 18 to 85 years: Normative values, reliability, and responsiveness. *Archives of Physical Medicine and Rehabilitation, 96*(3), 472-477.

Brosel, S., & Strupp, M. (2019). The vestibular system and ageing. *Sub-Cellular Biochemistry, 91*, 195-225. https://doi.org/10.1007/978-981-13-3681-2_8

Brown, C. S., Sloane, R., & Morey, M. C. (2020). Developing predictors of long-term adherence to exercise among older veterans and spouses. Journal of Applied Gerontology. *The Official Journal of the Southern Gerontological Society, 39*(10), 1159-1162. https://doi-org.dyc.idm.oclc.org/10.1177/0733464819874954.

Buchner, D. M., Cress, M. E., de Lateur, B. J., Esselman, P. C., Margherita, A. J., Price, R., & Wagner, E. H. (1997). The effect of strength and endurance training on gait, balance, fall risk, and health services use in community-living older adults. *The Journals of Gerontology. Series A, Biological Sciences and Medical Sciences, 52*(4), M218-M224.

Cauza, E., Hanusch-Enserer, U., Strasser, B., Ludvik, B., Metz-Schimmerl, S., Pacini, G., Wagner, O., Georg, P., Prager, R., Kostner, K., Dunky, A., & Haber, P. (2005). The relative benefits of endurance and strength training on the metabolic factors and muscle function of people with type 2 diabetes mellitus. *Archives of Physical Medicine and Rehabilitation, 86*(8), 1527-1533. https://doi.org/10.1016/j.apmr.2005.01.007

Centers for Disease Control and Prevention. (2003). General physical activities defined by level of intensity. https://www.cdc.gov/nccdphp/dnpa/physical/pdf/pa_intensity_table_2_1.pdf

Centers for Disease Control and Prevention. (2020a). Older adult fall prevention. https://www.cdc.gov/falls/index.html

Centers for Disease Control and Prevention. (2020b). Promoting health for older adults. https://www.cdc.gov/chronicdisease/pdf/factsheets/older-adults-H.pdf

Centers for Disease Control and Prevention. (2020c). STEADI Older adult fall prevention. https://www.cdc.gov/steadi/index.html

Charlier, R., Knaeps, S., Mertens, E., Van Roie, E., Delecluse, C., Lefevre, J., & Thomis, M. (2016). Age-related decline in muscle mass and muscle function in Flemish Caucasians: A 10-year follow-up. *Age, 38*(2), 36. https://doi.org/10.1007/s11357-016-9900-7

Chodzko-Zajko, W. J., Proctor, D. N., Fiatarone Singh, M. A., Minson, C. T., Nigg, C. R., Salem, G. J., & Skinner, J. S. American College of Sports Medicine. (2009). American College of Sports Medicine position stand. Exercise and physical activity for older adults. *Medicine and Science in Sports and Exercise, 41*(7), 1510-1530. https://doi.org/10.1249/MSS.0b013e3181a0c95c

Cohen, H., Burkhardt, A., Cronin, G. W., & McGuire, M. J. (2006). Specialized knowledge and skills in adult vestibular rehabilitation for occupational therapy practice. *American Journal of Occupational Therapy, 60*(6), 669-678. https://doi.org/10.5014/ajot.60.6.669

Combs, S. A., Diehl, M. D., Chrzastowski, C., Didrick, N., McCoin, B., Mox, N., Staples, W. H., & Wayman, J. (2013). Community-based group exercise for persons with Parkinson disease: A randomized controlled trial. *NeuroRehabilitation, 32*(1), 117-124.

Connors, B. P., McGlamery, J. N., & Stern, B. Z. (2019). Brief motivational interviewing: A tool for occupational therapy practitioners to support self-management. *SIS Quarterly Practice Connections, 4*(3), 16-18.

Craig, C. L., Marshall, A. L., Sjöström, M., Bauman, A. E., Booth, M. L., Ainsworth, B. E., Pratt, M., Ekelund, U., Yngve, A., Sallis, J.F., & Oja, P. (2003). International physical activity questionnaire: 12-country reliability and validity. *Medicine and Science in Sports and Exercise, 35*(8), 1381-1395.

D'Ascenzi, F., Anselmi, F., Fiorentini, C., Mannucci, R., Bonifazi, M., & Mondillo, S. (2019). The benefits of exercise in cancer patients and the criteria for exercise prescription in cardio-oncology. *European Journal of Preventive Cardiology*. https://doi.org/10.1177/2047487319874900

de Lacy-Vawdon, C. J., Klein, R., Schwarzman, J., Nolan, G., de Silva, R., Menzies, D., & Smith, B. J. (2018). Facilitators of attendance and adherence to group-based physical activity for older adults: A literature synthesis. *Journal of Aging and Physical Activity, 26*(1), 155-167. https://doi.org/10.1123/japa.2016-0363

de Waroquier-Leroy, L., Bleuse, S., Serafi, R., Watelain, E., Pardessus, V., Tiffreau, A. V., & Thevenon, A. (2014). The functional reach test: Strategies, performance and the influence of age. *Annals of Physical and Rehabilitation Medicine, 57*(6-7), 452-464.

Deshpande, N., Metter, J. E., Guralnik, J., Bandinelli, S., & Ferrucci, L. (2014). Sensorimotor and psychosocial determinants of 3-year incident mobility disability in middle-aged and older adults. *Age and Ageing, 43*(1), 64-69. https://doi.org/10.1093/ageing/aft135

Doherty, T. J., Vandervoort, A. A., & Brown, W. F. (1993). Effects of ageing on the motor unit: A brief review. *Canadian Journal of Applied Physiology, 18*(4), 331-358.

Duan, Y., Shang, B., Liang, W., Du, G., Yang, M., & Rhodes, R. E. (2021). Effects of eHealth-based multiple health behavior change interventions on physical activity, healthy diet, and weight in people with noncommunicable diseases: Systematic review and meta-analysis. *Journal of Medical Internet Research. 23*(2). https://doi.org/10.2196/23786

Duclos, M., Virally, M. -L., & Dejager, S. (2011) Exercise in the management of type 2 diabetes mellitus: What are the benefits and how does it work? *The Physician and Sports Medicine, 39*(2), 98-106. https://doi.org/10.3810/psm.2011.05.1899

Duncan, T. E., & McAuley, E. (1993). Social support and efficacy cognitions in exercise adherence: A latent growth curve analysis. *Journal of Behavioral Medicine, 16*(2), 199-218. https://doi.org/10.1007/BF00844893

Ehrlich, J. R., Hassan, S. E., & Stagg, B. C. (2019). Prevalence of falls and fall-related outcomes in older adults with self-reported vision impairment. *Journal of the American Geriatrics Society, 67*(2), 239–245.

El Ansari, W., Phillips, C. J., & Hammick, M. (2001). Collaboration and partnerships: Developing the evidence base. *Health & Social Care in the Community, 9*(4), 215-227.

Ershler, W. B. (2003). Cancer: A disease of the elderly. *Journal of Supportive Oncology, 1*, 5-10.

Fagard, R. (2001). Exercise characteristics and the blood pressure response to dynamic physical training. *Medicine and Science in Sports & Exercise, 33*, S484-S492.

Farrance, C., Tsofliou, F., & Clark, C. (2016). Adherence to community-based group exercise interventions for older people: A mixed-methods systematic review. *Preventive Medicine, 87*, 155-166.

Fakhari, M. (2017). Effects of Tai Chi exercise on depression in older adults: A randomized controlled trial. *Bali Medical Journal, 6*, 679.

Feltz, G., & Eichenauer, K. (2001). Psychosocial risk factor survey. https://psychosocialriskfactorsurvey.blogspot.com/

Ferrer-García, J. C., Sánchez López, P., Pablos-Abella, C., Albalat-Galera, R., Elvira-Macagno, L., Sánchez-Juan, C., & Pablos-Monzó, A. (2011). Benefits of a home-based physical exercise program in elderly subjects with type 2 diabetes mellitus. *Endocrinologia y Nutricion: Organo de La Sociedad Espanola de Endocrinologia y Nutricion, 58*(8), 387-394.

Fetters, A. (2017). How fit are you? Take this test. https://www.silversneakers.com/blog/fitness-test/

Franco, M. R., Tong, A., Howard, K., Sherrington, C., Ferreira, P. H., Pinto, R. Z., & Ferreira, M. L. (2015). Older people's perspectives on participation in physical activity: A systematic review and thematic synthesis of qualitative literature. *British Journal of Sports Medicine, 49*(19), 1268-1276. https://doi.org/10.1136/bjsports-2014-094015

Frei B. (1995). Cardiovascular disease and nutrient antioxidants: Role of low-density lipoprotein oxidation. *Critical Reviews in Food Science and Nutrition, 35*(1-2), 83-98. https://doi.org/10.1080/10408399509527689

Füzéki, E., Engeroff, T., & Banzer, W. (2017). Health benefits of light-intensity physical activity: A systematic review of accelerometer data of the National Health and Nutrition Examination Survey (NHANES). *Sports Medicine, 47*(9), 1769-1793. https://doi.org/10.1007/s40279-017-0724-0

Gallant, M. P., Tartaglia, M., Hardman, S., & Burke, K. (2019). Using Tai Chi to reduce fall Risk factors among older adults: An evaluation of a community-based implementation. *Journal of Applied Gerontology, 38*(7), 983-998. https://doi.org/10.1177/0733464817703004

Galloza, J., Castillo, B., & Micheo, W. (2017). Benefits of exercise in the older population. *Physical Medicine and Rehabilitation Clinics of North America, 28*(4), 659-669. https://doi.org/10.1016/j.pmr.2017.06.001

Greenberg, S., Almaro, N., Keren, G., & Sheps, D. (2004). The effect of spouse participation in cardiac rehabilitation program on patients' compliance and exercise level. *Harefuah, 143*(2), 99.

Health Foundation for Western and Central New York. (2014). Investing in better health for people and communities. Step Up to Stop Falls. https://www.health.ny.gov/health_care/medicaid/redesign/mrt8004/falls_prevention_docs/step_up.pdf

Health Foundation for Western and Central New York. (2021a). Step up to stop falls, overview. https://hfwcny.org/program/step-stop-falls/

Health Foundation for Western and Central New York. (2021b). Step up to stop falls toolkit. https://hfwcny.org/resource/step-stop-falls-toolkit/

Hlatky, M., Boineau, R., Higgenbotham, M., Lee, K. L., Mark, D., B., Califf, R. M., Cobb, F. R., & Pryor, D. B. (1989). A brief self-administered questionnaire to determine functional capacity (The Duke Activity Status Index). *American Journal of Cardiology, 64*, 651-654.

Horbinski, C., Zumpf, K. B., McCortney, K., & Eoannou, D. (2021). Longitudinal study of boxing therapy in Parkinson's Disease, including adverse impacts of the COVID-19 lockdown. Research Square. https://doi.org/10.21203/rs.3.rs-355283/v1

Hosseini, L., Kargozar, E., Sharifi, F., Negarandeh, R., Memari, A. H., & Navab, E. (2018). Tai Chi Chuan can improve balance and reduce fear of falling in community dwelling older adults: A randomized control trial. *Journal of Exercise Rehabilitation, 14*(6), 1024-1031. https://doi.org/10.12965/jer.1836488.244

Interprofessional Education Collaborative. (2016). Core competencies for interprofessional collaborative practice: 2016 update. Interprofessional Education Collaborative. https://hsc.unm.edu/ipe/resources/ipec-2016-core-competencies.pdf

Interprofessional Education Collaborative. (2021). What Is Interprofessional Education (IPE)? https://www.ipecollaborative.org/about-us

Janssens, J. P., Pache, J. C., & Nicod, L. P. (1999). Physiological changes in respiratory function associated with ageing. *The European Respiratory Journal, 13*(1), 197-205. https://doi.org/10.1034/j.1399-3003.1999.13a36.x

Janson, S. L., Cooke, M., McGrath, K. W., Kroon, L. A., Robinson, S., & Baron, R. B. (2009). Improving chronic care of type 2 diabetes using teams of interprofessional learners. *Academic Medicine, 84*(11), 1540-1548.

Janz, N. K., & Becker, M. H. (1984). The Health Belief Model: A decade later. *Health Education Quarterly, 11*(1), 1-47. https://doi.org/10.1177/109019818401100101

Jennings, S. C., Manning, K. M., Bettger, J. P., Hall, K. M., Pearson, M., Mateas, C., Briggs, B. C., Oursler, K. K., Blanchard, E., Lee, C. C., Castle, S., Valencia, W. M., Katzel, L. I., Giffuni, J., Kopp, T., McDonald, M., Harris, R., Bean, J. F., Althuis, K., & Morey, M. C. (2020). Rapid transition to telehealth group exercise and functional assessments in response to COVID-19. *Gerontology & Geriatric Medicine, 6*. https://doi.org/10.1177/2333721420980313

Jones, C. J., Rikli, R. E., & Beam, W. C. (1999). A 30-s chair-stand test as a measure of lower body strength in community-residing older adults. *Research Quarterly for Exercise and Sport, 70*(2), 113-119.

Joung, H. J., & Lee, Y. (2019). Effect of creative dance on fitness, functional balance, and mobility control in the elderly. *Gerontology, 65*(5), 537-546. https://doi.org/10.1159/000499402

Kaya, H. B. (2020). Effect of swimming exercise in old age on hopelessness and depression levels. *African Educational Research Journal, 8*, 353-359.

Kaya, R. D., Nakazawa, M., Hoffman, R. L., & Clark, B. C. (2013). Interrelationship between muscle strength, motor units, and aging. *Experimental Gerontology, 48*(9), 920-925. 10.1016/j.exger.2013.06.008

Keating, C. J., Párraga Montilla, J. Á., Latorre Román, P. Á., & Moreno Del Castillo, R. (2020). Comparison of high-intensity interval training to moderate-intensity continuous training in older adults: A systematic review. *Journal of Aging and Physical Activity, 28*(5), 798-807. https://doi.org/10.1123/japa.2019-0111

Klyczek, J. P., Bauer-Yox, N., & Fiedler, R. C. (1997) The Interest Checklist: A factor analysis. *American Journal of Occupational Therapy, 51*(10), 815-823. https://doi.org/10.5014/ajot.51.10.815

Ku, P. W., Steptoe, A., Liao, Y., Sun, W. J., & Chen, L. J. (2018). Prospective relationship between objectively measured light physical activity and depressive symptoms in later life. *International Journal of Geriatric Psychiatry, 33*(1), 58-65.

LaRoche, D. P., Millett, E. D., & Kralian, R. J. (2011). Low strength is related to diminished ground reaction forces and walking performance in older women. *Gait & Posture, 33*(4), 668-672. 10.1016/j.gaitpost.2011.02.022

Li, F., Harmer, P., Eckstrom, E., Fitzgerald, K., Chou, L. S., & Liu, Y. (2019). Effectiveness of Tai Ji Quan vs multimodal and stretching exercise interventions for reducing injurious falls in older adults at high risk of falling: Follow-up analysis of a randomized clinical trial. *JAMA Network Open, 2*(2), e188280. https://doi.org/10.1001/jamanetworkopen.2018.8280

Liston, M. B., Bamiou, D. E., Martin, F., Hopper, A., Koohi, N., Luxon, L., & Pavlou, M. (2014). Peripheral vestibular dysfunction is prevalent in older adults experiencing multiple non-syncopal falls versus age-matched non-fallers: A pilot study. *Age and Ageing, 43*(1), 38-43. https://doi.org/10.1093/ageing/aft129

Liu, C. J., Chang, W. P., & Chang, M. C. (2018). Occupational therapy interventions to improve activities of daily living for community-dwelling older adults: A systematic review. *American Journal of Occupational Therapy, 72*(4), 7204190060p1-7204190060p11. https://doi.org/10.5014/ajot.2018.031252

Liu, R. H. (2003). Protective role of phytochemicals in whole foods: Implications for chronic disease prevention. *Applied Biotechnology Food Science Policy, 1*, 39-46.

Liu, X., Shen, P. L., & Tsai, Y. S. (2021). Dance intervention effects on physical function in healthy older adults: A systematic review and meta-analysis. *Aging Clinical and Experimental Research, 33*(2), 253-263. https://doi.org/10.1007/s40520-019-01440-y

Looker, A. C. & Frenk, S. M. (2015). Percentage of adults aged 65 and over with osteoporosis or low bone mass at the femur neck or lumbar spine: United States, 2005-2010. *NCHS Data Brief*,(93), 1-8.

Mandel, D. R., Jackson, J. M., Zemke, R., Nelson, L., & Clark, F. A. (1999). *Lifestyle redesign: Implementing the Well elderly program.* American Occupational Therapy Association, Inc.

McKinnon, N. B., Montero-Odasso, M., & Doherty, T. J. (2015). Motor unit loss is accompanied by decreased peak muscle power in the lower limb of older adults. *Experimental Gerontology, 70*, 111-118. https://doi.org/10.1016/j.exger.2015.07.007

Mora, J. C., & Valencia, W. M. (2018). Exercise and older adults. *Clinics in Geriatric Medicine, 34*(1), 145-162. https://doi.org/10.1016/j.cger.2017.08.007

Myers, J., Sweeney, T., & Witmer, J. (2000). The wheel of wellness counseling for wellness: A holistic model for treatment planning. *Journal of Counseling and Development, 78*(3), 251-266.

Nagelkerk, J., Benkert, R., Pawl, B., Myers, A., Baer, L. J., Rayford, A., Berlin, S. J., Fenbert, K., Moore, H., Armstrong, M., Murray, M., Boone, P., Masselink, S., & Jakstys, C. (2018). Test of an interprofessional collaborative practice model to improve obesity-related health outcomes in Michigan. *Journal of Interprofessional Education & Practice, 11*, 43-50.

National Center for Injury Prevention and Control. (2015). *Preventing falls: A guide to implementing effective community-based fall prevention programs* (2nd ed.). Centers for Disease Control and Prevention.

National Council on Aging. (2021). Exercise programs that promote senior fitness. https://www.ncoa.org/center-for-healthy-aging/basics-of-evidence-based-programs/physical-activity-programs-for-older-adults/

National Institute on Aging. (2017). Short physical performance battery. https://www.sralab.org/rehabilitation-measures/short-physical-perfromance-battery

Oka, R. K., King, A. C., & Young, D. R. (1995). Sources of social support as predictors of exercise adherence in women and men ages 50 to 65 years. *Women's Health, 1*(2), 161-175.

Osuka, Y., Jung, S., Kim, T., Okubo, Y., Kim, E., & Tanaka, K. (2017). Does attending an exercise class with a spouse improve long-term exercise adherence among people aged 65 years and older: A 6-month prospective follow-up study. *BMC Geriatrics, 17*(1), 170. https://doi.org/10.1186/s12877-017-0554-9

Park, J., Gong, J., & Yim, J. (2017). Effects of a sitting boxing program on upper limb function, balance, gait, and quality of life in stroke patients. *NeuroRehabilitation, 40*(1), 77-86.

Pedrosa, H. G. (2009). Correlation between the walk, two-minute step test and TUG in hypertensive older women. *Brazilian Journal of Physical Therapy, 13*(3), 252-256.

Penn, I. W., Sung, W. H., Lin, C. H., Chuang, E., Chuang, T. Y., & Lin, P. H. (2019). Effects of individualized Tai-Chi on balance and lower-limb strength in older adults. *BMC Geriatrics, 19*(1), 235. https://doi.org/10.1186/s12877-019-1250-8

Philip, K. E., Katagira, W., & Jones, R. (2020). Dance for respiratory patients in low-resource settings. *Journal of the American Medical Association, 324*(10), 921-922.

Pizzi, M. (2001). The Pizzi Holistic Wellness Assessment, *Occupational Therapy in Health Care, 13*(3-4), 51-66. https://doi.org/10.1080/J003v13n03_06

Pizzi, M. (in press). Wellness and health promotion for people with physical disabilities. In H. Pendleton & W. Schultz-Krohn (Eds), *Pedretti's occupational therapy for physical dysfunction* (9th ed.). Elsevier.

Prochaska, J. O., & Velicer, W. F. (1997). The transtheoretical model of health behavior change. *American Journal of Health Promotion, 12*(1), 38-48. https://doi.org/10.4278/0890-1171-12.1.38

Podsiadlo, D., & Richardson, S. (1991). The timed "up & go": A test of basic functional mobility for frail elderly persons. *Journal of American Geriatric Society, 39*, 142-148.

Pollock, M. L., Gaesser, G. A., Butcher, J. D., Després, J. P., Dishman, R. K., Franklin, B. A., & Garber, C. E. (1998). ACSM position stand: The recommended quantity and quality of exercise for developing and maintaining cardiorespiratory and muscular fitness, and flexibility in healthy adults. *Journals AZ Medicine & Science, 30*, 6.

Pothula, V. B., Chew, F., Lesser, T. H. J., & Sharma, A. K. (2004). Falls and vestibular impairment. *Clinical Otolaryngology and Allied Sciences, 29*(2), 179-182. https://doi.org/10.1111/j.0307-7772.2004.00785.x

Powell, K. E., King, A. C., Buchner, D. M., Campbell, W. W., DiPietro, L., Erickson, K. I., Hillman, C. H., Jakicic, J. M., Janz, K. F., Katzmarzyk, P. T., Kraus, W. E., Macko, R. F., Marquez, D. X., McTiernan, A., Pate, R. R., Pescatello, L. S., & Whitt-Glover, M. C. (2018). The scientific foundation for the physical activity guidelines for Americans, 2nd Edition. *Journal of Physical Activity and Health, 16*(1), 1-11.

Qi, M., Moyle, W., Jones, C., & Weeks, B. (2020). Tai Chi combined with resistance training for adults aged 50 years and older: A systematic review. *Journal of Geriatric Physical Therapy, 43*(1), 32-41. https://doi.org/10.1519/JPT.0000000000000218

Rebuilding Together. (2012). Rebuilding together. https://www.aota.org/~/media/Corporate/Files/Practice/Aging/rebuilding-together/RT-Aging-in-Place-Safe-at-Home-Checklist.pdf

Rees-Punia, E., Evans, E. M., Schmidt, M. D., Gay, J. L., Matthews, C. E., Gapstur, S. M., & Patel, A.V. (2019). Mortality risk reductions for replacing sedentary time with physical activities. *American Journal of Preventive Medicine, 56*(5), 736-741.

Reguera-García, M. M., Liébana-Presa, C., Álvarez-Barrio, L., Alves Gomes, L., & Fernández-Martínez, E. (2020). Physical activity, resilience, sense of coherence and coping in people with Multiple Sclerosis in the situation derived from COVID-19. *International Journal of Environmental Research and Public Health, 17*(21). https://doi.org/10.3390/ijerph17218202

Rodrigues-Krause, J., Krause, M., & Reischak-Oliveira, A. (2019). Dancing for healthy aging: Functional and metabolic perspectives. *Alternative Therapies in Health and Medicine, 25*(1), 44-63.

Roman, M. A., Rossiter, H. B., & Casaburi, R. (2016). Exercise, ageing and the lung. *The European Respiratory Journal, 48*(5), 1471-1486. https://doi.org/10.1183/13993003.00347-2016

Roos, M. R., Rice, C. L., & Vandervoort, A. A. (1997). Age-related changes in motor unit function. *Muscle Nerve, 20*, 679-690. https://doi.org/10.1002/(SICI)1097-4598(199706)20:6<679::AID-MUS4>3.0.CO;2-5

Sanderson, B., & Bittner, V. (2006). Practical interpretation of 6-minute walk data using healthy adult reference equations. *Journal of Cardiopulmonary Rehabilitation, 26*(3), 167-171.

Schwartz, J., Rhodes, R., Bredin, S., Oh, P., & Warburton, D. (2019). Effectiveness of approaches to increase physical activity behavior to prevent chronic disease in adults: A brief commentary. *Journal of Clinical Medicine, 8*(3), 295. https://doi.org/10.3390/jcm8030295

Seidel, D., Brayne, C., & Jagger, C. (2011). Limitations in physical functioning among older people as a predictor of subsequent disability in instrumental activities of daily living. *Age and Ageing, 40*(4), 463-469. https://doi.org/10.1093/ageing/afr054

Serwe, K., Walmsley, A., & Pizzi, M.A. (2019). Reliability and responsiveness of the Pizzi Health and Wellness Assessment. *Annals of International Occupational Therapy, 3*(1), 7-13.

Shelkey, M., & Wallace, M. (2001). Katz Index of Independence in Activities of Daily Living. *Home Healthcare Nurse, 19*(5), 323-324.

Simonsick, E. M., Gardner, A. W., & Poehlman, E. T. (2008). Assessment of physical function and exercise tolerance in older adults: Reproducibility and comparability of five measures. *Aging, 12*(4), 274-280.

Singh, S., Morgan, M., Scott, S., Walters, D., & Hardman, A. E. (1992). Development of a shuttle walking test of disability in patients with chronic airways obstruction. *Thorax, 47*, 1019-1024.

Sousa, R. F., Gazzola, J. M., Ganança, M. M., & Paulino, C. A. (2011). Correlation between the body balance and functional capacity from elderly with chronic vestibular disorders. *Brazilian Journal of Otorhinolaryngology, 77*(6), 791-798.

Spitzer, R. L., Williams, J. B. W., & Kroenke, K. (1999). Patient Health Questionnaire-9. https://www.apa.org/depression-guideline/patient-health-questionnaire.pdf

Stathokostas, L., McDonald, M. W., Little, R. M., & Paterson, D. H. (2013). Flexibility of older adults aged 55-86 years and the influence of physical activity. *Journal of Aging Research*. https://doi.org/10.1155/2013/743843

Tivity Health. (2021). Silver Sneakers. https://www.silversneakers.com/learn-more/

Tomita, M., Saharan, S., Rajendran, S., Schweitzer, J., & Nochajski, S. (2014). Development, psychometrics and use of Home Safety Self-Assessment Tool (HSSAT). *American Journal of Occupational Therapy, 68*(6), 711-718.

U.S. Department of Health and Human Services. (2018a). 2018 Physical activity guidelines advisory committee scientific report. https://health.gov/sites/default/files/2019-09/PAG_Advisory_Committee_Report.pdf

U.S. Department of Health and Human Services. (2018b). Physical Activity Guidelines for Americans, 2nd edition. https://health.gov/sites/default/files/2019-09/Physical_Activity_Guidelines_2nd_edition.pdf

van der Zwan, J. E., de Vente, W., Huizink, A. C., Bögels, S. M., & de Bruin, E. I. (2015). Physical activity, mindfulness meditation, or heart rate variability biofeedback for stress reduction: A randomized controlled trial. *Applied Psychophysiology and Biofeedback, 40*(4), 257-268. https://doi.org/10.1007/s10484-015-9293-x

Wang, L. C., Ye, M. Z., Xiong, J, Wang, X. Q., Wu, J. W., Zheng, G. H. (2021). Optimal exercise parameters of tai chi for balance performance in older adults: A meta-analysis. *Journal of the American Geriatric Society, 69*, 2000-2010. https://doi.org/10.1111/jgs.17094

Warburton, D. E. & Bredin, S. S. (2016). Reflections on physical activity and health: What should we recommend? *Canadian Journal of Cardiology, 32*(4), 495-504.

Ware, J. E. & Sherbourne, C. D. (1992). The MOS 36-Item Short-Form Health Survey (SF-36) I. Conceptual framework and item selection. *Medical Care, 30*, 473-483.

Washburn, R. A., Smith, K. W., Jette, A. M., & Janney, C. A. (1993). The physical activity scale for the elderly (PASE): Development and evaluation. *Journal of Clinical Epidemiology, 46*, 153-162.

Whelton, P. K., Carey, R. M., Aronow, W. S., Casey, D. E., Collins, K. J., Himmelfarb, C. D., & Wright, J. T. (2018). 2017 ACC/AHA/AAPA/ABC/ACPM/AGS/APhA/ASH/ASPC/NMA/PCNA guideline for the prevention, detection, evaluation, and management of high blood pressure in adults: A report of the American College of Cardiology/American Heart Association Task Force on Clinical Practice Guidelines. *Journal of the American College of Cardiology, 71*(19), e127-e248.

World Health Organization. (2010). Framework for action on interprofessional education & collaborative practice. https://hsc.unm.edu/ipe/resources/who-framework-.pdf

World Health Organization. (2020). WHO guidelines on physical activity and sedentary behavior. https://apps.who.int/iris/bitstream/handle/10665/336656/9789240015128-eng.pdf?sequence=1&isAllowed=y

Yancik, R., & Ries, L. (2004). Cancer in older persons: An international issue in an aging world. *Seminars in Oncology, 31*, 128-136.

Yao, X., Hu, J., Kong, X., & Zhu, Z. (2021). Association between dietary calcium intake and bone mineral density in older adults. *Ecology of Food and Nutrition, 60*(1), 89-100. https://doi.org/10.1080/03670244.2020.1801432

Yerrakalva, D., Yerrakalva, D., Hajna, S., & Griffin, S. (2019). Effects of mobile health app interventions on sedentary time, physical activity, and fitness in older adults: Systematic review and meta-analysis. *Journal of Medical Internet Research, 21*(11), e14343. https://doi.org/10.2196/14343

Zalewski C. K. (2015). Aging of the Human Vestibular System. *Seminars in Hearing, 36*(3), 175-196. https://doi.org/10.1055/s-0035-1555120

Zigmond, A. S., & Snaith, R. P. (1983). The Hospital Anxiety and Depression Scale. *Acta Psychiatrica Scandinavica, 67*(6), 361-370. https://doi.org/10.1111/j.1600-0447.1983.tb09716.x

Part III

PROMOTING SOCIAL HEALTH

7

CHAPTER

Promoting Social Health

Children and Youth

Julie Kugel, OTD, OTR/L and Jennifer Crews, MA, CCC-SLP

Learning Objectives

At the end of this chapter, the reader will:

1. Be able to define social health and pragmatics (ACOTE B.1.2; SLP CAA Standards 3.1.2B)
2. Explain the five foundational social health categories (ACOTE B.1.2, B.1.3; SLP CAA Standards 3.1.1B)
3. Identify appropriate assessments to address social health (ACOTE B.4.4; SLP CAA Standards 3.1.4B)
4. Explore programming options for the different social health categories (ACOTE B.4.2, B.4.10; SLP CAA Standards 3.1.1B)

The ACOTE Standards used are those from 2018.

Key Words

Adverse Childhood Experiences, Pragmatics, Self-Esteem, Social Anxiety, Social Health

Case Study

Corry was an 11-year-old preteen who was diagnosed with autism at the age of 5. He was also diagnosed with ADHD and social anxiety by the age of 9 years old. He had received speech pathology and occupational therapy services through early intervention as an infant and partially through elementary school. He was often overwhelmed at school and had challenges in navigating the complexity of teacher instruction paired with the social expectations of an academic setting. At the age of 10 years old, Corry's family decided he would best benefit from a hybrid educational model. He was homeschooled as well as attended a unique program at a regional learning academy through his local public school district. The program offered home-based instruction through

Pizzi, M. A., & Amir, M. (Eds.). *Interprofessional Perspectives for Community Practice: Promoting Health, Well-Being, and Quality of Life* (pp. 123-137).

enrichment classes such as writing, chorus, and social skills. It also included resources for students such as time on campus, access to the school library, and social time with friends. Corry was enrolled in two classes on campus and completed the rest of his academic work online at home.

Corry managed well in social situations when interacting with just one person at a time. He used appropriate eye contact, body positioning, and was easily able to engage back and forth in conversation. He had plenty to talk about and initiated different topics of interest and asked appropriate questions when he became confused or was introduced to a topic that was unfamiliar to him. He understood the rules of turn taking in conversations and used active listening. He had great patience, and he knew how to bring humor and wit into his conversations. Because of his ability to use and apply basic social skills easily when interacting with a single person, it took Corry entering his preteen years before a gap in his social skills became noticeable.

When attending the regional learning academy, Corry's parents were expected to be on campus during his classes, either volunteering in the classroom or somewhere nearby. It was during this time on campus that Corry's mother witnessed the reality of her son's social struggles and angst. She watched how his social anxiety amplified when he had to interact with many peers at once. He was unable to follow the course of different conversations occurring simultaneously within small groups. He became flustered, at a loss for words, and felt hopeless and unsuccessful during these interactions. He could not handle when peers approached him in a direct manner, interacted with him quickly, and then walked away. He was unable to respond to the rapid fire of their questions or engage in their small talk. He became overwhelmed, agitated, and would yell or cry. At times he would literally run away from them and hide. This unpredictable behavior created distance and eroded any type of connection between Corry and his peers. Over time, Corry refused to attend his in-person classes, becoming more isolated at home. This was when his mom decided to seek additional help. Her primary concern was his inability to manage more complex social interactions as she observed regularly when he was at school.

Reflective Questions

1. What are the different variables and environments that impact the social health of children and youth?
2. What different variables and environments impacted the social health of Corry as an 11-year-old preteen?
3. What lights up a specific child, what inspires and motivates them, and how can personal motivation be utilized to improve the quality of their social relationships and social health?
4. What inspired and motivated Corry? What medical professional utilized his creative strengths to build positive social emotional health?
5. What resources and programs are available to families to improve a child's social health and well-being?
6. What programs were available for Corry in his community?

Social Health for Children and Youth

Social health is multifaceted and requires an intentional approach to best support the unique needs of youth. Corry struggled with more group based social situations even though he excelled in one-on-one interactions. He did not have the personal capacity to access appropriate social skills across different environments. **Social health** can be defined as the ability to create, sustain, and enjoy meaningful relationships in a variety of environments. These relationships have a substantial impact on our everyday behaviors, physical and mental health, and even our risk of illness and death (Umberson & Montez, 2010). Our feelings and the way we behave are largely impacted by our relationships with others, whether we are with them or not (Csikszentmihalyi, 1997). The quality of social relationships impacts health and well-being in both the short and long term indicating a strong need for public policies and programs to support social health (Umberson & Montez, 2010). Health and well-being are dynamic concepts that integrate mental, physical, and social factors and expand beyond just the absence of disease or illness (World Health Organization [WHO], 1986). Well-being is impacted by the quality of social relationships rather than quantity and having a supportive network can buffer the impact of a difficult relationship (Offer, 2020). Positive social health for youth is impacted by multiple environments including school, home, and the community. These environments can foster healthy relationships that allow emotional growth to take place (Delahooke, 2017) or they may be a source of stress and negativity.

Some scientists believe that emotional and social growth is directly impacted by neuroception (Porges, 2004), which involves the subconscious ability to quickly analyze risk in the environment (flight, fight, or freeze), and identify whether a person is safe and trustworthy or life threatening. For some children, especially those who are vulnerable, neuroception can become switched to the on position, identifying fear and dangers that do not really exist (Delahooke, 2017). An example of this may be a child starting school who defensively hits other children, grabs toys, or is reluctant to join in play, instead of safety this child may be feeling threatened (Delahooke, 2017). This may be impacted by developmental differences, sensory processing disorders, biomedical issues, and high levels of environmental or personal stress (Delahooke, 2017). Feeling safe in one's environment allows for learning, play, and engagement, which is essential for social development in youth (Delahooke, 2017). Observation of negative behaviors may be a cue to focus on neuroception and increase social and environmental support. Stressful environments can lead to maladaptive behaviors, impacting the child's participation and choices of activities.

Toxic stress is characterized by early exposure to chronic trauma and stress that impacts the developing nervous system and can lead to lifelong physical, mental, neurological, emotional, and social challenges (Gronski et al., 2013; Felitti et al., 1998; National Scientific Council on the Developing Child, 2012; Shonkoff et al., 2012). Childhood trauma includes witnessing, experiencing, or being threatened with physical, emotional, or sexual abuse, violence, extreme poverty and food scarcity, caregiver substance abuse, and parental depression (Gronski et al., 2013). Initial evidence identifying adverse childhood experiences (ACEs) and their impact on physical and mental health was first reported in the 1990s (Felitti et al., 1998). Systematic reviews and meta-analyses continue to support and build on that literature by identifying that beyond the physical health implications such as obesity and heart disease, outcomes associated with multiple ACEs include substance abuse, mental illness, and violence, representing a substantial public health crisis for future generations (Hughes et al., 2017).

Research overwhelmingly supports the critical role of early life experiences and that health professionals should be actively engaged in programming to provide preventative social based strategies and resilience building with youth and their families (Hughes et al., 2017). Collaborative, community-based solutions that involve a multidisciplinary team have the potential to profoundly impact the overall social health and well-being of youth and their families (Gronski et al., 2013). Occupational therapy practitioners can serve as members of these teams, focusing specifically on maximizing "health, well-being, and quality of life for all people, populations, and communities through effective solutions that facilitate participation in everyday living" (American Occupational Therapy Association, 2017, p. 1).

To help provide a foundation for understanding the complex and multidimensional factors of social health, the following categories were created by the authors of this chapter as a framework for understanding the literature, assessment, and intervention strategies provided in this chapter:

1. **Self-Esteem/Self-Advocacy:** To have confidence in one's own abilities and be able to speak up and ask for what you need, what you desire, and express what is necessary and important to you for your health and well-being.
2. **Creativity and Personal Expression**: "Creativity is sharing your inner world with the outer world" (Crews, 2014). It's taking personal inspiration and original ideas from within and bringing it out into the world.
3. **Physical Health**: Tuning into the state of your physical well-being and how well your body is functioning for daily living. These areas may include, but are not limited to, mental clarity, movement, balance, energy, mobility, and endurance.

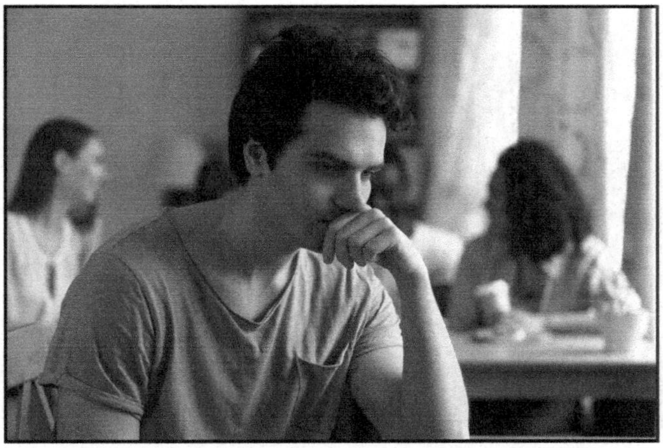

Figure 7-1. The impact of social participation on self-esteem. (iStock)

4. **Relational and Communication Skills**: The ability to interact, engage, communicate, and relate with others.
5. **Personal Values**: Self-determined values that guide one's actions based on what is important to an individual and living with a sense of integrity. For example, participating in environmental conservation, ethnic equality, and social justice.

Self-Esteem in Youth

Self-esteem can be defined as perception of value, worthiness, or an evaluation of self, it is subjective and often influenced by many factors in childhood and adolescence including competence and acceptance (Willoughby et al., 1996). Key factors for the development of high self-esteem across the life span include positive social support, positive relationships, and social acceptance (Figure 7-1; Harris & Orth, 2020). While high self-esteem and positive social support creates a positive loop that can continue throughout life, the opposite is also true for youth with low self-esteem who are more likely to experience poor relationships and decreased social support leading to a negative cycle of self-esteem development (Harris & Orth, 2020). Both negative and positive self-esteem may have a direct impact on resilience, social participation, and quality of life (QOL). Social participation can be defined as "activities that involve social interaction with others, including family, friends, peers, and community members, and that support social interdependence" (Bedell, 2012; Khetani & Coster, 2019; Magasi & Hammel, 2004 as cited in American Occupational Therapy Association, 2020, p. 34), it can be a direct indicator of overall daily functioning and QOL (Orsmond et al., 2013).

QOL for youth is complex and often involves the individual and family environment as well as the larger environment outside of the family including the community, schools, childcare, neighborhoods, and even local and national government policies (Pizzi & Renwick, 2010). Health care professionals can impact social health and self-esteem

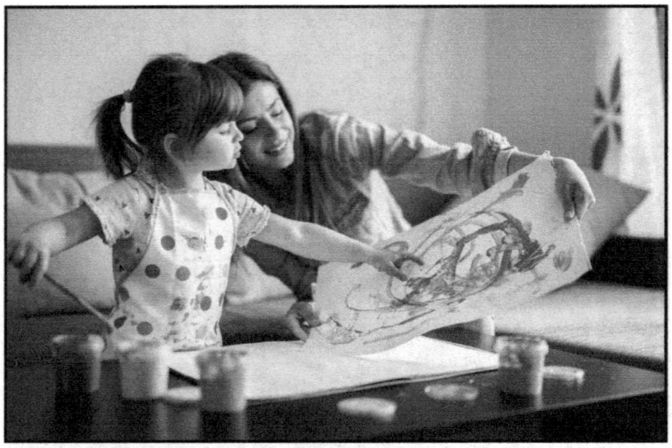

Figure 7-2. The intersection of social skills and creativity. (iStock)

in many different situations. Within the school setting, social participation and positive relationships with teachers and peers are so important that they can either hinder or support the ability to learn and achieve academic success (Leigers et al., 2016). Tinto's theory of departure confirms that attributes of social integration over time are intricately linked to whether or not a student will have success in higher education (1975; Choi et al., 2019). Students with disabilities are more likely to experience social isolation than their same age peers (Orsmond et al., 2013). Social participation can be addressed with initiatives led by occupational therapy practitioners that advocate for more inclusive physical and social environments both at school and in the surrounding community such as local parks, pools, and community centers (Leigers et al., 2016).

Social-emotional competence (SEC) as an outcome of social and emotional learning (SEL) is the ability to control cognitive processes, interact socially with others, and regulate behavior and emotion (Ahmed et al., 2020). These competencies not only promote healthy self-esteem, self-control, and social skills but academic success as well (Ahmed et al., 2020). Youth who are involved in violence often have a lack of social-emotional skills (Ahmed et al., 2020). Classroom students who were taught SEL skills such as understanding feelings and emotions, collaborating and negotiating with others, and learning about self-regulation had a significant difference in SEC as compared to a control group (Ahmed et al., 2020). SEL was developed from a deeper understanding of emotional intelligence (Goleman, 2005), which includes the areas of self-awareness, self-management, social awareness, and relationship management (Goleman, 2005; Bradberry & Greaves, 2009). Early social intervention targeting elementary school children has been shown to produce lasting changes into adulthood, with full intervention consisting of teacher development, child competencies including social skills training, and a parent workshop (Kosterman et al., 2019). With a focus on prosocial behaviors, positive health and well-being outcomes persisted more than 18 years after the intervention was provided (Kosterman et al., 2019).

Creativity and Personal Expression

Programming to teach children empathy skills during the school year found that compared to a control school, cognitive and emotional creative scores increased (78% higher than control), advocating the need for social and emotional learning integration along with the regular curriculum (Demetriou & Nicholl, 2021). The social skill of empathy can be described as "the ability to feel, share, imagine, project, identify, understand, or experience another's perspective through their feelings, thoughts, and actions" (Demetriou & Nicholl, 2021, p. 2). Empathy training for youth appears to be a strategy for not only promoting prosocial skills but also gives a boost in creativity that may lead to improved mental health and well-being (Figure 7-2).

A questionnaire examining children's perceived meaning of their everyday activities found that autonomy, perceived importance, level of challenge, and the perception of time all had an impact on meaning (Rosenberg et al., 2019). Perceived enjoyment of activities was strongly related to perceptions of time and whether it was going slowly or flying by (Rosenberg et al., 2019). Previous research has shown that engagement in creative and meaningful pursuits that are the "just right challenge" promote a feeling of flow that strongly contributes to overall health and well-being (Csikszentmihalyi, 1997; Larson, 2004). This flow is best found in activities such as art, sports, hobbies, and outdoor play that involve challenge, solving problems, and discovery (Csikszentmihalyi, 1997). Active games, sports, hobbies, and socializing provide three times more enjoyment than passive leisure such as television (Csikszentmihalyi, 1997) and yet the amount of time spent in sedentary and screen-based activities continues to increase to over 8 hours per day for many youth (de Moraes Ferrari et al., 2019). Of all screen-based activities, playing video games has been specifically linked to social isolation, social withdrawal, and depression (Guerrero et al., 2019) and higher screen time has been linked to lower self-esteem (Carson et al., 2016).

The combined impact of high screen time and a reduction in green time (time out in nature) may have an impact on mental health and well-being for youth (Oswald et al., 2020) in addition to decreasing overall health and increasing rates of overweight and obesity (Carson et al., 2016). Time spent outdoors not only contributes to the physiological regulation of heart rate and blood pressure, improving positive emotions, and decreasing negative emotions but it has also been shown to significantly improve creative performance and cognitive functioning (Yu & Hsieh, 2020; Williams et al., 2018). Decreasing sedentary time and increasing outdoor time has the potential to improve many areas of health.

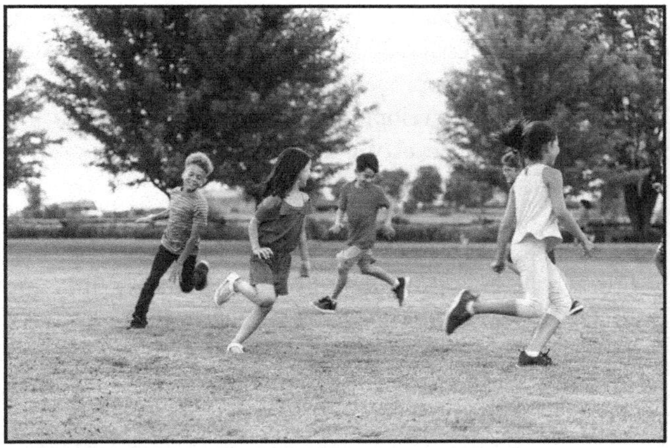

Figure 7-3. Physical health and social well-being. (iStock)

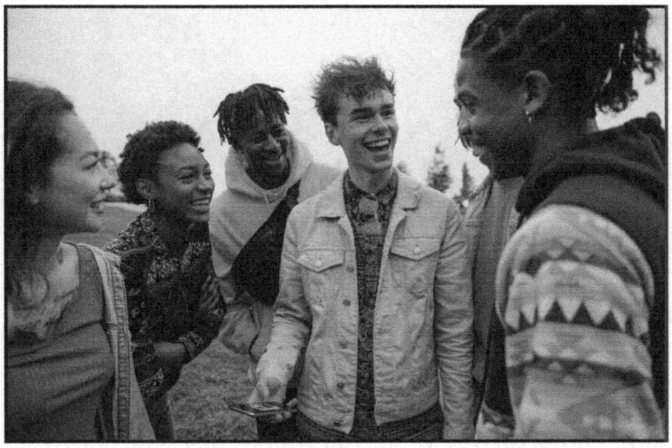

Figure 7-4. Developing social communication skills. (iStock)

Physical Health

Despite an extensive body of literature outlining the important role of physical activity for children, most youth do not get the recommended 60 minutes of exercise per day and rates of obesity in youth continue to increase (Hales et al., 2017; Andrie et al., 2021). Childhood obesity has a profound impact on "children's physical health, social, and emotional well-being, and self-esteem" (Sahoo et al., 2015, p. 187) and is considered a serious public health issue with devastating current and future implications. Anxiety, depression, poor school performance, and the absence of physical activity and sports involvement have all been associated with obesity (Andrie et al., 2021). Research on the recent impact of the COVID-19 lockdowns revealed significant increases in body mass index along with sedentary behaviors and substantial decreases in physical activity (Jia et al., 2021).

Participation in organized sports at school and in the community supports both physical and social well-being (Figure 7-3). A systematic review exploring occupation-based interventions to support positive behavior, mental health, and social participation for youth found strong evidence for sport interventions to support social participation and moderate evidence for yoga (Cahill et al., 2020). Yoga practice has been shown to decrease depression, anxiety, and body image disturbance for youth with eating disorders (Hall et al., 2016). A 14-week karate program for boys with autism spectrum disorder found significant reductions in communication and social skills deficits post-intervention and after a follow-up (Bahrami et al., 2016). In addition, a small feasibility study conducted by an occupational therapist found that taekwondo, a form of martial arts, may increase self-confidence in both physical and social abilities for children who have difficulty with social interaction (Calinog et al., 2021). Research suggests that engagement in physical activity with an emphasis on the mind-body connection, such as martial arts and yoga, is essential for youth as they develop social and emotional regulation skills (Cahill et al., 2020).

Relational and Communication Skills

Parents will first observe communication breakdowns in their child when interacting out in the community. At this point, speech-language pathologists are sought out by families to help with social language skills. It is through the avenue of communication or the lack thereof, where a child's social emotional health and well-being are often first identified. This typically occurs in early childhood or even infancy when the primary concern is around more basic communication within the family unit. The focus at that time is how the child interacts with other family members and can successfully request objects and actions in their environment to get their basic needs met. Families begin to develop a deep understanding of their child's communication at home and can easily work with the child during simple misunderstandings or miscommunications.

As children mature, however, they require more independent skills in social communication that extends beyond the family unit. This requires higher level communication and an overall understanding of how to navigate within a different social framework. This typically occurs around the age of 7 years and up into their preteen and teen years as we saw with Corry in the case study. At a time in life when relationships start to become more complex and multilayered, speech therapists and other health care professionals are approached for a second or third time due to parent's observations of difficult and painful interactions between their child and others in the community. This complexity is often due to the increased expectations in social situations combined with the simultaneous increased academic demands at school.

Social communication is the use of language in social contexts (Figure 7-4). It encompasses four areas—social interaction, social cognition, pragmatics, and language processing. "Social communication skills include the ability to vary speech style, take the perspective of others, understand

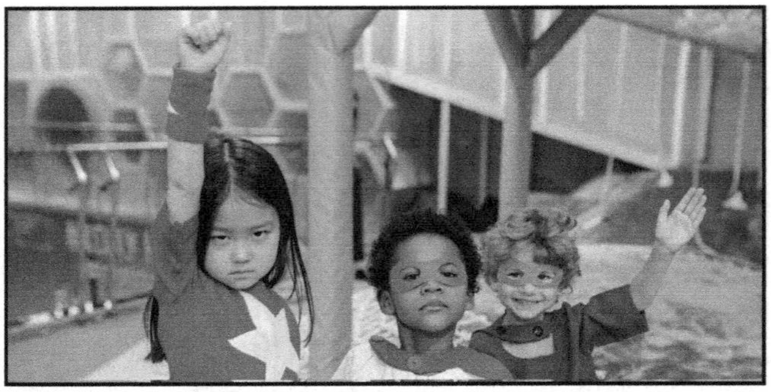

Figure 7-5. Social health and personal values. (iStock)

and appropriately use the rules for verbal and nonverbal communication, and use the structural aspects of language (e.g., vocabulary, syntax, and phonology) to accomplish these goals" (American Speech-Language-Hearing Association, n.d.). **Pragmatics** is one of the four components of social communication. As mentioned earlier, pragmatics are verbal and nonverbal communication skills necessary for positive social health in communication. Adriana Lavi wrote in the Clinical Assessment of Pragmatics (Lavi, 2019, p. 5) manual a brief literature review on the definition of pragmatics:

> Pragmatic language binds together semantics, morphology, syntax, and overall language comprehension and oral expression for the purpose of effective communication. It is the final element necessary for appropriate and effective communication to occur. Any deficit in pragmatics results in significant disruption of the communication process (Norbury, 2014). Hymes simply defines pragmatics as a student knowing when to say what to whom and how much. (Hymes, 1971)

There are many different approaches in best determining a child's strengths in the areas of social communication. These range from parent/teacher report, language sampling, naturalistic observation, peer/self-report, and formal assessments. In a survey of speech-language pathologists, it was determined that best practices for assessing social communication disorders were found in combining different approaches (Izaryk et al., 2021).

When a child is challenged in one or more of these areas of social communication it directly impacts all of their relationships and social interactions. It affects their self-confidence, their ability to build quality relationships, and their ability to maintain positivity in their lives. Any challenge in social communication, no matter what a child's diagnosis, will play a role in a child's social and emotional health and well-being.

Personal Values

Empowering youth to better understand their personal interests to improve meaningful social connections and relationships in all areas of their life is critical for developing strong personal values (Figure 7-5). For health care and school-based professionals it is important to recognize the need for a holistic approach that includes social and emotional health while developing strategies for engagement and involvement at each level of childhood with multicomponent interventions (Sancassiani et al., 2015).

When examined cross-sectionally and longitudinally, social isolation and loneliness increased the risk of mental health problems such as depression and anxiety, in some cases up to 9 years later (Loades et al., 2020). The COVID-19 pandemic caused an abrupt loss of social participation and community engagement for youth and their families within a very short period of time. Most school and community activities were prohibited, and social networks were moved into a virtual format. Virtual social networks present both positive and negative opportunities. An online social network allows youth to connect with family and friends near and far, but it has also been shown to increase the risk of cyberbullying, the risk of addiction, and a loss of privacy (García del Castillo et al., 2020). Online social networks can promote valuable social networks and positively impact health and well-being (García del Castillo et al., 2020). Health professionals have a role in developing these virtual social networks to meet the needs of youth who are increasingly accessing virtual resources. Focusing on the needs of youth and involving them in co-creating these virtual social networks may be a useful strategy for improving meaningful health promotion (García del Castillo et al., 2020). Table 7-1 includes examples of community participation and the impact on social health for self-esteem/self-advocacy, creativity and personal expression, physical health, relational and communication skills, and personal values.

Assessments

Corry's mother was significantly concerned about Corry's overall social communication and the direct impact his lack of skills had on his overall social and emotional health. She contacted Corry's physician, and a referral was made for a speech and language evaluation with an emphasis in social language. Corry started to receive weekly speech therapy sessions through a private practice within his community. Wanting to gain more insight into specifically what aspects of social communication and language were the most problematic for Corry, his new speech therapist asked his mom to fill out the Pragmatics Profile from the Clinical Evaluation of Language Fundamentals–Fourth Edition (CELF-4) assessment (Semel et al., 2003). The Pragmatics Profile provides a detailed in-depth outline of a student's social skills with a checklist of descriptive items in the following three areas:

1. Rituals and Conversational Skills
2. Asking For, Giving, and Responding to Information
3. Nonverbal Communication Skills

Table 7-1

Social Health Examples

CATEGORY	IMPACT ON SOCIAL HEALTH	COMMUNITY PARTICIPATION
Self-esteem/self-advocacy	Being able to ask for needs and wants. Self-esteem may have a direct impact on resilience, social participation, and QOL.	Self-esteem is promoted through engagement in community programs including youth confidence workshops, social skills development, and emotional intelligence training.
Creativity and personal expression	Creative pursuits and time in nature promotes physical health and emotional well-being.	Community theater, arts and crafts classes, music, dance, and outdoor recreation programs allow for creative expression and decrease sedentary time for youth.
Physical health	Sedentary behaviors are directly linked to depression, anxiety, and obesity in youth. Physical activity focusing on the mind-body connection, such as martial arts, and yoga impacts social and emotional regulation.	Local community sports activities are accessible year round. Health professionals can organize events and camps to enhance accessibility and integration.
Relational and communication skills	Social communication includes verbal and nonverbal skills for positive social health. Communication is foundational for positive social health.	Activities to promote communication skills include social skills groups, book clubs, and after school programming.
Personal values	Understanding personal interests allows for a client-centered focus when designing intervention strategies.	Social justice organizations, and conservation/ environmental groups promote civility, positive behavior, integrity, and a healthy lifestyle.

Pragmatic language are social language skills through both verbal communication and nonverbal communication that are used in our daily interactions with others. They are skills necessary for positive social health in communication. "Pragmatic language deficits translate into difficulty with correctly understanding and responding verbally to situations in a social context" (Lavi, 2019, p. 5).

Corry's scores indicated both strengths and weaknesses within all three sections. His strengths were understanding the rules in beginning and ending conversations, understanding jokes and humor, and appropriate communicative use of media such as text, email, and phone. He also excelled at responding well to interruptions and asking appropriate questions. These strengths gave him the tools to easily talk on the phone, text with a friend, and engage one on one with peers and adults in school and at home. These abilities were what carried him through his earlier years. His mother's current concerns became evident when further analyzing the responses on the CELF-4 pragmatics profile.

His scores indicated his greatest obstacles were when communicating in small group situations. He struggled with not knowing how to easily join or leave a group discussion. He was unable to interact in both structured and unstructured group activities and he had difficulty adjusting his speech to match or fit the current situation. This was when Corry would shut down in a conversation. He did not know what to say when agreeing or disagreeing with others and was unable to find the words to ask for clarification from his peers. He had not yet developed skills in knowing what to say to accept or reject invitations from friends, and often misinterpreted their body language and tone of voice in a group setting. Though Corry was a savant at talking with one person at a time, engaging with more than one person was scary and difficult for him and had a negative effect on his overall social, emotional, and mental well-being. In developing approaches to best assist Corry, his team saw strengths and challenges in four out of the five social health categories:

- Self-esteem/Self-advocacy
- Creativity and Personal Expression
- Relational and Communication skills
- Personal Values

They worked within these categories to inspire, motivate, and develop goals and interventions.

Assessing a child's ability in understanding social language, appropriate use of communication skills, levels of social anxiety, and the ability to read social cues in a wide variety of social situations are important key factors to determine what skills are present or absent for a child. The skills that directly affect their success within the context of social health. The following assessments are available across a wide variety of disciplines to best determine a baseline for both therapeutic interventions and/or community-based programming.

Assessments

- **Language Use Inventory**: A standardized parent-report questionnaire to assess pragmatic language in children 18 to 47 months of age. Fourteen subscales assess a child's communication in a wide range of settings for a broad variety of functions. Professional's score. (Pesco & O'Neill, 2012; O'Neill, 2009).
- **Pragmatic Language Skills Inventory (PLSI)**: The Pragmatic Language Skills Inventory (PLSI) is an easy-to-use, norm-referenced rating scale designed to assess children's pragmatic language abilities aged 5 to 0 through 12 to 11. Its 45 items can be administered in only 5 to 10 minutes. The PLSI has three subscales:
  1. Personal Interaction Skills - initiating conversation, asking for help, participating in verbal games, and using appropriate nonverbal communicative gestures.
  2. Social Interaction Skills - knowing when to talk and when to listen, understanding classroom rules, taking turns in conversations, and predicting consequences for one's behavior.
  3. Classroom Interaction Skills - using figurative language, maintaining a topic during conversation, explaining how things work, writing a good story, and using slang appropriately (Gilliam & Miller, 2007).
- **Children's Communication Checklist-2, U.S. Edition (CCC-2)**: A parent or caregiver rating scale based on the extensive research of author, Dr. Dorothy Bishop. CCC-2 helps rate aspects of communication, screens for general language, and identifies pragmatic language impairment for ages 4:0 to 16:11 years (Bishop, 2006).
- **Clinical Evaluation of Language Fundamentals – Fifth Edition (CELF-5)**: The CELF-5 is a flexible system of individually administered tests used to assist a clinician to accurately diagnose a language disorder in children and adolescents ages 5 through 21 years. Using the CELF-5's battery of structured tasks that test the limits of a student's language abilities as well as observation and interaction-based tasks, clinicians can effectively pinpoint a student's strengths and weaknesses to make appropriate placement and intervention recommendations. Test includes Pragmatics Profile and Pragmatics Activities Checklist (Semel, et al., 2013).
- **Test of Pragmatic Language-2 (TOPL-2)**: The TOPL-2 allows you to assess the effectiveness and appropriateness of a student's pragmatic language skills ages 6 to 18 to 11. Administered in approximately 45 to 60 minutes, it tests six core subcomponents of pragmatic language: physical setting, audience, topic, purpose (speech acts), visual-gestural cues, and abstraction (Phelps-Terasaki & Phelps-Gunn, 2007).
- **Clinical Assessment of Pragmatic (CAPS)**: Individually administered performance tests based on digital video scenes. Administered in 45 minutes to 1 hour for all six tests. For ages 7 to 18 years. Standard scores and percentiles for three index scores 1. Pragmatic Judgment 2. Pragmatic Performance 3. Paralinguistic and one overall score - Core Pragmatic Language Composite (Lavi, 2019).
- **Test of Integrated Language & Literacy Skills (TILLS)**: Test of Integrated Language & Literacy Skills is the reliable, valid assessment testing oral and written language skills in students ages 6 to 18 years. TILLS is a comprehensive, norm-referenced test that has been standardized for three purposes: To identify language/literacy disorders, to document patterns of relative strengths and weaknesses, and to track changes in language and literacy skills over time (Nelson et al., 2016).
- **Test of Problem Solving-2 Adolescent (TOPS-2)**: The TOPS 2: Adolescent uses a natural context of problem-solving situations related to adolescent experiences and assesses five different decision-making skill areas critical to academic, problem solving, and social success for ages 12 to 17:1. They include Making Inferences, Determining Solutions, Problem Solving, Interpreting Perspectives, and Transferring Insights (Bowers, et al., 2007).
- **Social Emotional Evaluation (SEE)**: The Social Emotional Evaluation (SEE) evaluates the social skills and higher-level language that students need to interact successfully in everyday situations at home, school, and in the community for ages 6 to 12:11.

The SEE presents typical social situations and common emotional reactions that elementary and middle school students frequently encounter. It is ideal for identifying social and emotional language needs of students with autism spectrum disorders, emotional disorders, learning disabilities, or attention deficit disorders (Wiig, 2008).

- **The Social Language Development Test–Elementary: Normative Update (SLDT-E: NU)** assesses language-based skills of social interpretation and interaction with friends, the skills found to be most predictive of social language development. Specifically, it measures the language required to appropriately infer and express what another person is thinking or feeling within a social context, to make multiple interpretations, take mutual perspectives, and negotiate with and support their peers. For ages 6 to 0 through 11 to 11. The test has four subtests, which require students to make inferences, interpret photographed scenes, and explain how they would resolve problems with peers (Bowers et al., 2016).
- **The Social Language Development Test–Adolescent: Normative Update (SLDT-A: NU)** assesses language-based social skills. Specifically, it measures students' ability to make inferences, and interpret and respond to social interaction for ages 12 to 0 through 17 to 11. The test has five subtests: Making Inferences, Interpreting Social Language, Problem Solving, Social Interpretation, and Interpreting Ironic Statements (Bowers et al., 2017).
- **Roberts Version of the UCLA Loneliness Scale**: This assessment measures how frequently an individual feels lonely and disconnected from others and was developed

to be used with adolescents. There is an 8-item short version that has been more widely studied with youth as well as a 20-item long version (Roberts et al., 1993).

- **KINDL Quality of Life Instrument**: This health-related QOL measure has been studied with a variety of populations and international groups and can be used with ages 3+ (Ravens-Sieberer & Bullinger, 1998).
- **The Peds QL**: This assessment measures health-related QOL with a brief parent and child instrument. It takes less than 4 minutes to complete, and it is considered reliable and valid to be used with ages 2 to 18 (Varni et al., 2001).
- **Social Connectedness Scale (SCS-R)**: This scale measures concepts of belonging, connectedness, and interpersonal closeness with an emphasis on the independent self (Lee et al., 2001).
- **The Children's Hope Scale (CHS)**: This scale is a six-item self-report measure that explores children's perception of whether or not their goals can be met. Internal consistency ranged from 0.72 to 0.86 (Snyder et al., 1997).
- **Coopersmith Self-Esteem Inventory:** Measures self-concept and intrapersonal competencies, there are five sub scores and an overall self-esteem score. This inventory has norm referenced scores and both a long and short form (Potard, 2017).
- **Social Anxiety Scale for Children-Revised (SASC-R)**: This 18-item self-assessment scale is specifically designed to examine the connection between social anxiety and youth friendships, peer relations, and social functioning. Higher levels of social anxiety are closely related difficulty with social functioning (La Greca & Lopez, 1998).
- **Pizzi Health and Wellness Assessment (PHWA)**: This self-assessment rates six categories of health including social, physical, family, occupational, emotional, and spiritual health. It is based on the premise that what we do every day impacts our health and well-being in a profound way. Intraclass correlation analysis showed good reliability (Serwe et al., 2019).
- **Work and Social Adjustment Scale for Youth**: This five-item scale is a self-report completed by youth that examines everyday activities and relationships within the context of how people behave, think or feel. There is also a parent version of the scale (De Los Reyes et al., 2019).

Interventions and Programs Promoting Social Health

In developing an intervention plan to assist Corry in his emotional and social health, his speech therapist decided to focus on Corry's strengths. Corry was extremely creative and talented. For example, Corry designed and created videos through an online app lip syncing his favorite songs and adding props and cartoon characters to his videos. He loved to take scenes from movies and rewrite them. He recreated each scene by adding new characters and developing new scenarios. He would write different endings to well-known movies for fun. When Corry was involved in creating or designing, he thrived. His speech therapist used these creative outlets and paired them with Corry's current social skill strengths as a springboard to improving his group pragmatic skills. Identifying Corry's passion for creativity was the gateway to moving him closer to learning and developing higher level social communication skills.

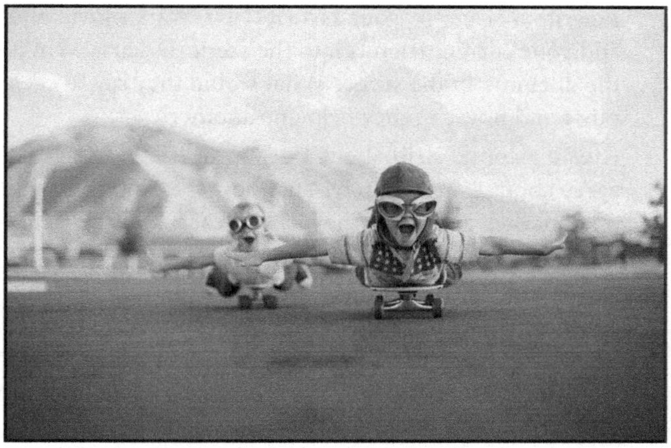

Figure 7-6. Developing social confidence. (iStock)

In order to do this, Corry, with the guidance of his therapist, developed three long-term goals that would help him be successful in group interactions:

1. Increase his communicative confidence.
2. Participate in a social skills group with at least three other peers.
3. Enroll in a large group activity.

His first long-term goal was to increase his communicative confidence. By strengthening this inner social muscle, he would eventually feel successful in approaching new people and making friends thus reducing his current isolation. As a result of this confidence, attending classes on campus would be less daunting. It would also promote self-advocacy both at school and at home and eventually be used when interviewing for future jobs and careers. Communicative confidence is a powerful cornerstone to an improved QOL. His therapist organized different activities that would focus on learning clarification skills, how to approach others, building vocabulary for better language use in collaboration skills, and developing ways to express himself nonverbally. Here are examples of the activities Corry focused on to meet his first long term goal of increasing communicative confidence (Figure 7-6):

- Plan a birthday party by assigning tasks to family members and friends. Make a list of action steps and items needed for the party. Collaborate with family members.

- Rewrite a scene in your favorite Star Wars movie and add your current friends into the scene. Discuss what is the dilemma in the scene? What would they say to each other and how can they help one another?
- Create a comic strip about a group of friends that disagree about something. Discuss how they interact with one another and what they say to each other. Discuss how they can say things differently.
- Watch your favorite movie with the sound off. Explore the body language of the main characters. What is their body language telling you? Discuss how they could change their body language to express something differently.
- Plan a family vacation. Take a survey of family members to determine their interests and where they would want to go.

Corry was highly motivated to complete these activities. He made the most progress in learning how to request clarification from others. He learned to repeat back to them what he heard and then ask, "Is this what you said?" and then give a final response of "Oh that's great, that will work well." or "I'm not understanding. Can you tell me that again?" He also gained confidence in reading the body language of his family members. His family responded positively to his new level of organization in planning activities, and this reenforced a natural safer space for him to communicate. He was therefore more at ease to engage because he could anticipate a level of communicative success, thus increasing his overall self-esteem. Through this first goal it became evident where Corry needed continued guidance; it was how he approached others. He was very task-driven, so he would approach his friends and family abruptly and immediately launch into his questions or the task at hand. This harsh approach was startling to his listeners and needed to be addressed. His therapist worked with him to have a gentler approach and to greet others first before diving into his agenda.

His second long-term goal was to participate in a social skills group with three other peers. To meet this goal Corry enrolled in an 8-week summer program held at the private practice where he attended his weekly speech sessions. The different skills targeted in this program included developing and growing friendships and identifying social blockers. This involved learning what behaviors help promote better connections with others such as approachability versus behaviors that may block the development of forming and maintaining friendships. Other topics included teamwork and sportsmanship and how to handle expected vs. unexpected words or actions from others. Lastly, the program covered the topics of conversational tools and conflict management in peer-, family-, and employment-related dynamics.

To encompass all these skills, a few of the many activities Corry participated in throughout the 8-week program are as follows:

- As a team, design something made with Legos. Work together to build it. Give a presentation to the therapist and parents about the design and how you made it.
- Using three different-sized large therapy balls, sit in a circle as a group and discuss various age-appropriate school based or family-based problems. Work as a team to determine if each one is a small, big, or huge problem. Each ball represents the different sizes. Once the team is in agreement as to the actual size of the problem, toss that particular sized ball around while developing a solution together.
- Write a brief play together on friendship. Assign roles, costumes, and lines. Perform the play for the therapist and parents.

Corry really shined during the summer program. The small group gave him an opportunity to apply the skills he learned in building his communicative confidence with his family and familiar individuals and then bridging those same skills into interactions with new and unfamiliar peers. His biggest challenge was navigating unexpected behaviors, words, and actions of the other members in the group. Their unpredictability was rattling at times for Corry. This is a common occurrence for many individuals learning social skill development. To be able to stay centered despite the unpredictability of others in one's environment cannot be emphasized enough as a precursor to strong social emotional health. Corry required consistent guidance in controlling his own words and actions while offering compassion for others in the group when they had difficulty controlling theirs.

Corry's third and last long-term goal was to enroll in a large group activity and attend it to full completion. Corry reported he was both excited and nervous about this goal. He knew he wanted to be with lots of his peers in one setting but was weary that he could maintain the interactions across an extended period of time. He knew his default was to shut down and then run and hide. Corry decided on his own to join his school's chorus. This was an easy transition for Corry because he could engage with his peers briefly in the beginning of class and then not have to communicate with them while they were singing. Everyone faced the same direction with all eyes on the chorus instructor, so he was not as overwhelmed with reading body language or facial expressions. Corry did on occasion have a few setbacks. Instead of running and hiding like before, he would just sit down in the middle of a conversation and cover his face with his hands. This was an improvement, because it provided his conversational partners with a question and by Corry remaining in close proximity gave them opportunities to help him. His peers were often willing to repair these communication breakdowns when he stayed physically within reach than when he would withdraw. Every week he reported back to his speech therapist as to what skills still needed developing and reflected on what social applications were learned and were deemed successful from his previous two goals.

One day Corry's school chorus was unexpectedly invited to sing for a local community theater. This particular event tested new opportunities for Corry. Though his family was concerned that it would be too overwhelming, he felt confident he could do it. Corry used previous reflection skills to remind his family of all the plays and scenes he had written over the years. He highlighted his skill in creating his own version of lyrics to various musicals and plays. He often shared these video creations with his peers in his social group as well as in his chorus class. They loved it and often gave him positive feedback and reinforcement. This naturally built his communication confidence. Corry proved to his family he could do it and successfully sang with his classmates at the local theater. Corry met his final goal. He attended a large group activity and completed the entire season.

In achieving all three long-term goals Corry demonstrated the ability to apply newly developed pragmatic skills across various settings. Though he still had occurrences of communication breakdowns when leaving or entering a group situation and ongoing challenges in reading the body language of people in a large group context, he was stronger and more confident in his approaches.

Participation in a social skills group, an active member of his school chorus, and a novice actor in his local community theater are just a few community-based programs that Corry was able to utilize and access. Fortunately, there are a wide variety of programs and interventions currently available to better establish social health for children and youth. The examples, listed under the five categories mentioned earlier, offer a variety of ideas for intervention and programming. Some of the programs could easily be listed under more than one category. The primary aspect in which the program or intervention targets was utilized to determine its main category. It is important to remember that when one or more of these five categories is out of balance, blocked, disrupted, disturbed, shut down, or dismissed, a child's overall social health is in jeopardy. It is our job as health professionals to observe these components in every child that crosses our path. To honor and recognize the gaps that may be occurring specific to every individual, which is not specific to a diagnosis.

1. **Self-Esteem/Self-Advocacy**
   - Emotional Intelligence Training for Children/Youth classes as well as certification programs are online through a variety of sources. Both self-paced and small group interactive are available.
   - Self-Esteem Training: Virtual youth confidence workshops and Youth Empowerment services are available online. Typically offered in small groups, interactive with 10 to 12 students.
   - Friendship Skills Development Programs: Online curriculums are available as well as online interactive programs. Check with local psychologists or speech pathologists for in person group programs.
   - Employment/Self Leadership: Interactive leadership training programs available online. Employment agencies for disabilities as well as the Department of Labor offer resources for classes and training.
   - Childhood Obesity: Local and national coalitions are available for membership. Advocacy training is available through the National Institute for Children's Health Quality in partnership with the Robert Wood Johnson Foundation and the American Academy of Pediatrics.
   - Anti-bullying initiatives: STOMP Out Bullying is a national nonprofit working to prevent and reduce all types of bullying. Campaigns and resources can be viewed online as well as a help chat line for kids and teens.
2. **Creativity and Personal Expression**
   - Community group classes: Art, writing, dance, music, pottery, and painting are often offered through local parks, community colleges, and recreation programs.
   - Craft classes are available at local craft stores such as Michael's as well as online.
   - Community theater and education programs provide year-round events and workshops.
   - Photography, videography, and media arts classes may be available at local community organizations, through local artists, and online.
3. **Physical Health**
   - Taekwondo and martial arts to support social and physical health.
   - Community gardens and farmers markets provide an opportunity for social interaction that may reinforce healthy eating habits.
   - Local Beekeepers' Association welcomes youth to events and workshops.
   - Local community sports are typically accessible year-round for a variety of athletic levels.
   - Yoga/Meditation/Mindfulness classes: there are many available YouTube videos and websites that provide free resources as well as local studios offering classes.
   - Summer and day camps may emphasize a specific skills/sport or provide a variety of fun activities to keep youth busy during the summer months.
   - The American Hiking Association helps to locate nearby trails as well as local groups and events.
4. **Relational and Communication Skills**
   - Social Skills groups are often offered both in person and virtually through private therapy clinics, public schools, and various national associations. These groups are typically led by a speech therapist, occupational therapist, psychologist, social worker, special education teacher, or guidance counselor. Other

resources are area human services agencies as well as nonprofit organizations.
- Social Emotional Health programs can be located through local mental health agencies.
- After school programs such as school paper, school podcast, or classroom blog are opportunities for strengthening communication.
- Boys & Girls Clubs of America is a national organization of local chapters that provide after-school programs.
- Community Robotics Programs can be located through 4-H clubs, after-school programs, summer camps, universities, and young engineer organizations. Online courses are available as well as nationwide robotic competitions.
- Book clubs for teens are offered through local libraries, community centers, and afterschool programs.
- Gaming clubs are available through a wide variety of resources. These include after school programs, online clubs for competitive gaming, cyber clubs through toy and gaming companies and online gaming design and development classes.

5. **Personal Values**
   - Executive Functioning Skills Program: Online curriculums are available as well as online interactive programs. Check with local learning centers, counselors, occupational therapists, or speech pathologists for in person group programs.
   - Journaling and writing courses are offered through bookstores, local libraries, community centers, community colleges as well as online classes.
   - Local conservation groups for nature and animal activism are local chapters that offer conservation programs for children such as the Sierra Club, the National Wildlife Foundation, and the Children and Nature Network to name just a few.
   - Recycling Programs can be found through school-based programs and nonprofit organizations. More resources can also be found through the Department of Energy and the Department of Ecology.
   - Social Justice organizations: The Be Kind People Project online offers resources for classrooms and communities that reinforces concepts of positive behavior, academic improvement, healthy lifestyles, and values of civility.

The next school year Corry substituted participation in chorus with joining his community theater. He surprised his entire family and therapeutic team with expanding his participation in school. He enrolled in more on campus classes, and more importantly, self-initiated auditioning for the local community theater. He practiced his audition during speech therapy, and he even requested input from his peers in the social group. Corry nailed his audition and got a small talking part in the play where he had three lines. This was a huge boost to his overall self-esteem and emotional health. He had accomplished more than he earlier believed was possible. He invited everyone from the social skills group to join his friends and family at the play.

Watching Corry on stage, emphasized the incredible achievement of accessing community services and programs, setting goals, and utilizing inner motivation and personal inspiration to move beyond obstacles and fears for improved social health. Corry was now able to move forward in expanding his own opportunities in the community fully empowered to embrace and maintain his own positive social emotional health. Social health and well-being requires the involvement of many disciplines and professionals working together. Seeing one's discipline as its own isolated entity when it comes to working with children and youth is nonproductive. It instead requires a recognition that professionals collaborate not only with a child's family and multidisciplinary team but also with a child's community-based programs.

Conclusion

The topic of social health for youth becomes increasingly more important with a deeper understanding of how our daily social interactions impact our health and well-being, both positively and negatively. It is easy to assume that different areas of health are more important to well-being. But when we are able to examine social health within a foundational context as in this chapter, we are able to see that positive social health promotes well-being, improves learning and academic participation, and decreases obesity and a host of other physical problems. Social health is also vitally important to self-esteem and self-concept, laying a foundation that can last throughout the life span. An interdisciplinary approach for youth ensures that collaboration is holistic, client-centered, and goal-specific.

Promoting social health for youth requires intentionally seeking out opportunities for collaboration with teams of health professionals and community agencies. Social health includes a complex and dynamic interaction between the person, community and the five categories described in this chapter: **Self-Esteem/Self-Advocacy, Creativity and Personal Expression, Physical Health, Relational and Communication Skills**, and **Personal Values**. It is essential to view each individual with a holistic lens understanding that through diverse approaches we can strengthen the social health of youth both today and for future generations.

References

Ahmed, I., Hamzah, A. B., & Abdullah, M. N. L. Y. B. (2020). Effect of social and emotional learning approach on students' social emotional competence. *International Journal of Instruction, 13*(4), 663-676. https://doi.org/10.29333/iji.2020.13441a

American Occupational Therapy Association. (2017). Vision 2025. *American Journal of Occupational Therapy, 71*, 7103420010. https://doi.org/10.5014/ajot.2017.713002

American Occupational Therapy Association (2020). Occupational therapy practice framework: Domain and process. (4th ed.) *American Journal of Occupational Therapy, 74*, 7412410010. https://doi.org/10.5014/ajot.2020.74S2001

American Speech-Language-Hearing Association (n.d.). Social Communication Disorder. (Practice Portal). https://www.asha.org/Practice-Portal/Clinical-Topics/Social-Communication-Disorder/

Andrie, E. K., Melissourgou, M., Gryparis, A., Vlachopapadopoulou, E., Michalacos, S., Renouf, A., Sergentanis, T. N., Bacopoulou, F., Karavanaki, K., Tsolia, M., Tsitsikam, A. (2021). Psychosocial factors and obesity in adolescence: A case-control study. *Children, 308*(8). https://doi.org/10.3390/children8040308

Bahrami, F., Movahedi, A., Marandi, S. M., & Sorensen, C. (2016). The effect of karate techniques training on communication deficit of children with autism spectrum disorders. *Journal of Autism and Developmental Disorders, 46*, 978-986. https://doi: 10.1007/s10803-015-2643-y

Bishop, D. (2006). *Children's Communication Checklist-2 | U.S. Edition. (CCC-2): Manual*. Pearson.

Bowers, L., Huisingh, R., & LoGiudice, C. (2007). *Test of Problem Solving 2: Adolescent: (TOPS-2: A): Examiners manual*. PRO-ED.

Bowers, L., Huisingh, R., & LoGiudice, C. (2016). *The Social Language Development Test–Elementary: Normative Update (SLDT-E: NU): Examiners manual*. PRO-ED.

Bowers, L., Huisingh, R., & LoGiudice, C. (2017). *The Social Language Development Test–Adolescent: Normative Update (SLDT-A: NU): Examiners manual*. PRO-ED.

Bradberry, T., & Greaves, J. (2009). *Emotional intelligence 2.0*. Talent Smart.

Cahill, S. M., Egan, B. E., & Seber, J. (2020). Activity and occupation-based interventions to support mental health, positive behavior, and social participation for children and youth: A systematic review. *American Journal of Occupational Therapy, 74*, 7402180020. https://doi.org/10.5014/ajot.2020.038687

Calinog, M., Kugel, J. D., Krpalek, D., & Salamat, A. (2021). The feasibility of taekwondo for addressing social interaction and social participation in children. *Open Journal of Occupational Therapy, 9*(2), 1-13, https://doi.org/10.15453/2168-6408.1768

Carson, V., Hunter, S., Kuzik, N., Gray, C. E., Poitras, V. J., Chaput, J-P., Saunders, T. J., Katzmarzyk, P. T., Okely, A. D., Gorber, S. C., Kho, M. E., Sampson, M., Lee, H., & Tremblay, M. S. (2016). Systematic review of sedentary behaviour and health indicators in school-aged children and youth: An update. *NRC Research Press, 41*(6), S240-S265. https://doi: 10.1139/apnm-2015-0630

Choi, A. N., Curran, G. M., Morris, E. J., Salem, A. M., Curry, B. D., Flowers, S. K. (2019). Pharmacy students' lived experiences of academic difficulty and Tinto's theory of student departure. *American Journal of Pharmaceutical Education 83*(10), 2150-2160. https:// 10.5688/ajpe7447

Council on Academic Accreditation in Audiology and Speech-Language Pathology. (2020). Standards for accreditation of graduate education programs in audiology and speech-language pathology (2017). http://caa.asha.org/wp-content/uploads/Accreditation-Standards-for-Graduate-Programs.pdf

Crews, J. (2014). The power of creativity. In D. J. Synder (Eds.), *Ignite calm: Achieving bliss in your work*. (pp. 125-128). Norlights Press.

Csikszentmihalyi, M. (1997). *Finding flow: The psychology of engagement in everyday life*. Basic Books.

De Los Reyes, A., Makol, B. A., Racz, S. J., Youngstrom, E. A., Lerner, M. D., & Keeley, L. M. (2019). The work and social adjustment scale for youth: A measure for assessing youth psychosocial impairment regardless of mental health status. *Journal of Child and Family Studies, 28*, 1-16. https://doi.org/10.1007/s10826-018-1238-6

de Moraes Ferrari, G. L., Pires, C., Solé, D., Matsudo, V., Katzmarzyk, P. T., Fisberg, M. (2019). Factors associated with objectively measured total sedentary time and screen time in children aged 9-11 years. *Jornal de Pediatria, 95*(1), 94-105. https://doi.org/10.1016/j.jped.2017.12.003

Delahooke, M. (2017). *Social and emotional development in early intervention: A skills guide for working with children*. PESI Publishing & Media.

Demetriou, H., & Nicholl, B. (2021). Empathy is the mother of invention: Emotion and cognition for creativity in the classroom. *Improving Schools*, 1-18, https://doi.org/10.1177/1365480221989500

Felitti, V. J., Anda R. F., Nordenberg, D., Williamson, D. F., Spitz, A. M., Edwards, V., Koss, M. P., & Marks, J. S. (1998). Relationship of childhood abuse and household dysfunction to many of the leading causes of death in adults: The Adverse Childhood Experiences (ACE) Study. *American Journal of Preventive Medicine, 14*, 245-258. https://doi.org/10.1016/s0749-3797(98)00017-8.

García del Castillo, J. A., García del Castillo-López, Dias, P. C., & García-Castillo, F. (2020). Social networks as tools for the prevention and promotion of health among youth. *Psicologia: Reflexão e Crítica, 33*(13). https://doi.org/10.1186/s41155-020-00150-z

Gilliam, J., & Miller, L. (2007). *Pragmatic Language Skills Inventory (PLSI)*. PRO-ED.

Goleman, D. (2005). *Emotional intelligence: Why it can matter more than IQ*. Bantam Dell.

Gronski, M. P., Bogan, K. E., Kloeckner, J., Russell-Thomas, D., Taff, S. D., Walker, K. A., & Berg, C. (2013). The Issue Is—Childhood toxic stress: A community role in health promotion for occupational therapists. *American Journal of Occupational Therapy, 67*, e148–e153. http://dx.doi.org/10.5014/ajot.2013.008755

Guerrero, M. D., Barnes, J. D., Chaput, J-L., Tremblay, M. S. (2019). Screen time and problem behaviors in children: Exploring the mediating role of sleep duration. *International Journal of Behavioral Nutrition and Physical Activity, 105*(16). https://doi.org/10.1186/s12966-019-0862-x

Hales, C. M., Carrol, M. D., Fryar, C. D., & Ogden C. L. (2017). Prevalence of obesity among adults and youth: United States, 2015-2016. U.S. Department of Health and Human Services. NCHS Data Brief, No. 288.

Hall, A., Ofei-Tenkorang, N. A., Machan, J., & Gordon, C. M. (2016). Use of yoga in outpatient eating disorder treatment: A pilot study. *Journal of Eating Disorders, 4*, 38. https://doi.org/10.1186/s40337-016-0130-2

Harris, M. A., & Orth U. (2020). The link between self-esteem and social relationships: A meta-analysis of longitudinal studies. *Journal of Personality and Social Psychology, 119*(6), 1459-1477. http://dx.doi.org/10.1037/pspp0000265

Hughes, K., Bellis, M. A., Hardcastle, K. A., Sethi, D., Butchart, A., Milton, C., Jones, L., Dunne, M. P. (2017). The effect of multiple adverse childhood experiences on health: A Systematic review and meta-analysis. *Lancet Public Health, 2*(8), e356-e366. https://doi.org/10.1016/S2468-2667(17)30118-4

Hymes, D. (1971). On communicative competence. In J. Pride & J. Holmes (Eds.), *Sociolinguistics*. Penguin.

Izaryk, K., Edge, R., & Lechwar, D. (2021). A survey of speech-language pathologists' approaches to assessing social communication disorders in children. *Perspectives - SIG 1 Language Learning and Education Perspectives Forum on Social Communication: Clinical Practice Issues, 6*(1), 1-17, https://doi.org/10.1044/2020_PERSP-20-00147

Jia, P., Zhang, L., Yu, W., Yu, B., Liu, M., Zhang, D., & Yang, S. (2021). Impact of COVID-19 lockdown on activity patterns and weight status among youths in China: The COVID-19 impact on lifestyle change survey (COINLICS). *International Journal of Obesity, 45*, 695-699. https://doi.org/10.1038/s41366-020-00710-4

Kosterman, R., Hawkins, J. D., Hill, K. G., Bailey, J. A., Catalano, R. F., & Abbott, R. D. (2019). Effects of social development intervention in childhood on adult life at ages 30 to 39. *Prevention Science, 20*, 986-995. https://doi.org/10.1007/s11121-019-01023-3

La Greca, A. M., & Lopez, N. (1998). Social anxiety among adolescents: Linkages with peer relations and friendships. *Journal of Abnormal Child Psychology, 26*(2), 83-94.

Larson, E. A. (2004). The time of our lives: The experience of temporality in occupation. *Canadian Journal of Occupational Therapy, 71*, 24-35. https://doi.org/10.1177/000841740407100107

Lavi A. (2019). *Clinical Assessment of Pragmatics (CAPs) [Manual]*. Western Psychological Services.

Lee, R. M., Draper, M., & Lee, S. (2001). Social connectedness, dysfunctional interpersonal behaviors, and psychological distress: Testing a mediator model. *Journal of Counseling Psychology, 48*(3), 310-318. https://doi.org/10.1037//0022-0167.48.3.310

Leigers, K., Myers, C., & Schneck, C. (2016). Social participation in schools: A survey of occupational therapy practitioners. *American Journal of Occupational Therapy, 70*, 7005280010. http://dx.doi.org/10.5014/ajot.2016.020768

Loades, M. E., Chatburn, E., Higson-Sweeney, N., Reynolds, S., Shafran, R., Brigden, A., Linney, C, McManus, M. N., Borwick, C., & Crawley, E. (2020). Rapid systematic review: The impact of social isolation and loneliness on the mental health of children and adolescents in the context of COVID-19. *Journal of the American Academy of Child & Adolescent Psychiatry, 59*(11), 1218-1239. https://doi: 10.1016/j.jaac.2020.05.009

National Scientific Council on the Developing Child. (2012). The science of neglect: The persistent absence of responsive care disrupts the developing brain (Working Paper 12). http://developingchild.harvard.edu/index.php/resources/reports_and_working_papers/working_papers/wp12/

Nelson, N., Plante, E., Helm-Estabrooks, N., & Hotz, G. (2016). *Test of Integrated Language & Literacy Skills (TILLS): Examiners manual*. Brookes Publishing.

Norbury C. (2014). Practitioner review: Social (pragmatic) communication disorder conceptualization, evidence and clinical implications. *Journal of Child Psychology and Psychiatry, 55*, 204-216.

O'Neill, D. K. (2009). *LUI Manual*. Knowledge in Development, Inc.

Offer, S. (2020). They drive me crazy: Difficult social ties and subjective well-being. *Journal of Health and Social Behavior, 61*(4), 418-436. https://doi.org/10.1177/002214652095276

Orsmond, G. I., Shattuck, P. T., Cooper B. P., Sterzing, P. R., & Anderson, K. A. (2013). Social participation among young adults with an autism spectrum disorder. *Journal of Autism and Developmental Disorders, 43*, 2710-2719. http://dx.doi.org/10.1007/s10803-013-1833-8

Oswald, T. K., Rumbold, A. R., Kedzior, S. G. E., & Moore, V. M. (2020). Psychological impacts of "screen time" and "green time" for children and adolescents: A systematic scoping review. *PLOS ONE* 15(9). e0237725. https://doi.org/10.1371/journal.pone.0237725

Pesco, D., & O'Neill, D. K. (2012). Predicting later language outcomes from the Language Use Inventory. *Journal of Speech, Language and Hearing Research, 55*, 421-434.

Phelps-Terasaki & Phelps-Gunn. (2007). *Test of Pragmatic Language-2* (TOPL-2) (2nd ed.). PRO-ED.

Pizzi, M. A., & Renwick, R. (2010). Quality of life and health promotion. In M. E. Scaffa, S. M. Reitz, & M. A. Pizzi (Eds.), *Occupational therapy in the promotion of health and wellness*. (pp. 122-134). F. A. Davis Company.

Porges, S. W. (2004). Neuroception: A subconscious system for detecting threats and safety. *Zero to Three, 24*(5), 19-24.

Potard, C. (2017). Self-esteem inventory (Coopersmith). In V. Zeigler-Hill, & T. K. Shackelford (Eds.), *Encyclopedia of personality and individual differences*. Springer International Publishing. https://doi.org/10.1007/978-3-319-28099-8_81-1

Ravens-Sieberer, U., & Bullinger, M. (1998). Assessing health related quality of life in chronically ill children with the German KINDL: First psychometric and content-analytical results. *Quality of Life Research, 7*(5), 399-407. https://doi.org/10.1023/a:1008853819715

Roberts, R. E., Lewinsohn, P. M., & Seeley, J. R. (1993). A brief measure of loneliness suitable for use with adolescents. *Psychological Reports, 72*, 1379-1391.

Rosenberg, L., Pade, M., Reizis, H., & Bar, M. A. (2019). Associations between meaning of everyday activities and participation among children. *American Journal of Occupational Therapy, 73*(6). 7306205030. https://doi.org/10.5014/ajot.2019.032508

Sahoo, K., Sahoo, B., Choudhury, A. K., Sofi, N. Y., Kumar, R., & Bhadoria, A. S. (2015). Childhood obesity: Causes and consequences. *Journal of Family Medicine and Primary Care, 4*(2), 187-192. https://doi: 10.4103/2249-4863.154628

Sancassiani, F., Pintus, E., Holte, A., Paulus, P., Moro, M. F., Cossu, G., Angermeyer, M. C., Carta, M. G., & Lindert J. (2015). Enhancing the emotional and social skills of the youth to promote their well-being and positive development: A systematic review of universal school-based randomized controlled trials. *Clinical Practice & Epidemiology in Mental Health, 11*, 21-40. https://doi.org/10.2174/1745017901511010021

Semel, E., Wiig, E. H., & Secord, W. A. (2003) Clinical Evaluation of Language Fundamentals - Fourth Edition (CELF - 4). The Psychological Corporation. Pearson.

Semel, E., Wiig, E. H., & Secord, W. A. (2013). *Clinical evaluation of language fundamentals* (5th ed.). The Psychological Corporation. Pearson.

Serwe, K. M., Walmsley, A. L. E., & Pizzi, M. A. (2019). Reliability and responsiveness of the Pizzi Health and Wellness Assessment. *Annals of International Occupational Therapy, 3*(1), https://doi.org/10.3928/24761222-20190910-04

Shonkoff, J. P., … Garner, A. S.; Committee on Psychosocial Aspects of Child and Family Health; Committee on Early Childhood, Adoption, and Dependent Care; Section on Developmental and Behavioral Pediatrics. (2012). The lifelong effects of early childhood adversity and toxic stress. *Pediatrics, 129*, e232-e246. https://doi.org/10.1542/peds.2011-2663

Snyder, C. R., Hoza, B., Pelham, W. E., Rapoff, M., Ware, L., Danovsky, M., Highberger, L., Rubinstein, H., & Stahl, K. J. (1997). The development and validation of the children's hope scale. *Journal of Pediatric Psychology, 22*(3), 399-421, https://doi.org/10.1093/jpepsy/22.3.399

Tinto, V. (1975). Dropout from higher education: A theoretical synthesis of recent research. *Review of Educational Research,* (45), 89-125. https://doi.org/10.3102/00346543045001089

Umberson, D., & Montez, J. K. (2010). Social relationships and health: A flashpoint for health policy. *Journal of Health and Social Behavior, 51*(S), S54-S66. https://doi.org/10.1177/0022146510383501

Varni, J. W., Seid, M., & Kurtin, P. S. (2001). The PedsQL 4.0: Reliability and validity of the Pediatric Quality of Life Inventory Version 4.0 Core Scales in healthy and patient populations. *Medical Care, 39*(8), 800-812. https://doi.org/10.1097/00005650-200108000-00006

Wiig, E. (2008). *Social Emotional Evaluation (SEE): Examiners manual.* WPS Publishing.

Williams, K. J. H., Lee, K. L, Hartig, T., Sargent, L. D., Williams, N. S. G., & Johnson, K. A. (2018). Conceptualising creativity benefits of nature experience: Attention restoration and mind wandering as complementary processes. *Journal of Environmental Psychology, 59*, 36-45. https://doi.org/10.1016/j.jenvp.2018.08.005

Willoughby, C., King, G., & Polatjko, H. (1996). A therapist's guide to children's self-esteem. *American Journal of Occupational Therapy, 50*(2), 124-132. https://doi.org/10.5014/ajot.50.2.124

World Health Organization. (1986). *Ottawa charter for health promotion.* Canadian Public Health Association.

Yu, C-P., & Hsieh, H. (2020). Beyond restorative benefits: Evaluating the effect of forest therapy on creativity. *Urban Forestry & Urban Greening, 51*, 126670. https://doi.org/10.1016/j.ufug.2020.126670

8

CHAPTER

Promoting Social Health

Adults

Jacqueline Kendona, OTD, OTR/L and Lucinda Acquaye-Doyle, PhD, MSW

Learning Objectives

At the end of this chapter, the reader will:

1. Discuss the role of social interaction on the health of an adult (ACOTE B.1.2, B.1.3; CSWE 6)
2. Describe types of social interactions adults engage in (ACOTE B.1.2, B.1.3; CSWE 6)
3. Discuss the environments where adults engage in social interactions (ACOTE B.1.2, B.1.3; CSWE 6)
4. Discuss interprofessional collaboration between practitioners (ACOTE B.4.25; CSWE 1)
5. Identify assessment tools used to measure adult social interactions (ACOTE B.1.2, B.1.3; CSWE 4, 7, 9)
6. Discuss interventions that support social health (ACOTE B.1.2, B.1.3; CSWE 8)
7. Apply understanding of professional standards to working with diverse communities (ACOTE B.4.25; CSWE 1, 3)

The ACOTE Standards used are those from 2018.

Key Words

Belonging, Cultural Humility, Interprofessional Collaboration, Social Capital, Social Participation

Pizzi, M. A., & Amir, M. (Eds.). *Interprofessional Perspectives for Community Practice: Promoting Health, Well-Being, and Quality of Life* (pp. 139-150).

Box 8-1: Case Study

Akua is a 38-year-old first-generation Ghanaian American female and is the oldest of three adult children. Her parents, both Ghanaian immigrants, split their year between Ghana and the United States. She lives on the same street as her younger brother who has two daughters and a son. Their younger sister is in graduate school.

Akua and her husband had a baby boy 6 months ago through in-vitro fertilization (IVF). She is trying to adjust to her new sleep schedule after returning to work. Akua works in a fast-paced engineering firm. She is one of two women in the electrical engineering department and the most senior engineer. She spent the past 10 years working long hours and attending after-work gatherings in local bars and restaurants. Akua returned to work 2 months ago but is unable to socialize as she did before she had her son. Due to the COVID-19 pandemic, Akua's parents were unable to travel to the United States to assist Akua with taking care of her son. As such, Akua's sister-in-law, a stay-at-home mom, helps with Akua's son when Akua is at work. However, due to a standing commitment, she expects Akua to pick up the baby after work by 5 pm. Akua's husband, a Ghanaian immigrant as well, is an operating room nurse. His work schedule is unpredictable as he is on the trauma team for his hospital. Akua feels trapped with her new role as a mother. She has been having difficulty sleeping, is increasingly irritable, and is having a hard time concentrating at work.

Active members of their community church, her husband asked her to talk to their pastor because he thinks she has not been herself lately. Akua does not think anything is wrong with her and rather fears that she no longer fits in at work because she cannot go out with her team after work for dinner and drinks.

REFLECTIVE QUESTIONS

1. With her inability to go out with her team after work, what is Akua's social capital at work after returning from maternity leave?
2. How does her sense of belonging at work affect her social capital with her new role as a mother?
3. Based on Akua's background, what cultural considerations would you need to consider if Akua was assigned to your caseload?
4. What data is of primary importance for the health care provider to collect from Akua?

The case study in Box 8-1 illustrates the multidimensional approach to working with adults toward socioemotional well-being including, but not limited to, cultural differences, family and work obligations, professional ethical standards, the complexities, and strengths of working collaboratively, and the role of interprofessionalism as it relates to overall community and population health.

Introduction

In the human nervous system, specific features of person-to-person interactions are innate triggers of adaptive biobehavioral systems, which in turn can support health and healing (Porges, 2011). Person-to-person interactions are essential for the health and well-being of adults as these are the years of work, getting married, starting a family, and contributing to the community. These interactions can be termed **social participation**, defined as "activities that involve social interactions with others, including family, friends, peers and community members, and that support social interdependence" (American Occupational Therapy Association, 2020a, p. 34).

Historically, scholars like Freud (1964), Erikson (1959), and Piaget (1957) have marked the adult life cycle as one tied to finding meaning and maintaining balance. Early adulthood (ages 18 to 40 years) and middle adulthood (ages 41 to 65 years) can be linked to significant transformative life experiences such as education completion, marriage, child-rearing, and career establishment and advancement. Fulfillment of these roles alongside engagement in social and civic responsibilities are synonymous with adult development. However, the management of these multiple roles can be complex. "The need to balance multiple roles and manage the conflicts that arise is a reality that is characteristic of middle age, regardless of one's specific lifestyle or circumstances" (Lachman, 2004, p. 304).

The World Health Organization (WHO; 1946) recognizes social participation as a social determinant of health that acts as a conduit to support one's health and well-being. Social interactions for the adult, be it with family, friends, or community, insulates them from various health conditions. Limited social interactions and decreased social support increases a person's mortality rate by two to four times compared to alcoholism, smoking, obesity, and physical inactivity (Kendona, 2017). Changes in cardiovascular risk and somatic symptoms like pain are linked to the quantity and quality of close social interactions (Zhaoyang et al., 2019). The bidirectional health benefits of social interactions are positive for the adult with subjective reports of decrease in physical symptoms (Zhaoyang et al., 2019). The physiological benefits of belonging and inclusion include a significant decrease in heart rate from baseline and an improvement in subjective positive mood (Begen & Turner-Cobb, 2015). There is an increase in self-reported psychopathology and decreased perceived physical health for persons with decreased perceived interpersonal social support compared to those with an increased perceived interpersonal social support (Moak & Agrawal, 2010). Health care professionals working with adults would better serve their client, which can be an individual, community, organization, or population, when they address barriers to social interactions, and consequently, the interventions that address such barriers.

The environments in which adults engage in social participation facilitates or inhibits their social health, including the social environment. The social environment can be defined as the neighborhoods in which we live, spaces where we have support from friends and family, groups, and organizations we belong to and the workplace (Jung et al., 2021; Mair et al., 2021). These environments consist of the spaces where they gather or congregate with others. They can be public, private, physical, or virtual such as their homes, places of work, worship, parks, coffee shops, restaurants, or stadiums to mention a few. It is important to understand the social environment where the adult engages socially, to help them optimize their social health.

The perceived absence of social participation or social connectedness can have a detrimental effect on the health of the adult. According to Walker et al. (2015), social support and social inclusion are powerful protective factors for health. In his groundbreaking book *The Polyvagal Theory*, Porges (2011) explains the neurophysiological effects of the social engagement system by discussing the neurophysiological benefits of a well-functioning social engagement system that allows for neuroception, and the effects on a person's health. Neuroception was coined by Porges (2011) to describe the subconscious process humans use to assess safety or threat in their environment. This subconscious detective system then gives way to physiological changes in the viscera that can impact a person's health and well-being. Porges (2011) emphasizes that the neurophysiological benefits of social connectedness as crucial to the well-being of humans.

The Importance of Interprofessional Collaboration

The therapeutic benefits of social interdependent relationships that occur during social participation can be harnessed during the person's encounter with health care professionals and the interprofessional team. The WHO (2010) defines interprofessional collaboration as, "when multiple health workers from different professional backgrounds work together with patients, families, [caregivers], and communities to deliver the highest quality of care" (p. 7). Through **interprofessional collaboration**, health care professionals can support adults in maximizing their health-related quality of life (QOL), using their social network.

Addressing issues in health care while seeking to strengthen patient health outcomes has been emphasized through interprofessional collaboration. Deemed Interprofessional Collaborative Practice (IPCP) by the WHO in 2010, this concept gained widespread recognition in its efforts to provide "safe, high-quality, patient-centered care" (McMorrow et al., 2017, p. 1). The call for multiple professions to collaborate by providing services that positively impact clients on the micro to macro level was actualized in 2011 through the formation of the Interprofessional Education Collaborative (IPEC Expert Panel; 2011), which originally represented dentistry, nursing, medicine, osteopathic medicine, pharmacy, and public health. In this collaboration, the health professions developed curricula that emphasized team-based care, while identifying a set of competencies for optimal care. "Health is increasingly understood as holistic well-being rather than simply the absence of disease" (Delavega et al., 2019, p. 556). In such a context, the role of health professions has achieved heightened importance. Occupational therapy and social work were later additions alongside seven other professional organizations in health care settings added to the collaborative in 2016.

The strengths of interprofessional collaboration are identified through Bronstein's Model of Interprofessional Collaboration (2003) and the competencies outlined by the IPEC (2011). Bronstein's framework highlights characteristics that demonstrate the benefits of interprofessional collaborations: interdependence, newly created professional activities, flexibility, collective ownership of goals, and reflection on the process (2003). The four domains created by the IPEC are values and ethics, roles and responsibilities, interprofessional communication, and teams and teamwork (2016). These domains emphasize recognition of the significance in our common values and ethical principles, celebrating the diversity of our professions and the strengths that come from each of our undergirded frameworks, developing strong communication skills by creating language and jargon that is universally recognized and respected, and fostering environments that appreciate the contributions of each group to the team and the interdependent relationships that are paramount to successful and effective teamwork (Wharton & Burg, 2017). Others have credited interprofessional collaboration with shared appreciation for collective knowledge, and a better appreciation for those in other professions (Miller et al., 2019; Kobayashi et al., 2019).

While there are clear indications for the need to incorporate interprofessional collaborations in health care settings, some institutions still struggle with barriers to sustaining collaborative initiatives and the practicality of providing space for interprofessional education and research due to the lack of flexibility in already strenuous curricula, competition for institutional resources, and the often unspoken hierarchical distinction amongst professions referred to as "profession-centrism" by Pecukonis et al. (2008). Nonetheless, through intentional development and training, we can eliminate the comfort of our discipline silos and "develop a health care practice built upon collaboration and interprofessional practice" (Pecukonis et al., 2008, p. 418).

To meet the social health needs of the adult client, health professionals must incorporate interprofessional collaboration into their practice. This allows for seamless transitioning of care and communication amongst health professionals as well as effective coordination of care for the adult client. In the case of Akua, a well-orchestrated collaboration between her physician, and allied health professionals would maximize health related QOL pertaining to her social health.

Person-in-Environment Framework

Humans influence and are influenced by the people, communities, and institutions they find themselves (Golden et al., 2015). The social environment influences healthy and unhealthy behaviors in humans such as the health choices a person makes (Hill et al., 2017). Understanding the person-in-environment perspective, professionals consider the diversity of systems that create barriers to fulfilling these obligations including micro- and macro-level factors such as oppression, social injustice, inequities, and physical and mental health deficits. Health care professionals must consider how these environmental factors impact a person's socioemotional well-being and overall health and aid the client in addressing these factors to achieve treatment goals. A person's social environment enhances or inhibits their health and well-being. A person can register a sense of safety in the social environment through neuroception, which can influence their social health (Porges, 2011). Akua's role as a mother is impacting her social environment at work. Motherhood has made it difficult for her to participate in afterwork social activities with her team. Akua's sense of safety within the team could be affecting her mood because of the lack of connectedness that socializing afterwork provided her before she became a mother.

The physical, cultural, and social environment plays a substantial role in the social health of adults. The environment includes the health care environment where health professionals encounter adults living with various health conditions. Living with and managing various health conditions can result in the development of a therapeutic relationship with health care providers, which can influence a person's health. The health care professional needs to understand the role the social environment plays in an adult's health to help maximize their health outcome. The social environments that have a significant impact on the health of adults include the home, workplace, and community.

An individual is a total sum of their lived experience. This includes their family history, formal and informal education, religious beliefs and practices, as well as inherited traditions and norms passed down over generations. All these cumulatively makes up their cultural environment. The effects of one's cultural environment on their health is all encompassing as it impacts their decision making that in turn impacts their social health. Wang and Langhammer (2018) note that culture "acts as an interpretive guide for the symbolic significance individuals attach to human behavior and human interactions" (p. 503). A person who grows up as a first-generation Muslim American of Albanian descent is going to have a different cultural environment compared to a first-generation Muslim American of Senegalese descent. A person's cultural environment affects their perceptions of how to relate to others. Some cultures value individualism while other cultures value interdependence, which affects how clients engage socially.

In the case of Akua, she chose to use IVF to assist her to become a parent. A person with a different cultural environment may not make the decision she made to use IVF. Akua also chose to go back to work, while her brother's wife chose to stay home with her children. The role one's cultural environment plays on their social health is multifaceted and the health care professional needs to factor the client's cultural environment into understanding of their clients. Understanding the reasons behind why a client like Akua may want to return to the social activities she engaged in before becoming a mother would help the health practitioner develop interventions to meet her social health needs.

When working with the adult client, the health care provider needs to consider the context in which they are encountering the adult. Health care providers can facilitate improved social health by first understanding the environment and the activities that the client engages in, to help the client, maximize their outcomes. The client in the case study has had changes in her home life that is impacting her work life. The interventions needed for a successful work life balance may require some changes in either her home environment or her work environment. As a new mother, she will need guidance from her health care practitioner (social environment) to identify the changes she needs to make, either at work or at home (physical environment) for her to experience satisfaction with her social health.

Family/Home

The family and home are the primary environments that people learn to engage in person-to-person interactions. The family structure can consist of a nuclear, blended, multigenerational, or foster family. Through the roles of spouse, parent, child, grandparent, aunt, uncle, cousins, niece, and nephew, humans learn and develop prosocial skills needed for social participation. The role a person plays in the family and home environment contributes to the skill set needed for person-to-person interactions outside the family and home environment. The social expectations for the various roles within the family vary, therefore health care practitioners should not have assumptions or stereotypes (Cole & Donohue, 2011). **Belonging** is defined as being accepted by others and feeling secure in relationships and connections to place (Scaffa & Rietz, 2020). Belonging stimulates a feeling of being inseparable, valuable, and participating in an environment or system that reinforces a person's sense of self (Işık &

Ergün, 2020). Regardless of the family structure, the family can contribute to a person's sense of belonging or lack thereof, which in turn affects the health of the person. The need to belong "is critical to healthy psychological well-being and physical functioning" (Begen & Turner-Cobb, 2015).

Hitch et al. (2014a) call attention to the multifaced nature of belonging. They highlight that "multiple belongings complicate attempts to categorize where a person belongs" (Hitch et al., 2014a). Nonetheless, a person's sense of belonging is linked to their doing, being, and becoming, which is expressed through engagement in activities that bring them a sense of connectedness and fuels their hopes and aspirations (Hitch et al., 2014b). This ultimately affects their social health and survival.

A person's sense of belonging within a family transcends the physical environment. According to Cole and Donohue (2011), home situations and contexts vary widely with culture. Having a strong sense of belonging has protective health benefits after a person moves away from home to college. Wakefield et al. (2016) found that greater family identification leads to better self-rated health over time. A decreased sense of belonging has a negative effect on the individual whereas an increased sense of belonging does the opposite (Cockshaw, 2013).

Workplace

The work environment can enhance a person's sense of belonging and facilitate their well-being and health. A healthy workplace supports the professional growth and development of the adult. Most adults spend a good amount of their waking hours in the workplace. According to Rydström et al. (2017), paid work is an activity that occupies most of a person's time in adult life. Martins (2015) notes that work increases a person's participation in activities to enhance their QOL. Work affords the adult the opportunity to interact with coworkers, managers, and depending on the type of work a person engages in, people outside the place of work. A person who works in a grocery store for example interacts with their peers, customers, and those who deliver the groceries that are sold in the store. Martins (2015) found that employment has the strongest correlation with life habits concerning social participation. A moderate correlation between social participation, employment, and self-efficacy was also found. This relationship in turn influences a person's perceived QOL and life satisfaction. Factors that can influence a person's health and well-being at work include social interactions, being accepted, being respected, a sense of support from coworkers and leaders as well as participation in valued and meaningful work (Rydström et al., 2017). These interactions insulate the adult's sense of well-being and health and is often seen as social capital.

The Oxford dictionary (Oxford University Press, n.d.) defines **social capital** as "the networks of relationships among people who live and work in a particular society, enabling that society to function effectively." A married person from a large family that serves on different teams at work, stays connected with their high school and college friends, participates in the parent teacher association of their children's school, is an active member of their church and in the choir is said to have good social capital. The relationships afforded this person through their social network fosters optimal health for the adult. According to the WHO (1998), social capital creates health because of the everyday interactions between people that results in strong bonds with mutual benefits. Social capital encompasses trust, support, and recognition. These are predictors of health and well-being in the work environment (Rydström et al., 2017).

People who work in environments with high social capital have a lower rate of health impairments. Having a strong sense of community in the workplace fosters productivity, morale, and makes the workplace enjoyable (Lampinen et al., 2017). Although a sense of belonging is contextual, Cockshaw et al. (2013) found that a decreased sense of belonging in the workplace can contribute to depression.

Community

Since belonging to a social group contributes to a sense of belonging and self-esteem, health care professionals need to understand the importance of this environment on a person's health and well-being (Jetten et al., 2017). Social participation in the context of a community is essential for the health and well-being of the adult. A community is an environment that facilitates person-to-person interactions beyond the home and workplace. People belong to a wide range of communities that includes variables such as geography, occupation, social, and leisure interest where they share a common culture, values, and norms (WHO, 1998).

A person may belong to the local parent-teacher association, a reggae band, and their professional association where they have a role as a political action advocate. As a result of belonging to multiple groups in the community, the person-to-person interactions that this person participates in enhances their sense of belonging and well-being. The social capital the various groups in the communities provide allows this individual to flourish (Jetten et al., 2017). The activities that a person engages in because of belonging to a community, contributions to the health and well-being of the individual. Belonging to a religious or spiritual community helps the adult navigate the various challenges of transitioning that this population encounters.

According to the Pew Research Foundation (2021), of 35,000 Americans surveyed in all 50 states, 70.6% identified themselves as Christian and 5.9% identified as belonging to a non-Christian faith such a Jewish, Muslim, Buddhist, or Hindi. Belonging to a faith-based, religious, or spiritual community insulates the adult during times of adversity due to the social capital these communities afford the adult. According to Mthembu et al. (2017), "spirituality shapes our relationships with others and our environments as well as our interconnectedness" (p. 16). The person-to-person interactions afforded adults by belonging to a religious or spiritual community is reported to insulate persons from depression and depressive symptoms (Cheadle & Dunkel Schetter, 2018).

The absence of a nurturing and supportive environment that a community affords can have detrimental effects on the person's physical, social, spiritual, and mental health (Jetten et al., 2017). It is unlikely that a community with which a person feels little sense of connection would provide the person with health benefits, regardless of the quantity of contact they have with their members (Wakefield et al., 2016). Therefore, it is important to understand a person's sense of connectedness within the community to which they belong.

The activities persons engage in during person-to-person interactions contribute to an improved health-related QOL. Interactions that take place among the family such as eating together, playing board games, and the mundane affairs of everyday activities of family interactions help insulate adults from various health conditions such as depression. Participating in family meals has positive health outcomes for parents (Didericken & Berge, 2015; Berge et al., 2012). Person-to-person activities that support health in the workplace may not be as obvious as those that take place in the home. A work environment that encourages employees to maximize their potential, the use of team-building activities, and facilitating a work-life balance all contribute to a sense of social health in the workplace (Lampinen et al., 2017).

Local communities such as the library, the YMCA, community centers, churches, and other religious organizations offer activities such as Mommy and Me for new parents and LIVESTRONG for cancer survivors (Lancaster Family YMCA, 2020). Some communities have found innovative ways to continue their social participation programs virtually, due to COVID-19 (Lancaster Family YMCA, 2020). The Lancaster Family YMCA continues to provide LIVESTRONG virtually to cancer survivors due to need for social distancing with COVID-19 (Lancaster Family YMCA, 2020). Activities such as yoga, meditation, and a variety of wellness education offered by the YMCA moved online because of the COVID-19 pandemic (Lancaster Family YMCA, 2020). There is emerging evidence to support the efficacy of these community social health programs. The findings from Vincenzo et al. (2021) offers some insight into the potential outcome of virtual community programs. The response of participants in the community to the virtual Otago fall prevention program demonstrates how "virtual health promotion programs can help mitigate the short- and long-term consequences of the pandemic" (Vincenzo et al., 2021).

Cultural Humility and Culturally Competent Practice

Culture is invisible to people that belong to a particular group in that they are not conscious of the social norms within their group (Cole & Donohue, 2011). The recognition of these cultural considerations in practice is contemporarily referred to as **cultural humility**, "a process of reflection and critique of one's own biases and an effort to recognize and rectify power imbalances in the helping relationship (Tervalon et al., 1998; as cited in Rosen et al., 2017, p. 291). Agner (2020) notes that cultural humility is a "lifelong learning-orientated approach" that is "a process-oriented, ongoing approach to interacting with, evolving culturally defined beliefs, ideas and behavior" (pp. 1-2).

Health professionals are encouraged to lean into cultural humility that transcends cultural competence because "culture is always in flux, cultural history inquiry is a helpful partner to social workers in their quest for cultural humility" (Sloane et al., 2018, p. 1015). This more appropriate term seeks to place the emphasis on the lifelong introspective work that is done through self-awareness and supportive interactions rather than simply focusing on a skill needed to work with various cultures (Rosen et al., 2017) while acknowledging that the client/patient is the "expert of their story" (Sloane et al., 2018, p. 1015). Although cultural humility is a more professionally acceptable term today, cultural competency is still used today.

Champions for cultural competency were known to come from the social work profession as they were cited as being "one of the first of the helping professions to begin to address the needs for culturally relevant programs, policies, and services" (Fong & Furuto, 2001, p. v). Current development of cultural competency has addressed the evolution of terms like diversity and the management of it. Cultural competence encompasses diversity and inclusion. A culturally competent health care practitioner needs to be familiar with inclusion and diversity. Taff & Blash (2017) view diversity as a construct that encompasses gender, disability, religious beliefs, race, ethnicity, and sexual orientation. The adult filters their person-to-person interactions, their social participation and social health, through these lenses.

Health care practitioners with an awareness of the invisible veil of culture are better equipped to meet the social health needs of their clients. In a world that is getting more accessible due to globalization and the world wide web, cultural competence is an essential tool for health care practitioners. For a practitioner to understand how an adult engages during social participation, they must first understand the lenses with which the adult sees the social environment. Subsequently, a practitioner with insight into their own culture and an awareness of the different cultures that exist will be better positioned to explore how to help their clients navigate the geopolitical constructs of their culture, as it relates to social participation and social health. Health care practitioners who embrace the diverse backgrounds of their clients have a better chance of meeting the health needs of these clients.

Assessments

Assessing social participation in clients is an important task that health care providers across the continuum need to incorporate into their practice. The WHO (1946) constitution postulates that "health is a state of complete physical, mental and social well-being not merely the absence of disease or infirmity." A person's sense of connectedness and belonging can lower their mortality rate (Wilks et al., 2020). Therefore, regardless of a person's disability or lack thereof, understanding their sense of belonging and social connectedness can help practitioners better meet the needs of their clients. Since intimacy is an important part of the adult years, health care providers need to assess and address barriers to successful engagement in social participation. Assessments that measure social connectedness and perceived social isolation would help practitioners better understand how the client's social health is influencing their well-being.

The assessments in Table 8-1 can help inform health care providers of their client's perceived social health and social participation. The assessments provided in Table 8-1 are intended to help the practitioner gain some insight into how the adult client perceives their social connectedness and their social health. Using self-assessments allows the client to reflect on their perceived social connectedness, free of outside influence. Health professionals can engage in follow-up discussions based on the responses provided by the client to better understand the client's areas of need.

The cultural competence assessment instrument is intended for use by practitioners. Exploring one's cultural competence will help practitioners remove barriers to understanding their clients' lived experiences. To transcend cultural competence and arrive at cultural humility, health care practitioners need to reflect and accept their position on culture to best meet the needs of their clients.

In the case of Akua, our aforementioned case study, there are several cultural considerations that a treatment team should take into account when working with her and her family. The practitioner must begin with acknowledgment of her ethnic origin, identifying as both Ghanaian and American as a starting place. Recognition of strengths, and an understanding of how her identity may impact her views on family, work, religious belief, marriage, and help-seeking behaviors will provide a foundation to provide appropriate and applicable recommendations that are ideal for her and her family, particularly in relation to social connectedness and social participation. It is important however to note that cultures are not monolithic. Not all Ghanaians may have the same beliefs or practices as this can be influenced by level of acculturation, educational level, personal and professional experiences, and community affiliation. Open communication and dialog with Akua and her family are the best way to obtain information that will be appropriate to her and her needs (Professional Reasoning Box A).

Interventions

Barriers to social participation for the adult include deficits in physical and mental function, unforeseen life stressors, transitions such as becoming a parent, or changes in jobs and lifestyle changes (Cole & Donohue, 2011). An evidence-informed and culturally sensitive intervention plan can yield the best outcome for the adult client. Interventions that enhance a person's sense of belonging at home, work, and in their community can improve the health and well-being of the adult. Meaningful interventions would best support their health and well-being.

Game nights, family walks, hikes, road trips, skiing, cycling, and family vacations are all activities that families can engage in to help improve the sense of belonging for the adult.

Team building activities that are person-centered can help create a social environment which is conducive to the health and wellness of the employees. Casucci et al. (2020) found that a gaming activity intended to decrease burnout in the workplace resulted in increased social participation. Community-based interventions that offer the adult opportunities for person-to-person interactions range from participating in a support group, religious activities, board games or bingo, taking cooking or quilting classes, and participating in advocacy through political activities (Cole & Donohue, 2011). Satten et al. (2016) found that participating in a church group weight loss program had positive outcomes for some participants. Although they identified social and cultural barriers to the success for some participants, they also noted that "an intensive faith-based lifestyle intervention can lead to significant reductions in weight" for the African American population studied (Satten et al., 2016, p. 95).

Collaborating with faith-based, religious, or spiritual communities offers the health professional an opportunity to help address the social health needs of adults. These communities may have existing infrastructure that can be used to address the social health needs of their members. Faith-based communities like the African American church has a history of providing spiritual and social support for their members with the aim of decreasing health disparities (Satten et al., 2016).

Table 8-1

Assessments Available for Interprofessional Teams

TOOL	DOMAINS	WHO COMPLETES ASSESSMENT	WHAT IS IT MEASURING
WHOQOL-BREF Available in 19 Languages (Skevington & McCrate, 2012)	• Physical health • Psychological • Social relationships • Environment	• Adult client • Self-assessment	An individual's perception of their QOL and health
Pizzi Health and Wellness Assessment (PHWA; Pizzi & Richards, 2017)	• Social • Physical • Family • Occupational • Mental • Emotional • Spiritual	• Adult client • Self-assessment	Six areas of health and well-being
Self-Reported Experiences of Activity Settings (SEAS) Persons using augmentative and alternative communication (King et al., 2014)	• Personal growth • Psychological engagement • Social belonging • Meaningful interactions • Choice and control	• Adult client • Self-assessment	Meaningful engagement, social connections, choice, and control
Patient Reported Outcome Measurements Information System (PROMIS) • Satisfaction with Participation in Discretionary Social Activities • Satisfaction with Social Roles and Activities • Satisfaction with Participation in Social Roles (National Institutes of Health, 2021)	• Physical, mental, and social health	• Adult client • Self-assessment	Function and well-being in physical, mental, and social domains of health
The Cultural Competence Assessment (CCA) instrument (Holstein et al., 2020)	• Cultural awareness • Sensitivity • Competence behaviors	• Health care practitioner • Self-assessment	To provide evidence of cultural competence among health care providers and staff

The 2020 COVID-19 pandemic mandated stay at home orders and changed how individuals engaged in social participation within the family, workplace, and community. COVID-19 brought us videoconferencing, also referred to as "zooming," a medium that allows for virtual social participation. Families have stayed connected using Zoom to host birthday parties, weddings, and funerals. Work that could be performed virtually such as team building activities, and meetings were performed from remote locations via online portals. Community activities such as support groups, health promotion activities such as group meditation classes continued virtually due to the public mandates of social distancing. A good working knowledge of how to use the various technologies available created new engagement opportunities that require specific skills but can still meet the social health needs of the adult client.

Professional Reasoning Box A

Max is a 44-year-old single man who suffered a spinal cord injury 3 years ago. Max was brought to the skilled nursing facility for therapy. It was determined unsafe for Max to return home due to lack of family and community support. Due to difficulty with finding him a safe discharge environment after he reached his maximum functional potential, he was transferred to a long-term care unit with mostly older adults. He currently shares a room with a 92-year-old man. Max spends most of his days in bed, refusing to attend any activity offered by the facility's recreation department. Max refused showers and was starting to develop a pressure ulcer when the occupational therapist was consulted for positioning. The occupational therapist noticed during the evaluation that Max was isolating himself. Max shared that he used to play chess with his dad growing up and wishes he could play chess again. The occupational therapist reached out to a local high school and was able to pair Max with a 16-year-old male who did not know how to play chess. Max was excited to learn he was going to share his chess skills with this teenager. Max's occupational therapist scheduled the visits with the high school student on days Max did not have scheduled therapy. The pair played chess in a room provided by the recreation department as the teenager could not go into the living area of the residents.

- Why did the occupational therapist pair Max with the high school student?
- What was the purpose of the chess game?
- Why were visits scheduled on days Max did not have therapy?

Ethical Considerations

When working with the adult population, health professionals must abide by the code of ethics of their profession at the forefront of their interactions. Adults who seek the services of professionals to improve their social health need to have confidence in the skill set of the health care provider to address the areas that need improvements. Understanding the person, the various environments in which they engage in person-to-person interactions, and the activities they engage in is essential to help them attain optimal social health.

The code of ethics for health professionals are congruent in their quest to place the needs of the client at the center. For example, the preamble of the National Association of Social Workers (NASW) is service, social justice, dignity and worth of the person, importance of human relationship, integrity, and competence (NASW, 2017). The seven core values that guide interactions between the occupational therapist and their clients are altruism, equality, freedom, justice, dignity, truth, and prudence (AOTA, 2020b). In addition to the seven core values, occupational therapists have six principles that guide ethical decision making. Using the principles of beneficence, nonmaleficence, autonomy, justice, veracity, and fidelity, occupational therapists can balance the needs of their clients against the backdrop of cultural beliefs, individual values, and organizational policies (AOTA, 2020a). Under their code of ethics, the American Physical Therapy Association (APTA) has eight principles of ethical obligations to guide physical therapists. The core values these principles imbue physical therapy practitioners with are compassion, caring, integrity, altruism, collaboration, duty, excellence, accountability, and social responsibility (APTA, 2020). These principles provide physical therapy practitioners guidance for ethical decision making when faced with challenges.

In the case of Akua, it is important for the health care practitioner to respect her autonomy and dignity with regard to wanting to be a mother and maintain her sense of belonging at work. Akua's need for belonging at work may not be congruent with the role of motherhood, however, ethical practice requires the health care practitioner to help her achieve this sense of belonging to improve her social health. The health care practitioner needs to remove all personal biases when evaluating and developing interventions to help Akua meet her social health needs. This can be achieved through collaborating with Akua using compassion and incorporating cultural humility into one's interactions. By doing this, the health care practitioner is practicing ethically while helping the client achieve optimal health.

Recommendations/Implications for Interprofessional Teams in the Community

Due to the lenses health professional have, they are uniquely positioned to address the social health needs of the adult population. Health professionals are well equipped to take a holistic approach to address the biopsychosocial needs of the persons they serve. By addressing the barriers to social participation, health professionals provide their clients the tools and resources needed to improve their social health and health-related QOL. An understanding of who the person is, the environment in which the person needs to engage in person-to-person activities, and the activities they engage in is necessary to help the adult maximize their social participation, thereby, improving their social health.

Using tools that allow clients to self-reflect and rate their perceived social connectedness would provide practitioners an understanding of where they need to focus interventions.

A shift toward cultural humility while adhering to the code of ethics allows practitioners great latitude in creating interventions that are client-centered and evidence-based. While health professionals can address the social participation needs of their clients for improved social health, they need to operate in an interprofessional environment, drawing on the skills of other practitioners. The richness of interprofessional collaboration in addressing the social health needs of the adult client must be harnessed to achieve optimal outcomes.

The Aim High support group is an example of a community program that benefit from interprofessional collaboration to meet the needs of caregivers and survivors of stroke and brain injury in York, Pennsylvania (American Stroke Association, 2021). The focus of the group is to provide social support, educational support, and in-person support (American Stroke Association, 2021). According to the Brain Injury Association of Pennsylvania (BIAPA), the Aim High support group provides education on topics like driving, cognitive ability, and how a stroke or brain injury impacts the lives of participants (n.d). This support group provides participants a supportive environment to share their feelings on various topics as well as their struggles and areas of interest. Participants find a sense of belonging and build social capital needed to navigate their journey of supporting a loved one or living with a brain injury or stroke.

Prior to the COVID-19 pandemic, the group met the second Wednesday of every month from 6:30 pm to 8 pm. Meetings have moved to a Zoom format, continuing to provide the much-needed support and sense of belonging to this population. According to the leader of the support group, S. Kurowski, OTR/L (personal conversation, August 22, 2021) it benefits from interprofessional collaboration to provide education for the group. Staff members from the hospital's physical therapy, occupational therapy, speech therapy, case management departments help provide education for the group. Community supports from Disability Rights Network of Pennsylvania, the Tri-State Advocacy Project, as well as a neuropsychologist, collaborate with the organizers to provide education for survivors and their caregivers (BIAPA, n.d.).

According to S. Kurowski, OTR/L (personal conversation, August 22, 2021) and current lead organizer of Aim High, the social bonds established at the support groups goes beyond the monthly meetings. Members stay connected through email and phone calls. They get together for other social events that goes beyond what is offered during the monthly support group meetings. Members engage in activities like line dancing, getting together for breakfast and have gone to the watch the local baseball team the York Revolutions (S. Kurowski, personal conversation August 22, 2021). The deep social bonds, sense of belonging, and social capital this group affords its members is one that health professionals looking to improve the social health of their clients. The Aim High support group is an example of how health care professionals collaborate to meet the social health needs of adults. This group uses the support group to provide a social environment and to create a safe and supportive environment that affords persons living with an acquired brain injury or stroke to connect with others and participate in the larger community.

Conclusion

Health professionals working with adults can help their clients thrive by weaving a thread of social health into their assessments and interventions. Understanding a client's social networks in the home, place of work, and the community will help health care professionals better address the health and well-being needs of their clients. Social health is essential for the health and well-being of the adult. Understanding where and how the adult engages in social participation, their sense of belonging and social capital is essential for those working with adults. Harnessing the benefits of interprofessional collaboration while practicing cultural humility is indispensable when addressing the social health needs of the adult. Professional organizations such as the AOTA and the NASW provides its members the tools and resources needed to better meet the needs of a culturally diverse population. Health care practitioners who seek to help their clients achieve optimal health need to be knowledgeable on the health benefits of addressing how their client engage in social participation. Addressing social health is not a luxury but a necessary catalyst to help clients achieve optimal health–related QOL.

References

Agner, J. (2020). Moving from cultural competence to cultural humility in occupational therapy: A paradigm shift. *American Journal of Occupational Therapy, 74*(4), 1-7. https://doi.org.libdb.dc.edu/10.5014/ajot.2020.038067

American Occupational Therapy Association. (2020a). Occupational Therapy Practice Framework: Domain and process - Fourth Edition. *American Journal of Occupational Therapy, 74* (Supplement 2). https://doi.org/10.5014/ajot.2020.74s2001

American Occupational Therapy Association. (2020b). Occupational Therapy Code of Ethics. (2020). *American Journal of Occupational Therapy, 74*, 1-13. https://doi.org.libdb.dc.edu/10.5014/ajot.2020.74S3006

American Physical Therapy Association. (2020). *Code of ethics for the physical therapist*. https://www.apta.org/siteassets/pdfs/policies/codeofethicshods06-20-28-25.pdf

Begen, F. M., & Turner-Cobb, J. M. (2015). Benefits of belonging: Experimental manipulation of social inclusion to enhance psychological and physiological health parameters. *Psychology & Health, 30*(5), 568-582. https://doi.org.libdb.dc.edu/10.1080/08870446.2014.991734

Berge, J. M., Wickel, K., Doherty, W. J., Berge, J. M., Wickel, K., & Doherty, W. J. (2012). The individual and combined influence of the "quality" and "quantity" of family meals on adult body mass index. *Families, Systems & Health: The Journal of Collaborative Family HealthCare, 30*(4), 344-351. https://doi.org.libdb.dc.edu/10.1037/a0030660

Brain Injury Association of Pennsylvania. (n.d.). Support group listing. https://biapa.org/programs/support-group-listing/

Bronstein, L. R. (2003). A model for interdisciplinary collaboration. *Social Work, 48*(3), 297-306. https://doi.org/10.1093/sw/48.3.297

Casucci, T., Locke, A. B., Henson, A., & Qeadan, F. (2020). A workplace well-being game intervention for health sciences librarians to address burnout. *Journal of the Medical Library Association, 108*(4), 605-617. https://doi.org.libdb.dc.edu/10.5195/jmla.2020.742

Cheadle, A. C. D., Dunkel Schetter, C., & The Community Child Health Network. (2018). Mastery, self-esteem, and optimism mediate the link between religiousness and spirituality and postpartum depression. *Journal of Behavioral Medicine, 41*(5), 711-721. https://doi.org.libdb.dc.edu/10.1007/s10865-018-9941-8

Cockshaw, W. D., Shochet, I. M., & Obst, P. L. (2013). General belongingness, workplace belongingness, and depressive symptoms. *Journal of Community & Applied Social Psychology, 23*(3), 240-251. https://doi.org.libdb.dc.edu/10.1002/casp.2121

Cole, M. B., & Donohue, M. V. (2011). *Social participation in occupational contexts: In schools, clinics and communities.* SLACK Incorporated

Delavega, E., Neely-Barnes, S. L., Elswick, S. E., Taylor, L. C., Pettet, F. L., & Landry, M. A. (2019). Preparing social work students for interprofessional team practice in health-care settings. *Research on Social Work Practice, 29*(5), 555-561. https://doi.org/10.1177/1049731518804880

Didericksen, K. W., & Berge, J. M. (2015). Modeling the relationship between family home environment factors and parental health. *Families, Systems & Health: The Journal of Collaborative Family HealthCare, 33*(2), 126-136. https://doi.org.libdb.dc.edu/10.1037/fsh0000115

Erikson, E. H. (1959). *Identity and the life cycle: Selected papers.* International Universities Press.

Fong, R., & Furuto, S. (2001). *Culturally competent practice: Skills interventions, and evaluations.* Allyn & Bacon.

Freud, S. (1964). *The Standard edition of the complete psychological works of Sigmund Freud.* (J. Strachey, Ed.). Macmillan.

Golden, S. D., McLeroy, K. R., Green, L. W., Earp, J. A. L., & Lieberman, L. D. (2015). Upending the social ecological model to guide health promotion efforts toward policy and environmental change. *Health Education & Behavior, 42*(1), 8S-14S. https://doi.org.libdb.dc.edu/10.1177/1090198115575098

Hill, P. L., Weston, S. J., & Jackson, J. J. (2017). Connecting social environment variables to the onset of major specific health outcomes. *Psychology & Health, 29*(7), 753-767. https://doi.org.libdb.dc.edu/10.1080/08870446.2014.884221

Hitch, D., Pépin, G., & Stagnitti, K. (2014a). In the footsteps of Wilcock, Part One: The evolution of doing, being, becoming, and belonging. *Occupational Therapy in Health Care, 28*(3), 231-246. https://doi.org.libdb.dc.edu/10.3109/07380577.2014.898114

Hitch, D., Pépin, G., & Stagnitti, K. (2014b). In the footsteps of Wilcock, part two: The interdependent nature of doing, being, becoming, and belonging. *Occupational Therapy in Health Care, 28*(3), 247-263. https://doi.org.libdb.dc.edu/10.3109/07380577.2014.898115

Holstein, J., Liedberg, G. M., Suarez-Balcazar, Y., & Kjellberg, A. (2020). Clinical relevance and psychometric properties of the Swedish version of the cultural competence assessment instrument. *Occupational Therapy International, 1*(10). https://doi.org.libdb.dc.edu/10.1155/2020/2453239

Interprofessional Education Collaborative. (2016). *Core competencies for interprofessional collaborative practice: 2016 update.* Interprofessional Education Collaborative.

Interprofessional Education Collaborative Expert Panel (2011). Core competencies for interprofessional collaborative practice: Report of an expert panel. Interprofessional Education Collaborative. http://www.aacn.nche.edu/education-resources/ipecreport.pdf

Işık, I., & Ergün, G. (2020). Hope and belonging in patients with schizophrenia: A phenomenological study. *Perspectives in Psychiatric Care, 56*(2), 235-242. https://doi.org.libdb.dc.edu/10.1111/ppc.12418

Jetten, J., Haslam, S. A., Cruwys, T., Greenaway, K. H., Haslam, C., & Steffens, N. K. (2017). Advancing the social identity approach to health and well-being: Progressing the social cure research agenda. *European Journal of Social Psychology, 47*(7), 789-802. https://doi.org.libdb.dc.edu/10.1002/ejsp.2333

Jung, S., Whittemore, R., Jeon, S., & Nam, S. (2021). Mediating roles of psychological factors and physical and social environments between socioeconomic status and dietary behaviors among African Americans with overweight or obesity. *Research in Nursing & Health, 44*(3), 513-524. https://doi.org.libdb.dc.edu/10.1002/nur.22130

Kendona, J. (2017). *Decreasing social isolation through an intergenerational social engagement program.* Doctor of Occupational Therapy Capstone Projects. Paper 5. http://hsrc.himmelfarb.gwu.edu/smhs_crl_capstones/5

King, G., Batorowicz, B., Rigby, P., McMain-Klein, M., Thompson, L., & Pinto, M. (2014). Development of a Measure to Assess Youth Self-Reported Experiences of Activity Settings (SEAS). *International Journal of Disability, Development & Education, 61*(1), 44-66. https://doi.org.libdb.dc.edu/10.1080/1034912X.2014.878542

Kobayashi, R., Schwartz, C. R., Willson, M. N., Clauser, J. M., Mann, D. P., Purath, J., Davis, A., Hahn, P. L., DePriest, D. M., Tuell, E. J., Odom-Maryon, T. L., Bray, B. S., & Richardson, B. B. (2019). Interprofessional Student Training: An Evaluation of Teaching Screening, Brief Intervention and Referral to Treatment (SBIRT). *Journal of Social Work Practice in the Addictions, 19*(1/2), 26-46. https://doi.org.libdb.dc.edu/10.1080/1533256X.2019.1589882

Lachman, M. E. (2004). Development in midlife. *Annual Review of Psychology, 55*, 305-331. https://doi.org/10.1146/annurev.psych.55.090902.141521

Lampinen, M.-S., Suutala, E., & Konu, A. I. (2017). Sense of community, organizational commitment and quality of services. *Leadership in Health Services 30*(4), 378-393. https://doi.org.libdb.dc.edu/10.1108/LHS-06-2016-0025

Lancaster Family YMCA. (2020). Community health programs. https://lancasterymca.org/livestrong-at-the-ymca/

Mair, C. A., Lehning, A. J., Waldstein, S. R., Evans, M. K., & Zonderman, A. B. (2021). Exploring neighborhood social environment and social support in Baltimore. *Social Work Research, 45*(2), 75-86. https://doi.org.libdb.dc.edu/10.1093/swr/svab007

Martins, A. C. (2015). Using the International Classification of Functioning, Disability and Health (ICF) to address facilitators and barriers to participation at work. *Work, 50*(4), 585-593. https://doi.org.libdb.dc.edu/10.3233/WOR-141965

McMorrow, S. L., DeCleene Huber, K. E., & Wiley, S. (2017). Capacity building to improve interprofessional collaboration through a faculty learning community. *Open Journal of Occupational Therapy, 5*(3), 1-11. https://doi.org.libdb.dc.edu/10.15453/2168-6408.1371

Miller, V. J., Murphy, E. R., Cronley, C., Fields, N. L., & Keaton, C. (2019). Student experiences engaging in interdisciplinary and interprofessional research collaborations: A case study for social work education. *Journal of Social Work Education, 55*(4), 750-766. https://doi.org.libdb.dc.edu/10.1080/10437797.2019.1627260

Moak Z. B., & Agrawal, A. (2010). The association between perceived interpersonal social support and physical and mental health: Results from the national epidemiological survey on alcohol and related conditions. *Journal of Public Health, 32*(2), 191-201. https://doi- org.libdb.dc.edu/10.1093/pubmed/fdp093

Mthembu, T. G., Wegner, L., & Roman, N. V. (2017). Spirituality in the occupational therapy community fieldwork process: A qualitative study in the South African context. *South African Journal of Occupational Therapy, 47*(1), 16-23. https://doi.org.libdb.dc.edu/10.17159/2310-3833/2016/v46n3a4

National Association of Social Workers (2017). Code of Ethics. https://www.socialworkers.org/About/Ethics/Code-of-Ethics/Highlighted-Revisions-to-the-Code-of-Ethics

National Institutes of Health. (2021). Patient reported outcome measure information system. https://www.healthmeasures.net/explore-measurement-systems/promis/intro-to-promis

Oxford University Press. (n.d.). Oxford learners dictionary. https://www.oxfordlearnersdictionaries.com/us/definition/english/social-capital

Pecukonis, E., Doyle, O., & Bliss, D. L. (2008). Reducing barriers to interprofessional training: promoting interprofessional cultural competence. *Journal of Interprofessional Care, 22*(4), 417-428.

Piaget, J. (1957). *Construction of reality in the child.* Routledge & Kegan Paul.

Pizzi, M. A., & Richards, L. G. (2017). Promoting health, well-being, and quality of life in occupational therapy: A commitment to a paradigm shift for the next 100 years. *American Journal of Occupational Therapy, 71*(4), 1-5. https://doi.org.libdb.dc.edu/10.5014/ajot.2017.028456

Porges, S. (2011). *The Polyvagal theory: Neurophysiological foundations of emotions, attachment, communication self-regulation.* W.W. Newton & Company Ltd.

Rosen, D., McCall, J., & Goodkind, S. (2017). Teaching critical self-reflection through the lens of cultural humility: an assignment in a social work diversity course. *Social Work Education, 36*(3), 289-298. https://doi.org/10.1080/02615479.2017.1287260

Rydström, I., Englund, L. D., Dellve, L., & Ahlstrom, L. (2017). Importance of social capital at the workplace for return to work among women with a history of long-term sick leave: A cohort study. *BMC Nursing, 16,* 1-9. https://doi.org.libdb.dc.edu/10.1186/s12912-017-0234-2

Satten, R., Williams, L., Dias, J., Garvin, J., Marion, L., Joshua, T., Kriska, A., Kramer, M., & Venkat Narayan, K. (2016). Community trial of a faith-based lifestyle intervention to prevent diabetes among African-Americans. *Journal of Community Health, 41*(1), 87-96. https://doi.org.libdb.dc.edu/10.1007/s10900-015-0071-8

Scaffa, M. E., & Reitz, S. M., (2020). *Occupational therapy in community and population practice* (3rd ed). F. A. Davis Company

Skevington, S. M., & McCrate, F. M. (2012). Expecting a good quality of life in health: assessing people with diverse diseases and conditions using the WHOQOL-BREF. *Health Expectations, 15*(1), 49-62. https://doi.org.libdb.dc.edu/10.1111/j.1369-7625.2010.00650.x

Sloane, H. M., David, K., Davies, J., Stamper, D., & Woodward, S. (2018). Cultural history analysis and professional humility: historical context and social work practice. *Social Work Education, 37*(8), 1015-1027. https://doi.org.libdb.dc.edu/10.1080/02615479.2018.1490710

Taff, S. D., & Blash, D. (2017). Diversity and inclusion in occupational therapy: Where we are, where we must go. *Occupational Therapy in Health Care, 31*, 72–83. https://doi.org/10.1080/07380577.2016.1270479

The Pew Research Foundation (2021). Religious landscape study. https://www.pewforum.org/religious-landscape-study

Vincenzo, J. L., Hergott, C., Schrodt, L., Rohrer, B., Brach, J., Tripken, J., Shirley, K. D., Sidelinker, J. C., & Shubert, T. E. (2021). Capitalizing on virtual delivery of community programs to support health and well-being of older adults. *Physical Therapy, 101*(4), 1-4. https://doi.org.libdb.dc.edu/10.1093/ptj/pzab001

Wakefield, J. R. H., Sani, F., Herrera, M., Khan, S. S., & Dugard, P. (2016). Greater family identification-but not greater contact with family members-leads to better health: Evidence from a Spanish longitudinal study. *European Journal of Social Psychology, 46*(4), 506-513. https://doi.org.libdb.dc.edu/10.1002/ejsp.2171

Walker, R., Koh, L., Wollersheim, D., & Liamputtong, P. (2015). Social connectedness and mobile phone use among refugee women in Australia. *Health & Social Care in the Community, 23*(3), 325-336. https://doi.org.libdb.dc.edu/10.1111/hsc.12155

Wang, R., & Langhammer, B. (2018). Predictors of quality of life for chronic stroke survivors in relation to cultural differences: A literature review. *Scandinavian Journal of Caring Sciences, 32*(2), 502-514. https://doi.org.libdb.dc.edu/10.1111/scs.12533

Wharton, T., & Burg, M. A. (2017). A mixed-methods evaluation of social work learning outcomes in interprofessional training with medicine and pharmacy students. *Journal of Social Work Education, 53.*

Wilks, S. E., Heintz, M. E., Lemieux, C. M., & Du, X. (2020). Assessing social connectedness among persons with schizophrenia: Psychometric evaluation of the perceived social connectedness scale. *Journal of Behavioral Health Services & Research, 47*(1), 113-125. https://doi.org.libdb.dc.edu/10.1007/s11414-019-09656-6

World Health Organization. (1946). Constitution of the world health organization. https://treaties.un.org/doc/Treaties/1948/04/19480407%2010-51%20PM/Ch_IX_01p.pdf

World Health Organization. (2010). Framework for action on interprofessional education and collaborative practice. http://apps.who.int/iris/bitstream/10665/70185/1/

World Health Organization Division of Health Promotion, Education, and Communication. (1998). Health promotion glossary. World Health Organization. http://apps.who.int/iris/handle/10665/64546

Zhaoyang, R., Sliwinski, M. J., Martire, L. M., & Smyth, J. M. (2019). Social interactions and physical symptoms in daily life: quality matters for older adults, quantity matters for younger adults. *Psychology & Health, 34*(7), 867-885.

9

CHAPTER

Promoting Social Health

Older Adults

Nicole A. Fidanza, OTD, OTR/L

Learning Objectives

At the end of this chapter, the reader will:

1. State the impacts of social participation, social isolation, and loneliness on health, well-being, and quality of life of older adults (ACOTE B.3.3)
2. List theories that postulate the social participation of older adults, explaining potential changes in their social behaviors and contact with others (ACOTE B.2.1)
3. Approach social participation from top-down and bottom-up lenses that look at both the issue itself and the underlying factors that influence it as foci of assessment and intervention (ACOTE B.3.2, B.3.6, B.4.3, B.4.4, B.4.9)
4. Understand the need for a public health approach to social participation, including multiple disciplines and tiers of action, to support healthy social aging of all seniors (ACOTE B.4.10, B.5.1, B.5.2)

The ACOTE Standards used are those from 2018.

Key Words

Frailty, Loneliness, Social Engagement, Social Isolation, Social Participation, Social Support

Case Study

Betty is a 76-year-old Black woman who lost her husband, Joe, 9 months ago. One month before Joe's unexpected passing, Betty and Joe had relocated to Florida, a lifelong dream. Their three adult children and their families all remained in the Northeast, and Betty connects with them via telephone several times every week. While Joe was more technologically savvy, Betty is uncomfortable with technology, despite her family's suggestions that she use her new iPad to FaceTime, email, and "follow" her grandchildren on social

Pizzi, M. A., & Amir, M. (Eds.). *Interprofessional Perspectives for Community Practice: Promoting Health, Well-Being, and Quality of Life* (pp. 151-174).

media. Betty does not have strong social ties in her new home state. Prior to his death, Betty and Joe had joined a local church congregation and signed up for a bowling league. While Betty does attend weekly religious services, she has lost interest in bowling without her beloved partner, as this was a hobby they shared together. Her excitement to relocate has turned into regret; she deeply misses Joe, their old home, and the family and friends they left behind.

Betty is independent with all daily tasks, both basic and instrumental, functional mobility, and driving. While accustomed to doing laundry and housework, she is concerned about managing the upkeep of their new home alone. She is in good health other than urinary stress incontinence (she typically wears an absorbent pad to prevent staining her clothing) and occasional memory complaints. Betty had an unexpected fall off a stepstool several weeks ago when attempting to change a lightbulb, landing on the shoulder of her right dominant arm. While she was able to get up without assistance, her shoulder pain persisted for over a week, especially when attempting to use the arm functionally. Her shoulder pain caused her to seek out a local physician, and after workup, she was diagnosed with a rotator cuff tear. Her son flew down for the surgical repair and stayed for a week post-operatively. Homecare services, including nursing, physical therapy, and occupational therapy, were referred as she is unable to drive for several weeks. When interacting with the homecare team, Betty appears sad and has trouble identifying functional goals for her therapies, as she "can't think of anything motivating without Joe."

When thinking about Betty's case:

1. What factors currently support and threaten Betty's social participation?
2. Which member(s) of the interprofessional team should be considering her social health as a priority of treatment?
3. What actions should be taken to support Betty's social participation?

Why the Social Health of Older Adults Is Important

Many seniors experience changes in physical and cognitive health, altered physical and social environments, role changes, and frailty with age, impacting their social functioning. Social isolation (an objective lack of social contact with others) and loneliness (the subjective feeling of being isolated) are serious public health risks associated with poor physical and mental health outcomes, including higher rates of mortality, depression, functional decline, and cognitive decline (National Academies of Sciences, Engineering, & Medicine [NASEM], 2020). There is substantial evidence that social isolation in later life is associated with a 25% increased risk for premature mortality from all causes (Holt-Lunstad et al., 2010). Evidence on loneliness is not as strong but is building. Chronic isolation and loneliness are associated with higher physician visits and resulting health care costs (Gerst-Emerson & Jayawardhana, 2015). In fact, an estimated $6.7 billion in annual federal spending is attributable to these categories of older adult (OA; AARP Research, 2018). Authorities expect the financial and public health impact of loneliness to increase as the nation's population ages. It is important for health professionals to consider isolation and loneliness as factors when engaging with older adult clients.

Introduction

Background

Almost every country in the world is experiencing growth in the size and proportion of persons aged 65 years and older in their population (United Nations, 2019). According to the United States Census Bureau's 2019 population estimates (2020), the nation's OA population age 65 years and older has grown by over a third (34%) over the past decade, and by 2060, nearly one quarter of Americans, or almost 95 million people, are estimated to be over the age of 65 years. Further, an estimated 16% of the global population, or one in six people, will be aged 65 or older (United Nations, 2019). OAs report that satisfying social relationships as critical to their well-being (Halaweh et al., 2018), and studies show that social activities are particularly important for OAs (Betts Adams et al., 2011). Social participation is an important determinant of health that must be taken seriously when considering healthy aging of this growing population.

The concept of social participation, for people of all ages, is multidimensional and often ambiguous, as it represents a continuum of activities from an individual level to societal level (Levasseur et al., 2010). Additionally, it is unique to each person based on personal characteristics and one's interactions with their living environments. For this chapter, **social participation** is defined as a person's involvement in activities that provide interactions with others in society or the community (Levasseur et al., 2010). **Social connectedness** encompasses the structural, functional, and quality aspects of how individuals connect to each other (NASEM, 2020). While often used interchangeably, social isolation and loneliness are two distinct conditions. **Social isolation** is the objective lack of or limited social contact with others (NASEM, 2020). **Loneliness** is the perception of social isolation or the subjective feeling of being lonely (NASEM, 2020). **Social support** is the actual or perceived availability of resources from others, typically within one's social network (NASEM, 2020).

It is estimated that more than one-third of adults aged 45 and older feel lonely, and almost one-fourth of OAs aged 65 and older are socially isolated (NASEM, 2020). While social isolation and loneliness (SI/L) are not medical conditions, they have reciprocal relationships with health (Prohaska et al., 2020). Perceived and objective SI/L increase the risk of mortality comparable with smoking and obesity (Holt-Lunstad et al., 2015). Poor social relationships are associated with a 50% increase in risk for dementia, a 29% increase in risk of coronary heart disease, and a 32% rise in the risk of stroke (AARP Research, 2018). Further, an annual mortality of 162,000 Americans is attributable to social isolation, exceeding the number of deaths from cancer or stroke (Veazie et al., 2019). With populating aging, the number of OAs experiencing SI/L is expected to increase, making these significant public health issues with the potential of becoming pandemics (Blazer, 2020; Gerst-Emerson & Jayawardhana, 2015, Jeste et al., 2020).

Call for Public Health/ Community Approaches

As social participation is a central aspect of health, a public health approach incorporating multiple perspectives is needed to benefit the social health of individuals and society (Prohaska et al., 2020). This the link between socialization and health has been recognized on global levels by the World Health Organization (WHO, 2002) and the United Nations (n.d.). Almost 2 decades ago, the WHO recognized social participation as a key influence of and direct consequence of health in its *Active Aging Policy Framework* (2002). As such, proposed enhancement of social participation was deemed a crucial component for healthy population aging. Social participation is a basic pillar of this *Framework*, which recommends strategies for decision makers, nongovernmental organizations, private industry, and health and social service professionals to foster social networks for OAs (WHO, 2002). These strategies include promotion of traditional societies and community groups run by/for OAs, volunteerism, neighborhood helping, peer mentoring and visiting, family caregivers, intergenerational programs, and outreach services to those who are isolated or lonely (WHO, 2002).

In 2015, the United Nations (UN) launched sustainable development goals (SDGs) as global aims to be a "blueprint to achieve a better and more sustainable future for all" (UN, n.d., para. 1). Goal 10 is centered on empowerment and promotion of social inclusion of all people, including OAs (UN, n.d.) Goal 11 is centered on provision on safe, inclusive, and accessible spaces, particularly for OAs and those with disabilities (UN, n.d.). Though the SDGs were intended to be achieved by the year 2030, the impact of the COVID-19 pandemic has delayed the progress of and deepened the need for most of these goals (UN, n.d.).

Importance of an Interprofessional Approach

Applying a public health approach to socialization of OAs requires a conceptualization of how an interprofessional team can serve all OAs, not just those who are socially isolated. This is achieved through adoption of the Interprofessional Education Collaborative's (IPEC) *Core Competencies for Interprofessional Collaborative Practice* (2016). It is crucial that each member of the team understands the roles and responsibilities of the different professionals on the team in providing safe and efficient social participation interventions. When working together to provide these interventions, the team must demonstrate mutual respect, trust, integrity, and high standards of ethics. Further, effective communication with each other, with clients, with families/caregivers, and with other stakeholders is needed. Lastly, the team must apply principles of team dynamics, process improvement, and conflict management to facilitate effective teamwork when providing social participation assessment and interventions to individuals, communities, and populations.

Evidence for Content

Theoretical Perspectives

There are several psychosocial theories focusing on OAs' social participation, its impact on their health and well-being, and changes to its quality and quantity over time (Havighurst, 1961; Cumming & Henry, 1961; Seiber, 1974; Atchley, 1989; Rowe & Kahn, 1997; Cartensen et al., 1999). The *Activity Theory of Aging* suggests that engaging in social activities buffers against negative consequences of aging on mental and physical health (Havighurst, 1961). Based on this theory, OAs stay active and healthy based on significant social engagement. Conversely, the *Disengagement Theory of Aging* suggests that aging is inevitable, and one's abilities, including those related to socialization and contact with others, reduce over time (Cumming & Henry, 1961). Based on this theory, OAs gradually lose connections with those in society, becoming inactive and lonely compared to younger cohorts. Though contradictory in nature, both theories have been supported by research (Arslantaş et al., 2015; Crewdson, 2016). It is suggested that both theories are valid based on specific socioeconomic and demographic factors of each older adult (Asiamah, 2017). The *Activity Theory of Aging* is likely supported in built, social, and economic environments that facilitate the social engagement of senior citizens.

Like the *Activity Theory of Aging*, the *Theory of Role Accumulation* suggests that having multiple roles and engaging in a variety of activities can benefit OAs' overall well-being (Seiber, 1974). This theory posits that any stress caused by role conflict or role overload is outweighed by overall gratification from holding a variety of roles. *Continuity Theory* emphasizes how OAs seek a consistent sense of self through continuing social roles, relationships, and activities (Atchley, 1989). Based on this theory, OAs attempt to preserve and maintain existing social connections tied to past experiences of their social world. This concept is further supported by Rowe and Kahn's *Model of Successful Aging* (1987, 1997), which emphasizes meaningful and purposeful social activities as one of four crucial factors in successful aging.

Comparable to the *Disengagement Theory of Aging*, the *Socioemotional Selectivity Theory* suggests that as people age, their focus shifts to time remaining in life, focusing on existing emotionally important relationships, and shifting attention away from new social contacts (Cartensen et al., 1999). This theory postulates that for OAs, new social relationships are less likely to provide quality connections. Both theories focus on decreased social networks with age, though for different causes (Atchley, 1989; Cartensen et al., 1999).

Understanding Social Participation

Just as many theories exist to explain the connections between aging and social participation, there is no current agreement around a common definition between medical, rehabilitative, and social fields (Aw et al., 2017; Douglas et al., 2017; Levasseur et al., 2010). According to the *Occupational Therapy Practice Framework: Domain and Process* (American Occupational Therapy Association [AOTA], 2020), social participation is one of the nine areas of occupation and is defined as the "activities that involve social interaction with others, including family, friends, peers, and community members, and that support social interdependence" (p. 34). The profession of occupational therapy further breaks social participation down into community participation, family participation, friendships, intimate partner relationships, and peer group participation. While this definition guides occupational therapy practice, it is not used by other disciplines whom occupational therapists work alongside in interprofessional teams. It is important for medical, rehabilitative, and social professionals to come to a consensus on a common definition to prevent communication difficulties and incomplete assessment and interventions for socialization (Levasseur et al., 2010).

It is crucial to consider that OAs participate in social participation in different ways, and the extent of this participation spans a full continuum of tasks (Levasseur et al., 2010) and connections to others (Aw et al., 2017). Levasseur et al. (2010) defines **social participation** as a person's involvement in activities that provide interactions with others in society or the community and created a six-level multidimensional taxonomy of social involvement based on the level of involvement of the individual with others, and the goals of these activities. Partaking in higher levels are allow one to influence and involve oneself in their community. The six levels with examples are:

1. Completing an activity in preparation for connecting with others (listening to the news in preparation to converse with others)
2. Being with others/alone but with people around (walking one's neighborhood)
3. Interacting with others (social contact) without doing a specific activity with them (conversing with a grocery store clerk)
4. Doing an activity with others/collaborating to reach the same goal (recreation sports)
5. Helping others (caregiving and volunteering)
6. Contributing to society (civic activities)

Aw et al. (2017) determined that the social participation of OAs in Singapore falls into a five-stage continuum based on individual, cultural, and policy contexts. While completed on a distinct population of OAs, parallels between this continuum and Levasseur et al.'s taxonomy exist, particularly related to higher levels of social participation. The five stages with examples are:

1. Social engagement (volunteering and helping others)
2. Expanding one's social network (participating in new social activities)
3. Seeking consistent social interactions (familiar faces, places, and activities only)
4. "Comfort-zoning alone" (solitary routines one has grown accustomed to)
5. Marginalization and exclusion (mistrust of others)

While no universal system exists to classify social participation, these frameworks should be used to address one's preferences and barriers to socialization. Not all OAs will be able or interested in moving up the continuum, and their preferences and barriers must be considered when attempting to provide appropriate social interventions. Participation at a given level is impacted by one's financial security, health status and management, psychosocial adjustment to social interactions (meeting new people, handing social conflict, etc.), family support/integration, culture, and public policy. For example, those with financial difficulties will prioritize resource utilization toward meeting their basic needs, and those with health issues may choose to simplify their social interactions instead of expanding them.

A social network is defined as "the array of social contacts that give access to social, emotional, and practical support" (Gray, 2009, p. 6). Networks with a wider range of social ties, such as diverse and friend-focused, are correlated with better physical and mental health outcomes, as well as subjective well-being. The restricted network with the most limited social ties is correlated with declining and poor health, the least physical activity, and greater mortality. Current evidence shows up to one-third of OAs falling into the restricted network type (Siette et al., 2020).

An analysis of social networks reveals men typically have more family-focused networks, and women have more diverse and friend-focused networks (Siette et al., 2020). This may be because women tend to innovate more than men in later life by being more receptive to new leisure activities, actively participating in social activities, and engaging at a greater frequency (Siette et al., 2020). Volunteering is also attributed to diverse social networks and its positive effects (Pilkington et al., 2012). Women are found to participate in religious, community, and volunteer activities more than men, except for sports (Levasseur et al., 2017).

Benefits of Social Participation to Older Adults

Psychosocial

Social participation is a protective factor against depression and other psychological distress (Choi et al., 2020; Mackenzie & Abdulrazaq, 2021; Park et al., 2018). Diversity of social activities is just as important as frequency in lowering one's depression risk (Choi et al., 2020). Participation in more social activities, and increased time spent in those activities, leads to more opportunities to form social relationships and exchange emotional intimacy, resulting in higher levels of perceived connectedness and lower levels of loneliness (Mackenzie & Abdulrazaq, 2021; Park et al., 2018). Further, perceived emotional support has been found to be a stronger buffer against depression more effective than self-care support, which may leave the OA feeling helpless (Jacobson et al., 2017). Lower rates of depression have been linked to social/communal activities and volunteering than with work or economic activities, particularly in women and those in urban settings (Choi et al., 2020; Mackenzie & Abdulrazaq, 2021; Miller et al., 2014).

Functional Ability

Social participation is associated with a lower likelihood of functional disability among older adults through psychosocial, behavioral, and physiological pathways (Gao et al., 2018; Glei et al., 2012; Kanamori et al., 2014; Li et al., 2014; Sakamoto et al., 2017). High levels of social participation allow an OA to take on multiple social roles, providing emotional support and psychologic benefit (Li et al., 2014). Further, it helps one to remain cognitively (Sakamoto et al., 2017; Wang et al., 2013) and physically active (James et al., 2011; Kanamori et al., 2014) and reduce the risk of functional decline (Tomioka et al., 2016). Social participation also has direct physiologic benefits such as increased immune functions and lowered biomarkers of disease risks (Glei et al., 2012). These connections vary based on the type of social activity, as each plays a different role in health promotion. For example, a leisure activity like golf will require more physical activity, strength, and activity tolerance than a book club discussion. Both regular engagement in organized social activities and active involvement in informal social interactions provide a buffer against functional decline (Gao et al., 2018; Tomioka et al., 2016), protecting against the risks of lengthy hospital stays (Newall et al., 2015), long-term care facility placement (Miller et al., 2014), and mortality (Haak et al., 2019).

Determinant Factors of Social Participation

Health Challenges and Chronic Conditions

While social participation can have positive impacts on health, physical, mental, and cognitive challenges associated with a decline in health with age pose challenges to one's social engagement (Ha et al., 2017). Issues such as urinary incontinence (more common in women; Nivestam et al., 2021; Vo et al., 2016), pain (Nivestam et al., 2021; Wilkie et al., 2016), impaired endurance (Nivestam et al., 2021), impaired vision, and dual-sensory loss (both vision and hearing; Mick et al., 2018) have been found to negatively impact OAs' social participation. Chronic conditions, alone or in combination, have also been tied to social withdrawal with age, particularly depression, diabetes, and osteoarthritis (Griffith et al., 2017). Overall, poor health is associated with decreased social contacts, decreased positive interactions with friends, and increased negative interactions with others (Ha et al., 2017).

Like physical capabilities, cognition is also a determinant factor for social participation. Older adults with subjective memory complaints and dementia are more likely to have difficulty in social activities compared to those with intact cognitive functioning (Lee & Park, 2020; Marioni et al., 2012). Recognizing these challenges often brings fear of social rejection and losing valued aspects of one's identity, causing withdrawal from social activities (Goll et al., 2015). Knowledge of these linkages allows for a public health approach in recognizing and treating these risks for SI/L (Griffith et al., 2017).

Functional Disability

Overall, OAs with fewer care needs and higher ability status report higher levels of social participation (Siette et al., 2020). In addition to and potentially because of the health challenges listed earlier, mobility challenges (Rosso et al., 2013), reduced gait speed (Warren et al., 2016), use of a mobility device (Nivestam et al., 2021), and fear of falling (Nilsson et al., 2015) are also associated with impaired social participation. During the aging process, inability to perform activities at a societal level are often the first indication of one's declining independence (Griffith et al., 2017). Social participation is often reciprocally tied to activities of instrumental activities of daily living (IADL) such as community mobility, financial management, and shopping, helping OAs to remain physically and cognitively active (Griffith et al., 2017). Those with IADL decline, particularly around managing transportation, are found to have lower rates of social participation in terms of diversity and frequency of social interactions (Nivestam et al., 2021). In Betty's case, her rotator cuff repair has caused pain and limited strength and mobility, negatively impacted her self-care and IADL functioning, including temporarily suspending her ability to drive. These factors also place her social functioning at risk.

Environmental Factors

Elements of one's physical, social, and virtual environments may support or inhibit social participation with age. Community belonging is shaped by feeling appreciated by the population, and adaptation of living environments to facilitate participation (Cao, 2019). The ability to access local stores, churches, and community centers has been deemed crucial to neighborhood participation (Duppen et al., 2020), and OAs living closest to social events and services reported higher levels of participation, particularly those who were no longer able to drive (Richard et al., 2013). Cost of community programs may lead one to decline participation if one is on a limited budget (Fischl et al., 2020). Changes in a spouse/partner's health, loss of family and friends, geographic relocation, and retirement may all limit one's social networks with age. Betty experienced several of these, impacting her social health. Further, aging peers may experience functional decline, limiting their contact with others. Disconnection based on technological advances and globalization have disrupted traditional social connections, which may restrict one's social participation (Jeste et al., 2020). If living alone and living in unsupportive/inaccessible environments, an OA's risk for decline is heightened (Park et al., 2018).

In a society that is becoming rapidly digitized, SP occurs increasingly more through digital technology, which enable people to connect with others and participate in society per their preference (Leist, 2013). Digital technologies include personal computers, smart telephones, computer tablets, software on these devices, internet, and the worldwide web. As of 2021 in America, over 75% of OAs have access to the internet, 61% of OAs own smart phones, and 45% of OAs report using social media (Pew Research Center, 2021a, 2021b, 2021c). Despite this, many OAs are classified as "digitally disengaged" with reduced or completely discontinued use of technology due to decreased capacity, increasing complexity of technology, and inadequate relevance of technology in their lives (Fischl et al., 2020). Betty likely falls into this category. Further, virtual connections may be superficial and sometimes harmful to OAs (Jeste et al., 2020). Design of usable digitalized services and facilitating satisfactory use of digital technology can support OAs' social participation through activities they find relevant (Fischl et al., 2020).

Social Isolation and Loneliness

Reduced or diminished social participation may lead to SI/L; both have been deemed threats to health and quality of life (QOL). While often used interchangeably, SI/L are two distinct conditions. **Social isolation** is the objective lack of or limited social contact with others, and **loneliness** is the perception of social isolation or the subjective feeling of being lonely (NASEM, 2020). Not all loneliness stems from social isolation; it may be specific to a certain type of relationship (Taylor, 2021). For example, one may long for a romantic relationship but actively participate in social activities with friends. In toxic relationships, such as those with family and friends, one may isolate from them but not feel loneliness due to the stress associated with them. These differences are based on the older adult's assessment of each relationship and the value it does/does not bring to their life. Social isolation can be operationalized using seven indicators as social isolation from: 1) adult children, 2) other family members, 3) friends, 4) living alone, 5) being unmarried, 6) not participating in social groups, or 7) religious activities. Increases in isolation based on combinations of these indicators are linked to increased loneliness. Support from a spouse/partner and friends alleviates loneliness more so than support from adult children and other family members (Chen & Feeley, 2014).

Consequences of loneliness include depression, noncommunicable disease, health behaviors like physical activity, stress, sleep, cognition, and premature mortality (Prohaska et al., 2020). Older adults with an older subjective age are more susceptible to depression (Shira et al., 2020). Further, higher loneliness in old age is linked to elevated stress markers, impaired sleep, and pro-inflammatory physiological effects, which may cause brain damage impacting emotional regulation and cognition (Hawkley & Cacioppo, 2010). Negative health outcomes linked to loneliness create a higher need for health care and are linked with higher utilization, especially among older adults who are more likely to be living with comorbidities (Gerst-Emerson & Jayawardhana, 2015). In fact, up to 1 in 10 OAs visit their doctor not because of a medical need but because they are lonely (Neill-Hall, 2013).

OAs vulnerable to SI/L include immigrants; lesbian, gay, bisexual, and transgender populations; minorities; and victims of elder abuse (NASEM, 2020). It is worth noting that significant gaps exist in "true" understanding of these conditions, as most research is focused on high-income countries (Prohaska et al., 2020). Further, SI/L are often stigmatizing conditions; one may not admit they are isolated or feeling lonely out of fear this reflects weakness or vulnerability. Socially isolated adults are less likely to participate in research studies and interventions meant to improve these conditions. More research needed on the intensity, frequency, and duration of OAs' loneliness, specifically.

Betty has several risk factors for decreased social participation and resulting SI/L, including being recently widowed, a recent geographic move, limited contact with peers in her new community, family and friends living out of state, discomfort with technology, and pain and functional disability stemming from her rotator cuff repair. Being African American, she is at higher risk of SI/L even without these other factors. In fact, she may already have developed these conditions based on the past 10 months of her life (particularly the move and loss of her spouse). If unaddressed, these issues place her overall health, well-being, and QOL at risk.

Social Participation in Assisted-Living and Long-Term Care Facilities

Despite public misconceptions, only about 5% of OAs reside in nursing homes and 2% reside in assisted living facilities (NASEM, 2010). Even though these OAs are surrounded by others, they have a low sense of belonging that leads to social isolation and a higher chance of experiencing depressive symptoms than those living at home (McLaren et al., 2013). In addition, over 50% of residents report loneliness and described their social relationships with other residents as lacking depth and connectedness despite having OAs living in the same facility. It is often difficult for OAs to adapt to a new environment after relocating to a long-term care facility, since they need to meet other residents, create social networks, and experience continuity of lifestyle to maintain their social participation (Hersch et al., 2012). A lack of transition services can lead to problems with participation in meaningful occupations, including social participation (Orentlicher et al., 2017). Functional disability has been associated with decreased social participation and elevated signs of depression because of social withdrawal from activities offered within these facilities (Bekhet & Zauszniewski, 2014; Beuscher & Dietrich, 2016). Although residents with functional disabilities are sometimes limited in their abilities to actively interact with others during social activities, opportunities for social engagement brings notable psychological benefits to these individuals (Koehn et al., 2016).

Assessment

Occupational Profile

First and foremost, an occupational profile should be completed by an occupational therapist to understand the OA's social history including their meaningful occupations, patterns of daily living, interests, roles, values, and beliefs (AOTA, 2020). This information is vital to understanding the impact one's socialization has on their health and QOL and can be used to determine goals and intervention strategies, using probing questions, along with discovering frequency of contact with others, and context of interactions (live or virtual). Changes in one's social functioning with age should also be explored to determine the level of impairment present, if any. Learning this information about Betty would be incredibly helpful in alerting the team to her social decline of late.

Top-Down Assessment Tools

Going beyond the occupational profile, top-down assessment of social participation can also include standardized assessments that focus on socialization, interests, and psychosocial functioning. Some are based on observations of the client when engaged in group activity, while others are based on self-reported data to generate one's social history. Some are focused on social health directly, while others can be linked to one's success or impairments in social functioning. Top-down assessments focused on social network size, subjective social supports, and SI/L can also be used to gather information on an OAs' social health. The information generated by these assessments may be used to add more depth to the Betty's occupational profile. Please see Tables 9-1, 9-2, and 9-3 for a comprehensive list of top-down assessment tools.

Bottom-Up Assessment Tools

To holistically assess an OAs' social health, looking at the client through a bottom-up lens is crucial to understanding the underlying factors that support and inhibit the client's

Table 9-1

Focus Area: Social Participation

ASSESSMENT	FOCUS AREAS	OUTCOMES
Social Profile, Adult/Adolescent Version (Donohue, 2013)	Observation of: • Activity participation • Social interaction • Group membership/social roles • Level of participation in social group	Client placed in one of the following social participation levels: • Parallel • Associative • Basic cooperative • Supportive cooperative • Mature
Assessment of Communication & Interaction Skills (Forsyth et al., 1998)	Observation of: • Physicality (e.g., gestures, gazes) • Information exchange (e.g., speaks, asks) • Relations (e.g., respects, relates)	Performance of each skill rated as: • Competent • Questionable • Ineffective • Deficient
Role Checklist Version 3: Participation and Satisfaction (Scott, 2019)	Self-assessment of role performance in 10 areas, including: • Worker • Family member • Friend	Each role is assessed for: • Participation in • Satisfaction with participation • Rationale for noncompletion
Modified Interest Checklist (Keilhofner & Neville, 1983)	Self-assessment of leisure interests that influence activity choices, many of which have a social component	Data on a client's interest and engagement in 68 activities in the past, presently, and in the future
Activity Card Sort, 2nd Edition (Baum & Edwards, 2008)	Self-report of a client's: • Occupational, social, and leisure activities • Reflection of engagement history including changes in activity with rationale Three versions exist based on client's health status: 1. Healthy 2. Sick/In an institution 3. Recovering	Information obtained from these self-reported surveys can provide insight into the OAs' social priorities and interests
The Medical Outcomes Study 36-Item Short-Form Health Survey (Ware & Sherbourne, 1992)	Self-assessment of eight health concepts within a 4-week window, including: • Social functioning and limitations in social activities due to physical or emotional problems • Roles—both physical and emotional—and limitations in usual role activities due to physical or emotional problems	Clients are asked to answer yes/no questions or to rate their responses to open-ended questions based on a Likert scale. All items are scored so that a high score defines a more favorable health state.

(continued)

Table 9-1 (continued)

Focus Area: Social Participation

ASSESSMENT	FOCUS AREAS	OUTCOMES
Social Adjustment Scale Self-Report (Weissman & Bothwell, 1976)	Self-assessment of the following within the past 2 weeks: • Work • Social & leisure activities • Relationships with extended family • Relationships with spouse (if applicable) • Parental role (if applicable) • Role within the family unit	Each item is rated on a 5-point scale, with higher scores indicating greater impairment in functioning. An overall adjustment score is obtained by adding the sum of all items and dividing by the number of items, with higher scores indicating greater impairment in functioning.
Social Functioning Questionnaire (Tyrer et al., 2005)	Self-assessment of the following within the past 2 weeks: • Work and home task completion • Economic stability • Close interpersonal relationships • Sexual activity • Loneliness & isolation	Each item is rated on a 4-point scale, with higher scores indicating greater impairment in functioning. An overall adjustment score is obtained by adding the sum of all items, with higher scores indicating greater impairment in functioning.
Life Satisfaction Index for the Third Age (Barrett & Murk, 2006)	Self-reflection on: • Zest vs. apathy • Resolution and fortitude • Congruence between desired and achieved goals • Self-concept • Mood tone	Clients are asked to agree or disagree to a series of statements about their life, attitudes, and outlook. Positive well-being is indicated by one taking pleasure in daily activities, finding meaning in life, reporting feelings of success in achieving life goals, an optimistic attitude, and positive self-image.

Table 9-2

Focus Area: Social Supports

ASSESSMENT	FOCUS AREAS	OUTCOMES
Lubben Social Network Scale (Lubben et al., 2006)	Self-report of: • Type, size, closeness, and frequency of social contact with family and friends • Perceived social support from social contacts	Each item is rated on a 6-point scale, with higher scores indicating more social engagement. An overall score is obtained by adding the sum of all items, with higher scores indicating more social engagement.
Duke-UNC Functional Social Support Questionnaire (Broadhead et al., 1988)	Measures the strength of one's social support in different situations, such as: • When one is ill • When one is having financial trouble	Each item is rated on a 6-point scale, with higher scores indicating greater social support. An overall score is obtained by adding the sum of all items, with higher scores indicating greater social support.
Duke Social Support Index (Koenig et al., 1993)	Simplified version of the Duke-UNC Functional Social Support Questionnaire specifically designed for chronically ill OAs, measuring two subscales: • Social interactions • Satisfaction with social support	Each item is rated with higher scores indicating greater social support. Items in each subscale are added with higher scores indicating greater social support. An overall score is obtained by adding the sum of both subscales, with higher scores indicating greater social support.

Table 9-3

Focus Area: Social Isolation/Loneliness

ASSESSMENT	FOCUS AREAS	OUTCOMES
UCLA (University of California, Los Angeles) Loneliness Scale (Version 3) (Russell, 1996)	• 20-item measure of subjective feelings of SI/L • Participants rate items on scale of "never" to "often"	Each item is rated on a four-point scale with higher scores indicating a greater expression of loneliness or social isolation.
De Jong Gierveld Loneliness Scale (De Jong & Van Tilburg, 2006)	Developed for OAs to assess: • "Emotional loneliness" related to intimate relationships • "Social loneliness" related to a wider social network	Scores, ranging from 0 to 11, are based on summing dichotomous item scores. The total loneliness score can be categorized as one of four levels: not lonely, moderate loneliness, severe loneliness, and very severe loneliness.
Social Isolation Scale (Nicholson et al., 2020)	Developed for OAs to assess: • Frequency of contact • Depth of connection • Feelings of belonging and inclusion	Frequency items based on a Likert scale of "none" to 6x or more. Connection items based on Likert scale from "strongly disagree" to "strongly agree." Results speak to objective "connectedness" and subjective "belongingness."

social participation. This bottom-up approach focuses on the specific underpinnings that influence social participation. For OAs, these include motor, sensory, cognitive, psychosocial, self-care, and health-related factors. Taking in the "big picture" through these siloed factors, as well as through the interplay between them, will enable the interprofessional team to improve one's social participation, functional independence, and overall QOL. In some cases, impaired social functioning is directly linked to impairments in these areas, which causes the OAs to socially withdraw. There are several ways to assess social participation from the bottom-up, including functional observation, self-assessments, and objective testing.

Physical, mental, and social changes are gradual and usually not problematic to the person experiencing them, often exacerbated by lifestyle choices and environmental factors. Those living with health conditions may experience these changes quicker and more drastically based on their specific disease process. It is imperative that both age and medical history be considered when assessing the OAs via the bottom-up approach.

Motor

From a motor perspective, clients with strength, range of motion, or balance impairments may withdraw from participating in social activities not because they are not interested in the activity, but because they are limited in their abilities to physically participate in them successfully, if at all. For example, an OA with muscle weakness may lack the strength and/or stamina to engage in leisure pursuits that provide social interactions with others or an OA with a history of falls may be hesitant to dine out with neighbors due to feelings of instability, fear of another fall, or both. Motor impairments may be evaluated by physical therapists, occupational therapists, or both professions depending on the setting and diagnosis of the client. Some suggested assessments include:

- Gross or isolated muscle testing
- Goniometry or functional assessment of range of motion
- Berg Balance Scale (Berg et al., 1992)
- Functional Reach Test (Weiner et al., 1992)
- Timed Up and Go (TUG; Podsiadlo & Richardson, 1991)
- Activities-Specific Balance Confidence Scale (Powell & Myers, 1995)

In Betty's case, her rotator cuff repair has caused temporary impairments in shoulder strength and range of motion. Clear and timely interprofessional communication amongst the care team is needed to convey results and discuss implications these impairments are having on one's current functioning, including social functioning.

Sensory

Sensory impairments including hearing, vision, and pain may also negatively impact one's social health. Clients with impaired hearing may withdraw from social activities due to difficulties with engaging in conversation and tuning out background noise, leading to frustration and discomfort. Within the interprofessional team, an audiologist can screen individuals to confirm if a hearing loss is present, determine the kind and degree of loss, and provide treatment for the hearing loss which may include custom-fit hearing aids. Once hearing impairment is addressed, OAs may feel more comfortable engaging in social activities, particularly those in crowded or noisy environments.

Visual impairments may negatively impact an OA's social health due to difficulties taking in their environment, including the faces and nonverbal communication of others. Visual impairments may also lead to difficulty reading printed materials used in a social activity, such as a church hymnal or a restaurant menu, and safely navigating crowded environments. Therefore, visual deficits may cause an OA to withdraw from previously enjoyable social activities due to feelings of frustration and discomfort. Within the interprofessional team, an optometrist or ophthalmologist can provide evaluation and treatment of the client's vision based on their medical history. For some, once their visual impairment is addressed, they may feel more comfortable engaging in social activities.

Pain may also cause an OA to withdraw from social activities. Pain may be underlying during all functional activity, including social activity, or may be exacerbated by activities that provide the opportunity to socialize, such as an exercise class, recreation sports league, or knitting group. Pain is multidimensional and should be evaluated as such, including the intensity, location, duration, description, impact on activity, and factors that influence pain perception. These factors include social supports available and current level of social functioning. Initial pain screenings assessment can be done by anyone in the interprofessional team, including physicians, specialists, nurses, rehabilitative professionals, and social workers. Self-report is the most common approach to identifying pain; it is crucial that the client is directly asked about pain (e.g., "Do you have any pain?") instead of general well-being (e.g., "How are you doing?"; Booker & Herr, 2016). Further, open-ended questions provide a better response, and allow the client to explain their pain in their own words. It is important to note that clients with cognitive, sensory, and language deficits may be unable to accurately engage in this type of assessment. The best assessments for pain intensity for OAs include:

- Numeric Pain Rating Scale (Stratford & Spadoni, 2001)
- Faces Pain Scale-Revised (Hicks et al., 2001)

Based on the client's responses, referrals can then be made to the appropriate health care professional(s) to address pain management. In Betty's case, her rotator cuff repair has caused shoulder pain that may be addressed by a physical therapist, occupational therapist, or physician.

Cognitive

While cognitive changes are be seen in healthy aging, these changes are typically not problematic to the OA, though they can be exacerbated by lifestyle choices and environmental factors, such as tobacco, alcohol, and substance abuse, a sedentary lifestyle, lack of cognitive stimulation from daily tasks, and social isolation (Mayo Clinic, 2020). Medical conditions can also impact an OA's cognitive abilities. Many disease processes that affect cognition are more common in OAs than in persons who are younger, including neurocognitive disorders (both major and minor), cardiac disease, cerebrovascular diseases, and diabetes mellitus. It is crucial to note the potential lifestyle, environmental, and medical influences on one's abilities when screening and evaluating for cognitive impairment.

Cognitive impairments including attention, memory, language, and executive functions may also negatively impact one's social health. Clients who recognize the presence of a mild cognitive impairment may withdraw to avoid potential difficulties with social activities and changes in others' perceptions of them. Clients with more pronounced cognitive impairment may not recognize their limitations but struggle to engage in social activities because of them. Assessment of cognition can be assessed through functional observation, self-report, or standardized evaluation. Self-report of cognitive abilities should be only one piece of the puzzle, though, as one may have difficulty judging their own cognitive capacities. Recommended cognitive assessments for OAs include:

- Mini Mental State Exam (MMSE; Folstein et al., 1975)
- Montreal Cognition Assessment (MoCA; Nasreddine et al., 2005)
- Saint Louis University Mental Status (SLUMS; Tariq et al., 2006)

Many members of the interprofessional team can assess an OA's cognition using the tools above. A supplement to these tools is the report of a knowledgeable observer to provide insight into an OA's daily functioning. This observer may be a spouse, family member, friend, home health provider, or skilled nursing home staff member.

Psychosocial

Psychosocial issues including depression and anxiety may also have significant negative impact on an OA's socialization as they may lead to withdrawal from previously enjoyed activities and interactions. Suggested assessments for OA include:

- Geriatric Depression Scale (GDS; Brink et al., 1982; Sheikh & Yesavage, 1986)
- Geriatric Anxiety Scale (Segal et al., 2010)
- Adult Manifest Anxiety Scale-Elderly (Reynolds et al., 2003)

These tools can be completed by any interprofessional team member, including other caregivers. It is important to note that they are meant to screen for these mental health conditions and further diagnostic inquiry is needed to formally diagnose one with depression or anxiety. Nonetheless, these tools can provide useful information to the interprofessional team to initiate the next steps of psychosocial treatment, and to monitor the impact of treatment over time, once initiated. Betty has several risks for depression including relocation, widowhood, and recent functional decline. The interprofessional team should screen for depression and make appropriate referrals if needed.

Activities of Daily Living

Clients in need of assistance with activities of daily living (ADLs) may also experience negative impacts on their social health, should the ADL difficulties correlate to social engagement. Clients who recognize the ADL impairment may withdraw to avoid potential difficulties during social activities and changes in others' perceptions of them. Examples of this may be feeding or using the restroom during a meal in a restaurant or being able to successfully dress and groom in prep for a trip into the community. OAs who rely on the assistance of others, such as those in assisted-living and skilled-nursing environments, may be delayed from engaging in social opportunities if ADL assistance is not timely. Suggested assessments include:

- Barthel Index (BI; Mahoney & Barthel, 1965)
- Modified Barthel Index (MBI; Shah et al., 1989)
- Functional Independence Measure (FIM; Keith et al., 1987)

Health-Related Factors

Older adults living with medical conditions, particularly when mismanaged or during an exacerbation, may experience difficulties engaging in social activity, causing them to withdraw. For clients with cardiopulmonary diagnoses, poor activity tolerance and endurance may limit one's abilities to engage in functional activities, especially those with aerobic components. Functional activity tolerance can be evaluated by physical and occupational therapists through timed observation of one's completion of functional activities, noting how many minutes the OA is able to tolerate each activity (such as self-care tasks) and how many rest breaks, with rest break duration, are needed during each activity. The Borg Rating of Perceived Exertion Scale (Borg, 1982) can be used to assess one's perceived exertion and fatigue, or how hard one thinks their body is working, during a specific task.

Incontinence of bowel or bladder may cause OAs to withdraw from social opportunities due to fear or embarrassment over a potential accident, noticeable odor emitted from their person, and/or difficulty managing their toileting routine, including absorbent undergarments. While Betty previously was able to manage her urinary stress incontinence without difficulty, her recent rotator cuff surgery may impact this, indirectly impacting her social health. From a medical perspective, review of one's medical, surgical, neurologic, obstetric, and mental health history, as well as one's current medications, should be included in an incontinence evaluation (National Institute for Health and Care Excellence [NICE], 2015). Quality of life questionnaires can be used to determine the severity of incontinence symptoms impacting one's daily life. Suggested assessments include:

- Bristol Female Lower Urinary Tract Symptoms Questionnaire (Jackson et al., 1996)
- Fecal Incontinence and Constipation Questionnaire (Wang et al., 2014)

Intervention

As socialization is a determinant of health, and SI/L have been deemed public health issues, a public health approach to interventions addressing the social participation of OAs is needed to maximize healthy aging of individuals and society (Gerst-Emerson & Jayawardhana, 2015; Prohaska et al., 2020). With regards to social health, this multitiered approach includes primary, secondary, and tertiary levels of interventions designed to meet the OAs where they fall on the continuum of social functioning. The continuum of social functioning spans from social isolation to active social engagement (Aw et al., 2017). Applying a public health approach to socialization calls for all members of the interprofessional team to include promotion and prevention in addition to remediation of problems. This shift in thinking requires a conceptualization of how the team can serve all OAs, not just those who are socially isolated. A continuum of services aimed at the promotion of social health, prevention of risk factors of social withdrawal, early detection of risks, and intervention is needed.

Just as the detection and assessment of threats to one's social functioning involves all members of the interprofessional team, interventions to improve socialization are also interprofessional in nature. Further, interventions may take a top-down or bottom-up approach to improving social participation, based on the client's distinct impairments, functional status, and goals. Based on their scopes of practice, different members of the team may take one or both approaches when caring for the client through a public health lens in all settings across the continuum of health care.

Primary Prevention

Adopted from the field of public health, primary interventions involve wide-scale initiatives that promote positive social health. At this tier, promotion interventions are aimed at the public and implemented before threats to social health occur. With regard to social health, promotion efforts should focus on facilitating social connections and designing built and social environments to keep OAs socially active (Chen & Feeley, 2014). Within these efforts, OAs themselves should be educated on the importance of staying socially active. Further, they should be encouraged to maintain active social engagement as a part of their daily routine and provided with strategies to maintain positive social interactions with existing close contacts. Contacts of OAs should also be educated on this topic, and encouraged to provide companionship, make home visits, and send caring or supportive messages. Primary interventions may occur at global, national, state, and local levels, and may involve policy and services geared toward promoting social health of seniors.

Public Health Campaigns

Public health campaigns are used to help all people, including health care professionals and the general public make informed decisions about their health and the health of their patients (National Institutes of Health, 2020). In 2019, the AARP Foundation launched a campaign, Connect2Affect, to address SI/L (AARP Foundation, 2021). The major goal of the campaign is to create a network of resources that meets the needs of anyone who is SI/L and that helps build the social connections that OAs need to thrive. The campaign has helped to increase awareness of the impact of SI/L on OAs, to provide information on service and training resources, and to create networks. In the United Kingdom, the Campaign to End Loneliness was founded in 2011 with the goal of connecting individuals and communities through shared research, evidence, and knowledge (2021). The campaign created a series of toolkits, research briefs, and public events to raise awareness about the health impacts of SI/L.

Age-Friendly Community Guidelines

The WHO's *Global Age-friendly City Guide* (2007) provides an outline for cities to become more accessible to and inclusive of OAs of all abilities; these include built and social environments. The guide provides eight domains that support successful aging within a community, including social participation and social inclusion. In the United States, these guidelines have been adopted by AARP to develop a network of *Age-Friendly States and Communities* (2012). The creation of these communities is dependent on collaboration between elected officials, partner organizations, local leaders, and OAs themselves. Based on their knowledge and expertise, these initiatives should include team members representing the medical, rehabilitative, and social disciplines discussed in this chapter.

Recommendations for age-friendly cities to promote the social participation of OAs include hosting events that are in a convenient and accessible location for those of varying abilities, offered at low or no cost, and offered during the day as this is often most convenient for this demographic (AARP, 2012; WHO 2007). To facilitate social inclusion of OAs, the WHO (2007) and AARP (2012) recommend anti-ageism education to reduce negative and inaccurate stereotypes of OAs, training staff to respond to the needs of older clientele, promotion of intergenerational activities, and consideration of older people as partners in making community decisions.

Within these primary intervention initiatives, the other six domains of age-friendly communities are transportation, outdoor buildings and spaces, community support and health services, communication and information, civic participation and employment, and housing (AARP, 2012; WHO, 2007). When considering social health from a bottom-up perspective, all play a role in either supporting or inhibiting a senior's social engagement. Considerations for how to foster participation and connection amongst members of a social group can be found in Box 9-1.

Secondary Prevention

Secondary prevention involves more targeted interventions for those at-risk for social isolation, with risk being physical, psychological, psychiatric, cognitive, social, cultural, or environmental. See Box 9-2 for examples within each category of risk. While one OA may present with one risk, they are often interconnected, so another may present with several. Betty currently falls in this tier based on multiple risks. Early prevention programs may focus on screening for and elimination of risk factors that negatively impact socialization, and promotion of protective factors in place that foster socialization. NASEM (2020) recommends careful consideration of these risk factors when working with each OA the care team encounters. An understanding of the risk factors followed by timely identification of at-risk OAs will then allow for referral to the appropriate medical, rehabilitative, and social preventative interventions needed.

Once risks are identified, education should be given to the senior on the risk, the potential connection to and adverse outcomes associated with SI/L, and the recommended next step(s). As an example, functional impairment is associated with SI/L. In this case, a referral should be made to occupational and physical therapy. Any number of interprofessional team members can be involved in promoting social health through secondary prevention. Efficient communication between them is crucial to ensure that all threats are

Box 9-1: Risks for Social Isolation and Loneliness

- Physical: Chronic disease such as stroke or cancer; functional impairment in gait and/or ADL; hearing or vision impairment; pain
- Psychological/Psychiatric: Major depression, generalized anxiety disorder, social anxiety disorder
- Cognitive: Alzheimer's and other dementias; subjective memory complaints
- Personal: Living alone, being unmarried (single, divorced, widowed), bereavement, no participation in social groups, strained relationships, sex, recent retirement, recent geographic move, socioeconomic status, driving status, education status
- Cultural: Immigrant status, LGBTQ+ status; minority status
- Community Environmental: Access to community transportation, housing status, geographic location, community safety, design of built environment, civic spaces, community engagement opportunities, access to activities
- Social: Public policies, public discourse, dominant political ideologies that influence society, social media, increased use of internet for goods and services

Adapted from National Academies of Sciences, Engineering, and Medicine. (2020). *Social isolation and loneliness in older adults: Opportunities for the health care system*. The National Academies Press. https://doi.org/10.17226/25663, Health Resources & Services Administration. (2019). *The "Loneliness Epidemic."* https://www.hrsa.gov/enews/past-issues/2019/january-17/loneliness-epidemic, and Prohaska, T., Burholt, V., & Burns, A. (2020). Consensus statement: Loneliness in older adults, The 21st century social determinant of health? *BMJ Open, 10*, e034967. https://doi.org/10.1136/bmjopen-2019-034967.

Box 9-2: Key Disciplines Involved in Promoting Social Health By Risk Factor*

- Physical - medical physicians (both generalists and specialists), audiologists, optometrists, ophthalmologists, occupational therapists, physical therapists, speech-language pathologists, nurses, physician assistants, CNAs, social workers
- Psychological/Psychiatric - psychologists, psychiatrists, occupational therapists, social workers
- Cognitive - neurologists, occupational therapists, social workers, speech-language pathologists
- Community Environmental - lawmakers and elected officials, civic engineers, occupational therapists, senior centers, churches, community centers
- Social - lawmakers and elected officials, business owners

* Not all discussed at length in this chapter

being addressed, to prevent duplication of services, and to provide updates on the efficacy of each intervention. At this tier, strong evidence exists to support the social engagement of OAs through leisure education, chronic disease self-management, and physical activity interventions (Franke et al., 2021; Smallfield & Molitor, 2018).

Further, NASEM (2020) recommends that health care providers periodically perform a SI/L assessment for those at risk, using a validated tool (see assessment section for some examples), to identify if these issues are present. While there is limited evidence to determine how to implement these tools in clinical settings, it is recommended that within an organization, one tool or set of tools is selected and used universally, and that this information be included in one's electronic health records. Each organization would determine who should conduct the assessment, at what frequency, and with what follow-up recommendations (NASEM, 2020; Prohaska et al., 2020). The tool should be given as intended and in entirety, as editing by the evaluator will render findings invalid and confusing. Should the team not recognize Betty's SI/L risks, having a system in place that screens all OAs would detect any threats to her social health.

Tertiary Prevention

Tertiary prevention is a reactionary approach after SI/L has occurred, which aims to prevent further impacts of this issue and restore the OA to an optimal state of social functioning. There is no cookie-cutter approach to addressing SI/L, and the approach to intervention should be tailored to meet the needs and goals of each individual client (Franke et al., 2021; Jeste et al., 2020). At this level of intervention, services pay particular attention to the causes and consequences of SI/L. Understanding the root cause(s) will then lead to referral to the appropriate medical, rehabilitative, and social interventions. As an example, functional impairment is associated with hearing loss. In this care, a referral should be made to an audiologist. Once causes are identified, education should be given to the senior on the cause and its link to their current impairments. Further, understanding the consequences of one's SI/L will also lead to referral to the appropriate medical, rehabilitative, and social interventions needed. For example, seniors who are isolated may become depressed over time. While the depression may not have been the initial cause of the isolation, its presence may likely cause one to withdraw further socially. It is therefore critical that the effects of the mental health disorder be diminished to promote the overall health and well-being of the client.

Intervention at this level should also focus on strategies to increase opportunities for social interaction, enhance social support, and potentially improve social skills (Jeste et al., 2020). These may include home visits, daily contact programs with outreach in person or via technology, and engagement in community-based groups. Exploration of one's activity history and current interests, as well as available offerings within the community, should occur in collaboration with the client, with the end goal of identifying programming that is accessible to and of interest to the client. Underlying factors that limit accessibility at individual (e.g., poor balance or functional activity tolerance) and community levels (e.g., lack of community transportation) should be discussed. Interventions to remediate or compensate for these factors should then be explored based on the client's specific situation.

For group programming, should clients choose these, careful consideration should go into the group structure and leadership to best promote relationship building amongst participants. The group leader should be personable, positive, motivating, and accommodating. Opportunities to share information and experiences, and to learn from others, should be provided. These include providing personal introductions, use of paired and group discussions to promote interactions between participants, and encouraged exchange of contact information (Franke et al., 2021). As participants may feel more comfortable and supported when they are with others who they perceive to be similar (Bennett et al., 2018), frequent opportunities to engage with others of familiar backgrounds and experiences is recommended.

Interprofessional Perspectives

As social participation of OAs is multifaceted, an interprofessional team involving rehabilitative, medical, and social disciplines is needed to best address the unique and holistic needs of each client. SI/L OAs are not often identified in their communities, but almost all interact with the health care system (Blazer, 2020). Therefore, health care providers are in a strong position to identify those at risk and those living with SI/L. They care for the health issues that may cause or result from these conditions. SI/L are similar but distinct conditions, and clinicians must understand how they differ to provide the best possible treatment (Taylor, 2021). As they often influence each other, many OAs experience both conditions simultaneously.

Applying a public health approach to the promotion of socialization calls for all members of the team to include promotion and prevention in addition to remediation of problems. Further, awareness of the top-down and bottom-up approaches to social health are needed by each team member to timely identify, evaluate, and intervene in this arena. Threats to social health may be uncovered by any member of the team, at any time, and in any setting across the continuum of care. Prompt communication and collaboration are needed to ensure that referrals are being made to the proper professional to address each specific need related to social health. In Betty's case, each interaction with her physician, surgeon, therapists, nurses, and other members of the team is an opportunity for her social health to be addressed.

In addition to keeping a close eye on the supports and barriers to one's social health, each member of the care team may also be considered a member of a client's social network based on the frequency, duration, and depth of their interactions with the client. For OAs in subacute rehabilitation following an injury or illness, for those who are homebound receiving homecare services, and for those who reside in skilled-nursing facilities, care team members often provide the bulk of their meaningful daily social interactions. For isolated and lonely OAs residing in the community, research shows they are more likely to seek medical assistance to satisfy needs for interaction and interpersonal stimulation, as the doctor-patient relationship provides social support (Gerst-Emerson & Jawawardhana, 2015). All health professionals should be aware of, and take into consideration, loneliness as a factor when engaging with clients.

Rehabilitative

Occupational therapists and occupational therapy assistants are experts in human functioning across the life span, and they have a distinct role in addressing social health in comparison to the interprofessional disciplines involved in this arena. Occupational therapists and occupational therapy assistants understand their clients through a holistic approach that focuses on the use of functional activity as both an intervention process and an end goal (AOTA, 2020). Training in social skills, group dynamics, and client-centered modes of communication exemplifies their expertise in social health.

Speech-language pathologists and speech-language pathology assistants are experts in communication who address speech, language, vocal quality, fluency, and swallowing (American Speech-Language-Hearing Association, n.d.a, b). Like occupational therapy, this rehabilitative field also looks at social health through top-down and bottom-up approaches, but in this case the focus is on communication vs. functional independence, from producing clear speech (bottom-up) to social communication and social interactions (top-down).

Physical therapists and physical therapy assistants are movement experts who address motion, pain, and function through prescribed exercise, hands-on care, and patient education (American Physical Therapy Association, n.d.). With regards to social functioning of an OA, these rehabilitative professionals take a bottom-up approach focused primarily on the motor components of social functioning: strength, range of motion, balance, gait, and stair negotiation.

Medical

Physicians may specialize in a specific patient population, such as geriatricians who care for OAs, general practitioners who care for patients of all ages, and general internists who care for adults. These doctors practice primary care, or the day-to-day care that is one's first contact with the health care system (American Academic of Family Physicians, n.d.). Primary care physicians are often the first to recognize a health issue. Upon doing so, they may order diagnostic tests and/or make referrals to medical or rehabilitative specialists based on the issue at hand. Physicians take a bottom-up approach to social participation by addressing the underlying medical issues that limit one's social independence. For example, a client may report poor balance and fear of falling that stops them from community outings, prompting a physician referral to physical and occupational therapy. In addition to physicians, there are other members of the medical team that are crucial in the care of OAs' social health that include nurses and physician assistants.

In homecare, assisted living facilities, and skilled nursing homes, certified nursing assistants, home health aides, and homemakers may help with vital sign monitoring, self-care, functional mobility, home management, and community mobility tasks and provide companionship to their clients (United States Bureau of Labor, 2021a, 2021b). They are crucial members of the interprofessional team as they have consistent contact with OAs who are at risk for social isolation due to medical complexities and functional impairment. These professionals can observe the fluctuations in the patients' physical conditions and the subtle changes in their emotional states, thereby allowing them to relay this information to upper levels of the health care team and contribute to furthering optimal treatment and healing.

Social

Social workers are professionals who focus on enhancing the well-being of people and communities by addressing social injustices and other threats to this well-being (National Association of Social Workers, 2021). Clinical social workers can diagnose and treat mental, behavioral, and emotional issues. They work with clients to change behavior or cope with difficult situations, such as transitioning from the hospital back to their homes and managing a new chronic illness. Social workers may clients to other resources, such as support groups or other health professionals. They may work in a variety of specialties including geriatrics. Social workers can address OAs' social health through a top-down approach based on counseling, advocacy, and referrals to other disciplines.

Community Program

The Towers at Tower Lane (also known as The Towers) is a senior housing community in New Haven, Connecticut. It is home to over 300 older adults. This not-for-profit site provides moderate to low-income housing to a diverse population age 62 or older, with an average age of 83 years. The Towers offers different models of care including independent living, assisted living, and Connecticut Homecare for Elders Program (Connecticut Department of Social Services, 2021) services, and has contracts with local primary care physicians, geriatric psychiatrists and other specialists, and rehabilitative services. Seventy percent of residents at the site need hands-on personal care for one or more activities of daily living and 45% report no routine contact with family. Recognizing that their residents were at risk for social isolation and functional decline, they sought partnership with Quinnipiac University's Department of Occupational Therapy. A qualitative study on social participation was the first step in improving and/or developing systems to better promote their health and independence, prevent functional and medical decline, and enhance their overall QOL (Fidanza et al., 2018).

This revealed a lack of support for newly transitioned residents, making it challenging for these residents to develop a sense of belonging and connect with others upon move in (Fidanza et al., 2018). Many participants spoke to feeling alone after moving in, despite positive impressions before making the transition (Fidanza et al., 2018). Further, most residents did not see offered recreational activities as sources of socialization and reported little autonomy over the topics or frequency of these activities (Fidanza et al., 2018). Activity leaders were often volunteering and lacked training in group dynamics, or in how to foster conversations and build relationships among people (Fidanza et al., 2018). Observations showed that most socialization was spontaneous, short, and superficial (Fidanza et al., 2018). Suggestions were provided to the facility on ways to improve the resident socialization, including a revised assessment protocol for use upon move-in to gather beneficial data on new residents, changes to currently offered programming and systems, and improved education for those running groups.

The results of this study lead to the development of two programs: one within the profession of occupational therapy and the other within the site itself. *Opportunity to Thrive: The Fidanza Method to Enrich Older Adult Social Health* (referred to as *Opportunity to Thrive*) was created for occupational therapists to address the underliers of social health and QOL within a senior living establishment (Fidanza et al., 2018, 2020 ,2021a) at The Towers. This program is organically evolving and currently includes a resident assessment to detect current risk factors, pathways to ensure parity of care between residents, educational handouts for residents who are considered at risk, and educational materials for staff and volunteers, particularly those involved in group programming at the site. This program is a part of The Towers' Proactive Partner Model, which places the resident at the center of services designed to meet their needs and goals at no extra cost to the resident.

The first step of *Opportunity to Thrive* program is the *Opportunity to Thrive Resident Assessment*, a mixed-methods intake tool that holistically evaluates each new resident upon their move into the facility, and quarterly thereafter to track changes in status over time (Fidanza et al., 2019). This assessment is used generate key data on each resident to enhance their sense of belonging within the facility while also identifying potential threats to their physical health, mental health, and QOL. The assessment revamped the site's original intake procedure, which was often subjective and lacked standardization. The original intake also had gaps in identifying pertinent information about the resident.

The *Opportunity to Thrive Resident Assessment* is twofold. Upon move-in, an occupational profile interview is conducted to gather background information on the resident. This includes their life story, such as what their life was like growing up, family, friends, school/college, marriage, work, children, and hobbies; why they moved to The Towers; which daily activities they require assistance with; their functional and community mobility; how they spend their time; how often they socially interact with others; and activities they are/would like to be involved in at The Towers. This interview helps to gain the trust of the residents, as well as understand more about their life to provide them with social activities that meet their preferences. These social activities may be participation in group programs, connections with fellow residents and/or volunteers who share similar interests/backstories, and potential leadership opportunities such as Resident Council.

The second part of the *Opportunity to Thrive Resident Assessment* evaluation assesses the resident for frailty. **Frailty** is defined as "a clinically recognizable state of increased vulnerability resulting from aging-associated decline in reserve and function across multiple physiologic systems such that the ability to cope with every day or acute stressors is comprised" (Xue, 2011, p. 1). The *Opportunity to Thrive* program looks at frailty through an occupational therapy lens, adapted from Fried et al. (2001; Fidanza et al., 2019). Specifically, new residents are assessed in five main areas: physiology, physical function, cognitive function, psychosocial function, and ADLs. The instruments chosen to assess each frailty subcomponent were based on the following criteria: standardization (administered, scored, and interpreted in the same way for all test-takers), ease of administration (they do not require complex setup or many materials), duration of administration (most take less than 10 minutes), and strong reliability and validity data (they are proven to measure the intended subject). Within the *Opportunity to Thrive* program, this assessment package is given on admission and again every 120 days to track changes in frailty over time.

Physiology is assessed by weight loss, which is self-reported during the initial assessment. The resident is also weighed for future reference (with consent). Criteria for frailty includes unintentional loss of 10 pounds or more in the last year, or unintentional weight loss of 5% of body weight or more in the last year. Physical function/strength is assessed using the Timed Up and Go (TUG) and Jamar Dynamometer. The TUG is used to identify if a resident is a fall risk (Podsiadlo & Richardson, 1991). Criterion for frailty is completion of the TUG in 12 seconds or longer (Podsiadlo & Richardson, 1991). The Jamar Dynamometer is used to identify grip strength in the participants' right and left hands (Bohannon et al., 2006). Criteria for frailty are numbers below average for age and gender (Bohannon et al., 2006). Participants with poor balance (as observed by the evaluator) are not asked to step onto the sale during the physiology evaluation. Similarly, for physical function/strength assessment, participants who were observed with poor balance were only given the Jamar Dynamometer test.

ADL is assessed using the *Barthel Index* to identify how independent participants are when taking care of themselves (Mahoney & Barthel, 1965). Criterion for frailty includes a score of 90 or less (Mahoney & Barthel, 1965). Psychosocial function is assessed using the *Geriatric Depression Scale, short form*, which is used to identify participants at risk for developing depression or who are showing depressive symptoms (Burke et al., 1991). Criteria for frailty is a score of five or higher (Burke et al., 1991). Cognition is assessed using the *Mini Mental State Evaluation* (Folstein et al., 1975). The *Mini Mental State Examination* is used to identify cognitive impairment via the domains of orientation, attention, visual-spatial skills, memory, and language. A criterion for frailty is a score of 24 or less (Folstein et al., 1975).

During the intake assessment, each of the quantitative assessments is per the assessment itself. See Table 9-4 for the specific criteria for frailty, based on the assessment itself. Based on the results of these quantitative assessments, participants are classified for frailty as follows: Not Frail/Green if 0 criteria for frailty are present; Pre-Frail/Yellow if 1 to 2 criteria for frailty are present; and Frail/Red if 3 or more criteria for frailty are present. Upon completion of the *Opportunity to Thrive* assessment, all quantitative information is documented in an electronic spread sheet to determine the residents' category of frailty, and to track changes in one's frailty scores over time. Further, each occupational profile is saved to the resident's electronic case file for administration to review as needed.

Analysis of the quantitative component of the *Opportunity to Thrive Resident Assessment* frailty component reveals that upon move into The Towers, most residents are Pre-Frail or Frail, placing their health, QOL, and occupational engagement at risk (Fidanza et al., 2019). Once one's specific risk factors are identified, The Towers then *Opportunity to Thrive Care Pathways*, created by occupational therapy students, to standardize the process of addressing residents' needs (Fidanza et al., 2021a). The pathways were designed to create a plan of action that enables opportunities

Table 9-4

Focus Area: Social Isolation/Loneliness

CATEGORY	ASSESSMENT	CRITERIA FOR FRAILTY
Physiology	Weight loss-self reported and current weight taken	Unintentional loss of 10 pounds or more in the last year, OR unintentional weight loss of 5% of body weight or more in the last year
Physical function/strength	Timed Up and Go Jamar Dynamometer	Completion in 12 seconds or longer Below average for age and gender norms
ADLs	Barthel Index	Score of 90 or less
Psychosocial	Geriatric Depression Scale, short form	Score of 5 or higher
Cognition	Mini Mental Status Examination	Score of 24 or less

for improved health and well-being, and to provide equitable intervention opportunities to all those in need, via secondary prevention (Fidanza et al., 2021a).

Based on a resident's frailty risk factors, *Opportunity to Thrive Care Pathways* contain interventions specific to each area of concern available at The Towers. These pathways include participation in evidence-based group programming, referrals to doctors and other health care professionals (such as nutritionists, occupational therapists, and physical therapists), one-on-one visits with volunteers, and client/caregiver/family education. The group programs listed in the pathways are often evidence-based and include *A Matter of Balance* (Tennstedt et al., 1998), *Jewish Aging Mastery* (National Council on Aging, 2012), *Music and Memory* (Music and Memory Inc., 2021), and *Opening Minds Through Art* (Opening Minds Through Art, Inc., 2021). Non-evidence–based group programs include arts and crafts, brain teasers (e.g., jeopardy, word searches, sudoku, etc.), reminiscing, movement programs (e.g., tai chi, yoga, etc.), and client education (e.g., fall prevention, coping strategies, etc.). The process of categorizing currently offered programs based on frailty category allowed the site to identify which risk factors are robustly covered vs. which need more programming/support. Research into evidence-based programming, referral sources, and other possible additions to these care pathways is ongoing, with the goal of adding to the pathways over time to best meet the needs of residents with that specific area of concern.

Concurrent to the use of care pathways by The Towers' staff after the *Opportunity to Thrive Resident Assessment* is completed, residents who flag in a specific frailty category are given educational handouts on that risk factor (Fidanza et al., 2021b). These handouts were created by occupational therapy students based on *Federal Plain Language Guidelines* (Plain Language Action and Information Network, 2011), the Centers for Disease Control and Prevention (CDC) *Clear Communication Index* (CDC, 2014), and Centers for Medicare and Medicaid Services (CMS) *Toolkit for Making Written Material Clear and Effective* (CMS, 2010). One handout was made for each of the five frailty categories. Each of the five frailty handouts was created with a specific format and layout to ensure easy readability for the residents.

Each handout has a title bolded at the top of the page, specific to the frailty category that is being addressed. Handout titles use simple language and are clearly stated so that the reader can be oriented and prepared for what the following information entails. The title is followed by a short introduction that gives a brief overview of the frailty assessment. A short statement is included stating what the results of the assessment showed for the specific frailty category the handout was addressing. The information on each handout was separated into three categories. This first section of information is titled "Why It's Important" and included what health factors the resident is at risk for or more likely to experience. The next section is titled "What to Look Out For" and included information about what signs and symptoms to be aware of. The last section is titled "What to Do" and included information on preventative measures that could be taken in order to slow or decrease the progression of the frailty factor. Every handout included one picture that was relevant to the information as well as a short wrap-up sentence to encourage residents to discuss available programs with their resident service coordinator (Fidanza et al., 2021b).

Within the *Opportunity to Thrive Program*, education has also been provided to The Towers staff and volunteers who run group programs to facilitate both resident participation and social connections within a given group. A tip was created by occupational therapy students that focuses on the following areas: group format, group dynamics, forming connections, and making activities easier/harder. These strategies align with WHO's (2007) and AARP's (2012) *Age-Friendly* suggestions. See Box 9-3 with for the tips provided. This handout was presented in an in-service to current staff and volunteers and is being used to educate new staff and volunteers on an as-needed basis. Education has also been given on group programming ideas, based on informal surveys of The Towers' residents, to better address the variety of interests present amongst them. Two successful programs that have stemmed from the informal surveys include a reminiscing group and a men's group.

Box 9-3: Strategies to Facilitate Participation and Social Connections Within a Group Activity

GROUP FORMAT

Your group should be broken into different parts, including:

- Introduction (have members introduce themselves)
- Main activity (an activity that involves the theme of the group)
- Discussion about activity (help residents apply the theme to their lives)
- Conclusion (wrap up the activity and thank people for coming)

Make sure you have a set time for how long each part of the group should last. This way, you'll be able to keep all group members on track and be able to progress through the group.

GROUP DYNAMICS

- It is important to consider varying personalities while running a group.
- Some residents are more easygoing while others are more apprehensive to the group process.
- The way that these personalities interact greatly impacts how the group runs, and the impact of the group on each resident.
- It is okay to pause the group to direct a resident who starts to speak off topic/speaks for too long.
- If a resident is not participating, kindly ask them if they have anything to share. If they do not wish to participate, it is okay. Allow them to observe the group.
- If a conflict arises between residents, remain neutral as the leader. Step in kindly to remind residents that the expectation is to be respectful to one another.

FORMING CONNECTIONS

- Groups are used as a form of social participation and connection for residents who may not get out of the facility often.
- It is important as the group leader to try and find common themes between the residents that they can bond over during and after the group.
- Beginning the group by going around in a circle and having introductions of each group member will allow the residents to make connections with familiar and unfamiliar faces.
- Try to address the residents by name so that you produce an overall feeling of inclusivity within the group.

MAKING ACTIVITIES EASIER/HARDER

- Many residents have different strengths and weaknesses that can be apparent within a group setting.
- Different abilities can influence the group process, as well as individual participation.
- Providing group members with modified activities will enable them to feel more successful.
- Consider breaking the activity down into simple steps, and give one clear direction for each step, one step at a time.
- Provide one on one assistance during the group if a resident is struggling with an activity.
- Consider making worksheets with larger print for those with visual impairments, and seat residents with hearing impairments closer to the group leader.
- If the individual is still unable to participate fully within the activity, don't worry! The resident is participating in a social experience which is the most important thing

The *Opportunity to Thrive* program continues to organically develop as it identifies resident needs regarding socialization and frailty. Partnership between The Towers providing learning opportunities to occupational therapy students through the Quinnipiac University Master of Occupational Therapy curricula, including service learning, Capstone projects, and level II fieldwork experiences. There is opportunity for other disciplines to be involved in this program, particularly social workers and physical therapists, to support residents from declining functionally while living at The Towers. *Opportunity to Thrive* can be replicated in other senior housing facilities; please contact this author for further discussion at nicole.fidanza@quinnipiac.edu.

Conclusion

Addressing the social participation of OAs is a key factor in successful aging. As the world population ages, more attention is being paid to supporting older adults to remain connected to and contributing members of their communities. Targeting social participation may present one of the greatest opportunities to improve OAs' general health and will also generate societal benefits by increasing community contributions from this group (Douglas et al., 2017). A clear understanding of the concepts included in social participation, how they are related, and how they combine to produce improved health outcomes enables health professionals to understand how they can intervene to improve the health of an aging population. The health care system must play a role in helping reduce both the incidence and the negative health impacts of social isolation and loneliness among older adults.

Currently, the systems in which OAs engage have untapped potential to identify these risk factors and prevent the health detriments associated with them. An interprofessional public health approach to addressing these social determinants of health is needed to serve all older adults, not just those who are socially isolated. Using the *Core Competencies for Interprofessional Collaborative Practice* (IPEC, 2016), interprofessional teams are poised to address social health of individuals, communities, and populations. Services should promote social health, prevent the risk factors of social withdrawal, detect risks for social isolation and loneliness in a timely manner, and remediate these issues if present.

References

AARP. (2012). Introducing the Age-Friendly Network. https://www.aarp.org/livable-communities/network-age-friendly-communities/info-2014/an-introduction.html.

AARP Foundation. (2021). Connect 2 Affect. https://connect2affect.org

AARP Research. (2018). Loneliness and social connections: A national survey of adults 45 and older. https://connect2affect.org/wp-content/uploads/2018/09/AARP-740C-Loneliness-Report-v3-with-LOGO-TAG.pdf/

American Academy of Family Physicians. (n.d.). Primary care. https://www.aafp.org/about/policies/all/primary-care.html

American Occupational Therapy Association. (2020). Occupational therapy practice framework: Domain and process (4th ed.). *American Journal of Occupational Therapy, 74*(Suppl. 2), 7412410010. https://doi.org/10.5014/ajot.2020.74S2001

American Physical Therapy Association. (n.d.). What physical therapists do. https://www.apta.org/your-career/careers-in-physical-therapy/becoming-a-pt

American Speech-Language-Hearing Association. (n.d.a). Social communication. https://www.asha.org/public/speech/development/Social-Communication/

American Speech-Language-Hearing Association. (n.d.b). Who are speech-language pathologists? https://www.asha.org/public/who-are-speech-language-pathologists/

Arslantaş, A., Adana, F., Ergin, F. A., Kayar, D., & Acar, G. (2015). Loneliness in elderly people, associated factors and its correlation with quality of life: A field study from Western Turkey. *Iranian Journal of Public Health, 44*, 43-50.

Asiamah, N. (2017). Social engagement and physical activity: Commentary on why the activity and disengagement theories of ageing may both be valid. *Cogent Medicine, 4*(1), 1-3. https://doi.org/10.1080/2331205X.2017.1289664

Atchley, R. C. (1989). A continuity theory of normal aging. *The Gerontologist, 29*(2), 183-190. https://doi.org/10.1093/geront/29.2.183

Aw, S., Koh, G., Oh, Y. J., Wong, M. L., Vrijhoef, H. J. M., Harding, S. C., Geronimo, M. B., Lai, C. Y. F., & Hildon, Z. J. L. (2017). Explaining the continuum of social participation among older adults in Singapore: From 'closed doors' to active ageing in multi-ethnic community settings. *Journal of Aging Studies, 42*, 46-55. https://doi.org/10.1016/j.jaging.2017.07.002

Barrett, A., & Murk, P. (2006, October 4-6). Life Satisfaction for the Third Age (LSITA): A measurement of successful aging [Conference presentation]. Midwest Research-to-Practice Conference in Adult, Continuing, and Community Education, St. Louis, MO, United States.

Baum, C. M., & Edwards, D. (2008). *Activity card sort* (2nd ed.). American Occupational Therapy Association.

Bekhet, A. K., & Zauszniewski, J. A. (2014). Chronic conditions in elders in assisted living facilities: Associations with daily functioning, self-assessed health, and depressive symptoms. *Archives of Psychiatric Nursing, 28*, 399-404. http://dx.doi.org/10.1016/j.apnu.2014.08.013

Bennett, E. V., Clarke, L. H., Wolf, S. A., Dunlop, W.L. et al. (2018). Older adults' experiences of group-based physical activity: A qualitative study from the 'GOAL' randomized controlled trial. *Psychology of Sport and Exercise, 39*, 184-192. https://doi.org/10.1016/j.psychsport.2018.08.017

Berg, K. O., Wood-Dauphinee, S. L., Williams, J. I., & Maki, B. (1992). Measuring balance in the elderly: Validation of an instrument. *Canadian Journal of Public Health, 83*(Suppl 2), S7-S11.

Betts Adams, K., Leibbrandt, S., & Moon, H. (2011). A critical review of the literature on social and leisure activity and well-being in later life. *Ageing & Society, 31*, 683-712. https://doi.org/10.1017/S0144686X10001091

Beuscher, L., & Dietrich, M. (2016). Depression training in an assisted living facility. *Journal of Psychosocial Nursing, 54*(5), 25-31. https://doi.org/10.3928/02793695-20160201-01

Blazer D. G. (2020). Social isolation and loneliness in older adults: A mental health/public health challenge. *JAMA Psychiatry, 77*(10), 990-991. https://doi.org/10.1001/jamapsychiatry.2020.1054

Bohannon, R.W., Bear-Lehman, J., Desrosiers, J., Massy-Wastropp, N., & Mathiowetz, V. (2006). Average grip strength: A meta-analysis of data obtained with a Jamar dynamometer from individuals 75 years or more of age. *Journal of Geriatric Physical Therapy, 30*(1), 28-30.

Booker, S. Q., & Herr, K. A. (2016). Assessment and measurement of pain in adults later in life. *Clinics in Geriatric Medicine, 32*(4), 677-692. https://doi.org/10.1016/j.cger.2016.06.012

Borg, G. A. (1982). Psychophysical bases of perceived exertion. *Medicine and Science in Sports and Exercise, 14*, 377-381.

Brink, T. L., Yesavage, J. A., Lum, O., Heersema, P. H., Adey, M., & Rose, T. L. (1982). Screening tests for geriatric depression. *Clinical Gerontologist, 1*(1), 37-43. https://doi.org/10.1300/J018v01n01_06

Broadhead, W. E., Gehlbach, S. H., De Gruy, F. V., & Kaplan, B. H. (1988). The Dune-UNC Functional Social Support Questionairre: Measurement of social support in family medicine patients. *Medical Care, 26*(7), 709-723.

Burke, W. J., Roccaforte, W. H., & Wengel, S. P. (1991). The short form of the Geriatric Depression Scale: A comparison with the 30-item form. *Topics in Geriatrics, 4*(3), 173-178. https://doi.org/10.1177/089198879100400310

Campaign to End Loneliness. (2021). About the campaign. https://www.campaigntoendloneliness.org/about-the-campaign

Cao, Q., Dabelko-Schoeny, H. I., White, K. M., & Choi, M. S. (2020). Age-friendly communities and perceived disconnectedness: the role of built environment and social engagement. *Journal of Aging and Health, 32*(9), 937–948. https://doi.org/10.1177/0898264319865421

Carstensen, L. L., Isaacowitz, D. M., & Charles, S. T. (1999). Taking time seriously: A theory of socioemotional selectivity. *American Psychologist, 54*(3), 165-181. https://doi.org/10.1037/0003-066X.54.3.165

Centers for Disease Control and Prevention. (2014). Clear Communication Index. https://www.cdc.gov/ccindex/index.html

Centers for Medicare and Medicaid Services. (2010). Toolkit for Making Written Materials Clear and Effective. https://www.cms.gov/Outreach-and-Education/Outreach/WrittenMaterialsToolkit/ToolkitTableOfContents

Chen, Y., & Feeley, T. H. (2014). Social support, social strain, loneliness, and well-being among older adults: An analysis of the Health and Retirement Study. *Journal of Social and Personal Relationships, 31*(2), 141-161. https://doi.org/10.1177/0265407513488728

Choi, E., Han, K., Chang, J., Lee, Y. J., Choi, W. W., Han, C., & Ham, B. (2020). Social participation and depressive symptoms in community-dwelling older adults: Emotional support as a mediator. *Journal of Psychiatric Research, 137*, 589-596. https://doi.org/10.106/j.psychires.2020.10.043

Connecticut Department of Social Services. (2021). Connecticut Homecare Program for Elders. https://portal.ct.gov/DSS/Health-And-Home-Care/Connecticut-Home-Care-Program-for-Elders/Connecticut-Home-Care-Program-for-Elders-CHCPE

Crewdson, J. A. (2016). The effect of loneliness in the elderly population: A review. *Healthy Aging & Clinical Care in the Elderly, 8*, 1-8. http://dx.doi.org/10.4137/HACCE

Cumming, E., & Henry, W. E. (1961). *Growing old*. Basic Books.

De Jong, J., & Van Tilburg, T. (2006). 6-item scale for overall, emotional, and social loneliness: Confirmatory tests on survey data. *Research on Aging, 28*(5), 582-598. https://doi.org/10.1177/0164027506289723

Donohue, M. V. (2013). *Social profile: Assessment of social participation in children, adolescents, and adults*. AOTA Press.

Douglas, H., Georgiou, B. A., & Westbrook, J. (2017). Social participation as an indicator of successful aging: An overview of concepts and their associations with health. *Australian Health Review, 41*(4), 455-462. http://doi.org/10.1071/AH16038

Duppen, D., Lambotte, D., Dury, S., Smetcoren, A., Pan, H., & De Donder, L. (2020). Social participation in the daily lives of frail older adults: Types of participation and influencing factors. *The Journals of Gerontology. Series B, Psychological Sciences and Social Sciences, 75*(9), 2062. https://doi.org/10.1093/geronb/gbz045

Fidanza, N., Baker, N., Brown, R., Gallagher, H., & Godusky, K. (2019, October). Determining the needs of newly transitioned residents in a senior living facility: A mixed-methods assessment [Conference presentation]. Connecticut Public Health Association Annual Conference, Plantsville, CT, United States.

Fidanza, N., Baker, N., Brown, R., Gallagher, H., & Godusky, K. (2020, April). Determining the needs of newly transitioned residents in an assisted living facility: A mixed-methods assessment [Conference presentation]. AOTA 2020 Annual Conference & Expo (cancelled), Boston, MA, United States.

Fidanza, N., Kowal, J., & Bondoc, S. (2018, March). Exploring social isolation versus participation amongst older adults in assisted living facilities. [Short course]. Connecticut Occupational Therapy Association Annual Conference, Wallingford, CT, United States.

Fidanza, N., Kowal, J., & Bondoc, S. (2021a). An exploration of social participation amongst older adults in assisted living facilities. [Poster presentation]. AOTA 2021 Inspire Conference, Virtual, United States.

Fidanza, N., Kowal, J., McLoone, M., Nelson, H., & Vendetti, A. (2021b). Addressing new resident frailty through pathways and education [Poster presentation]. AOTA 2021 Inspire Conference, Virtual, United States.

Fischl, C., Lindelof, N., Lindgren, H., & Nilsson, I. (2020). Older adults' perceptions of contexts surrounding their social participation in a digitized society: An exploration in rural communities in Northern Sweden. *European Journal of Ageing, 17*, 281-290. https://doi.org/10.1007/s10433-020-00558-7

Folstein, M. F., Folstein, S. E., & McHugh, P. R. (1975). "Mini mental state": A practical method for grading the cognitive state of patients for the clinician. *Journal of Psychiatric Research, 12*(3), 189-198. https://doi.org/10.1016/0022-3956(75)90026-6

Forsyth, K., Salamy, M., Simon, S., & Keilhofner, G. (1998). *Assessment of communication and interaction skills, Version 4.0* (ACIS). Model of Occupation Clearinghouse.

Franke, T., Sims-Gould, J., Nettlefold, L., et al. (2021). "It makes me feel not so alone": features of the Choose to Move physical activity intervention that reduce loneliness in older adults. *BMC Public Health, 21*(312), 1-15. https://doi.org/10.1186/s12889-021-10363-1

Fried, L., Tangen, C., Walston, J., Newman, A., Hirsch, C., Gottdiener, J., & McBurnie, M. (2001). Frailty in older adults: Evidence for a phenotype. *The Journals of Gerontology, 56* (3), 146-157. https://doi.org/10.1093/gerona/56.3.m146

Gao, M, Zhihong, S., Li, Y., Zhang, W., Tian, D., Zhang, S., & Gu, L. (2018). Does social participation reduce the risk of functional disability among older adults in China? A survival analysis using the 2005-2011 waves of the CLHLS data. *BMC Geriatrics, 18*(1), 224. https://doi.org/10.1186/s12877-018-0903-3

Gerst-Emerson, K., & Jayawardhana, J. (2015). Loneliness as a public health issue: The impact of loneliness on health care utilization among older adults. *American Journal of Public Health, 105*(5), 1013-1019. https://doi.org/10.2105/AJPH.2014.302427

Glei, D. A., Goldman, N., Ryff, C. D. Lin, Y., & Weinstein, M. (2012). Social relationships and inflammatory markers: An analysis of Taiwan and the U.S. *Social Science & Medicine, 74*(12), 1891-1899. https://doi.org/10.1016/j.socscimed.2012.02.020

Goll, J. C., Charlesworth, G., Scior, K., & Stott, J. (2015). Barriers to social participation among lonely older adults: The influence of social fears and identity. *PLOS ONE, 13*(7), e0201510. https://doi.org/10.1371/journal.pone.0201510

Gray, A. (2009). The social capital of older people. *Ageing and Society, 29*, 5-31. Https://doi.org/10.1017/s0144686x08007617

Griffith, L. E., Parminder, R., Levasseur, M., Sohel, N., Payette, H., Tuokko, H., van den Huevel, E., Wister, A., Gilsing, A., & Patterson, C. (2017). Functional disability and social participation restriction associated with chronic conditions in middle-aged and older adults. *Journal of Epidemiology and Community Health, 71*(4), 381-389. 10.1136/jech-2016-207982

Guo, Q., Bai, W., & Feng, N. (2018). Social participation and depressive symptoms among Chinese older adults: A study on rural-urban differences. *Journal of Affective Disorders, 239*, 124- 130. https://doi.org/10.1016/j.jad.2018.06.036

Ha, J., Khang, S. K., & Choi, N. (2017). Reciprocal effects between health and social support in older adults' relationships with their children and friends. *Research on Aging, 39*(2), 300–321. https://doi.org/10.1177/0164027515611182

Haak, M., Löfqvist, C., Ullén, S., Horstmann, V., & Iwarsson, S. (2019). The influence of participation on mortality in very old age among community-living people in Sweden. *Aging Clinical and Experimental Research, 31*, 265-271 (2019). https://doi-org./10.1007/s40520-018-0947-4

Halaweh, H., Dahlin-Ivanoff, S., Svantesson, U., & Willén, C. (2018). Perspectives of older adults on aging well: A focus group study. *Journal of Aging Research*, 9858252. https://doi.org/10.1155/2018/9858252

Havighurst, R. J. (1961). Successful aging. *The Gerontologist, 1*, 8-13. http://dx.doi.org/10.1093/geront/1.1.8

Hawkley, L. C., & Cacioppo, J. T. (2010). Loneliness matters: A theoretical and empirical review of consequences and mechanisms. *Annals of Behavioral Medicine, 40*(2), 218- 227. http://dx.doi.org/10.1007/s12160-010-9210-8

Health Resources & Services Administration. (2019). The "Loneliness Epidemic." https://www.hrsa.gov/enews/past-issues/2019/january-17/loneliness-epidemic

Hersch, G., Hutchinson, S., Wilson, C., Maharaj, T., & Watson, K. B. (2012). Effect of an occupation-based cultural heritage intervention in long-term geriatric care: A two-group control study. *American Journal of Occupational Therapy, 66*, 224-232. https://doi.org/10.5014/ajot.2012.002394

Hicks, C. L., von Baeyer, C. L., Spafford, P. A., van Korlaar, I., & Goodenough, B. (2001). The Faces Pain Scale-Revised: Toward a common metric in pediatric pain measurement. *Pain, 93*(2), 173-183. https://doi.org/0.1016/S0304-3959(01)00314-1

Holt-Lunstad, J., Smith, T. B., & Layton, J. B. (2010). Social relationships and mortality risk: A meta-analytic review. *PLOS Medicine 7*(7), e1000316. https://doi.org/10.1371/journal.pmed.1000316

Interprofessional Education Collaborative. (2016). Core Competencies for Interprofessional Collaborative Practice. https://healthipe.utexas.edu/core-competencies-interprofessional-collaborative-practice

Jackson, S., Donovan, J., Brookes, S., Eckford, S., Swithinbank, L., & Abrams, P. (1996). The Bristol Female Lower Urinary Tract Symptoms questionnaire: Development and psychometric testing. *British Journal of Urology, 77*(6), 805-812. https://doi.org/10.1046/j.1464-410x.1996.00186.x

Jacobson, N. C., Lord, K. A., & Newman, M. G. (2017). Perceived emotional support in bereaved spouses mediates the relationship between anxiety and depression. *Journal of Affective Disorders, 211*, 83-91. https://doi.org/10.1016/j.jad.2017.01.011

James, B. D., Boyle, P. A., Buchman, A. S., & Bennett, D. A. (2011). Relation of late-life social activity with incident disability among community-dwelling older adults. *The Journals of Gerontology. Series A, Biological Sciences and Medical Sciences, 66*(4), 467-473. https://doi.org/10.1093/gerona/glq231

Jeste, D. V., Lee, E. E., & Cacioppo, S. (2020). Battling the Modern Behavioral Epidemic of Loneliness: Suggestions for Research and Interventions. *JAMA Psychiatry, 77*(6), 553-554. https://doi.org/10.1001/jamapsychiatry.2020.0027

Kanamori, S., Kai, Y., Aida, J., Kondo. Kawachi, I., Hirai, H., Shirai, K. Ishikawa, & Suzuki, K. (2014). Social participation and the prevention of functional disability in older Japanese: The JAGES cohort study. *PLoS One 9*(6), https://doi.org/10.1371/journal.pone.0099638.

Keith, R. A., Granger, C. V., Hamilton, B. B., & Sherwin, F. S. (1987). The functional independence measure: A new tool for rehabilitation. *Advances in Clinical Rehabilitation, 1*, 6-18.

Kielhofner, G., & Neville, A. (1983). *Modified interest checklist*. Model of Occupation Clearinghouse.

Koehn, S. D., Mahmood, A. N., & Stott-Eveneshen, S. (2016). Quality of life for diverse older adults in assisted living: The centrality of control. *Journal of Gerontological Social Work, 59*(7-8), 512-536. https://doi.org/10.1080/01634372.2016.1254699

Koenig, H. G., Westlund, R. E., George, L. K., Hughes, D. C., Blazer, D. G., & Hybels, C. (1993). Abbreviating the Duke Social Support Index for use in chronically ill elderly individuals. *Psychosomatics, 34*, 61-69.

Lee, C. D., & Park, S. (2020). Subjective memory complaints (SMC) as a determinant factor of social participation among community-dwelling older adults. *American Journal of Occupational Therapy, 74*(S1), 7411505185. https://doi.org/10.5014/ajot.2020.74S1-PO6605

Leist, A. K. (2013). Social media use of older adults: A mini-review. *Gerontology 59*, 378-384. https://doi.org/10.1159/000346818

Levasseur, M., Dubois, M. F., Généreux, M., Menec, V., Raina, P., Roy, M., Gabaude, C., Couturier, Y., & St-Pierre, C. (2017). Capturing how age-friendly communities foster positive health, social participation and health equity: A study protocol of key components and processes that promote population health in aging Canadians. *BMC Public Health, 17*(1), 502. https://doi.org/10.1186/s12889-017-4392-7

Levasseur, M., Richard, L., Gauvin, L., & Raymond, E. (2010). Inventory and analysis of definitions of social participation found in the aging literature: proposed taxonomy of social activities. *Social Science & Medicine, 71*(12), 2141-2149. https://doi.org/10.1016/j.socscimed.2010.09.041

Li, Y., Xu, L., Chi, I., & Guo, P. (2014). Participation in productive activities and health outcomes among older adults in urban China. *The Gerontologist, 54*(5), 784–796. https://doi.org/10.1093/geront/gnt106

Lubben, J., Blozik, E., Gillmann, G., Iliffe, S., von Renteln Kruse, W., Beck, J. C., & Stuck, A. E. (2006). Performance of an abbreviated version of the Lubben Social Network Scale among three European Community–dwelling older adult populations. *Gerontologist, 46*(4), 503-513. http://dx.doi.org/10.1093/geront/46.4.503

Mackenzie, C. S. & Abdulrazaq, S. (2021). Social engagement mediates the relationship between participation in social activities and psychological distress among older adults. *Aging & Mental Health, 25*(2), 299-305. https://doi.org/10.1080/13607863.2019.1697200

Mahoney, F. I., & Barthel, D. (1965). Functional evaluation: The Barthel Index. *Maryland State Medical Journal, 14*, 56-61.

Marioni, R. E., van den Hout, A., Valenzuela, M. J., Brayne, C., Matthews, F. E., & MRC Cognitive Function and Ageing Study. (2012). Active cognitive lifestyle associates with cognitive recovery and a reduced risk of cognitive decline. *Journal of Alzheimer's Disease, 28*(1), 223. https://doi.org/10.3233/JAD-2011-110377

Mayo Clinic. (2020). Mild cognitive impairment—Symptoms and causes. https://www.mayoclinic.org/diseases-conditions/mild-cognitive-impairment/symptoms-causes/syc-20354578

McLaren, S., Turner, J., Gomez, R., McLachlan, A. J., & Gibbs, P. M. (2013). Housing type and depressive symptoms among older adults: A test of sense of belonging as a mediating and moderating variable. *Aging & Mental Health, 17*(8), 1023-1029. https://doi.org/10.1080/13607863.2013.805402

Mick, P., Parfyonov, M., Wittich, W., Phillips, N., Guthrie, D., & Kathleen Pichora-Fuller, M. (2018). Associations between sensory loss and social networks, participation, support, and loneliness: Analysis of the Canadian Longitudinal Study on Aging. *Canadian Family Physician, 64*(1), e33-e41.

Miller, L. M., Dieckmann, N. F., Mattek, N. C., Lyons, K. S., & Kaye, J. A. (2014). Social activity decreases placement in a long-term care facility for a prospective sample of community-dwelling older adults. *Research in Gerontological Nursing, 7*(3), 106-112. https://doi.org/10.3928/19404921-20140110-02

Mitchell, A. J., Bird, V., Rizzo, M., & Meader, N. (2010). Diagnostic validity and added value of the geriatric depression scale for depression in primary care: A meta-analysis of GDS30 and GDS15. *Journal of Affective Disorders, 125*(1-3), 10-17. https://doi.org/10.1016/j.jad.2009.08.019

Music and Memory, Inc. (2021). Music and memory. https://musicandmemory.org/

Nasreddine, Z. (2021). About MoCA. https://www.mocatest.org/about/

Nasreddine, Z. S., Phillips, N. A., Bédirian, V., Charbonneau, S., Whitehead, V., Collin, I., Cummings, J. L., & Chertkow, H. (2005). The Montreal Cognitive Assessment, MoCA: A brief screening tool for mild cognitive impairment. *Journal of the American Geriatrics Society, 53*(4), 695-699. https://doi.org/10.1111/j.1532-5415.2005.53221.x

National Academies of Sciences, Engineering, and Medicine. (2010). Size and demographics of aging populations. https://www.ncbi.nlm.nih.gov/books/NBK51841/

National Academies of Sciences, Engineering, and Medicine. (2020). *Social isolation and loneliness in older adults: Opportunities for the health care system*. The National Academies Press. https://doi.org/10.17226/25663.

National Association of Social Workers. (2021). About social workers. https://www.socialworkers.org/News/Facts/Social-Workers

National Council on Aging. (2012). What is the aging mastery program? https://www.ncoa.org/article/what-is-the-aging-mastery-program

National Institutes of Health. (2020). NIH public health campaigns. https://prevention.nih.gov/research-priorities/dissemination-implementation/nih-public-health-campaigns

National Institute for Health and Care Excellence. (2015). Urinary incontinence in women. https://www.nice.org.uk/guidance/qs77

Neill-Hall, J. (2013). Family doctors ill-equipped for loneliness epidemic. Campaign to End Loneliness. https://www.campaigntoendloneliness.org/wp-content/uploads/downloads/2013/11/FINAL-GP-Polling-PR-15.11.13.pdf

Newall, N., McArthur, J., & Menec, V. H. (2015). A longitudinal examination of social participation, loneliness, and use of physician and hospital services. *Journal of Aging and Health, 27*(3), 500-518. https://doi.org/10.1177/0898264314552420

Nicholson, N. R., Feinn, R., & Dixon, J. (2020). Psychometric evaluation of the Social Isolation Scale in older adults. *The Gerontologist, 60*(7), e491-e501. https://doi.org/10.1093/geront/gnz083

Nilsson, I., Nyqvist, F., Gustafson, Y., & Nygård, M. (2015). Leisure engagement: Medical conditions, mobility difficulties, and activity limitations-A later life perspective. *Journal of Aging Research, 2015*, 610154. https://doi.org/10.1155/2015/610154

Nivestam, A., Westergren, A., Petersson, P., & Haak, M. (2021). Promote social participation among older persons by identifying physical challenges—An important aspect of preventive home visits. *Archives of Gerontology and Geriatrics, 93*, 104316. https://doi.org/10.1016/j.archger.2020.104316

Opening Minds Through Art, Inc. (2021). Opening Minds Through Art. https://www.scrippsoma.org/about/

Orentlicher, M., Case, D., Podvey, M., Myers, C., Rudd, L., & Schoonover, J. (2017). Frequently asked questions (FAQ): What is occupational therapy's role in transition services and planning? https://www.aota.org/~/media/Corporate/Files/Secure/Practice/Children/FAQ-What-is-OTs-Role-in-Transition-Services-and-Planning-20170530.pdf

Park, M. J., Park., N. S., & Chiriboga, D. A. (2018). A latent class analysis of social activities and health among community-dwelling older adults in Korea. *Aging & Mental Health, 22*(5), 625–630. https://doi.org/10.1080/13607863.2017.1288198

Pew Research Center. (2021a). Internet fact sheet. https://www.pewresearch.org/internet/fact-sheet/internet-broadband/

Pew Research Center. (2021b). Mobile fact sheet. https://www.pewresearch.org/internet/fact-sheet/mobile/

Pew Research Center. (2021c). Social media fact sheet. https://www.pewresearch.org/internet/fact-sheet/social-media/

Pilkington, P., Windsor, T.D., & Crisp, D. (2012). Volunteering and subjective well-being in midlife and older adults: The role of supportive social networks. *The Journals of Gerontology Series B Psychological Sciences and Social Sciences, 67*(2), 249-260. https://doi.org/10.1093/geronb/gbr154

Plain Language Action and Information Network. (2011). Federal plain language guidelines. https://www.plainlanguage.gov/guidelines/

Podsiadlo, D., & Richardson, S. (1991). The Timed "Up & Go": A test of basic functional mobility for frail elderly persons. Journal of the *American Geriatrics Society, 39*(2), 142- 148. https://doi.org/10.1111/j.1532-5415.1991.tb01616.x

Powell, L. E., & Myers, A. M. (1995). The Activities-Specific Balance Confidence (ABC) Scale. *Journals of Gerontology Series A: Biological Sciences & Medical Science, 50A*(1), M28-M34. https://doi.org/10.1093/gerona/50a.1.m28

Prohaska, T., Burholt, V., & Burns, A. (2020). Consensus statement: Loneliness in older adults, The 21st century social determinant of health? *BMJ Open, 10*, e034967. https://doi.org/10.1136/bmjopen-2019-034967

Reynolds, C., Richmond, B., & Lowe, P. (2003). *The adult manifest anxiety scale-elderly version (AMAS-E).* Western Psychological Services.

Richard, L., Gauvin, L., Kestens, Y., Shatenstein, B., Payette, H., Daniel, M., Moore, S., Levasseur, M., & Mercille, G. (2013). Neighborhood resources and social participation among older adults: Results from the VoisiNuage study. *Journal of Aging and Health, 25*(2), 296-318. https://doi.org/10.1177/0898264312468487

Rosso, A. L., Taylor, J. A., Tabb, L. P., & Michael, Y. L. (2013). Mobility, disability, and social engagement in older adults. *Journal of Aging and Health, 25*(4), 617-637. https://doi.org/10.1177/0898264313482489

Rowe, J. W., & Kahn, R. L. (1987). Human aging: Usual and successful. *Science, 237*(4811), 143-149.

Rowe, J. W., & Kahn, R. L. (1997). Successful aging. *Gerontologist, 37*(4), 433-440.

Russell, D. (1996). UCLA Loneliness Scale (Version 3): Reliability, validity, and factor structure. *Journal of Personality Assessment, 66*, 20-40.

Sakamoto, A., Ukawa, S., Okada, E., Sasaki, S., Zhao, W., Kishi, T., Kondo, K., & Tamakoshi, A. (2017). The association between social participation and cognitive function in community-dwelling older populations: Japan Gerontological Evaluation Study at Taisetsu community Hokkaido. *International Journal of Geriatric Psychiatry, 32*(10), 1131–1140. https://doi.org/10.1002/gps.4576

Scott, P. (2019). *Role checklist version 3: Participation and satisfaction (RCv3).* Model of Occupation Clearinghouse.

Segal, D. L., June, A., Payne, M., Coolidge, F. L., & Yochim, B. (2010). Development and initial validation of a self-report assessment tool for anxiety among older adults: The Geriatric Anxiety Scale. *Journal of Anxiety Disorders, 24*(7), 596-603. https://doi.org/10.1016/j.janxdis.2010.05.002

Sieber, S. D. (1974). Toward a theory of role accumulation. *American Sociological Review, 39*(4), 567-578. https://doi.org/10.2307/2094422

Siette, J., Berry, H., Jorgensen, M., Brett, L., Georgiou, A., McClean, T., & Westbrook, J. (2020). Social participation among older adults receiving community care services. *Journal of Applied Gerontology: The Official Journal of the Southern Gerontological Society,* 733464820938973. Advance online publication. https://doi.org/10.1177/0733464820938973

Shah, S., Vanclay, F., & Cooper, B. (1989). Improving the sensitivity of the Barthel Index for stroke rehabilitation. *Journal of Clinical Epidemiology, 7*, 42, 703-709.

Sheikh, J. I., & Yesavage, J. A. (1986). Geriatric Depression Scale (GDS). Recent evidence and development of a shorter version. In Brink T. L. (Ed.), *Clinical gerontology: A guide to assessment and intervention* (pp. 165-173). The Haworth Press, Inc.

Shira, A., Hoffman, Y., Bodner, E., & Palgi, Y. (2020). Covid-19-related loneliness and psychiatric symptoms among older adults: The buffering role of subjective age. *American Journal of Geriatric Psychiatry, 28*(11), 1200- 1204. doi: 10.1016/j.jagp.2020.05.018

Smallfield, S., & Molitor, W. L. (2018). Occupational therapy interventions supporting social participation and leisure engagement for community-dwelling older adults: A systematic review. *American Journal of Occupational Therapy, 72*(4), 7204190020p1-7204190020p8. https://doi.org/10.5014/ajot.2018.030627

Stratford, P. W., & Spadoni, G. (2001). The reliability, consistency, and clinical application of a numeric pain rating scale. *Physiotherapy Canada, 53*(2), 88-91.

Tariq, S. H., Tumosa, N., Chibnall, J. T., Perry III, M.H., & Morley, J. E. (2006). Comparison of the Saint Louis University Mental Status Examination and the Mini-Mental State Examination for detecting dementia and mild neurocognitive disorder: A pilot study. *The American Journal of Geriatric Psychiatry, 14*(11), 900. https://doi.org/10.1097/01.JGP.0000221510.33817.86

Taylor, H. O. (2021). Social isolation's influence on loneliness among older adults. *Clinical Social Work Journal, 48*(1), 140-151. https://doi.org/10.1007/s10615-019-00737-9

Tennstedt, S., Howland, J., Lachman, M., Peterson, E., Kasten, L., & Jette, A. (1998). A randomized, controlled trial of a group intervention to reduce fear of falling and associated activity restriction in older adults. *The Journals of Gerontology: Series B, 52B*(6), 384-392. https://doi.org/10.1093/geronb/53B.6.P384

Tyrer, P., Nur, U., Crawford, M., Karlsen, S., McLean, C., Rao, B., & Johnson, T. (2005). The social functioning questionnaire: A rapid and robust measure of perceived functioning. *International Journal of Social Psychiatry, 51*(3), 265-275. https://doi.org/10.1177/0020764005057391

United Nations. (n.d.). Sustainable Development Goals. https://www.un.org/sustainabledevelopment/sustainable-development-goals/

United Nations, Department of Economic and Social Affairs, Population Division (2019). World population ageing 2019: Highlights (ST/ESA/SER.A/430).

United States Bureau of Labor. (2021a). Nursing assistants and orderlies. https://www.bls.gov/ooh/healthcare/nursing-assistants.htm#tab-2

United States Bureau of Labor. (2021b). Home health and personal care aides. https://www.bls.gov/ooh/healthcare/home-health-aides-and-personal-care-aides.htm#tab-2

United States Census Bureau. (2020). 65 and older population grows rapidly as Baby Boomers age. https://www.census.gov/newsroom/press-releases/2020/65-older-population-grows.html

Veazie, S., Gilbert, J., Winchell, K., Paynter, R., & Guise, J. M. (2019). Addressing social isolation to improve the health of older adults: A rapid review. Agency for Healthcare Research and Quality (US).

Vo, K., Forder, P. M., & Byles, J. E. (2016). Urinary incontinence and social function in older Australian women. *Journal of the American Geriatrics Society, 64*(8), 1646-1650. https://doi.org/10.1111/jgs.14250

Wang, H. X., Jin, Y., Hendrie, H. C., Liang, C., Yang, L., Cheng, Y., Unverzagt, F. W., Ma, F., Hall, K. S., Murrell, J. R., Li, P., Bian, J., Pei, J. J., & Gao, S. (2013). Late life leisure activities and risk of cognitive decline. *The Journals of Gerontology. Series A, Biological Sciences and Medical Sciences, 68*(2), 205-213. https://doi.org/10.1093/gerona/gls153

Wang, Y. C., Deutscher, D., Yen, S. C., Werneke, M. W., & Mioduski, J. E. (2014). The self-report fecal incontinence and constipation questionnaire in patients with pelvic-floor dysfunction seeking outpatient rehabilitation. *Physical Therapy, 94*(2), 273-88. https://doi.org/10.2522/ptj.20130062

Ware, J. E., & Sherbourne, C. D. (1992). The MOS 36-item Short-Form Health Survey (SF-36): I. Conceptual framework and item selection. *Medical Care, 30*, 473-83.

Warren, M., Ganley, K. J., & Pohl, P. S. (2016). The association between social participation and lower extremity muscle strength, balance, and gait speed in US adults. *Preventive Medicine Reports, 4*, 142-147. https://doi.org/10.1016/j.pmedr.2016.06.005

Weiner, D. K., Duncan, P. W., Chandler, J., & Studenski, S. A. (1992). Functional reach: A marker of physical frailty. *Journal of the American Geriatrics Society, 40*(3), 203-207.

Weissman, M. M., & Bothwell, S. (1976). Assessment of social adjustment by patient self-report. *Archives of General Psychiatry, 33*(9), 1111-1115. https://doi.org/10.1001/archpsyc.1976.01770090101010

Wilkie, R., Blagojevic-Bucknall, M., Belcher, J., Chew-Graham, C., Lacey, R. J., & McBeth, J. (2016). Widespread pain and depression are key modifiable risk factors associated with reduced social participation in older adults: A prospective cohort study in primary care. *Medicine, 95*(31), e4111. https://doi.org/10.1097/MD.0000000000004111

World Health Organization. (2002). Active aging: A policy framework. https://www.who.int/ageing/publications/active_ageing/en/

World Health Organization. (2007). Global age-friendly cities: A guide. https://www.who.int/ageing/projects/age-friendly-cities-communities/en/

Xue, Q. L. (2011). The frailty syndrome: Definition and natural history. *Clinics in Geriatric Medicine, 27*(1), 1-15. https://doi.org/10.1016/j.cger.2010.08.009

Part IV

Promoting Occupational Health and Productivity

10

CHAPTER

Promoting Occupational Health and Productivity

Children and Youth

Madalynn Wendland, PT, DPT, ATP, Board-Certified Pediatric Clinical Specialist; Kelle DeBoth Foust, PhD, OTR/L; and John M. Schaefer, PhD, BCBA-D

Learning Objectives

At the end of this chapter, the reader will:

1. Define play and the ultimate results from successfully participating in play including fun, fulfillment, friendship, freedom, and preparation for the future (OT B.1.1, PT 7D21, PT 7D31; CEC 5.2)
2. Differentiate indirect and direct determinants for participation in play experiences in the community setting (OT B.4.23, OT B.4.27, PT 7D8, PT 7D10, PT 7D34; CEC 5.6)
3. Describe a structural paradigm for play using an enriched environment to optimize participation and stimulate development across multiple domains (OT B.5.1, PT 7D11, PT 7D27, PT 7D39; CEC 5.5, CEC 5.6)
4. Reflect on the unique and overlapping roles and responsibilities of different members of an interprofessional team and the importance of collaboration to promote quality play experiences for children and youth (OT B.4.19, OT B.4.23, OT B.4.25, PT 7D7, PT 7D16, PT 7D17, PT 7D24, PT 7D28, PT 7D37, PT 7D39)

The ACOTE Standards used are those from 2018.

Key Words

Activity, Autonomy, Competence, Enriched Environment, Freedom, Friendships, Fulfillment, Fun, Function, Interprofessional Collaborative Practice, Just-Right Experiences, Participation, Relatedness

Pizzi, M. A., & Amir, M. (Eds.). *Interprofessional Perspectives for Community Practice: Promoting Health, Well-Being, and Quality of Life* (pp. 177-194).

An Introduction to Occupational Health of Children and Youth

Childhood activities are personally valued activities and tasks that relate to self-care, education, and play (Lim et al., 2016) and promote occupational health. Occupational health is being productive, engaged, and participatory in activities that promote one's health and well-being. Participation in play is integral in optimizing health and developmental outcomes for children and youth (Kolehmainen et al., 2011). By promoting play in an enriched environment, children and youth can experience fun, freedom, fulfillment, and friendship while transitioning to their future roles as competent and autonomous individuals who situationally relate to their family and peers (Kolehmainen et al., 2011; Palisano et al., 2011; Powrie et al., 2015). An enriched environment is defined as "...interventions that aim to enrich at least one of the motor, cognitive, sensory, or social aspects of the environment for the purposes of promoting learning" (Morgan et al., 2013, p. 737). Play is also essential to successful participation in meaningful activities and is therefore an important component of child health. Unfortunately, a lack of community-based participation and play can have long-term consequences including impaired competence with activities and reduced physical and mental health and potentiation of passive dependency or learned helplessness that can be detrimental to one's autonomy and sense of self as well as impede feelings of social relatedness and the development of friendships (Longo et al., 2013). An absence of play experiences can be even more prevalent in populations of children and youth who present with developmental disabilities where physical, sensory, cognitive and/or speech and language function may be impaired. In such cases, practitioners can create available, accessible, affordable, and adaptable community spaces that have been intentionally and interprofessionally designed to facilitate "just-right" experiences to help augment a child's functional performance based on environmental and/or personal factors and optimize opportunities for engagement in meaningful play.

Play as the Central Activity of Children and Youth

The occupational health and productivity of children and youth centers around an ability and opportunity to play while interacting with peers and family and learning within a variety of environments. In fact, the position of both the Association for Childhood Education International and the American Occupational Therapy Association (AOTA) is that play is a critical component to the health and well-being of children as they grow and develop (AOTA, 2012; Brown & Thyer, 2020; Essame, 2020). Sheridan chronicled her thoughts on play, which she described as active engagement in a physical or mental task that is emotionally satisfying (Sheridan, 2011). Garvey (1990), further operationalized play in four central tenets:

1. That play creates joy and is positively perceived by its participants
2. The motivation to play is intrinsic, meaning there is no predetermined or desired outcome or product other than the pleasure that is to be experienced
3. The choice to play is both voluntary and spontaneous
4. That participants must be actively engaged in the play task or behavior

The International Classification of Functioning, Disability and Health-Children and Youth (ICF-CY) classifies health status across three main areas: body structures and **function**, **activity**, and **participation** (WHO, 2007). Function reflects the impact of a child's health condition(s) on their physical abilities and impairments. Activity refers to the tasks that the child is presented with across their environments across their day while participation refers to the domains in which the child needs to be able to engage (WHO, 2007). Play is both an action and a process (Sheridan, 2011) dependent upon successful functioning, activity selection, and participation. Play is also dynamic, meaning that the level at which a person engages in an activity can ebb and flow, with play often perceived differently among individuals or by a single individual at different points in time (Sheridan, 2011). Contextualized environmental factors, including both *physical* and *attitudinal* features, the availability of materials, and the players who are present and involved can influence play (Brown & Thyer, 2020; Imms et al., 2015; Sheridan, 2011; Willis et al., 2018a, 2018b). And, while beyond the scope of this chapter, there are various types and stages of play that emerge at age-specific points in time including unoccupied behaviors, solitary play, onlooker behavior, parallel play, associative play, and then finally cooperative play (Sheridan, 2011). It is also important to highlight the iterative nature of play, which reflects a child's current abilities while stimulating the acquisition of new skills that will expand a child's overall performance across developmental domains (Brown & Thyer, 2020; Law, 2002; Sheridan, 2011). In contrast, an absence of adequate play experiences can hinder children's health and well-being, and negatively impact their quality of life (QOL).

Even though enabling successful participation is a complex and multidimensional undertaking, the desire to play is innate to most children (Coussens et al., 2021; Imms et al., 2015; Palisano et al., 2011; Willis et al., 2017). Kolehmainen et al. (2011) outlined five distinctive steps to be used when attempting to optimize participation: 1) identification of impairments, 2) identification of child-specific beliefs and preferences, 3) identification of parent-specific beliefs and preferences, 4) selection of evidenced-based interventional strategies to support participation, and 5) identification of strategies to promote behavior change to sustain engagement

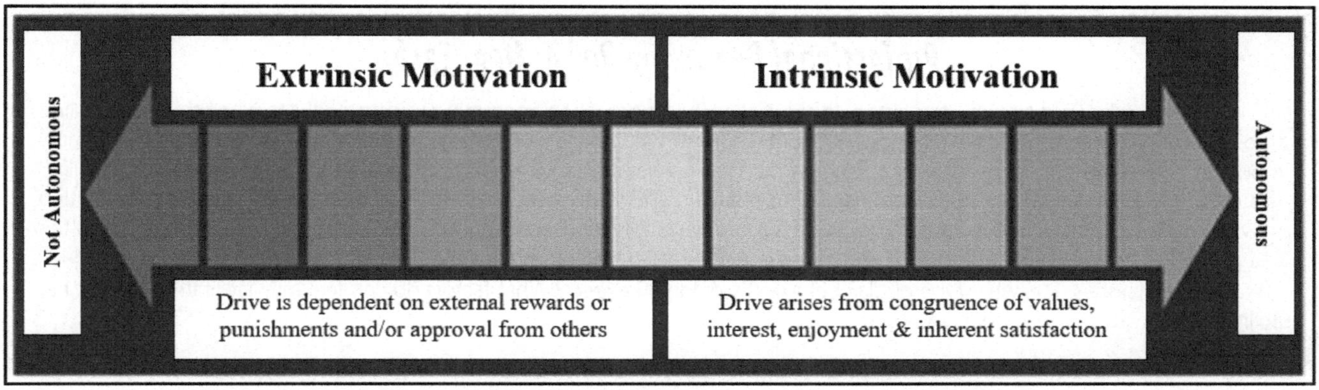

Figure 10-1. The Influence of Motivation on Autonomy. (Data source: Ryan, A. & Deci, A. [2000]. Self-determination theory and the facilitation of intrinsic motivation, social development and well-being. *American Psychologist,* 55[1], 68-78.)

in activities. According to the Self-Determination Theory, this engagement (or motivation) is driven by the basic physiological needs of **competence** (i.e., ability to perform a desired task), **autonomy** (i.e., volitional choice making that aligns with one's sense of self), and **relatedness** (i.e., connectedness with others and/or a community; Powrie et al., 2015; Reedman et al., 2019). These constructs correspond to the objectives and ultimate desired outcomes of play with a plethora of evidence supporting the notion that the act of playing helps children acquire and refine task performance (competence), learn personal independence (autonomy), and understand their role within their family, school, and community (relatedness) as well as enhance their overall QOL. Specific to the construct of autonomy, there is a greater chance for perseverance and continuation of play behaviors when children are internally motivated as opposed to being extrinsically enticed to earn a reward or deterred to avoid punishment (Figure 10-1; Powrie et al., 2015; Reedman et al., 2019; Willis et al., 2017). Moreover, sustained participation in activities has been shown to have significant benefits on overall health, including improvements in sense of self and connections with others, decreased incidence of depression, increased educational achievement and meaningful contributions to society, and higher overall QOL (Anaby et al., 2014; Law, 2002; Palisano et al., 2012).

An example of how motivational constructs impact play is if the goal is to spur autonomy, opportunities that are intrinsically motivating to children and youth should be cultivated (Professional Reasoning Box A). Professionals should also intentionally match activities to each child's abilities and preferences, which in turn, minimizes the likelihood that children become sad, frustrated, or disengaged; become too physically or mentally taxed to allow for engagement; or motivation that can perpetuate passive-dependency or learned helplessness (Anaby et al., 2021; Coussens et al., 2021; Law, 2002; Longo et al., 2013). This **just-right experience** manifests itself as a task that does not cause undue stress but is appropriately challenging (physically and/or mentally) with mastery attainable, which can then amplify intrinsic motivation as well as the enjoyment and satisfaction experienced through play, and thus, optimize occupational productivity (Case-Smith & Arbesman, 2008; Law, 2002; Reedman et al., 2019; Willis et al., 2018b). Finally, by engaging in play within a variety of environments, children begin to make sense of a broader world while building and practicing context-specific skills that are specific to how personal factors and sensorimotor, cognitive, language, and social-emotional abilities intersect with environmental factors (Sheridan, 2011; Willis et al., 2017, 2018b).

A Paradigmatic Structure for Play in an Enriched Environment

There is no widely accepted or standardized process for implementing play activities that can guarantee that experiences will be pleasurable. One reliable method of increasing the likelihood that a child finds something engaging and enjoyable to interact with is by facilitating a naturally **enriched environment**. In a community setting, maintaining an enriched environment requires incorporating sensorimotor, cognitive, social, and/or communicative stimuli that are accessible to all children throughout the environment (Professional Reasoning Box B). Research supports environmental enrichment as a potential mechanism to promote engagement, learning, and foster overall health and development for children and youth (Anaby et al., 2020; Coussens et al., 2021; Law, 2002; Morgan et al., 2013).

In addition to enriching the environment, tasks that elicit learning should be intentionally embedded or situated into an activity to optimize neurophysiological development and improve functional performance through experience- (or use) dependent practice (Kolehmainen et al., 2011; Morgan et al., 2013; Nithianantharajah & Hannan, 2006; Sale et al., 2014; Willis et al., 2018b). Standardizing how play activities are implemented in an enriched environment should be intentionally structured to include: a *ceiling* that contains the ultimate desired results; *pillars* that support domain-specific experiences and outcomes; and, a *foundation* where

Professional Reasoning Box A: Meet Sasha

Sasha is a 7-year-old girl who presents with significant challenges when attempting to communicate with others or mobilize through an environment. She has a diagnosis of Gould syndrome with a history of bilateral intraventricular hemorrhage. Her primary mode for expressing her needs is through laughing or crying. She also requires full assistance for all instrumental and mobility-related activities of daily living due to an inability to maintain antigravity head and trunk control and difficulty in coordinating movements in her arms and legs for walking. Sasha is a happy, socially motivated young girl, but her play behaviors are most often categorized as spectator/onlooker due to underlying impairments in her communication and physical function.

Based on Sasha's age, what type of play behaviors would you expect? What factors do you feel may facilitate or hinder her ability to fully participate in cooperative play?

Professional Reasoning Box B: Sasha Engaging in an Enriched Environment

On a class field trip, Sasha and a group of her classmates with significant disabilities visit a typical exhibit at a local zoo. The class comes to the first exhibit, some ringtail lemurs, that has not made an effort to enrich the environment. Some of the children look through the glass at the animal playing, eating, or sleeping. Depending on how active the animals are, these visual stimuli might temporarily hold the attention of an average child without a visual impairment for time. However, for Sasha and her classmates who have a range of intensive needs, the lemur exhibit is not very engaging. By contrast, in the next exhibit, the orangutans, the zoo has planned several additional sensory experiences. Sasha can touch a facsimile of the orangutan's fur or manipulate a model of the animal's skeleton. She can push a button and hear the orangutan's call. She can place her hand in the paw print of the orangutan. Each of these additional stimuli enrich the environment and make it more likely Sasha will be engaged.

determinants of participation are identified and addressed (Figure 10-2).

Seminal work by Powrie et al. (2015) uncovered four *ceiling* effects or overarching themes that result from meaningful play experiences: 1) **fun**, or the pleasure experienced; 2) **freedom**, or having the ability to choose if and how to participate without constraint; 3) **fulfillment**, or being able to discover and explore the environment while developing and displaying one's occupational potential and level of fitness; and 4) **friendships**, or feeling a sense of social connectedness and belonging (Professional Reasoning Box C).

Although it can be challenging to meet the needs of a diverse population of children with and without disabilities in a community context, considering each component of an enriched environment provides an opportunity to present activities and options for different types of play where children can choose what best meets their needs and desires. These mechanisms and outcomes are then encircled by a cultural context where the use of family-centered programming promotes safe (physical and emotional) learning and social interactions (Willis et al., 2018a). For example, interprofessional teams can consider unique influences that a family's cultural background has over the roles of different family members, and what activities they prioritize as a family. By taking into consideration factors such as maternal and paternal roles, religious or spiritual affiliations, and shared activities, the team can design interventions and supports that enhance participation for the child.

The *pillars* of domain-specific experiences should be formed with activities that stimulate competence in skills across domains (e.g., sensorimotor, cognitive, social, and language) and enhance a child's autonomy and relatedness (i.e., sense of self) to improve physical and mental well-being and overall health (Coussens et al., 2021; Kaelin et al., 2021; Kolehmainen et al., 2011; Morris et al., 2018; Palisano et al., 2012; Willis et al., 2018b). As the context reflecting a child's ability to perform a task within a specific environment can vary, barriers and facilitators should be considered and addressed to optimize how full populations of children and youths can effectively participate in play (Golden & Walsh, 2013; Palisano et al., 2011; Willis et al., 2018a). "Just-right" experiences that match a child's capabilities and are enriched through stimulation of sensorimotor, cognitive, social, and language-related functions help buttress the *pillars* with the purpose of supporting overarching participation goals (i.e., fun, freedom, fulfillment, friendship, and future). Moreover, because each individual may present with different strengths or limitations, professionals should compile a wide repertoire of adaptable activities within each pillar that can be selectively implemented to compliment a child's competence while eliminating discrepancies between a child's capacity and performance during community play (Golden & Walsh, 2013; King et al., 2006; Palisano et al., 2011). For children who lack age-expected competencies, the severity of their delays can also impact participation, although it is important to realize that emphasizing activities focusing on "fixing" body functions and structural impairments may or may not change performance or participation (Maxwell et al., 2012; Reedman et al., 2019; Professional Reasoning Box D).

In a study by King et al. (2006), physical ability was found to predict a child's initial level of involvement in an activity, although motoric function was not associated with changes

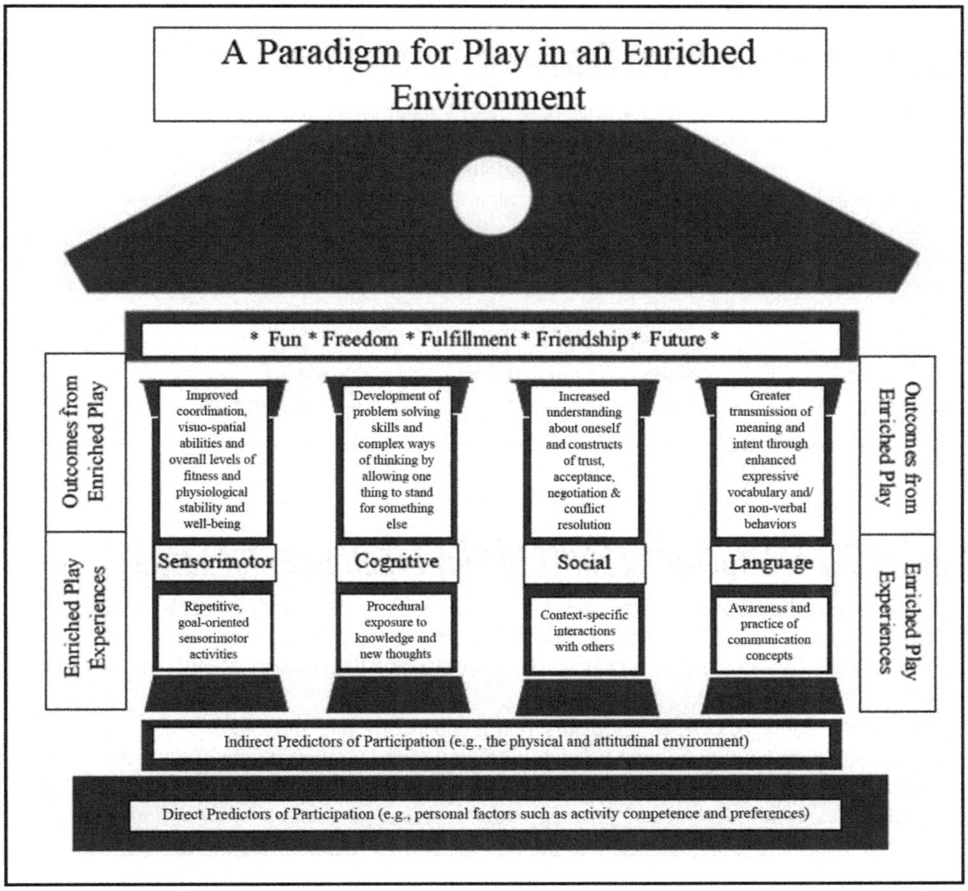

Figure 10-2. A paradigmatic structure for play in an enriched environment.

Professional Reasoning Box C: Using Predictors to Plan for Engagement

Fiona is a 3-year-old girl with cerebral palsy who struggles with truck and head stability and who has difficulty bearing weight through her legs. When planning a therapy session for Fiona, the team uses their assessment data from previous sessions to plan a multitude of sensory experiences that Fiona can engage in independently and socially. Fiona is first placed in a harness system that counterbalances much of her body weight and supports her trunk so that she can work on her head stability and movement of her limbs. The team places several items within her reach, but far enough away to require some stretch and intentional movement. Several of the items light up or make noise, which Fiona has shown a preference for in the past. When Fiona reaches for the ball lighting up the team member scripts the interaction to continue to engage her cognitively and socially, "I see you want to play with the ball, let's play." Fiona laughs with excitement, to which the team member responds verbally, "You are excited to play; me too," approximating a social communicative exchange. One team member sits opposite Fiona and gently rolls the ball toward Fiona aiming it toward her nondominant arm. Another team member sits behind Fiona and helps physically prompt her to cross her midline with her dominant had to push the ball. The team member assisting has to also push the ball to roll it back Fiona's play partner, but the play partner verbally praises Fiona for the effort, "Yay! You rolled the ball back, let's play again." After several turns Fiona begins to whine quietly and shuffle her feet, which the team recognizes as a sign of fatigue to resistance. They chose a couple of high-preference toys that use switches to play songs and place them closer to Fiona making it more likely she will engage even when she is starting to fatigue.

in participation behaviors over a trajectory of time. In fact, utilizing play experiences that are designed to help a child's sense of self flourish (by integrating features of autonomy or relatedness) may be more impactful than building activity competence (via impairment-based interventions) for some children (Kaelin et al., 2021; King et al., 2006; Kolehmainen et al., 2011; Palisano et al., 2012; Powrie et al., 2015; Reedman et al., 2019; Willis et al., 2018a). Nurturing the development of a sense of self necessitates that professionals consciously consider personal factors including a child's interests and preferences while ensuring they feel comfortable, motivated, and confident about their ability to autonomously engage in play and promote perseverance (Kaelin et al., 2021; Reedman et al., 2019).

Finally, understanding the determinants of participation for children and youth helps tailor activities to match a child's capabilities and select additional resources or support to optimize the frequency and sustainability of attendance

Professional Reasoning Box D: Enhancing Participation

Samuel is a 5-year-old boy who presents with poor fine motor skills that affect his handwriting. He struggles with writing activities in the classroom and frequently avoids or refuses to complete these tasks. His kindergarten teacher has provided some fine motor strengthening activities (e.g., putty, mini pull-apart toys) along with additional drawing and handwriting exercises. His grasp strength and stamina have improved slightly over the last few months, but minimal improvements in overall handwriting skills are noted. The teacher refers him to the school occupational therapist. Working with Samuel and his family to better understand his preferences and interests, the occupational therapist begins to incorporate race cars (Samuel's favorite) and large gross motor play activities into intervention sessions targeting prewriting and writing skills. Samuel enjoys these activities immensely, and even requests to play the race car shaving cream letter game when he arrives for therapy. Over time, Samuel is less resistant to handwriting activities in the classroom, feeling more competent, and both the occupational therapist and his teachers observe marked improvements. Samuel even volunteers to write on the board in front of the class and is able to participate more fully in the classroom setting. He feels more confident and connected to his peers, improving his occupational health and well-being.

Professional Reasoning Box E: Structuring Enriched Play Experiences for Sasha

Sasha loves to dance! She enjoys being with others and is eager to engage in social situations. Her family is not just committed to finding and having Sasha attend events that are fun and fulfilling but has also strongly advocated for additional resources and support to ensure they have the financial means to maximally support Sasha's freedom when participating in activities in her home, school, and community environments.

Question(s): Based on Sasha's preferences, what types of activities (***pillars***) might you incorporate into play experiences? From these activities, what ultimate outcomes (***ceiling***) do you hope Sasha will achieve? How might you adapt activities to emphasize activity competence that addresses Sasha's direct and indirect determinants of participation (***foundation***)? How might you adapt activities to enhance her sense of self that addresses Sasha's direct and indirect determinants of participation (***foundation***)?

and intensity of involvement (Anaby et al., 2021; Bedell et al., 2013; Coussens et al., 2021; Kaelin et al., 2021; King et al., 2006; Majnemer et al., 2008; Palisano et al., 2011; Reedman et al., 2019; Willis et al., 2018b). The influence of potential barriers or facilitators can be direct or indirect (Anaby et al., 2014; Bult et al., 2011; Kaelin et al., 2021; Palisano et al., 2011). A child's age, functional ability, and preferences along with the history of familial participation and family values/cultural orientation can directly impact if and how a child engages in play (Anaby et al., 2014; Kolehmainn et al., 2011; Majnemer et al., 2008; Morris et al., 2018; Palisano et al., 2011).

Availability, accessibility, affordability, and adaptability of the environment indirectly affect participation (Bedell et al., 2013; Imms et al., 2015; Palisano et al., 2011). Participation can be facilitated by professionals trained to support meaningful play in the community (Maxwell et al., 2012), while participation can be impeded by perceived or actual environmental barriers (physical or attitudinal), a physically or emotionally enfeebled caregiver, inadequately coordinated health-related services, and lower household income levels that prohibit equal access to for-cost community activities and reliable transportation (Anaby et al., 2014; Bedell et al., 2013; Brown & Thyer, 2020; Bult et al., 2011; Coussens et al., 2021; King et al., 2006; Majnemer et al., 2008; Palisano et al., 2011; Willis et al., 2018b).

Ultimately, it is important to realize that participation is impacted by a confluence of direct and indirect factors, which may or may not be modifiable (Brown & Thyer, 2020; Bult et al., 2011; King et al., 2006). It is necessary to deliberately establish a paradigmatic structure for play to ensure children and youth have opportunities to participate in activities that will help them become competent, autonomous, and relatable adults who are productive members of society (King et al., 2006; Schmidt et al., 2020; Professional Reasoning Box E).

Policies and Practices for Participation

The ICF-CY framework depicts the interdependence of biological, personal, and social perspectives that influence health status as children grow and develop (Bult et al., 2011; Kolehmainen et al., 2011; Reedman et al., 2019; WHO, 2007). This framework is not discipline-specific within the health care field and helps to establish a common language when classifying a child's function through three core components: 1) health condition, 2) body function and structures, activity, and participation and 3) environmental and personal factors (Bult et al., 2011; Kolehmainen et al., 2011;

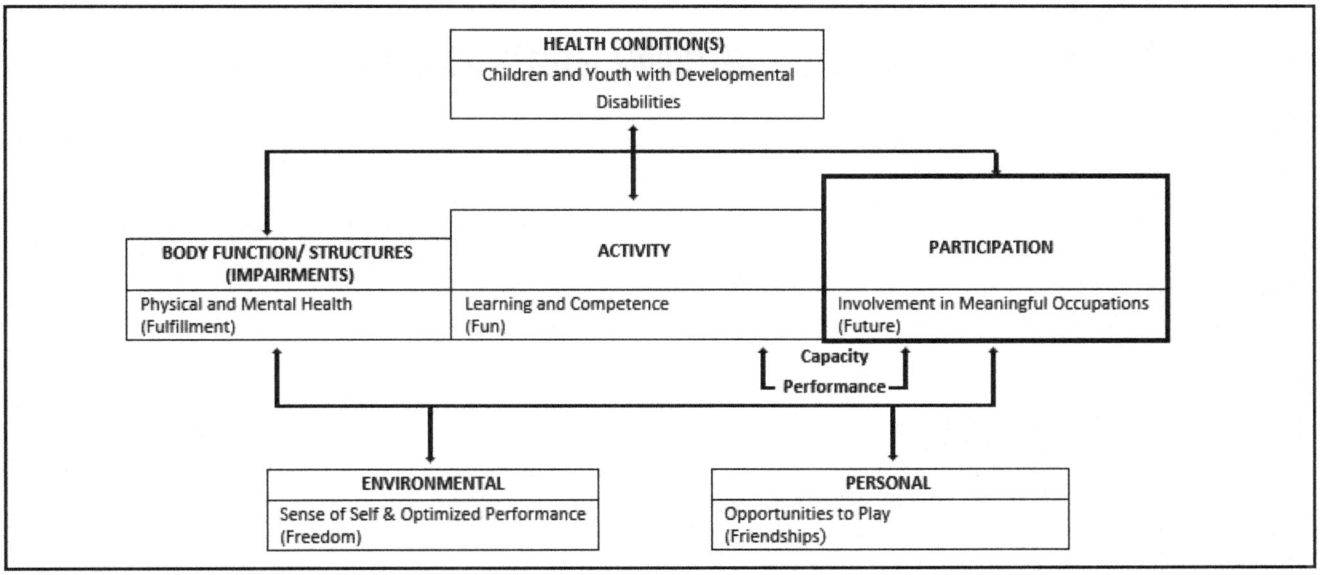

Figure 10-3. The multidimensional confluence of factors impacting meaningful participation. (Adapted from Rosenbaum, P. & Gorter, J. W. [2011]. The 'F-words' in childhood disability: I swear this is how we should think! *Child: Care, Health and Development, 38*[4], 457-463 and Willis, C., Girdler, S., Thompson, M., Rosenberg, M., Reid, S., & Elliott, C. [2017]. Elements contributing to meaningful participation for children and youth with disabilities: A scoping review. *Disability and Rehabilitation, 39*[17], 1771-1784.)

WHO, 2007). For example, activities are defined as "the execution of specific tasks or actions by an individual" (WHO, 2007 p. 9). Whereas participation has been defined as a person's "involvement in a life situation" (WHO, 2007 p. 9). How an individual chooses to become involved in a life situation often reflects personal factors (e.g., values, preferences, and cultural identity) and/or environmental factors such as enabling or impeding aspects of a physical space, the social climate and/or how the person or activity is perceived (Anaby et al., 2020; Bedell et al., 2013; Coussens et al., 2021; Kaelin et al., 2021; Imms et al., 2015; King et al., 2006; Majnemer et al., 2008; Morris et al., 2018; Palisano et al., 2011; WHO, 2002). Likening the ICF-CY model to a paradigmatic structure for enriched play further demonstrates the multidimensionality of meaningful participation (Rosenbaum & Gorter, 2011; Willis et al., 2017). Regardless of underlying health conditions or impairments in body function or structures, the *Community-Based Rehabilitation Guidelines* (WHO, 2010a) proclaim that people of all ability levels should be enabled to participate in play, sport, recreation, and leisure activities within their home, school/work, and/or community (Figure 10-3),

The importance of meaningful participation is further supported in section 300.34 of the Individuals with Disabilities Education Act (IDEA, 2017) that highlights children and youth should be supported to engage in recreation and leisure activities within the school and community as part of their right to related services. As play, sport, recreation, and leisure activities can improve a person's physical and mental health and well-being, successful participation is being increasingly regarded as the ultimate health outcome (Bult et al., 2011; Coussens et al., 2021; FitzGerald et al., 2018; Imms et al., 2015; Majnemer et al., 2008; Morris et al., 2018; Powrie et al., 2015; Willis et al., 2017). Additional health benefits (e.g., improvements in neuromuscular strength and cardiovascular endurance) and prevention of comorbid conditions (e.g., hypertension and obesity) have also been associated with routine participation in physical activity (Morris et al., 2018; Willis et al., 2018a).

According to Article 30 in the United Nations Convention on the Rights of Persons with Disabilities (2008), all persons, regardless of ability level, should not only have equal access to, but also be encouraged to participate to the fullest extent possible in inclusive and disability-specific activities. **Inclusion** can be viewed as a matter of social justice achieved through active and equal participation in shared learning activities, supporting those with disabilities across environments as full members of the community (Cologon, 2013). Inclusion requires we ensure not only that everyone is treated fairly or equitably, but also that all individuals have the same opportunities to participate in the naturally occurring activities of society, including play (Ideishi et al., 2010). Professionals have to consider play determinants that influence attendance and a child's physical and/or mental involvement, which are the two essential criteria that epitomize participation (Coussen et al., 2021; Imms et al., 2015).

For a child with a disability, collaborative interprofessional care becomes even more imperative as various disciplines, family members, and the child work jointly to explore and holistically support engagement in activity that supports a child's occupational health. These efforts should be combined across settings and environments so that a child engaged in play or establishing friendships in, for instance, the school setting, can generalize skills and interactions to play contexts with friends in the community setting. The unique perspectives of each team member can help to analyze a child's strengths, challenges, and appropriate environmental and sensory-based modifications that make optimal engagement and participation possible.

Professional Reasoning Box F: Describing Sasha's Function Using the ICF-CY

Sasha was diagnosed with Gould syndrome with a history of bilateral intraventricular hemorrhage diagnosed in utero at 6 months post-menstrual age. Impairments in her body functions and structures (e.g., the presence of spasticity, cortical visual impairment, and decreased strength) limits her ability to complete activities and fully participate in a variety of environments with assistive technology (i.e., functioning at Gross Motor Function Classification System [GMFCS] Level V). Sasha's family wants her to be able to play with her peers and to increase the frequency of attending events within the community that requires exploration of available programs as well as that intensifies her level of involvement by improving the accessibility and adaptability of the physical and attitudinal aspects of community environments. See Professional Reasoning Box G.

Assessment

There is no single tool or biomarker that can accurately predict or track a child's ability to participate in play, sport, recreation, and leisure activities. Rather, fully engaging with and getting the most out of play, sport, recreation, and leisure, requires a child to use an array of physical, cognitive, communicative, and social skills. To best assess all of the needs of the child, we recommend practitioners approach new clients using ICF-CY model (WHO, 2007; Professional Reasoning Box F).

To examine children and youth who wish to participate in community activities, a comprehensive battery of validated tools that address different constructs of body structures/ function, activity, and/or participation is warranted. In addition, practitioners should also administer assessment tools that examine and objectify direct and indirect determinants to participation, motivation, and engagement. To place a child within the ICF-CY model and get a better understanding of their strengths and needs in functionality, activity, and participation many teams begin a larger-scale developmental inventory assessment. This is often administered or led by a psychologist. For school-aged children, an intervention specialist working on the students Individualized Education Program (IEP) team may also administer or support a developmental inventory assessment. Most assessments in this class tend to involve numerous item questionnaires answered by parent, caregiver, or teacher with or without direct observation by the psychologist administering the test. These assessments are generally divided into domains and subdomains, including cognitive (e.g., reasoning, base academic skills), communication skills (e.g., receptive, expressive), functional skills (e.g., personal care, community engagement), social skills (e.g., interpersonal relationships, self-regulation and coping skills), and motor functioning (e.g., gross motor movement, fine motor movement). Two common examples of well-validated developmental inventories are the Battelle Developmental Inventory, second edition (BDI-2) and the Vineland Adaptive Behavior Scales, third edition (VABS-3).

Developmental inventories are often confused with screening tools that school programs use to screen all children whose development may be delayed in one or more areas. The Ages and Stages Questionnaire (ASQ-3) or Devereux Early Childhood Assessment (DECA) are common examples of such screeners used in early childhood settings.

Communication

For many children with severe impairments, teams may want to continue with more specialized assessments after establishing where the child lies within the ICF-CY continuum. The first most common barrier to children's participation and engagement is deficits in communication skills, specifically those with language disorders. The classic example is a child with autism spectrum disorder who only speaks in one- or two-word phrases for requesting.

The first area to assess more deeply, might be measuring the child's receptive vocabulary (i.e., what word the child recognizes). Here, a team might choose an assessment like the Peabody Picture Vocabulary Test Fifth Edition (PPVT-5; Dunn, 2018).

Motor Function

Motor function is another area that can present significant barriers to participation. When assessing how motor function affects engagement in activities, specific validated assessments like the Gross Motor Function Measure (GMFM; Russell et al., 2002) or the Peabody Developmental Motor Scales, second edition (PDMS-2; Folio & Fewell, 2000) could be used. As an example, the GMFM-88 (Russell et al., 2002) is a valid, criterion-referenced tool that can be used for children between 5 months and 16 years of age. For students with obvious motor impairments in specific areas or with specific profiles, a range of specialized assessments are also available. Similarly, categorizing a child's function using the GMFCS (Palisano et al., 2007) levels (I: independent with few limitations to V: fully dependent) can help to establish performance expectations and the need for assistive technology (e.g., mobility devices) when completing different activities (Longo et al., 2013).

Participation and Engagement

Assessing participation and engagement in meaningful activities is also important for the interprofessional team to consider in their overall evaluation plan.

Using Goal Attainment Scaling (GAS; Kiresuk & Sherman,1968; Kiresuk et al., 2014) is also an effective means to track and measure changes in outcome areas that are otherwise difficult to capture with standardized assessments because norm-referenced assessments typically measure developmental changes over longer periods of time. GAS uses a client's unique, individualized goals and provides a means to uniformly score and track changes and progress over shorter periods that are meaningful for the intervention process. GAS scoring (ranging from -2 current level to +2 highest possible level, with 0 being expected achievement) essentially describes the extent to which a client is achieving their goals (Kiresuk et al., 1994; Willis, 2017). For example, SwimSations is an aquatic therapy program developed by Dr. Kristen Pataki at Cleveland State University in Cleveland, Ohio. SwimSations is an 8-week program integrating aquatic therapy with occupational therapy to provide a sensory-enriched play-based experience that focuses not only on motor skills and tolerating sensory input, but also play skills, communication, leisure activities, and self-esteem. After the first baseline session, three goals are developed for each child in the areas of sensory processing, behavior, and participation/engagement using GAS. Sensory goals primarily relate to tolerating water and sensory activities in the water, as well as seeking out tools to self-regulate. Behavioral goals include observable behaviors such as transitioning in and out of the pool, following directions, and staying on task. Examples of participation goals include engaging in weekly activities and interacting with peers. Standardized developmental assessments would not typically be sensitive enough to detect changes in these types of activities and goals, and therefore, GAS offers an evidence-based alternative to measurement.

Behavior

Another important consideration for some children is the assessment of interfering and challenging behavior. This may be more common with certain disability categories, for example, a child with autism may struggle with minor interfering behavior like stereotypy or echolalia that can break a child's concentration or distract from engagement in an activity. Some children may also have more significant challenging behaviors (e.g., self-injurious or physical aggression) that can present a significant barrier to participation. Some developmental inventories, like the VABS-3 include an assessment of interfering and challenging behavior that can help a team assess the scope of the challenge. If behavioral problems are identified, a Functional Behavior Assessment (FBA) is the next level of assessment that may or may not require a Functional Analysis. The FBA is a process of evaluation more than one specific assessment tool with the purpose to identify functions of behavior and their antecedents in order to develop a behavioral modification plan. These assessments often involve trial-based evaluation of student behavior that is considerably more in depth than conducting observation in a child's natural environment and asking caregivers to respond to a questionnaire. To effectively conduct, interpret, and use the results of an FBA in program planning, a team should include a Board-Certified Behavior Analyst. One possible alternative to using a battery of assessments focusing more in depth on specific domains is using targeted assessments for specific disability groups. The most well-developed line of assessments for specific disabilities is for children with autism. Assessments like the Assessment of Basic Language & Learning Skills (ABLLS; Partington, 2010) are frequently used in school-based and clinical practice.

Child Preferences

Considering the child's motivation to engage with the activities the team presents is important when attempting to determine how to structure a "just-right" experience for a child. Assessing preferences can be as simple as asking the child or their caregivers about the things the child seems to like engaging with. One validated questionnaire to examine preferences is the Reinforcer Assessment for Individuals with Severe Disability (RAISD; Fisher et al., 1996). For students with more severely impactful disabilities, teams might want to consider testing preferences using a validated protocol like the multiple stimulus without replacement (MSWO), paired stimulus, or free operant methods or assessing preferences.

Occupational Health

QOL and well-being measures should also be incorporated into the holistic battery of assessments selected to evaluate a child's occupational productivity. For instance, the Pediatric Quality of Life Inventory (Varni et al., 1999) is a brief, standardized assessment that systematically assesses patients' and parents' perceptions of health-related QOL (HRQOL) in pediatric patients with chronic health conditions. This type of assessment takes specific health conditions into consideration and can evaluate how they affect overall QOL. Other tools such as the Well-Being Indicator Tool for Youth (WIT-Y) can further examine related constructs such as well-being. The WIT-Y evaluates physical, cognitive, and mental health in addition to community, relationships, purpose, environment, and safety and security. These tap into additional constructs from the ICF-CY, environment and personal factors, that help complete the overall picture of health and functioning in children and youth (Professional Reasoning Box G).

Professional Reasoning Box G: Assessing Sasha

Sasha has received various assessments across settings and practices (e.g., outpatient therapy and school-based) that have helped to identify her current abilities and areas where she is limited. For example, using the GMFM (Russell et al., 2002) her total score = 16.4%, with her strengths in lying and rolling (Dimension A). In addition, through the use of the Canadian Occupational Performance Measure (COPM; Law et al., 1990), Sasha's family indicated that while she may be limited in her productivity in play/school, active recreation, and social activities, these are the outcomes they most desire Sasha to be able to achieve.

Thinking of a child who is familiar to you, what types of assessments might you utilize to examine and measure the success of engagement in a community program? Are there certain assessment tools that should be used for every child? How might your assessment choice and technique vary for children with different underlying impairments or who have different participation goals?

Intervention

Findings gathered during the assessment process should be used to guide intervention selection and implementation in an attempt to optimize occupational health and participation outcomes (Kaelin et al., 2021). Intervention decisions should also incorporate applicable information from current evidence, the child's/family's preferences and goals, and the expertise of the professional who is implementing play activities in a community setting (Case-Smith & Arbesman, 2008; Palisano et al., 2012). Maximizing engagement, productivity, and health can require strategies directed at the level of the individual, organization/community site, and/or society (Ideishi et al., 2010; Kaelin et al., 2021). It is common practice to implement multimodal interventions targeting various domains (i.e., sensory-motor, cognitive, social-emotional, and language) and areas of function (i.e., body structures, activity, and participation). In addition to providing opportunities for play in an enriched environment, there are two other categories of intervention that are particularly relevant to maximizing participation outcomes: 1) child- and family-centered education to empower individuals and ensure opportunities for play in the community, and 2) universally designed environments that foster "just-right" experiences used to acquire new skills or refine competence and improve performance (which may require modifications to the environment). The ultimate goal of interventions should be to reduce or eliminate modifiable barriers while promoting children and youth to develop competence, autonomy, and relatedness that results in functional gains and optimizes occupational health.

Child- and Family-Centered Education

Interventions that involve education, coaching, and providing family-centered care are strongly recommended, effective interventions (Novak & Honan, 2019). Alarmingly, only 15.7% of children with special health care needs tend to receive services in a family-centered, comprehensive, and coordinated system (Office of Disease Prevention and Health Promotion [ODPHP], 2020). Family-centered practices have recognized the parent as the expert with a need to understand the child's and family's goals and preferences for health-related care (Law, 2002; Novak & Honan, 2019; Palisano et al., 2012). A family's ethnicity, values, and other sociodemographic characteristics should be considered by professionals before making recommendations to avoid imposing unwelcomed interventions (Brown et al., 2016; Case-Smith & Arbesman, 2008; Coussens et al., 2021). Novak and Honan (2019) highlighted that strategies used to educate families should incorporate sharing of information about a child's condition and options for interventions, providing necessary resources for families to access services, while addressing overall family health and well-being (e.g., advising about coping when familial stress is reported). Moreover, it is also critical to engage children and youth when making decisions about the care they will receive, while being responsive to their activity preferences to ensure enjoyment and task perseverance (Law, 2002; Morris et al., 2018; Palisano et al., 2011, 2012). Education using a philosophy of family-centered care can help to optimize a child's participation in play, increase a family's satisfaction with services, and decrease feelings of parental burden or stress that may be heightened in families caring for a child with a developmental disability (Coussens et al., 2021; Jansen et al., 2003; Law, 2002; Palisano et al., 2011; Willis et al., 2018a).

Coaching, for example, can help optimize long-term functional outcomes and overall occupational health by empowering children and families to manage their own circumstances (Coussens et al., 2021; Kahjoogh et al., 2019). This technique engages children and families in systematic, collaborative goal-setting that coincides with exchange of information, a structured problem-solving process, and emotional support (Kahjoogh et al., 2019). Another emphasis is to build capacity, no matter the level of ability or disability (Anaby et al., 2021; Coussens et al., 2021). This requires flexible, and at times, innovative thinking and reflection, and should consider not just the child's capacity but how an activity can be adapted to "real-life" scenarios to optimize performance (Anaby et al., 2021). Coaching can also help identify environmental constraints (i.e., physical or attitudinal barriers) that could hinder a child's performance in home, school, or community spaces (Lim et al., 2016). For example, if a child with autism spectrum disorder is limited in their ability to participate in community events or settings (such as at the science museum or local farmers markets) due to hypersensitivity to sensory stimuli, coaching can help derive family-oriented goals to increase participation in several ways. An interprofessional team can help educate the family on techniques to mitigate overstimulation, selecting specific sites and devising environmental modifications, fully considering all activities in a community setting without limiting selections based on feared behaviors, and working through perceived attitudinal barriers that have historically hindered participation. Approaching this as a team can help the parents feel more competent and confident venturing out into the community and give both parents and children tools to manage unexpected circumstances.

Environments

Considering environmental design in preparation for community participation can help ameliorate contextualized restrictions in participation or can improve how an individual performs a task by minimizing physical and attitudinal barriers. Setting the scene can help individuals feel better prepared for community events (Kaelin et al., 2021) by preemptively communicating event expectations to attendees using social stories, sensory guides, or simply talking about different activities and adapting them to match the users' needs (Case-Smith & Arbesman, 2008; DeBoth et al., 2021; Fletcher, 2014; Silverman & Carr Tyszka, 2017). Professionals and community organizers running community programs should predetermine tasks required to effectively play and who will be available to help support play opportunities (which can then enhance the likelihood that participation outcomes are achieved; Kaelin et al., 2021). For example, having a trusted adult who can provide positive reinforcement and encouragement during play or engaging a peer role model who can demonstrate desired behaviors dually targets development of a child's sense of self while breaking down attitudinal barriers and creating positive social interactions (e.g., friendship; Kaelin et al., 2021; Powrie et al., 2015; Willis et al., 2018a). Professionals should also present activities in a way that give children and youth a choice on if and how to play in addition to devising alternative activities or segmenting a task into more manageable "just-right" experiences that are fun and fulfilling (Case-Smith & Arbesman, 2008; Kaelin et al., 2021; Powrie et al., 2015).

Lobbying for environments that mediate the types and amount of sensory stimulation and/or having access to assistive technologies (e.g., augmentative and alternative communication or mobility devices) can help to augment a child's sensorimotor, cognitive, or communication capabilities to enhance independent exploration and prevent maladaptive behaviors and ill health (Bult et al., 2011; Lobo et al., 2013; Gannotti, 2017; Palisano et al., 2011). While advancements have been made in the recent past, many cultural centers/informal learning centers (e.g., museums, libraries, zoos, science centers), parks, playgrounds, sporting fields, and fitness centers remain physically inaccessible (Langa et al., 2013). These barriers can deter families of children with developmental disabilities from even attempting to play in these environments (Kaelin et al., 2021; Morris et al., 2018). A child's or family's preferences may inspire them to take a chance given adequate information about potential adaptations thoughtfully designed, including the creation of activities that support participation goals (Bult et al., 2011; Morris et al., 2018; Kaelin et al., 2021; Rimmer et al., 2016). Modifying these physical spaces has been associated with significant gains in how a child performs a task and ultimately participates (Bult et al., 2011; Kramer, 2018).

Finally, the costs associated with attending events should also be considered as part of the overall environment. More than 50% of parents who are caring for children with cerebral palsy have indicated needing help finding appropriate programs within the community, expanding the variety of opportunities for play that are available, affordable, and accessible may require advocacy at a systems level to trigger regulation and reform of legislation (Coussens et al., 2021; Longo et al., 2013; Palisano et al., 2012). Even though laws exist, (e.g., 2010 ADA Standards for Accessible Design and the 1999 Olmstead decision) society needs to be pushed to ensure equal and inclusive participation in any community setting, that allow for physical, cognitive, and social engagement regardless of a child's ability level or personal constraints (Coussens et al., 2021; Lussenhop et al., 2016; Pendo & Iezzoni, 2020; Rimmer et al., 2016). In fact, nearly 50% of interventions used by parents/caregivers to assist children's meaningful play engagement target contextual or environmental features (Kaelin et al., 2021).

Effectively implemented environmental modification strategies not only enhance participation outcomes but also promote optimal physical and mental health and well-being while reducing summative health-related costs (Bedell et al., 2013; Coussens et al., 2021; Gannotti, 2017; Ideishi et al., 2010; Kolehmainen et al., 2011; Kramer, 2018; Palisano et al., 2011). Ideally, a team of individuals who have lived experiences as users of assistive technology (i.e., persons with

Professional Reasoning Box H: Let's Play Ball!

Sasha has two older brothers, one of whom is an avid baseball player. During the spring and summer months, this family spends many nights at the ballfield. When asked, Sasha's family reported that their ultimate goal would be for Sasha to be able to participate in play with her peers and family members without restrictions in any community setting. Because of this, Sasha's family has piloted the use of a multidirectional, over-ground, hands-free harness system (MoH; see Figure 10-4), which they set up right next to the bleachers. This assistive device allows Sasha to have greater independence in her mobility while watching her brother pitch his team to victory. In addition, Sasha's family has attempted to break down attitudinal barriers, as Sasha's mom sends notes to all the players' families, sharing a little about Sasha's abilities including that she is very social and to encourage the players' siblings to come and play with her during the game.

For families who may face financial constraints, what strategies could you employ to ensure children have access to performance-enhancing assistive technology to optimize participation in play? Thinking of a community space you enjoy visiting, and what types of physical and/or attitudinal barriers are present that could limit meaningful participation for children and youth?

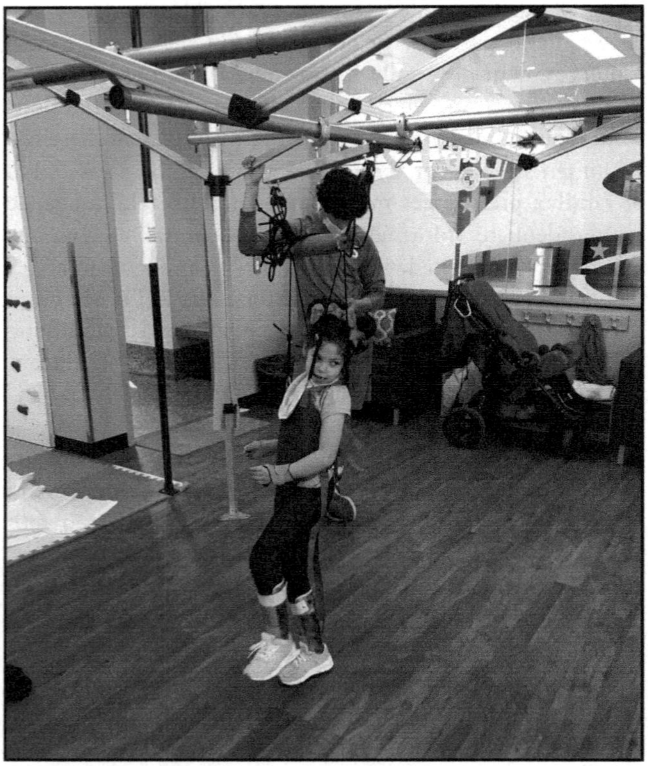

Figure 10-4. Child in multidirectional overground harness (MOH) system.

disabilities) and/or have specific expertise in universal environmental design and prescribing assistive technology should be involved from the conception of spaces intended to be built for children and their families in order to be fully inclusive. However, this may not always be possible and therefore if such teams are willing to think creatively, interventions can be recommended and implemented that improve attitudinal and physical barriers within existing community environments (Law, 2002; Palisano et al., 2011). For example, older cities tend to have more buildings that do not meet current ADA standards for accessibility. Professionals such as physical therapists, occupational therapists, design experts, and engineers can work together with children with disabilities and their families to modify physical barriers in community spaces that prohibit participation. This may include expanding doorways, adding ramps, textured walkways, colorful covers for fluorescent lighting, or adding sound-absorbing panels to large, open spaces. These modifications can greatly increase access and promote well-being and enhance QOL (Professional Reasoning Box H). For individuals wishing to learn more about designing accessible programs there are various organizations and resources available, including the National Center on Accessibility (available at: https://ncaonline.org/) with design standards available through the Americans with Disability Act's website (available at: https://www.ada.gov/regs2010/2010ADAStandards/2010ADAstandards.htm).

Interprofessional Perspectives

We are in an era with an increased urgency for team-based models of care due to a shortage of 4.3 million health care professionals worldwide. This has impacted the ability of our health care system to deliver quality, cost effective care for populations that are faced with health issues that are becoming increasingly complex (Abu-Rish et al., 2012; Frenk et al., 2010; Health Professions Accreditors Collaborative [HPAC], 2019; Institute of Medicine of the National Academies [IOMNA], 2015; Reeves et al., 2016; WHO, 2010a). These evolving challenges can be met by opportunities for improvement, including a vision outlined by the Institute of Medicine that involves teaching and supporting the next generation of health care providers to serve as members of interprofessional teams. **IPCP** is characterized by "multiple health workers from different professional backgrounds working together with patients, families, carers, and communities to deliver the highest quality of care" (WHO, 2010a, p. 13). The Interprofessional Education Collaborative (IPEC) has further defined four competencies for education and practice that, when present, reflect the skills necessary for team-based practice (HPAC, 2019; IPEC, 2016). These IPEC competencies are:

Professional Reasoning Box I: The Roles of Interprofessional Players to Enhance Sasha's Play Experience

Sasha has a motivated, informed, and prepared set of team members (including her parents, primary care provider, neurologist, physiatrist, outpatient occupational, physical, and speech therapists, school-based occupational, physical and speech therapists, intervention specialist, vision specialist, orientation and mobility specialist, aquatic therapy instructor, and home nursing).

Based on her impairments in body functions and structures and activity competence, who do you believe are the most essential team members to collaboratively create meaningful play experiences for Sasha and why? Who do you believe is the best equipped to lead Sasha's team and why? How might you address conflict that arises when team members disagree on how to best support Sasha's participation in play?

1. Values and Ethics: maintaining a climate of mutual respect and shared values
2. Roles and Responsibilities: using the knowledge of one's own role and those of other professions to appropriately assess and address the health care needs of patients
3. Interprofessional Communication: promoting, maintaining, and supporting practices that foster continuity of patient care, and
4. Team and Teamwork: optimizing team dynamics to most effectively plan, deliver, and evaluate patient care.

The benefits of having collaborative, workforce-ready, team-oriented practitioners that promote the continuity of care between professionals include minimizing clinical error rates and improving patient outcomes while enhancing team functioning and personal job satisfaction (Abu-Rish et al., 2012; HPAC, 2019; IOMNA, 2015; Reeves et al., 2016; WHO, 2010b). In addition, linking efforts of the traditional health care team with the work being conducted by childcare providers/educators and professionals of community programs has the potential to accentuate the beneficial effects on health outcomes while optimizing meaningful participation for children and youth (WHO, 2010b; Professional Reasoning Box I).

Community Programs for All

There have been numerous reports of partnerships between health/educational institutions and community entities (e.g., fitness facilities, museums, and aquariums, Ideishi et al., 2010; Langa et al., 2013; Leichtman et al., 2014; Lussenhop et al., 2016; Richards et al., 2015). The driving force to establish these collaborations is centered around visions to enhance the participation of children and youth with sensory-processing deficits and/or mobility impairments. Use of enriched play experiences in the community is less well described in the literature. However, an exemplar program, Participation in Leisure Allowing Access for Everyone on the Move (PLAAY on the Move), is a community-based initiative that is organized through Cleveland State University and travels to a variety of local museums and community spaces. Its mission is to support the engagement of children of all ability levels in enriching and stimulating activities using low-cost technologies to minimize barriers that limit participation. While trained faculty, therapists, and university students attend these events and often assist children to mobilize through the environment, PLAAY on the Move, unlike conventional therapy, is a play experience with an emphasis on providing assistance in a way that aligns with overarching participation goals of fun, freedom, fulfillment, friendship, and future. PLAAY on the Move events are designed for children 5 months through 8 years of age with programming that includes interactive crafts while promoting exploration of different community spaces. As many existing community programs are geared for school-age children with 39.3% of preschoolers in the United States reporting difficulties when attempting to participate in activities outside the home (Lim et al., 2016), PLAAY on the Move fills an unmet need, by designing interactive crafts and activities that promote exploration for a younger population of children and youth (ages 5 months through 8 years of age). When considering developmental and neuromaturational processes, capturing and engaging young children in participation endeavors is critical to ensure appropriate levels of experience- (or use) dependent practice (Gannotti, 2017; Kolehmainen et al., 2011; Morgan et al., 2013; Nithianantharajah & Hannan, 2006; Sale et al., 2014)

PLAAY on the Move runs with a no-cost registration process with minimal fees associated with parking and transportation. Depending on the size of the community space, 7 to 12 children with mobility and/or sensory-based impairments typically attend these events that occur approximately 10 times each year. Many families also bring typically developing siblings and peers that are welcomed to participate in the activities provided. PLAAY on the Move events are also unique in that they facilitate access to an array of kid-friendly, low-cost assistive technologies and adaptive sensory experiences that can be used to help facilitate attendees to engage with toys, exhibits, and each other. For example, 6- or 12-volt battery-powered modified ride-on cars (ROCs) that have been specially adapted to promote independent use and exploration (through replacement of the foot pedal activator with a low-profile switch that can be moved anywhere on the car) are available for use in the community during

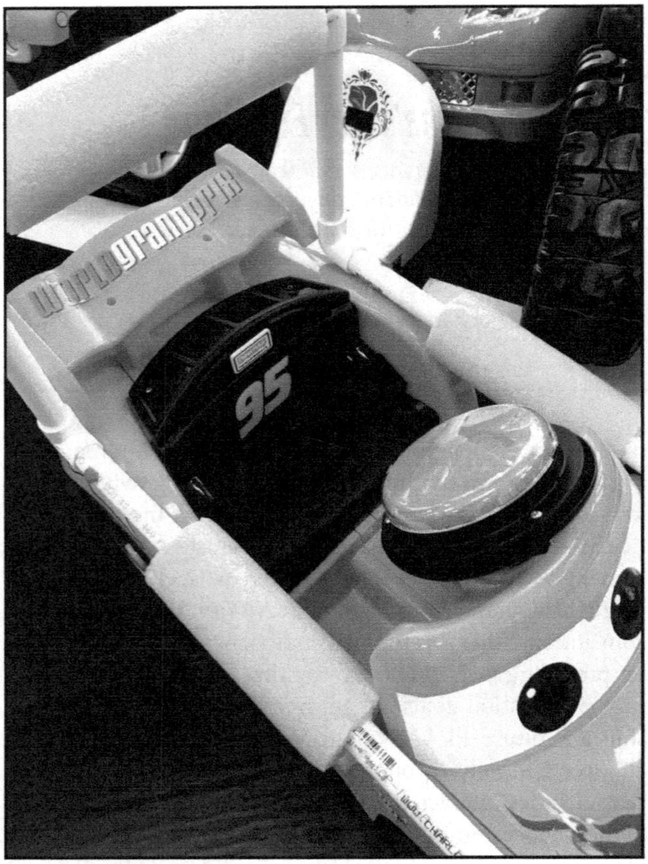

Figure 10-5. Adapted car.

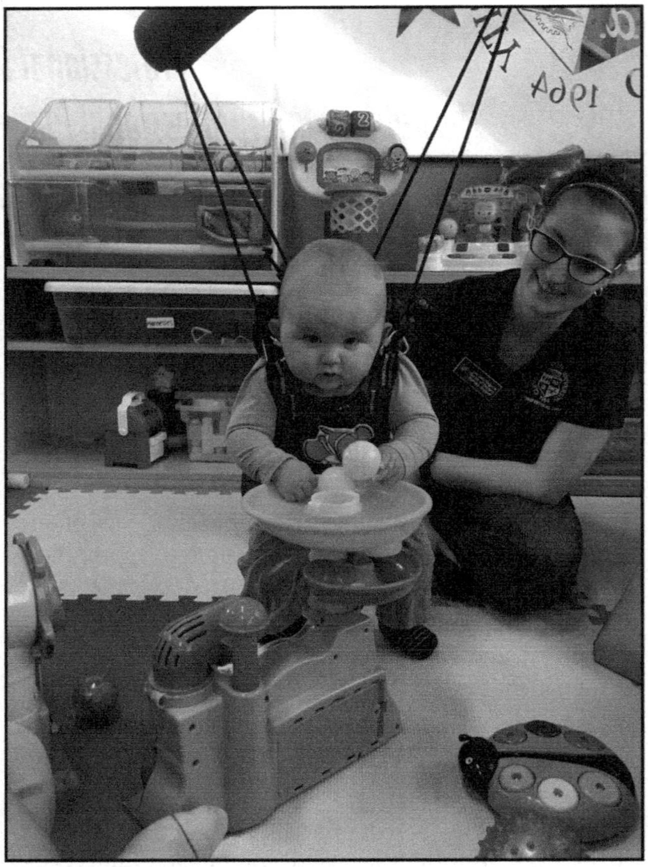

Figure 10-6. Child in bungee system.

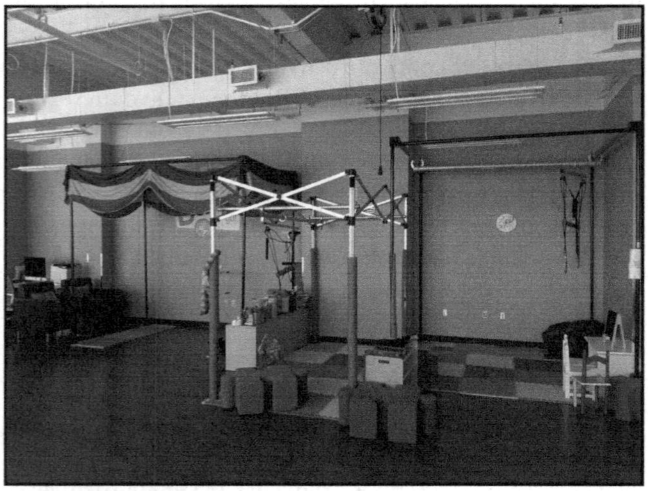

Figure 10-7. MOH systems.

PLAAY on the Move events (Huang et al., 2018; Logan et al., 2016; DeBoth et al., 2021). PVC piping covered with pool noodles or kickboards, Velcro chest straps and seatbelts, and airplane neck pillows can be added (or removed) to support optimal seating postures (Figure 10-5; Logan et al., 2016; DeBoth et al., 2021). Another mobility aid used during PLAAY on the Move (PoM) events is a portable MOH. This FDA-registered, body-weight support system (Enliten, LLC) allows for 360 degrees of real-world mobility within a collapsible frame, with the standard size encompassing a 10' x 10' area, although sizes can be customized to fit almost any physical space (DeBoth et al., 2021; Kokkoni et al., 2020). Two types of suspension are available. The first option connects a harnessed child to a movable rail structure that slides along the metal frame via bungee cords (Figures 10-6 and 10-7; Kokkoni et al., 2020). A secondary function of the bungee system is that it can elicit a sensory response as the cords give and take when a child loads the system by moving up or down. The second counterweight system, allows children to move vertically, which can be particularly helpful working on transitions or when wanting to move up and down different surface levels to participate in a play activity (Kokkoni et al., 2020). Because of its portability, this device can be moved almost anywhere in the environment to maximize independent, multisensory, self-selected engagement with activities or exhibits. Additionally, the inherent adaptability of MOHs can be used to support a child in a variety of positions while facilitating a "just-right" experience while sitting, creeping, standing, walking, or climbing (DeBoth et al., 2021; Kokkoni et al., 2020; Professional Reasoning Box J).

Professional Reasoning Box J: Sasha at PLAAY on the Move

While Sasha participates in various therapy-related activities, she is limited in her abilities to independently explore and play in a community setting. Having access to a MOH during PoM helps to augment her physical capabilities and maximize her participation. This freedom, along with her ability to have fun, feel fulfillment, and develop friendships requires a team-based approach to optimize the setup of the equipment and environment to foster opportunities for Sasha to move independently and facilitate social interactions during age-appropriate play activities that are "just-right."

What training may be required of PoM staff to ensure they are prepared to safely support participation of children and youth attendees? How might multiple team members use their discipline-specific skills to implement an enriched dance party for Sasha?

Conclusion

Participation-related services provided to children and youth, particularly those with developmental disabilities, are at a turning point due to escalating health care costs, limited access to adequately trained professionals, and a push for interprofessional collaborative practices that emphasize participation-based health promotion in the community. Intentional, universally designed community-based programs that embody "just-right" play experiences in an enriched environment while promoting ultimate participation-related outcomes (fun, freedom, fulfillment, friendship, and future) can not only improve overall health and mental well-being, but can develop the competence, autonomy, and relatedness, and thus, occupational health for children and youth of all abilities. Moreover, the planning, implementation, and evaluation of experiences that promote child-centered play can be enhanced by creating a community-oriented home where an interprofessional team of professionals understand each other's role, responsibilities, and scopes of practice, work synergistically so that children and their families receive the quality of services they deserve. Through these efforts to maximize participation, all children—those with and without disabilities—will have access to opportunities that promote learning, support development, provide novel experiences, and build relationships. Interprofessional teams are critical for understanding and assessing these needs and existing barriers while also developing appropriate and effective interventions. By doing so, this can lead to better QOL and greater sense of well-being, critical components for optimizing occupational health in children and youth.

References

Abu-Rish, E., Kim, S., & Choe, L., et al. (2012). Current trends in interprofessional education of health sciences students: a literature review. *Journal of Interprofessional Care, 26*, 444-451.

American Occupational Therapy Association. (2012). Tips for living life to its fullest: Learning through play. https://www.aota.org/-/media/Corporate/Files/Practice/Children/Browse/Play/Learning%20Through%20Play%20tip%20sheet.pdf

Anaby, D., Avery, L., Gorter, J. W., Levin, M. F., Teplicky, R., Turner, L., Cormier, I., & Hanes, J. (2020). Improving body functions through participation in community activities among young people with physical disabilities. *Developmental Medicine and Child Neurology, 62*(5), 640-646. https://doi.org/10.1111/dmcn.14382

Anaby, D., Law, M., Coster, W., Bedell, G., Khetani, M., Avery, L., & Teplicky, R. (2014). The mediating role of the environment in explaining participation of children and youth with and without disabilities across home, school, and community. *Archives of Physical Medicine and Rehabilitation, 95*(5), 908-917. https://doi.org/10.1016/j.apmr.2014.01.005

Anaby, D., Ryan, M., Palisano, R. J., Levin, M. F., Gorter, J. W., Avery, L., Cormier, I., Teplicky, R., Coulter, J., & Hanes, J. (2021). Participation during a pandemic: Forging new pathways. *Physical & Occupational Therapy in Pediatrics*. https://doi.org/10.1080/01942638.2021.1875739

Bedell, G., Coster, W., Law, M., Liljenquist, K., Kao, Y. C., Teplicky, R., ... Khetani, M. A. (2013). Community participation, supports, and barriers of school-age children with and without disabilities. *Archives of Physical Medicine and Rehabilitation, 94*(2), 315-323. https://doi.org/10.1016/j.apmr.2012.09.024

Bult, M. K., Vershuren, O., Jongmans, M. J., Lindeman, E., & Ketellar, M. (2011). What influences participation in leisure activities of children and youth with physical disabilities? A systematic review. *Research in Developmental Disabilities, 32*, 1521-1529. https://doi.org/10.1016/j.ridd.2011.01.045.

Brown, H. E., Atkin, A. J., Wong, G., Chinapaw, M. J. M., Sluijs, E. M. F. (2016). Family-based interventions to increase physical activity in children: a systematic review, meta-analysis and realist synthesis. *Obesity Reviews, 17*, 345-360. doi: 10.1111/obr.12362.

Brown, T., & Thyer, L. (2020). The convergent validity of the Children's Leisure Assessment Scale (CLASS) and Children's Assessment of Participation and Enjoyment and Preferences for Activities of Children (CAPE/PAC). *Scandinavian Journal of Occupational Therapy, 27*(5), 349-363. https://doi.org/10.1080/11038128.2019.1672784

Case-Smith, J., & Arbesman, M. (2008). Evidence based review of interventions for autism used in or of relevance to occupational therapy. *American Journal of Occupational Therapy, 62*(4), 16-429. https://doi.org/10.5014/ajot.62.4.416

Cologon, K. (2013). Inclusion in education: Towards equality for students with disability (Issues Paper). Children with Disability Australia. https://apo.org.au/sites/default/files/resource-files/2013-10/apo-nid36129.pdf

Coussens, M., Vitse, F., Desoete, A., Vanderstraeten, G., Van Waelvelde, H., Van de Velde, D. (2021). Participation of young children with developmental disabilities: Parental needs and strategies, a qualitative thematic analysis. *BMJ Open, 11*, e042732. https://doi.org/10.1136/bmjopen-2020-042732.

DeBoth. K., Wendland, M., Bilinovic, T., & Sanford, C. (2021). Caregiver perceptions of child participation in sensory friendly community events. *Journal of Occupational Therapy, Schools & Early Intervention*. https://doi.org/10.1080/19411243.2020.1862729.

Dunn, D. M. (2018). *Peabody picture vocabulary test* (5th ed.). NCS Pearson.

Essame, C. (2020). Developmental play: A new approach to understanding how all children learn through play. *Childhood Education, 96*(1), 14-23.

Fisher, W. W., Piazza, C. C., Bowman, L. G., & Amari, A. (1996). Integrating caregiver report with a systematic choice assessment. *American Journal on Mental Retardation, 101*, 15-25.

FitzGerald, T. L., Kwong, A. K. L., Cheong, J. L. Y., McGinley, J. L., Doyle, L. W., & Spittle, A. J. (2018). Body structure, function, activity, and participation in 3- to 6-year-old children born very preterm: An ICF-based systematic review and meta-analysis. *Physical Therapy, 98*(8), 691-704.

Fletcher, T. (2014). Supporting individuals with special needs at the Dallas Museum of Art. *OT Practice, 19*(5), 12-20.

Frenk, J., Chen, L., Bhutta, Z. A., et al. (2010). Health professionals for a new century: transforming education to strengthen health systems in an interdependent world. *The Lancet, 376*, 1923-1958.

Folio M., & Fewell, R. F. (2000). *Peabody developmental motor scales* (2nd ed.). Austin: Pro-Ed.

Gannotti, M. E. (2017). Coupling of intervention with dose to optimize plasticity and participation in pediatric neurologic populations. *Pediatric Physical Therapy, 29*, S37-S47.

Garvey, C. (1990). *Play*. Harvard University Press.

Golden, T., & Walsh, L. (2013). Play for all at Chicago Children's Museum: A history and overview. *Curator, 56*(3), 337-347. https://doi.org/10.1111/cura.12032

Health Professions Accreditors Collaborative. (2019). Guidance on developing quality interprofessional education for the health professions. https://healthprofessionsaccreditors.org/wp-content/uploads/2019/02/HPACGuidance02-01-19.pdf

Huang, H. H., Chen, Y. M., Huang, H. W., Shih, M. K., Hsieh, Y. H., & Chen, C. L. (2018). Modified ride-on cars and young children with disabilities: Effects of combining mobility and social training. *Frontiers in Pediatrics, 5*, 299. https://doi.org/10.3389/fped.2017.00299

Ideishi, R. I., Willock, C., & Thach, K. (2010). Participation of children with special needs at the aquarium. *Developmental Disabilities Special Interest Section Quarterly, 33*(2), 1-4.

Imms, C., Adair, B., Ullenhag, A., Rosenbaum, P., & Granlund, M. (2015). 'Participation': a systematic review of language, definitions, and constructs used in intervention research with children with disabilities. *Developmental Medicine & Child Neurology, 58*, 29-38. https://doi.org/10.1111/dmcn.12932

Individuals with Disabilities Education Act: Sec. 300.34 Related services. (2017). US Department of Education. Retrieved from: https://sites.ed.gov/idea/regs/b/a/300.34

Institute of Medicine of the National Academies. (2015). Measuring the impact of interprofessional education on collaborative practice and patient outcomes. National Academies of Sciences.

Interprofessional Education Collaborative. (2016) *Core competencies for interprofessional collaborative practice*. Interprofessional Education Collaborative.

Jansen, L. M. C., Ketelaar, M., & Vermeer, A. (2003). Parental experience of participation on physical therapy for children with physical disabilities. *Developmental Medicine & Child Neurology, 45*, 58-69. https://doi.org/10.1017/S0012162203000112.

Kaelin, V. C., Bosak, D. L., Villegas, V. C., Imms, C., & Khetani, M. A. (2021). Participation-focused strategy use among caregivers of children receiving early intervention. *American Journal of Occupational Therapy, 75*(1), 1111. https://doi.org/10.5014/ajot.2021.041962

Kahjoogh, M. A., Kessler, D., Hossini, S. A., Rassafiani, M., Akbarfahimi, N., Khaney H. R., Biglarian, A. (2019). Randomized controlled trial of occupational performance coaching for mothers of children with cerebral palsy. *British Journal of Occupational Therapy, 82*(4), 213-219. https://doi.org/10.1177/0308022618799944

King, G., Law, M., Hanna, S., King, S., Hurley, P., Rosenbaum, P., … Petrenchik, T. (2006). Predictors of leisure and recreation participation of children with physical disabilities: A structural equation modeling analysis. *Children's Health Care, 35*(3), 209-234. https://doi.org/10.1207/s15326888chc3503_2

Kiresuk, T. J., & Sherman, R. E. (1968). Goal attainment scaling: A general method for evaluating comprehensive community mental health programs. *Community Mental Health Journal, 4*(6), 443-453.

Kiresuk, T. J., Smith, A., & Cardillo, J. E. (Eds.). (1994). *Goal attainment scaling: Applications, theory, and measurement*. Lawrence Erlbaum Associates, Inc.

Kiresuk, T. J., Smith, A., & Cardillo, J. E. (2014). *Goal attainment scaling: Applications, theory, and measurement*. Psychology Press.

Kokkoni, E., Mavroudi, E., Zehfroosh, A., Galloway, J. C., Vidal, R., Heinz, J., & Tanner, H. G. (2020). GEARing smart environments for pediatric motor rehabilitation. *Journal of Neuro Engineering and Rehabilitation, 17*(1), 16. https://doi.org/10.1186/s12984-020-0647-0

Kolehmainen, N., Francis, J. J., Ramsay, C. R., Owen, C., McKee, L., Ketelaar, M., & Rosenbaum, P. (2011). Participation in physical play and leisure: Developing a theory-and evidence-based intervention for children with motor impairments. *BMC Pediatrics, 11*(1), 1-8.

Kramer, J. M. (2018). The pathways and resources for participation and engagement (PREP): methodological contributions to environment-focused interventions. *Developmental Medicine & Child Neurology, 60*, 436-444. https://doi.org/10.1111/dmcn.13725

Langa, L. A., Monaco, P., Subramaniam, M., Jaeger, P. T., Shanahan, K., Ziebarth, B. (2013). Improving the museum experiences of children with autism spectrum disorders and their families: An exploratory examination of their motivations and needs and using web-based resources to meet them. *Curator, 56*(3), 323-335.

Law, M. (2002). Participation in the occupations of everyday life. *American Journal of Occupational Therapy, 56*(6), 640-649.

Law, M., Baptiste, S., McColl, M., Opzoomer, A., Polatajko, H., & Pollock, N. (1990). The Canadian occupational performance measure: An outcome measure for occupational therapy. *Canadian Journal of Occupational Therapy, 57*(2), 82-87.

Leichtman, J., Palek-Zahn, C., Tung, V., Becker, S., & Jirikowic, T. (2014). Developing inclusive museum environments for children with autism spectrum disorder and their families. *Developmental Disabilities Special Interest Section Quarterly, 37*(1), 1-4.

Lim, C.Y., Law, M., Khetani, M., Pollock, N., & Rosenbaum, P. (2016). Participation in out-of-home environments for young children with and without disabilities. *OTJR, 36*(3), 112-125. https://doi.org/10.1177/1539449216659859.

Lobo, M. A., Harbourne, R. T., Dusing, S. C., & McCoy, S. W. (2013) Grounding early intervention: physical therapy cannot just be about motor skills anymore. *Physical Therapy, 93*(1), 94-103.

Logan, S. W., Feldner, H. A., Galloway, J. C., & Huang, H. H. (2016). Modified ride-on car use by children with complex medical needs. *Pediatric Physical Therapy, 28*(1), 100-107. https://doi.org/10.1097/PEP.0000000000000210

Longo, E., Badia, M., & Orgaz, B. (2013). Patterns and predictors of participation in leisure activities outside of school in children and adolescents with Cerebral Palsy. *Research in Developmental Disabilities, 34*(1), 266. https://doi.org/10.1016/j.ridd.2012.08.017

Lussenhop, A., Mesiti, L. A., Cohn, E. S., et al. (2016). Social participation of families with children with autism spectrum disorder in a science museum. *Museums & Social Issues, 11*(2), 122-137. https://doi.org/10.1080/15596893.2016.1214806

Majnemer, A., Shevell, M., Poulin, C., Birnbaum, R., Chilingaryan, G., Rosenbaum, P., & Poulin, C. (2008). Participation and enjoyment of leisure activities in school-aged children with cerebral palsy. *Developmental Medicine & Child Neurolology, 50*(1), 751-758. https://doi.org/10.1111/j.1469-8749.2008.03068.x

Maxwell, G., Augustine, L., & Granlund, M. (2012). Does thinking and doing the same thing amount to involved participation? Empirical exploration for finding a measure of intensity for a third ICF-CY qualified. *Developmental Neurorehabilitation, 15*(4), 274-283.

Morgan, C., Novak, I., & Badawi, N. (2013). Enriched environments and motor outcomes in cerebral palsy: Systematic review and meta-analysis. *Pediatrics, 132*, e735-746. https://doi.org/10.1542/peds.2012-3985.

Morris, A., Imms, C., Kerr, C., & Adair, B. (2018). Sustained participation in community-based physical activity by adolescents with cerebral palsy: A qualitative study. *Disability and Rehabilitation, 41*(25), 3042-3051. https://doi.org/10.1080.09638288.2018.1486466.

Nithianantharajah, J., & Hannan, A. J. (2006). Enriched environments, experience-dependent plasticity and disorders of the nervous system. *Nature Reviews Neuroscience, 7*(9), 697-709.

Novak, I., & Honan, I. (2019). Effectiveness of paediatric occupational therapy for children with disabilities: a systematic review. *Australian Occupational Therapy Journal, 66*, 258-273. https://doi.org/10.1111/1440-1630.12573

Office of Disease Prevention and Health Promotion. (2020). Healthy People 2030- MICH-20. https://health.gov/healthypeople/objectives-and-data/browse-objectives/health-care/increase-proportion-children-and-adolescents-special-health-care-needs-who-have-system-care-mich-20

Palisano, R., Rosenbaum, P., Bartlett, D., & Livingston, M. (2007). *Gross motor function classification system expanded and revised.* CanChild Centre for Childhood Disability Research, McMaster University.

Palisano, R. J., Chiarello, L. A., King, G. A., Novak, I., Stoner, T., & Fiss, A. (2012). Participation based therapy for children with physical disabilities. *Disability and Rehabilitation, 34*(12), 1041-1052. https://doi.org/10.3109/09638288.2011.628740

Palisano, R.J., Chiarello, L.A., Orlin, M., et al. (2011). Determinants of intensity of participation in leisure and recreational activities by children with cerebral palsy. *Developmental Medicine & Child Neurology, 53*(2), 142-149.

Partington, J. W. (2010). *The assessment of basic language and learning skills, revised.* P Behavior Analysts, Inc.

Pendo, E., & Iezzoni, L. I. (2020). The role of law and policy in achieving healthy people's disability and health goals around access to health care, activities promoting health and wellness, independent living and participation, and collecting data in the United States. Department of Health and Human Services, Office of Disease Prevention and Health Promotion. https://www.healthypeople.gov/sites/default/files/LHP_Disability-Health-Policy_2020.03.12_508_0.pdf

Powrie, B., Kolehmainen, N., Turpin, M., Ziviani, J., & Copley, J. (2015). *Developmental Medicine & Child Neurology, 57*, 993-1010.

Reedman, S. E., Boyd, R. N., Trost, S. G., Elliott, C., & Sakzewski, L. (2019). Efficacy of participation-focused therapy on performance of physical activity participation goals and habitual physical activity in children with cerebral palsy: A randomized controlled trial. *Archives of Physical Medicine and Rehabilitation, 100*, 676-686. https://doi.org/10.1016/j.apmr.2018.11.012

Reeves, S., Fletcher, S., Barr, H., et al. (2016). A BEME systematic review of the effects of interprofessional education: BEME Guide No. 39. *Medical Teacher, 38*(7), 656-668.

Richards, K. A. R., Eberline, A. D., Padaruth, S., & Templin, T. J. (2015). Experiential learning through a physical activity program for children with disabilities. *Journal of Teaching in Physical Education, 34*, 165-188. https://doi.org/10.1123/jtpe.2014-0015

Rimmer, J. H., Padalabalanarayanan, S., Malone, L. A., & Mehta, T. (2016). Fitness facilities still lack accessibility for people with disabilities. *Disability and Health Journal, 10*, 214-221. https://doi.org/10.1016/j.dhjo.2016.12.011

Rosenbaum, P., & Gorter, J. W. (2011). The 'F-words' in childhood disability: I swear this is how we should think! *Child: Care, Health and Development, 38*(4), 457-463.

Russell, D. J., Rosenbaum, P., Wright, M., & Avery, L. M. (2002). *Gross motor function measure (GMFM-66 & GMFM-88) users manual.* Mac Keith Press.

Ryan, A., & Deci, A. (2000). Self-determination theory and the facilitation of intrinsic motivation, social development and well-being. *American Psychologist, 55*(1), 68-78.

Sale, A., Berardi, N., & Maffei, L. (2014). Environment and brain plasticity: Towards an endogenous pharmacotherapy. *Physiological Reviews, 94*(1), 189-234.

Schmidt, A. K., van Gorp, M., van Wely, L., Ketelaar, M., Hilberink, S. R., Roebroeck, M. E., Tan, S. S., van Meeteren, J., van der Slot, W., Stam, H., Dallmeijer, A. J., de Groot, V., Voorman, J. M., Smits, D. W., Wintels, S. C., Reinders-Messelink, H. A., Gorter, J. W., & Verheijden, J. (2020). Autonomy in participation in cerebral palsy from childhood to adulthood. *Developmental Medicine and Child Neurology, 62*(3), 363-371. https://doi.org/10.1111/dmcn.14366

Sheridan, M. D. (2011). *Play in early childhood* (3rd ed.). Revised and updated by Howard, J. & Alderson, D. Routledge.

Silverman, F. & Carr Tyszka, A. (2017). Centennial topics—supporting participation for children with sensory processing needs and their families: Community-based action research. *American Journal of Occupational Therapy, 71*(4), 7104100010. https://doi.org/10.5014/ajot.2017.025544

United Nations. (2008, May 3). United Nations Convention on the Rights of Persons with Disabilities. https://www.un.org/disabilities/documents/convention/convoptprot-e.pdf

Varni, J. W., Seid, M., & Rode, C. A. (1999). The PedsQL™: measurement model for the pediatric quality of life inventory. *Medical Care*, 126-139.

Willis, C., Nyquist, A., Jahnsen, R., Elliott, C., & Ullenhag, A. (2018a). Enabling physical activity participation for children and youth with disabilities following a goal-directed, family-centered intervention. *Research in Developmental Disabilities, 77*, 30-39. https://doi.org/10.1016/j.ridd.2018.03.010

Willis, C. E., Reid, S., Elliott, C., Rosenberg, M., Nyquist, A., Jahnsen, R., & Girdler, S. (2018b). A realist evaluation of a physical activity participation intervention for children and youth with disabilities: What works, for whom, in what circumstances, and how? *BMC Pediatrics, 18*(1), 1-15.

Willis, C., Girdler, S., Thompson, M., Rosenberg, M., Reid, S., & Elliott, C. (2017). Elements contributing to meaningful participation for children and youth with disabilities: A scoping review. *Disability and Rehabilitation, 39*(17), 1771-1784.

World Health Organization. (2007). International classification of functioning, disability, and health: children and youth version. WHO Press. https://apps.who.int/iris/bitstream/handle/10665/43737/9789241547321_eng.pdf?sequence=1&isAllowed=y

World Health Organization (WHO). (2010a). Recreation, leisure and sports. In Khasnabis, C., Heinicke Motsch, K., Achu K., et al. *Community-based rehabilitation: CBR guidelines*. WHO Press. https://www.ncbi.nlm.nih.gov/books/NBK310922/

World Health Organization; Hopkins D. (2010b). Framework for Action on Interprofessional Education & Collaborative Practice. Health Professions Network Nursing and Midwifery Office within the Department of Human Resources for Health. WHO Press. https://apps.who.int/iris/bitstream/handle/10665/70185/WHO_HRH_HPN_10.3_eng.pdf

World Health Organization. Noncommunicable Diseases and Mental Health Cluster. (2002). Innovative care for chronic conditions: building blocks for actions: Global report. World Health Organization. https://apps.who.int/iris/handle/10665/42500

CHAPTER 11

Promoting Occupational Health and Productivity

Adults

Deirdre Daley, PT, DPT, MSHPE and Ann Marie Dale, PhD, OTR/L

Learning Objectives

At the end of this chapter, the reader will:

1. Articulate the unique and collaborative contributions of common stakeholders in occupational health promotion and protection (ACOTE B.4.25, B.4.26; CAPTE 7D7, 7D16, 7D28, 7D34, 7D35, 7D39)
2. Understand the impact of integrated health and safety systems in workplace to promote worker health, well-being, and productivity (ACOTE B.4.18, B.4.19, B.4.20, B.4.23; CAPTE 7C, 7D6, 7D12, 7D36, 7D37)
3. Discuss a systematic approach to performing an occupational health needs assessment, planning and intervention by an interprofessional team (ACOTE B.4.27, B.5.1; CAPTE 7A, 7D1, 7D12, 7D17, 7D19, 7D20, 7D23, 7D29)
4. Describe the unique opportunities and competencies relevant for practice in the occupational environment (ACOTE B.3.2, B.3.4, B.4.1, B.4.3, B.4.4, B.4.5, B.4.10; CAPTE 7B, 7D8, 7D10, 7D16, 7D19h, 7D20, 7D26, 7D27, 7D31, 7D32, 7D33, 7D34, 7D35, 7D41, 7D43)

The ACOTE Standards used are those from 2018.

Key Words

Absenteeism, Accommodation, Americans with Disabilities Act, Ergonomic/Safety Team, Ergonomics, Health and Safety Professionals, Hierarchy of Controls, Job Analysis, Occupational Health, OSHA First Aid, Presenteeism, Primary, Secondary, Tertiary Prevention, Total Worker Health, Transitional or Modified Work, Workers' Compensation

Pizzi, M. A., & Amir, M. (Eds.). *Interprofessional Perspectives for Community Practice: Promoting Health, Well-Being, and Quality of Life* (pp. 195-215).

Introduction

As of April 2021, 125 million adults between the ages of 18 to 65 years were employed full-time in the United States. These adults engage in earning a living wage, as well as gaining personal gratification from active participation in work (Statista, 2021). While workplaces may vary in form and function, the defined nature and structure of each workplace presents a unique opportunity to influence health and well-being at the organization and larger social community level. The significant portion of daily hours spent at work provides an opportunity for employers and medical providers to proactively address occupational and personal health issues.

Individuals who engage in the worker role can include those who are able bodied or disabled, those who are involved in paid or unpaid work (volunteers) and those who engage in seasonal, temporary, part-time, or full-time employment. Workers with physical, psychosocial, mental, or cognitive disabilities are not excluded from work and many laws protect employees from discrimination to allow individuals equal access to all the benefits and privileges of employment, similar to individuals without disabilities (U.S. Equal Employment Opportunity Commission, 2008).

This chapter will introduce the reader to the dynamic interface between work, the worker role, health, productivity and well-being, as well as how the interprofessional health team can positively influence health and productivity outcomes.

Occupational Health and Productivity

Work is an important part of our everyday life. **Occupational health** traditionally refers to the health of the workforce and work-related exposures that can have negative and positive impact on worker health. It can also mean the level of productive activity in one's daily life, which can include being productive as a worker. The work role in an adult's life is an important role that contributes to one's health and well-being. The role of worker also provides economic stability for oneself and/or one's family. Workers derive physical and mental health benefits through economic, social, and physical engagement at work (Waddell & Burton, 2006). Workers in poor health are unable to function to the best of their ability. The World Health Organization (WHO) linked health status as a predictor of economic growth (WHO, 1999), and therefore a company's productivity is similarly dependent on the health of their workforce.

Individuals function most efficiently and effectively when their body is in its healthiest state. Acute as well as chronic disease often create reduced functional capability, and this may impact work and personal productivity. Worker health is also influenced by the social, psychological, and cultural aspects of the workplace. Companies that address health and safety risks through policies, programs, and practices, as well as provide health-promoting wellness programs and services can build a workplace culture focused on health and well-being. There are significant benefits of integrating health, safety, and wellness to produce positive outcomes for workers, businesses, and communities.

The workplace provides an ideal environment to foster health, deliver health information, improve access to health services, and availability of programs to promote healthy living. Research continues to support an interplay between work, health, and productivity. Delivery of health services at the workplace can improve access for workers and promote better health and wellness during work and at the home-work interface (Chari et al., 2018; Colombo et al., 2018; Garcia-Gomez et al., 2008; Hamar et al., 2015; Harvard University T.H. Chan School of Public Health, 2016; Health Productivity and Performance Study Committee, 2015; Horst et al., 2014; Isham et al., 2020; Pelkowski & Berger, 2004; Rodriguez-Alvarez & Rodriguez-Gutierrez, 2018; Schaller & Stevens, 2015). The large number of hours spent at work make the workplace a good environment to promote healthy behaviors to help support overall wellness. Interprofessional engagement and therapeutic interactions with workers can help workers achieve a healthy lifestyle to enjoy a state of health and well-being.

Benefits and Risks of Work

Work promotes many positive aspects of health by providing financial compensation, a sense of accomplishment, pride, meaning, socialization, and in many cases, access to health insurance and pensions (Waddell & Burton, 2006). Yet work may also expose workers to potentially health-harming physical or psychosocial stressors (Burgard & Lin, 2013). Physical hazards in work tasks may cause chronic musculoskeletal disorders (Marras, 2006). Psychosocial stressors of work such as job strain, effort-reward imbalance, job insecurity, and low support may contribute to poor mental health (Stansfeld & Candy, 2006). Work organization of demanding schedules and inefficient work processes may add to work stress. The rise in nonstandard work hours and shift to a 24/7 economy has been linked to sleep disorders and physical health problems such as coronary artery disease and peptic ulcers (Lin et al., 2019; Presser, 2005). Technological advancements, outsourcing, and globalization have contributed to the decline of traditional work, job insecurity, and poor mental health (Landsbergis et al., 2014). Economic events such as the recession of 2008 and furlough and job loss during the COVID-19 pandemic have created profound financial strain on workers and their families (Hertz-Palmor et al., 2021).

Prevailing chronic disease trends and economic pressures present significant challenges for employers and employees, yet most employers provide limited programs and health promotions for their workforce (Kirsten, 2010). This inactivity may be due to lack of awareness of work-related health issues, or lack of knowledge of how and what to change to promote worker health. There are many aspects of work that may contribute to poor worker health and health disparities. Changes in employment conditions have disproportionately affected workers in lower socioeconomic or social class positions including racial and ethnic minorities and immigrants (Landsbergis et al., 2014).

The *International Classification of Functioning, Disability and Health* (ICF) is a classification system that considers the health and function of individuals in multiple domains and environments (WHO, 2001), including the work environment. The ICF model considers the health conditions, activities, and capacity of an individual, including work participation. The workplace can have a positive impact on worker's physical and mental health through ergonomic programs, supportive work environments, and return to work or stay at work policies following illness or injury. Alternatively, stressful work conditions or exposures to physically forceful work, demanding supervisors and aggressive schedules, and coworker bullying may present barriers to health, negatively impacting work and productivity.

The Interprofessional Team in the Workplace

Many health and non-health professionals can be involved in various aspects of occupational health services in the workplace. Occupational health professionals differ by training, scope of work, and roles. An example of an interprofessional team focused on providing health and safety in the workplace may include human resource professionals that consider job placement and work compatibility; operations and safety professionals that address work flow, productivity, and work hazards; occupational health nurses that focus on injury response, health and hazard detection; and physical and occupational therapists that focus on human performance in the context of prevention and minimizing work disability. Each professional's role can have a direct or indirect effect on worker health.

Other on-site medical team members may include part-time, full-time, or contracted health professionals or providers such as nurses, medical doctors or physician assistants, exercise physiologists, athletic trainers, wellness coaches, and other specialty providers (i.e., nutritionists, occupational psychologists). Nonmedical workplace professionals that may be involved in health and safety include environment specialists, industrial hygienists, and human factors engineers, training and development personnel, and union representatives.

Workplace **health and safety professionals** (or **health and safety team**) bring significant experience in the areas of safety, training, regulation and standards, operational processes, and group dynamics. They are valuable partners to a collaborative interprofessional team that drives successful implementation of health and safety programs. Each team member brings their individual expertise, personal strengths, work experience, unique training, and background that allows them to provide key insights into operations and practical ideas for change. Supervisors and management are key stakeholders regarding operations, resource allocation and coordination of productivity, and process considerations in their respective areas of responsibility. Engineers and industrial hygienists provide insights into planning, workplace equipment, and the work environment. Human resource personnel have expertise in regulatory, benefits, and sustainability of the workforce (human) resources. Individual team members generally do not have expertise in all areas of occupational health. Developing a collaborative working relationship allows for contributions from each team member and helps create positive worker health outcomes (Interprofessional Education Collaborative, 2016).

Over the past decade, there has been a significant shift in understanding the benefits and need for population health. Changes in health care education competencies, health delivery, and collaboration between medical providers and other fields are part of the framework for realizing those outcomes (Association of Schools & Programs of Public Health, 2015; Berwick et al., 2008; Fox & McCorkle, 2018; Interprofessional Education Collaborative, 2016). Developing community partnerships, such as those between health and business professionals, are an important part of improving health outcomes through interprofessional practice. Key elements of interprofessional practice include shared values and ethics, mutual role understanding and integration, communication, and teamwork (Interprofessional Education Collaborative, 2016).

The Role of Prevention in Health and Safety

Optimal health is obtained and maintained through prevention. Prevention is a collection of activities or interventions intended to eliminate or reduce risks associated with the development of disease (Centers for Disease Control and Prevention [CDC], 2013). There are three phases of the "Levels of Prevention" shown in Figure 11-1. **Primary prevention** aims to prevent disease or injury before disease develops. **Secondary prevention** aims to detect disease in its earliest form at the time of mild symptoms and prevents disease progression or complications of health conditions. **Tertiary prevention** aims to reduce the effects of disease on the functional performance of the person (CDC, 2013). Related to one's occupational/productive health status and worker role, primary prevention may include increasing resilience and altering unhealthy behaviors by improving knowledge of healthy behaviors through workshops

Before Evidence of Disease or Injury	Disease Onset / Clinical Diagnosis	Established Disease/Problem
Primary Prevention	**Secondary Prevention**	**Tertiary Prevention**
Injury prevention, health promotion, avoid injury reduce or modify risk/s	Early detection and treatment, prevent progression	Supportive and rehabilitative services to minimize morbidity and maximize quality of life
Organizational and Department Level	Department and Worker Level - People at early stage of disease	Worker Level - People with symptomatic or advanced disease

Figure 11-1. Levels of prevention strategies. (Adapted from Centers for Disease Control and Prevention. [2013]. *NCD prevention and control.* U.S. Department of Health and Human Services. https://www.cdc.gov/globalhealth/healthprotection/fetp/training_modules/3/Prevention-and-Control_FG_Final_09262013v2.pdf)

on-site (e.g., proper diet, exercise routines, avoid smoking). Secondary prevention may include symptom management and identifying hazards at work and changing work methods. Tertiary prevention may include activities that help people manage complex health conditions such as chronic diseases like diabetes or rheumatoid arthritis.

Historically, workplace wellness programs reflected on-site health and safety teams targeting primary prevention and basic health surveillance that may have involved nursing and other medical professionals. More modern models of care involve safety and health professionals across the spectrum of care—with medical professionals contributing to safety's understanding of human performance and behavior, and safety personnel contributing to post-injury return to work plans. When workers interface with an interprofessional team, the health, well-being, and quality of life of the workforce is enhanced.

Therapists as Part of Work Communities

As a member of the interprofessional team, therapists have unique training in function, psychosocial interactions, and human-environment interface that empowers them with knowledge to enhance the optimal recovery of individuals with injury or illness. Therapists are valuable members of a medical team that may help efforts go beyond reactive (post-injury care) to address risks and population health in an effort to prevent injury or minimize disability and ill health costs. The routine presence of physical and occupational therapists in a workplace gives the therapists an opportunity to develop a deep understanding of the interactions between workers and their work activities as well as the organizational, cultural, and environmental factors that can act as barriers and facilitators to improving the worker-environment setting. Therapists can use their understanding of workers, job demands, and health risks to guide prevention and maximize human performance in a work setting.

Therapists offer value along the full continuum of employment from "hire to retire" and can meet the needs of all individuals, regardless of their personal, physical, or mental limitations. During the application and new hire phases of employment, therapy services may include post-offer employment testing and new hire conditioning (i.e., helping ensure workers can meet the physical demands of a job). During the active work phase, services may include **job analysis** (describing the functions, tasks, and/or demands of the job), ergonomics, pre-shift warm up or exercise, education, health fairs, health consultation and coaching, and other prevention services. When a worker experiences a work-limiting injury or illness, therapy services may include triage, first aid, job coaching, clinical intervention, performance assessment, job matching, return to work recommendations, problem-solving communication, and/or care coordination. Situations of limited work participation may be mitigated by a therapist consultation regarding temporary work modifications or permanent job accommodations.

Many rehabilitation providers' first exposure to the field of occupational health and prevention occurs when they treat a worker who was injured at work as a patient in an outpatient setting and who is unable to perform their usual work activities. Some therapists interact with a company by making a single visit to the worksite to conduct an **ergonomic evaluation** for an injured worker to improve return to work transition by optimizing the interface between a worker and their work, or to collect critical job demand information for creation of a company job specific functional testing. However, therapists who are contracted and physically located on site can become more integrated into the operations of the company and provide a greater number of services to the company and their workers.

Work Injury: Secondary Prevention Level

This section will focus on the individual worker as a component of a work community and the interaction of the interprofessional team in that context. The following case presents a common type of work injury that results in relatively minor work restrictions where the worker is likely to return to full duty in about 2 weeks.

Case Study: Matt—Part 1

Matt Freeman is a 42-year-old machine operator who has been employed in a box manufacturing plant for 15 years. His job involves loading box materials into the machine and monitoring or maintaining machine operation.

Over the past week, Matt started to experience right shoulder pain while working on the box machine. The machine had jammed several times just prior to ending the last shift of his work week. Matt had to forcefully push and pull the stock by hand to release the jam, reset the machine, and then restock the machine. Matt felt he had sprained his shoulder. He thought it would resolve over the weekend, but he continued to have difficulty lifting objects above shoulder level and moving heavy objects when he returned to work. Matt spoke to his supervisor about his problem since he felt he could not keep up with expected production on the box machine when he returned to work after the weekend.

Recently, the production department combined several jobs from different assembly lines within the department under the job title of machine operator.

Matt lives and works in an economically depressed, rural area. He is part of a group of workers who share a commuting van, traveling 45 minutes to work. Things are stressful at home and money is tight. His daughter and son-in-law recently moved in with Matt and his wife, and his daughter announced there was a new baby on the way. He is worried his injury may not allow him to continue to do his job. He had a shoulder injury about 7 years ago and missed work, which strained the family financially.

Interprofessional Team

Human resources, supervisor, nurse, physical or occupational therapist, safety manager, engineer, ergonomist, physician, counselor.

Health Assessment

This case is classified at the secondary level of prevention. After Matt told his supervisor about his painful shoulder, his supervisor contacted human resources to complete the initial injury reporting and to have an assessment of his condition by a nurse, physical therapist, or occupational therapist. If the medical providers were not on site, Matt may have been seen by an on-site first aid team who may have recommended sending him to a local urgent care or medical facility.

In this case, the occupational health nurse collects work history and medical information, performs an examination, obtains injury-related data reports, and refers Matt to an on-site therapist for an evaluation and intervention. The role of the therapist in work-focused health care involves addressing the worker and work tasks during the examination, and establishing the prognosis, goal development, and interventions. The examination should include information about the interplay between the worker, work tasks, and work life; assess for pain and disability in the course of work; worker beliefs about work and prognosis; and the types of supports that are available (Hutting et al., 2020).

The physical exam may initially involve obtaining self-reported health measures, examination of body functions and structures, functional activity tolerance, and assessment of performance capabilities. His presentation of shoulder pain and strength deficits with resisted overhead movements may be determined to have minimal physical limitations. Screening for biopsychosocial risks may be critical to understand Matt's behaviors and beliefs about his injury. Factors such as fear avoidance, catastrophizing, and perceived lack of work support are important to assess as these issues may interfere with treatment progression and Matt's state of mental well-being. Identifying potential risks for delayed return to work can help the on-site therapist target appropriate interventions in the plan of care (Burton, 2015).

Job Assessment

During the job assessment, Matt reports that his physical problems are from pushing and pulling stock to unjam the box machine and that these jams have occurred more than usual in the past few weeks despite putting in several maintenance calls. By conducting an assessment of Matt's health condition, presentation, and the physical demands of his regular job as well as the other jobs on the line, the therapist has the necessary information to make the most appropriate recommendations.

It will be important to compare Matt's capabilities to the specific demands of his job and provide the most relevant education and return to work recommendations. To help determine the best options to support Matt's work participation, the therapist may consider whether Matt could perform the physical demands of another job position in his work area. The therapist or safety manager would coordinate with a supervisor and workers who perform the job to gather information and assess the physical demands (postural assessment, loads, forces, repetition of movements and duration of tasks) of the other machine operator positions on the line as well as the layout of equipment and materials. Safety personnel, an industrial hygienist, and training and development personnel may also assist in studying the work area.

Job match tables, with elements similar to that found in Table 11-1, can be reviewed to identify which jobs Matt can perform and/or how they can be modified. The health and safety team may be able to identify tasks that can be modified temporarily to allow Matt to continue to function in his usual work area. Ideally, members from medical, safety, and the supervisor work together as a team to develop a plan to help the worker, their peers, and other stakeholders integrate changes to the workplace in a manner that respects worker privacy and team cohesion while minimizing the creation of risk for other workers.

Encouraging Matt to perform work tasks within his abilities, while limiting overhead activities, can help keep him engaged at work, continue his commuting plan and social interactions, and allow for continued productive work while he regains his strength. Matt's situation of working on a production line with many different positions under a single job title (and being cross-trained) provides the opportunity to discuss options with the supervisor and safety team of having Matt temporarily assigned to alternative jobs with machines that do not require strenuous shoulder use.

The therapist may conduct a worksite ergonomics assessment and ask for input from both Matt and from safety and engineering on the recent problem with the machine operation. Ideally, the box machine is regularly maintained as part of an engineering ergonomic control to eliminate the cause of stock jams, but getting the machine serviced by maintenance may take some time. An administrative ergonomic control may be a short-term solution, such as rotating the workers between the problem machine and other positions to reduce the overall physical risk level of all workers. (See A Deeper Look Box).

Since Matt had no lost time from work, his case may be considered first aid only. Workers like Matt with transient, mild symptoms may benefit from learning self-management interventions such as thermal care (heat or ice) and education about self-care, pain education, activity management, and body mechanics as well as information and problem-solving skills on how to address potential flare ups (Hutting et al., 2019; Industrial Insurance Medical Advisory Committee & Industrial Insurance Chiropractic Advisory Committee, 2019; Linton et al., 2016; Occupational Safety and Health Administration, n.d.b). If more formal medical evaluation and specific clinical manual therapy or exercise treatment was indicated, the situation or claim may have needed more than first aid, and therefore would need to be reported to the company's workers' compensation insurer (and logged as an OSHA recordable).

First aid assessment may occur at the workers' workstation or in a clinical setting depending on the worker presentation and need. Some clinicians practice in a shared space with nursing or first aid with access to a private exam room, others may be integrated into a worksite health center that has a full suite of equipment and/or includes a space that also serves as a fitness center. In Matt's case education, self-management, and thermal modalities generally don't require significant space. Clinical spaces in the workplace vary in size and scope, similar to other outpatient facilities, with the biggest difference often being access for workers in their work environment.

Safety Risk Assessment

While regulatory guidance and administrative requirements provide a framework for medical care after a work-related injury, safety and risk management analyses are also important to consider as potentially contributing factors to the injury (North Carolina State University, n.d.; Occupational Safety and Health Administration, n.d.a). In the earlier example, the box machine had repeated mechanical problems resulting in stock jams. Employers generally employ preventive maintenance by the engineering department to ensure operational continuity, as well as a report process for poor performing equipment or equipment failures such as stock jams. When machines do not function properly or have repeated mechanical breakdowns, an investigation or safety review can help identify problems.

While Matt's recent shoulder discomfort may be associated with mechanical failure of the equipment, the safety team may interview Matt and consider the reason for the jams. The safety team in this case may check to see if the machine set up was problematic, the quality of the material was out of standard thus leading to more jams than usual, or if the appropriate processes were followed and if the operator was

Table 11-1

Job-Specific Functional Testing and Gap Analysis Based on Job Descriptions

PHYSICAL DEMAND	SUMMARY WORK DEMANDS	SUMMARY PHYSICAL PERFORMANCE	JOB MATCH	RECOMMENDATIONS
Lifting	10 to 45 lbs. (O) 18 to 60 in.	25 lbs. maximum to 60 in. 45 lbs. to 48 in.	No	Limit set up tasks above shoulder or rotate to another positions during machine/product changeovers (able to meet demands of print setup)
Carrying	10 to 45 lbs. (S) 18 to 72 in.	20 lbs. to 72 in. 45 lbs. to 48 in.	No	Break up loads to 20# if start or end height of a carry exceeds a height of 48 in.
Push/Pull	10 to 50 lbs. (O)	55 lbs.	Yes	Regular job demands only, not upset conditions of jams requiring maintenance
Reaching	18 to 66 in. (O)	Able	Yes	Gradually return to operation and QA starting with 3 to 4 hours per day and increasing 2 hours per week depending on response

Physical demand frequency categories: (C) continuously - more than 2/3 of the shift, (F) frequently - 1/3 to 2/3 of shift. (O) occasionally - up to 1/3 of shift; (S) seldom 1% to 2% of the shift.
Data source: U.S. Bureau of Labor Statistics. (2021). *Occupational requirements survey: Handbook of methods.* United States Department of Labor. https://www.bls.gov/opub/hom/ors/pdf/ors.pdf

A Deeper Look: Human Factors Engineering and Ergonomics

Human factors and ergonomics is an area of study that designs tools, equipment and activities based on the psychological and physiological capabilities of the human. Ergonomics in the workplace may include physical and cognitive solutions applied to an individual or group of workers (Human Factors and Ergonomics Society, n.d.; World Health Organization, 2016).

There are many professionals that work in the field of ergonomics including Human Factors engineers (for tool, equipment, and systems design), cognitive engineers (to monitor mental processes, memory, reasoning, and motor reactions), industrial engineers (to study system designs of tasks in an organization), and psychologists (to study the social connectedness of individuals and culture of the organization).

Ergonomic designs focus on users with normal capabilities. Most ergonomists with engineering backgrounds have little or no training in anatomy, kinesiology, or disease to understand how health conditions may impact normal body function and recovery. Ergonomists view problems at a macro or systems level to be solved for a population or group of people rather than an individual. Physical and occupational therapists focus on micro-level problems for an individual worker and sometimes a work group or department. Therapists may use similar methods of assessment to ergonomists including task analysis, modifications to design, and intervention development. Therapists can also provide assessments on individuals with health concerns, assess activity limitations and make recommendations on possible modifications, and communicate with the team on the expected course of recovery.

One important ergonomics tool is the Hierarchy of Controls (HOC) that prioritizes controls based on providing the greatest benefit to the workers (Centers for Disease Control and Prevention, 2018). The most effective control is "elimination" that describes a change in the process, so the task is no longer performed. "Substitution" replaces the task with a solution such as automating the process. "Engineering" is a mid-level modification to the process or machine, so the workers have limited or no exposure to the hazard. "Administrative controls" change the way people work to reduce the risk such as rotating workers, training workers on better methods, or providing ergonomically designed tools. The least effective control is to use "personal protective equipment" that places a barrier between the hazard and the worker.

familiar with the usual operational procedure. Identifying operational problems that contribute to the worker's physical discomfort can help prevent another worker from experiencing a similar problem, while also improving the machine performance and operational productivity.

Intervention

Matt's case will require only temporary accommodations as his symptoms will likely resolve in a short period of time. Ergonomic work modifications such as decreased loads, changing work heights, providing mechanical assists, and carts or transfer equipment to move loads may make it possible for workers like Matt to return to work more quickly. Temporary job modification will allow Matt to continue work participation and productivity while improving his job satisfaction and well-being with minimal life interruptions.

From a safety assessment or a worksite ergonomic evaluation, the box stock jamming and need to push/pull the stock from the machine would be identified as the likely cause of Matt's shoulder discomfort. One recommendation may seek to engage with facility engineers and the maintenance department to produce a long-term solution.

If the department did not have workers cross-trained and regularly rotate to different positions on the line, then Matt would be the only worker trained to work the box machine job which would be considered an essential task of his machine operator job. However, Matt's job title of "machine operator" is the same job title as other positions on the production line so a temporary reassignment is possible and, in most cases, psychologically and economically beneficial.

Part of the therapist's role is to educate Matt about the expected rate of healing, so he has a realistic understanding about his recovery time. It may be necessary to explore options to help Matt manage his personal stress as this may manifest in attitudes, beliefs, and/or behaviors that may contribute to delayed recovery or return to usual activities. Matt's concern over his family's finances, and concern about the temporary change in work activities of coworkers within his work group may contribute to mental stress. The therapist may use a psychologically informed practice approach and provide information on stress reduction activities as part of Matt's care plan. The therapist may seek acceptance and support from the work group and from Matt's supervisor for the work change. Helping Matt find meaning and a sense of accomplishment in his work and to seek assistance for stress may be part of his treatment plan depending on his response to care. If Matt needs more support, the nurse and therapist could discuss referral to a counselor, social services, or psychologist with the referring provider or Matt's general medicine doctor and appropriate patient consent as discussed later in this chapter.

Workers' Compensation: Injury Requiring Care Beyond First Aid (Secondary Prevention Level)

Case Study: Matt—Part 2

The case study would be somewhat different if Matt presented with a longstanding shoulder impingement or tendonitis problem that went beyond first aid as a recordable injury that was covered under Workers' Compensation insurance.

Interprofessional Team

Human resources, supervisor, nurse, physician, physical or occupational therapist, workers compensation case manager, safety manager, engineer, ergonomist, counselor.

Assessment

A more detailed evaluation may be needed to assess the extent, acuity, and severity of his presentation, the work and home activity limitations, participation restrictions, and/or health or social complications. Findings from the assessment would determine treatment and the extent of work modifications that may be needed. More restrictive work duties should be discussed with the medical team and appropriate workplace stakeholders such as the supervisor, and the health and safety manager.

Functional testing based on the impacted area, which in Matt's case is the shoulder and upper extremity, and the activities of the job tasks (i.e., push/pull, lift, carry, reaching) can provide valuable information for progress notes and return to work recommendations in an efficient way. Comparing the worker's ability to the job demands allows therapists to share information on performance gaps as well as condition-specific information, and functional and environmental barriers and facilitators to aid decision-making by other medical providers such as occupational nurses, physicians, case managers, or adjusters.

Intervention

Condition-specific strengthening, job coaching, problem-solving and psychologically informed practice may be the indicated treatments, along with condition-specific exercise, manual therapy, and thermal modalities consistent with evidenced-based clinical practice guidelines (American Physical Therapy Association, n.d.). The therapist may recommend using work activity as graded exercise or conditioning depending on the nature and severity of the injury.

Delays in return to work or repeated work absences can have a negative impact on work engagement and productivity. Communication and care coordination require a team effort from medical, insurance, supervisor, safety, and human resources to minimize unnecessary time away from work. Post-injury return to work is optimized when the medical providers understand the job demands and provide guidance on work abilities, and employers provide return to work policies and foster transitional or modified work that adapts work tasks to allow workers to remain engaged in work with the goal of progressing to a prior or higher level of functional performance. Engaging workers in planning and formulating goals related to work participation and return to work helps foster a therapeutic alliance, development of problem-solving abilities, and strengthening of self-management strategies (Shaw et al., 2011).

There can be high human and monetary costs from delayed return to work, extensive medical care, or surgery. Sustaining health and promoting injury prevention can have cost saving impact on the corporate bottom line as discussed at the end of this chapter. Surveillance and prevention activities that help avoid problems or foster early interventions to avoid costly problems, disability and suffering associated with work injury is discussed in further detail later in this chapter.

Personal Health Condition: Working With a Chronic Disease (Tertiary Prevention Level)

Onsite clinical care can also involve tertiary prevention, with a goal of helping workers manage the impact of individual chronic conditions so they may remain engaged in work for the economic, social, and personal benefits of work.

Case Study: Matt—Part 3

In this case, we assume that Matt sought onsite health services for his personal health condition after learning about onsite health services while attending a company health fair, or after seeing an educational notice on the bottom of a cafeteria television monitor that plays during lunch time. Matt presents to the health clinic with a 5-year history of diabetes, hoping to obtain help from the medical staff on how to become more active, eat better, and feel better. This case study presents a worker with an existing medical condition that is not considered work-related; however, the condition may impact the worker's ability to stay at work.

Matt notes he is worried about his declining health, lack of exercise, and says he knows he isn't eating right. He is experiencing early symptoms of foot neuropathy and worries that he will have to retire early or be limited playing with his grandchild if he doesn't change his lifestyle. He feels more tired after work and struggles with motivation to exercise.

Interprofessional Team

Nurse, physical or occupational therapist, nutritionist, physician, behavioral health practitioner, safety manager, engineer, ergonomist, counselor (perhaps an endocrinologist and/or pharmacist).

Assessment

The occupational health nurse reviewed Matt's medical history, general health goals, and medication record and offered to do a health risk assessment with him. She also asked Matt if he received routine physician exams and has had nutritional education for his diabetic condition. Interprofessional care goals may focus on improving self-management, function, vitality, and well-being. The nurse reviewed some options for care; she offered to help Matt with monitoring his food diary and to set up nutritional education through the onsite medical team or through a virtual consultation with a nutritionist in the community. The nurse recommended Matt receive a general wellness evaluation from the onsite physical or occupational therapist. Connecting Matt to the workplace and community services allows him to have more intervention options and support to help meet his needs.

The therapist conducted a body systems review, an assessment of readiness for change, and a biopsychosocial screening. The use of motivational interviewing or psychologically informed practice may help guide Matt's goal setting and explore his understanding for management of his medical condition, nutrition, and exercise in addition to his potential fears and barriers to participation in a health program. The interview may extend to exploring his work, social, and family goals, what he has tried in the past, and whether he felt he succeeded or not in his prior self-management.

Intervention

Health service interventions for Matt may involve elements of education, supported problem solving, and behavioral change. Specific services may include having the occupational nurse help Matt review his glucose monitoring and activity log and working with the therapist to explore options for a diabetes appropriate progressive exercise program that he may find enjoyable. The onsite medical team may offer social support initially until Matt finds ways to build supports through other means in his lifestyle. This may include using a social services referral depending on his level of need and success with his program.

Matt's case is a good example of how workers (or patients) want to receive lifestyle advice to help meet their health needs. Interventions designed to improve physical activity through work may include: 1) providing information and using self-motivating approaches to improve knowledge, skills and attitudes; 2) providing supportive resources; 3) reinforcing desired behavior via social and reward mechanisms to establish new norms; 4) using policy or administrative actions to support change; or 5) making environmental changes in the workplace (Jirathananuwat & Pongpirul, 2017). Depending upon how comfortable Matt feels with the interprofessional and onsite care team, services may go beyond short-term education and extend into workplace modifications should his health decline.

If Matt finds he is beginning to experience functional limitations at work, he may agree to having a functional test by a physical therapist (workers not under workers compensation or medical care may not be required to take a medical test unless there is cause to suspect threat or it is required due to business necessity; The U.S. Equal Employment Opportunity Commission, n.d.). The information may foster collaborative discussions and problem-solving with his physician, the company nurse, his supervisor, or human resources on ideas for work modifications. Translating physical abilities and limitations into functional language may allow supervisors, workers, the medical team, and human resources to explore options for sustained work participation. Communication and care coordination brings together team members to leverage their knowledge and to find options for work modification to benefit the worker and the workplace.

Case Study Questions

The earlier case introduces Matt and the manufacturing department. Although the case is presented in the context of a manufacturing environment, the process to identifying problems and solutions may apply to any environment and industry (Professional Reasoning Box A). Consider the following questions:

1. What are Matt's needs?
2. What interprofessional team would you consider coordinating with and why?
3. How do health services/occupational systems integrate for the best outcome?
4. What prevention or intervention strategies would you use in this case?

Group Level: Prevention Program (Primary Prevention Level)

Physical or mental health issues can occur when individuals engage productively in the worker role, but there are times when several workers in one area experience physical or mental health issues. Several workers with the same job title may experience similar injuries or have similar complaints of discomfort or pain. These complaints may directly relate to recent work activities, a change in work processes, or mandatory overtime. There may be many workers in an area with similar demographics such as advancing age or obesity and also struggle with chronic health conditions. Conducting a group wide assessment provides an opportunity to explore the health needs of a larger number of workers and implement interventions (CDC, 2015a, 2016).

Health, health care costs, injury incidence, and injury risk may all be positively impacted through primary prevention programs directed at employees and their families. Programs may be targeted at the group and department level or the organizational level. Workplace needs and worker priorities vary, so assessment of workplace needs and worker priorities are often used to develop the best intervention strategies to help achieve the largest impact (CDC, 2015a, 2016). Common workplace prevention programs may focus on improving physical and mental health and wellness, reducing risk, early detection, available services and benefits, supportive environmental supports, community programs and partnerships using screening, informational, and/or skill-building approaches. This section will introduce the reader to group- or departmental-level prevention programs and later introduce the role of health professionals in organizational-level prevention programs.

Case Study: Matt—Part 4

With recent changes in the manufacturing department, workers have noted they are working more hours and their health behaviors are impacted. Discussion between the supervisor, safety manager, nurse, and therapist resulted in a goal to look at the health and prevention needs of the department as part of a health and safety initiative. The safety supervisor also notes a previous ergonomics team became idle about 1 year ago.

Professional Reasoning Box A
A Deeper Look: The Americans with Disabilities Act and Amendment

Individuals with permanent disabilities or progressively debilitating chronic conditions may face the possibility they will not be able to return to their prior job without modification.

The goal of the **Americans with Disabilities Act (ADA)** of 1990, and the broadened definition under the Americans with Disabilities Act Amendments Act (ADAAA) of 2008 (U.S. Equal Employment Opportunity Commission, 2008), is to help individuals with disability have the opportunity to participate in work and social activities. Part of the Act requires employers to provide reasonable accommodations for qualified employees who have a disability that may impact job performance. Readers are encouraged to learn more about ADA/ADAAA as part of their professional development; however, a basic overview of the interactive accommodation process (referred to as ADA in the following text) is provided here:

- ADA laws and regulations becomes relevant when a disability impacts a worker's job performance—the disability is often recorded by a physician based on a diagnosis, impairment, or limitation that results in a work disability. If an individual cannot fully participate in work, the worker may seek an accommodation.
- Workers may approach their supervisor using lay person language requesting a work adjustment, or access company policies and procedures to submit a request for accommodation.
- The worker may be asked to disclose the nature of the disability (what tasks are limited or the type of impairment), but the individual is not required to disclose a specific diagnosis. Employers must engage in an interactive process to provide a "reasonable accommodation" that bridges work performance gaps.
- The "interactive process" generally involves the worker and workplace representative working together to determine if the worker can return to work with some type of modification or reassignment. An employee may be asked to suggest the type of accommodation that may help them participate in work.
- Decisions related to accommodations are made between the worker and workplace representative. Therapists may be asked to consult on options, benefits, and estimating the costs of accommodations. Employers are not required to select accommodations that pose undue hardships such as accommodations that would change the nature of the job or are unduly expensive. It is the employer's choice to make decisions if there are multiple viable options available.
- Consider an individual with arthritis who is finding it difficult to stay at work and is beginning to take time off from work due to pain and limited work tolerance. In this situation, ergonomics or work modifications may allow the individual to remain working and avoid the decline in work engagement associated with absence.

Case Study Questions

Until now, the case examples in this chapter have focused on the individual worker; however, when many individuals in an area or department report health problems, the group of workers in the area should be reviewed. The case questions in this scenario are similar to previous questions except these apply to the work group in the department rather than a single worker.

1. What are the needs of the group of workers in Matt's department?
2. What interprofessional team would you consider coordinating with?
3. How do health services/occupational systems integrate for the best outcome?
4. What prevention/intervention strategies would you use in this case?

Health and Prevention for Workers

While prior elements of the case study have given specific examples of problems, this section will present a broader look at some of the common health behavior and health problems that are commonly addressed with prevention programs. Research done in collaboration with groups such as the National Institute for Occupational Safety and Health (NIOSH), the CDC and **Total Worker Health®** has led to the development of a number of health factors that are commonly considered as part of workplace assessment and development of prevention programs (Center for the Promotion of Health in the New England Workplace, 2014; CDC, 2019b; Chari et al., 2018). Based on worker symptoms and complaints of fatigue or less healthy lifestyle behaviors in this case, needs related to musculoskeletal disorders, nutrition/eating habits, physical activity, weight management, tobacco and other substance use, sleep and fatigue, and stress/mental health may be areas to consider as part of investigation and assessment regarding where to focus prevention efforts. The instruments often cover other areas that have been identified to impact occupational health such as policy and benefit availability, health risk screening for cancer and early disease detection, blood pressure and heart disease, diabetes, maternal health and lactation support, work/environmental supports, depression, flu shots and vaccines, financial health, and social/community engagement.

Interprofessional Team

- Human resources, safety, supervisor, human resources, risk manager, training team/coaches, industrial hygienist, physical or occupational therapist, nurse, engineer, workers.

Groups or Organizations as Clients

Most health professionals begin their careers working with individuals or single patients to address wellness goals or assess ill health; however, the health provider can have a broader impact by assessing a group of workers. Creating awareness and engagement on the diverse drivers of health prior to injury is a significant opportunity to educate, impact behavior, and correct misinformation while learning about the impact of life roles and environmental considerations that can be found in community practice. Health providers in the workplace often have a broad understanding of the health care system to help refer workers to appropriate providers in a timely manner. The role of providers in primary prevention in the workplace is often situational and depends on the goals and priorities of the group or organization.

When addressing health promotion and prevention, many workplace teams or groups follow a series of common process improvement steps to solve a problem or implement change. As described in the CDC Workplace Health Model, the steps of a process include 1) assessment, 2) planning and management, 3) implementation, and 4) evaluation (CDC, 2016). The assessment step involves clearly defining the problem or problems. This often requires collecting data to understand the scope and context of the problem, synthesize the data, and summarize the factors related to the problem to share with the team. The next step involves planning for management of the problem. At this step, the team must define the goal, brainstorm interventions, prioritize interventions, decide on the preferred plan, and select the interventions for implementation. Implementation includes the activities and strategies that will be used to deliver the intervention.

The following sections provide an overview of the way that organizations can identify and respond to the specific health and safety needs of a group level in a participatory manner to improve overall health and well-being.

Group-Level Assessment: Assembling an Interprofessional Team

Primary prevention at a group level may include a wide range of health and safety objectives and interventions—identifying the best interventions should be based on an analysis of need, potential benefit, cost, and willingness of the group to invest in the interventions. The goal of assessment for groups often involves determining the perceived needs, or potential risks to worker health and function related changes in work process that may manifest as an increase in worker complaints, degrading performance or injuries. These investigations should always consider input from the workers, whether that is by having them serve as active members of the investigative team or by asking them to provide their input through surveys and focus groups.

Conducting the needs analysis and gathering relevant company data for the CDC Workplace Health Model process includes assembling the appropriate assessment team. The individuals needed for the team will depend upon the nature of the problem but should always include a person from safety and management, a member of the operational team such as a supervisor, and various consultants from groups like engineering and medical. It is recommended that one or more members are front-line workers with institutional knowledge about the work processes and culture of the work area. The interprofessional team will benefit from having members with expertise on different topics related to the issues. Table 11-2 is the list of professionals with knowledge on various topics that may be beneficial to include on various interprofessional assessment teams.

All team members can provide input into outlining the safety and wellness needs, goals, and contributing factors used to develop the team's plan. As the company's traditional safety and health efforts become broadened to incorporate workplace health, wellness, and well-being initiatives, the company may benefit from developing a steering committee of middle and upper management to review plans from the assessment team and ensure ongoing coordination and alignment of the plans with corporate efforts. Having regular meetings and accountability ensures the team is working together. Ongoing communication guided by an assessment/action plan helps to integrate health and safety workplace efforts with the operational policies and procedures of the company and to promote the best level of health of the workforce through the company processes (McLellan et al., 2017; Punnett et al., 2020; Sorensen et al., 2016).

The assessment phase includes a review of data to fully understand the problem. Data may come from required documentation of injury reports and business operations and production reports (U.S. Bureau of Labor Statistics, 2013), but it should include data of the real and perceived needs of the workers from across a work area or the organization. Historical injury data looks backward; it is often considered "lagging" data because the event or injury has already

Table 11-2

Team Members With Knowledge on Various Topics Related to Workplace Problems

TOPICS	TEAM MEMBERS WITH KNOWLEDGE ON TOPICS
Staffing needs and turnover, hiring, orientation and training, organizational behavioral needs for transitioning work teams	Human Resources, Training Team/Coaches, Supervisors
Operational metrics, incentive programs	Human Resources, Safety, Supervisor
Injury logs, near miss data, de-identified data on worker health, disability claim trends	Human Resources, Safety, Risk, Industrial Hygienist, Supervisor
Health risk assessment, surveys, and surveillance data	Physical Therapist, Occupational Therapist, Risk, Safety, Workers, Occupational Nurse,
Job analysis, ergonomics	Physical Therapist, Occupational Therapist, Safety, Engineer, Workers

Professional Reasoning Box B: A Deeper Look

Individual Health Risk Assessments to Create Aggregate Group Data

Organizations may offer health risk assessments to establish a baseline of workers general health status and to determine the health needs of the workforce. Health information may be collected by surveys, biometric testing, or a combination of the two. Biometric data is more objective than surveys but has a higher cost and is more time consuming to collect on a large group. Both methods rely on workers to participate and often requires an incentive to get adequate participation to make the data representative of the workgroup. Workplace health risk information may guide wellness efforts and the need for intervention on topics such as stress, sleep, nutrition, movement, and disease. These health initiatives may be combined with efforts to reduce workplace risks as part of ergonomic and safety programs or separate for wellness initiatives.

happened so the injury can't be prevented. This may include injury logs, workers' compensation and disability claims data, and safety audits. In contrast, "leading indicators" are data from activities that can identify potential risks before a problem occurs. Examples of leading indicators include ergonomic assessments, early symptom reporting, near miss tracking, hazard audits, worker surveys, and health risk assessments that aggregate worker data that can be used to objectively describe or benchmark program problems and outcomes (Inouye, 2015; Karimi et al., 2021; Sheehan et al., 2016).

Surveys of workers are a good way to evaluate the health, physical and psychosocial risks—asking about pain or discomfort, performance challenges, productivity demands, health behaviors, or other problems in their job (Magnavita, 2018; National Institute for Occupational Safety and Health, 2021a, 2021b; Washington State Department of Labor & Industries, 2021). Issues that are identified through surveys or surveillance may be precursors to future injuries or indicate a change in work culture, engagement and satisfaction. Aggregate productivity and health data of the work group can be used to monitor changes in risks and well-being (Professional Reasoning Box B).

Planning and Interventions

Developing a plan of action includes identification of appropriate objectives, interventions, and implementation activities (Lee et al., 2016; NIOSH, 2021b; Peters et al., 2018; Peters et al., 2020). After assessing data and understanding needs, the health and safety team will begin to set clear objectives and prioritize them based on the potential impact to address reduce risk and promote worker health. Next, the team will brainstorm to generate a number of possible interventions to meet the objectives. The interventions should be clearly defined and include the required resources of time, money, equipment, as well as the knowledge, skills, and personnel needed to accomplish the objective(s) (CDC, 2015b; Occupational Safety and Health Administration, 2016; University of Massachusetts Lowell, n.d.).

Once the team has agreed on a plan and selected the interventions to implement (CDC, 2015), the team must choose the strategies or methods they plan to use to deliver the interventions or to make changes in the work area. The implementation strategies must include a communication plan to show how and to whom the activity will be communicated (Kent et al., 2016). Communication may need to be done in many forms with the same information or using similar messages. Formal communication may be provided in written form through email or visual signs with reminders about critical information such as start dates, and information offered through trainings or given during regular meetings such as safety briefings. Informal communications should be given by the supervisors, management team, and all others who interact with the affected workers on a daily basis.

Group and Organizational Intervention Initiatives

The business, cultural, and personnel dynamics of each workplace as well as the wide range of health and safety considerations mean that the methods of addressing group or organizational needs may differ under different conditions. For example, health initiatives at one location may be oriented to immunizations, health trackers, and insurance rebates while another organization may choose bottom-up participatory initiatives where one to two initiatives are selected in each department. The following are some group and organizational interventions initiatives that could be implemented as part of health and prevention activities in a group or organizational level process.

- Participatory Teams: teams that include worker representatives have the distinct advantage to more quickly identify the cause of problems, identify viable solutions, and gain buy-in from the workers. Mixed teams of workers and professionals must develop trust to function effectively, so the workers feel comfortable sharing ideas (Newman et al., 2020; Nobrega et al., 2017).
- Health and Preventive Activities: activities may include exercise facilities, yoga classes, sports and walking programs, nutrition, health screenings, joint protection programs, mindfulness, relaxation, smoking cessation, sleep hygiene awareness and coping and communication skill development (Abdin et al., 2018; Berry & Mirabito, 2011; Grimani et al., 2019; Jirathananuwat & Pongpirul, 2017; Mattke et al., 2013; White et al., 2016).
- Ergonomics, Engineering, or Process Changes: based on the hierarchy of controls, interventions can be aimed at eliminating problematic tasks, substitution, or use of an alternative process will reduce the risks of the job. Machine modifications, new equipment purchases, and revamping tasks and processes are all possible changes that may involve assessment group investigation and prioritization (Nobrega et al., 2017; van Eerd et al., 2010; Williams-Whitt et al., 2015).
- On-Site or Near-Site Fitness: the job tasks in most positions do not provide an adequate amount of daily activity to maintain physical fitness. All workers may benefit from having access to formal fitness and conditioning facilities and gyms. Sites may integrate conditioning into the first 4 to 8 weeks of employment. Companies may offer discounts or reimburse health plan costs for gym memberships or wellness programs (Mattke et al., 2013; Proper & van Oostrom, 2019).

Role of the Therapist in Prevention Programs

Therapists in an occupational health setting may be actively involved with group or departmental assessments and implementing interventions. The role of on-site therapists to the assessment team will depend upon the company structure, culture, and needs as well as the knowledge of the therapist. This role may require conducting an assessment of the physical, social, and environmental factors of the workforce that goes beyond the entry-level training received by most physical and occupational therapists. Yet the opportunity to be involved with prevention in a group of workers can allow therapists to positively impact worker health and well-being, minimize potential work limiting risks, and optimize work participation in larger numbers of workers, with intervention earlier in the course of the disease (Donovan et al., 2021; Jaegers et al., 2020; Prall & Ross, 2019).

The therapist may be asked to serve periodically or in an ongoing capacity as a consultant to the team or as a facilitator (Adam et al., 2010; Eagers et al., 2020; McMenamin et al., 2021; Reitz et al., 2020). In these roles, the therapist can provide more insight into the health of the workforce, express concern or insights about potential interventions, and assist with implementation strategies to deliver the interventions. The therapist has a unique knowledge base that can be very useful to the team; however, team members may not know about the therapist's expertise and what they may offer. Therapists who have the opportunity to serve on teams to promote worker health should learn about the organizational structure and business operations as well as the importance of organizational culture.

A Deeper Look: Professional Development and Competencies in Occupational Health

Physical and occupational therapists' initial professional training and practical experience does not generally include collaboration with non-health professionals in safety and engineering. Competencies in the area of occupational health have been described in a number of articles including those for therapists new to work-related practice (Adam et al., 2013), "cross cutting" occupational health and safety competencies that span multiple disciplines (Olson et al., 2005), and Total Worker Health competencies aimed at reducing work injury and disability while sustaining and improving

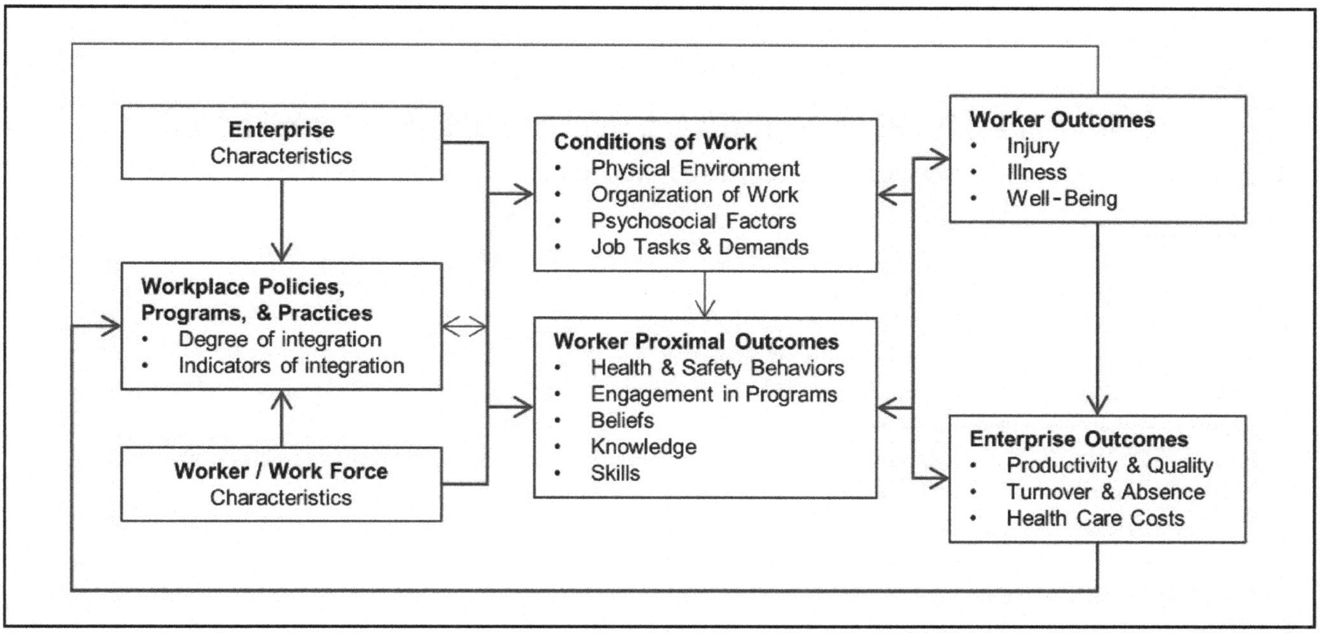

Figure 11-2. Conceptual model for integrated approaches to the protection and promotion of worker health and safety. (Studies conducted in Boston and Minnesota [2009-2015]. Data source: Sorensen et al., [2016].)

worker health and well-being (Newman et al., 2020). Areas for development in occupational health commonly include work injury and illness prevention, familiarity with occupational factors, workplace systems and culture, health promotion and public health, data gathering and analysis, cross-discipline teaming, and communication. Regardless of training and expertise, physical and occupational therapists must learn to work and coordinate with a team of other professionals within and outside of the health care system.

Making the Case for Organizational Integrated Services: A Total Worker Health Model

Work-related injuries continue to challenge organizations bottom line, costing more than $170.8 billion in 2018, with the highest cost coming from direct and indirect costs related to wages and productivity costs (31%), medical expenses (20%), and administrative expenses (34%; National Safety Council, 2018). An economic evaluation based on information from work site managers identified the organizational costs of lost productivity due to absence (**absenteeism**) or reduced productivity due to **presenteeism** exceeded wages—so each day a worker was absent cost the company 1.97 times wages in lost productivity (Strömberg et al., 2017). Absenteeism and presenteeism costs arise from the underlying health of the workforce.

To help organizations create a comprehensive and integrated occupational health, safety and wellness program for worker well-being, NIOSH established the Total Worker Health (TWH) program (Punnett et al., 2020). TWH emphasizes the use of organizational policies, programs, and practices to provide comprehensive support for worker health. Program components includes operational coordination, policy changes, and participatory engagement of workers. Results of TWH studies have shown positive return on investment (ROI), such as workers being 28% less likely to be injured on the job when provided paid sick leave compared to those without sick leave (CDC, 2018).

The Harvard TWH Center proposed a conceptual model to illustrate the factors involved with creating an integrated approach consistent with TWH (Figure 11-2). An integrated approach considers all levels of the organization in all decisions (leadership, middle management, safety, supervisors, and front-line workers). The outcomes of worker health are influenced by the 1) conditions of work and 2) factors such as personal behaviors and engagement in workplace programs. This means production and safety decisions consider the input from workers and the effects on worker health, creating a more cohesive workforce; improving employee health and well-being; and the financial state of the company (Sorensen et al., 2016).

Over the past decade, a number of evaluation instruments have been developed to assess multiple dimensions of organizational culture in a comprehensive manner that spans worker and worksite health. Research into tools such as the CDC Worksite Health Scorecard and the Harvard T.H. Chan Workplace Integrated Safety and Health Assessment seek to provide a way to frame dimensions of health to promote awareness, planning, implementation, and changes in health outcomes at a comprehensive level (CDC, 2019a;

Professional Reasoning Box C: Additional Resources for Regulatory, Ergonomics, and Total Worker Health

WORKPLACE SAFETY, ERGONOMICS, AND TOTAL WORKER HEALTH

- Job Accommodation Network. https://askjan.org/
- National Institute for Occupational Safety and Health. NIOSH Total Worker Health. https://www.cdc.gov/niosh/twh/
- National Institute for Occupational Safety and Health. Workplace Safety & Health Topics. Ergonomics and Musculoskeletal Disorders https://www.cdc.gov/niosh/topics/ergonomics/default.html
- Occupational Requirements Survey. https://www.bls.gov/ors/
- Occupational Safety and Health Administration. Recommended Practices for Safety and Health Programs. https://www.osha.gov/safety-management
- University of Massachusetts Lowell. IDEAS Tool. https://www.uml.edu/Research/CPH-NEW/Healthy-Work-Participatory-Program/generate-solutions/default.aspx
- University of Massachusetts Lowell. New Online Toolkit to Improve Employee Health, Safety and Well-being. https://www.uml.edu/research/cph-new/news/newtoolkit.aspx

LEGAL AND REGULATORY

- Federal Motor Carrier Safety Administration. Fmcsa.dot.gov
- Mine Safety & Health Administration. msha.gov
- OSHA Laws and Regulations. https://www.osha.gov/laws-regs
- U.S. Bureau of Labor Statistics. Injuries, Illnesses and Fatalities. www.bls.gov/iif/
- Washington State Labor & Industries. Get Started with Safety & Health. https://lni.wa.gov/safety-health/preventing-injuries-illnesses/get-started-with-safety-health/

Harvard University T.H. Chan School of Public Health, n.d.). Workplace integration of health professionals, prevention, and health and safety services often contribute significantly to positive scores.

Exemplary Organizations

Exemplary organizations have strong, proactive workplace health and safety cultures. The key elements for these organizations are well-known: leadership and management commitment, worker participation, hazard identification and effective implementation of controls, injury management and disability prevention, safety and health training, and planning and evaluation (Occupational Safety and Health Administration, 2016). Proactive organizations use continuous process improvement, always trying to adapt to the changes in their system to maintain optimal performance. The continuous improvement model uses the same steps outlined in the department case—assessment of the problem, plan for action, implement for change, and review the results. There are many characteristics of exemplary organizations with robust and proactive continuous improvement models. These organizations conduct regular review of policies, programs, and operational work practices (NIOSH, 2021a; Schwatka et al., 2021); ensure worker benefits and incentives align with the policies, programs, and practices; support worker health so the overall mission of the organization can be achieved; and proactive health and safety and ergonomic teams.

Exemplary organizations with strong organizational cultures also support the health culture of their workers. The health of the workers extends beyond the concern for injury on the job but includes the overall health of the workers in all business decisions, both on and off the job (Professional Reasoning Box C).

Conclusion: Take-Home Message

Physical and occupational therapists are traditionally trained to maximize functional ability for individuals suffering from acute and chronic conditions through clinical treatment and disability management. However, the unique training offered through these therapeutic programs provides knowledge and skills that can be applied in many more areas of society including community practice in the workplace. Working on site at the workplace gives therapists the opportunity to tailor treatments to incorporate the worksite, enables access to workers to monitor progress, and to participate in overall health management of the workforce through interprofessional teams. Interprofessional teams may convene professionals with medical expertise (nursing, therapy, physicians, industrial hygienists) or from the organization (human resources, operations, safety, engineering, and ergonomics) to have the relevant knowledge and decision makers to solve problems for worker health and well-being. The therapist may use their clinical skills in treatment of injured workers, but their professional training and experience sets them up to become a critical asset to employers, on-site medical teams, workplace operations, and workers. Therapists actively present in the workplace can fill many gaps in the operations side of the business. Therapist's knowledge of the abilities and limitations of the human body can help managers make the best operational decisions involving their workers. As therapists become familiar with the work world, business operations, and worker issues, they may expand their role in the workplace to focus on prevention health programs and resolving system level problems that contribute to injury risk. Therapists can help organizations achieve and continuously improve their work process to maintain this exemplary status, and the healthiest workforce possible.

Review Questions

1. Describe two ways health can be positively impacted by work and two ways health can be negatively impacted by work.

Work contributes to positive aspects of health by providing:

- Financial compensation to provide for self/family
- Access to health insurance and pensions
- Sense of accomplishment, pride, meaning
- Socialization

Work may expose workers to potentially health-harming physical or psychosocial stressors:

- Exposure to chemical and biological hazards
- Physical injuries from falls or being struck by objects
- Repeated and cumulative physical exposures in work tasks
- Psychosocial stressors of work may contribute to poor mental health
- How tasks are delegated may contribute to health concerns
- Nonstandard work hours has been linked to sleep disorders and physical health problems
- Job insecurity has been linked to poor mental health
- furlough and job loss during the COVID-19 pandemic has created profound financial strain

2. Describe the Hierarchy of Controls (HOC) and give an example of each of the five levels of controls.

HOC that prioritizes controls based on providing the greatest benefit to the workers. The most effective control is "elimination" that describes a change in the process, so the task is no longer performed. "Substitution" replaces the task with a solution such as automating the process. "Engineering" is a mid-level modification to the process or machine, so the workers have limited or no exposure to the hazard. "Administrative controls" change the way people work to reduce the risk such as rotating workers, training workers on better methods, or providing ergonomically designed tools. The least effective control is to use "personal protective equipment" that places a barrier between the hazard and the worker.

3. Describe the interactive process within the context of a worker seeking job accommodation under the Americans with Disabilities Act and Amendment.

Workers may approach their supervisor using lay person language requesting a work adjustment, or access company policies and procedures to submit a request for accommodation.

The worker may be asked to disclose the nature of the disability (what tasks are limited or the type of impairment), but the individual is not required to disclose a specific diagnosis. Employers must engage in an interactive process to provide a "reasonable accommodation" that bridges work performance gaps.

The "interactive process" generally involves the worker and workplace representative working together to determine if the worker can return to work with some type of modification or reassignment. An employee may be asked to suggest the type of accommodation that may help them participate in work.

Decisions related to accommodations are made between the worker and workplace representative. Therapists may be asked to consult on options, benefits, and estimating the costs of accommodations.

4. How does the role of the physical and occupational therapist change when workplace health services expand beyond treatment or secondary prevention of individual workers to primary prevention for a department or organizational level?

Secondary prevention aims to detect new disease in its earliest form, typically at the time of mild symptoms to prevent progression of disease or complications to health conditions or injuries. Early intervention can help minimize the impact of workplace risks and reduce the duration of medical care and related costs following injury. Secondary prevention may include treatment of new symptoms or injuries and management of identified work hazards (e.g., alternative methods to avoid manually lifting heavy materials).

Primary prevention may include increasing resilience and altering unhealthy behaviors by improving knowledge of risks, management to prevent the spread of infectious disease, and increase knowledge of the benefits of healthy and safe behaviors (e.g., proper diet, exercise routines, avoid smoking). This may also include routine health checks. Assessments at the primary level identify risks or hazards and remove them before they can have a negative impact on the health of workers in the department or work group.

Therapists may be a part of team or more of a consultative role for primary prevention as part of program design, support, or delivery of primary health interventions such as education, surveillance, and skill development. In secondary prevention or post-injury services, the therapist may have more of a service coordination role and communication driver.

5. Give an example of how physical and occupational therapists work together in a complementary manner with workplace safety professionals for 1) worker/worksite assessment and 2) implementation of health interventions.

Each member of an integrated health and safety team brings their individual expertise, personal strengths, and work experience based on their unique training and background. Occupational health nurses and therapists bring a health, wellness, treatment, and medical perspectives and skills. Supervisors and management are knowledgeable on operations, resource allocation and coordination of productivity, and process considerations in their respective areas of responsibility. Engineers and industrial hygienists provide key insights into planning and workplace equipment. Human resource personnel have expertise in regulatory, benefits, and sustainability of the workforce (human) resources. Developing a working knowledge and relationship for all team members who can contribute to integrated safety and health team, helps strengthen positive outcomes and efficacy.

The Workplace Health Model process must include multiple professions working together as part of an assessment team. The individuals needed for the team will depend upon the nature of the problem but should always include a person from safety and management and likely a person from operations and from ergonomics and/or medical. It is also recommended that one or more members are front-line workers with institutional knowledge about the work processes and culture from the work area. The interprofessional team will benefit from having members with expertise on topics related to the issues.

The following table should encompass many examples provided to answer this question.

ASSESSMENT TOPICS (NEEDS ANALYSIS, ROOT CAUSE ANALYSIS)	INTERVENTIONS/TYPES OF INTERVENTIONS	TEAM MEMBERS COLLABORATING
Injury logs, near miss data, de-identified data on worker health, disability claim trends	Operational supports and interventions (work hours, breaks, overtime, schedule, supply, and availability on the jobsite of equipment and tools, training, supervisory leadership, etc.)	Human Resources, Safety, Risk, Industrial Hygienist, Supervisor, Consultant Therapist
Health risk assessment, surveys, and surveillance data (safety teams)	Health and prevention activities and participatory teams promoting personal health, education, supporting physical activity and exercise, nutrition, mindfulness, relaxation, well check visits, sleep hygiene, and supporting/coping communication, new hire or post hire on-site/near-site fitness and conditioning	Physical Therapist, Occupational Therapist, Risk, Safety, Workers, Occupational Nurse,
Job analysis, ergonomics assessment (ergonomics team)	Task or engineering changes (equipment, machine, layout)	Physical Therapist, Occupational Therapist, Safety, Engineer, Workers

References

Abdin, S., Welch, R. K., Byron-Daniel, J., & Meyrick, J. (2018, Jul). The effectiveness of physical activity interventions in improving well-being across office-based workplace settings: a systematic review. *Public Health, 160*, 70-76. https://doi.org/10.1016/j.puhe.2018.03.029

Adam, K., Gibson, E., Lyle, A., & Strong, J. (2010). Development of roles for occupational therapists and physiotherapists in work related practice: An Australian perspective. *Work, 36*(3), 263-272. https://doi.org/10.3233/wor-2010-1028

Association of Schools & Programs of Public Health. (2015). Framing the Future: Population Health across All Professions Expert Panel Approach. https://aspph-wp-production.s3.us-east-1.amazonaws.com/app/uploads/2015/02/PHaAP.pdfpublis

Berry, L. L., & Mirabito, A. M. (2011, Apr). Partnering for prevention with workplace health promotion programs. *Mayo Clinic Proceedings, 86*(4), 335-337. https://doi.org/10.4065/mcp.2010.0803

Berwick, D. M., Nolan, T. W., & Whittington, J. (2008). The triple aim: care, health, and cost. *Health Affairs (Project Hope), 27*(3), 759-769. https://doi.org/10.1377/hlthaff.27.3.759

Burgard, S. A., & Lin, K. Y. (2013, Aug). Bad jobs, bad health? How work and working conditions contribute to health disparities. *The American Behavioral Scientist, 57*(8). https://doi.org/10.1177/0002764213487347

Burton, A. K. (2015). The Psychological Flags Framework: Overcoming Obstacles to Work. In Current Thinking in Back Pain Management. Henry Stewards Talks Ltd. http://hstalks.com/?t=BL1983919-Burton

Centers for Disease Control and Prevention. (2013). NCD prevention and control. U.S. Department of Health and Human Services. https://www.cdc.gov/globalhealth/healthprotection/fetp/training_modules/3/Prevention-and-Control_FG_Final_09262013v2.pdf

Centers for Disease Control and Prevention. (2015a). Organizational level assessment. U.S. Department of Health and Human Services. https://www.cdc.gov/workplacehealthpromotion/model/assessment/assessment-interview.html

Centers for Disease Control and Prevention. (2015b). Workplace health improvement plan. U.S. Department of Health and Human Services. https://www.cdc.gov/workplacehealthpromotion/planning/action-plan.html

Centers for Disease Control and Prevention. (2016). Workplace health model. U.S. Department of Health and Human Services. https://www.cdc.gov/workplacehealthpromotion/model/index.html

Centers for Disease Control and Prevention. (2018). Total Worker Health®a New Model For Well-being at Work. U.S. Department of Health and Human Sevices. Retrieved December 27, 2023 from https://www.cdc.gov/workplacehealthpromotion/initiatives/resource-center/pdf/WHRC_Total_Worker_Health_Brief_2018-3-508.pdf

Centers for Disease Control and Prevention. (2019a). CDC Worksite Health ScoreCard Manual. U.S. Department of Health and Human Services. https://www.cdc.gov/workplacehealthpromotion/initiatives/healthscorecard/pdf/CDC-Worksite-Health-ScoreCard-Manual-Updated-Jan-2019-FINAL-rev-508.pdf

Centers for Disease Control and Prevention. (2019b). Worksite ScoreCard. U.S. Department of Health and Human Services. https://www.cdc.gov/workplacehealthpromotion/initiatives/healthscorecard/worksite-scorecard.html

Center for the Promotion of Health in the New England Workplace. (2014). Healthy Workplace All Employee Survey. University of Massachusetts Lowell. https://www.uml.edu/docs/All%20Employee%20Survey_tcm18-147258.pdf

Chari, R., Chang, C. C., Sauter, S. L., Petrun Sayers, E. L., Cerully, J. L., Schulte, P., Schill, A. L., & Uscher-Pines, L. (2018, Jul). Expanding the paradigm of occupational safety and health: A new framework for worker well-being. *Journal of Occupational and Environmental Medicine, 60*(7), 589-593. https://doi.org/10.1097/jom.0000000000001330

Colombo, E., Rotondi, V., & Stanca, L. (2018). Macroeconomic conditions and health: Inspecting the transmission mechanism. *Economics and Human Biology, 28*, 29-37. https://doi.org/10.1016/j.ehb.2017.11.005

Donovan, M., Khan, A., & Johnston, V. (2021, Mar). The contribution of onsite physiotherapy to an integrated model for managing work injuries: A follow up study. *Journal of Occupational Rehabilitation, 31*(1), 207-218. https://doi.org/10.1007/s10926-020-09911-0

Eagers, J., Franklin, R. C., Broome, K., Yau, M. K., & Barnett, F. (2020, Nov 2). Current occupational therapy scope of practice in the work-to-retirement transition process: An Australian study. *Scandinavian Journal of Occupational Therapy*, 1-16. https://doi.org/10.1080/11038128.2020.1841286

Fox, K., & McCorkle, R. (2018). an employee-centered care model responds to the triple aim: Improving employee health. *Workplace Health & Safety, 66*(8), 373-383. https://doi.org/10.1177/2165079917742663

Garcia-Gomez, P., Jones, A. M., & Rice, N. (2008). Health effects on labour market exits and entries. Health, Econometrics and Data Group: University of York. https://www.york.ac.uk/media/economics/documents/herc/wp/08_03.pdf

Grimani, A., Aboagye, E., & Kwak, L. (2019, Dec 12). The effectiveness of workplace nutrition and physical activity interventions in improving productivity, work performance and workability: a systematic review. BMC Public Health, 19(1), 1676. https://doi.org/10.1186/s12889-019-8033-1

Hamar, B., Coberley, C., Pope, J. E., & Rula, E. Y. (2015). Well-being improvement in a midsize employer: changes in well-being, productivity, health risk, and perceived employer support after implementation of a well-being improvement strategy. *Journal of Occupational and Environmental Medicine, 57*(4), 367-373. https://doi.org/10.1097/jom.0000000000000433

Harvard University T.H. Chan School of Public Health. (n.d.). Workplace Integrated Safety and Health (WISH) Assessment. Northeastern University. http://centerforworkhealth.sph.harvard.edu/resources/workplace-integrated-safety-and-health-wish-assessment

Harvard University T.H. Chan School of Public Health. (2016). The Workplace and Health. https://www.rwjf.org/content/dam/farm/reports/surveys_and_polls/2016/rwjf430330.

Health Productivity and Performance Study Committee. (2015). Exploring the Value Proposition for Workforce Health Business Leader Attitudes about the Role of Health as a Driver of Productivity and Performance. https://www.shrm.org/ResourcesAndTools/hr-topics/benefits/Documents/HPP-Business-Leader-Survey-Full-Report_FINAL.pdf

Hertz-Palmor, N., Moore, T. M., Gothelf, D., DiDomenico, G. E., Dekel, I., Greenberg, D. M., Brown, L. A., Matalon, N., Visoki, E., White, L. K., Himes, M. M., Schwartz-Lifshitz, M., Gross, R., Gur, R. C., Gur, R. E., Pessach, I. M., & Barzilay, R. (2021, Aug 1). Association among income loss, financial strain and depressive symptoms during COVID-19: Evidence from two longitudinal studies. *Journal of Affective Disorders, 291*, 1-8. https://doi.org/10.1016/j.jad.2021.04.054

Horst, D. J., Broday, E. E., Bondarick, R., Serpe, L. F., & Pilatti, L. A. (2014). Quality of working life and productivity: An Overview of the conceptual framework. *International Journal of Managerial Studies and Research, 2*(5), 87-98.

Hutting, N., Boucaut, R., Gross, D. P., Heerkens, Y. F., Johnston, V., Skamagki, G., & Stigmar, K. (2020). Work-focused health care: The role of physical therapists. *Physical Therapy, 100*(12), 2231-2236. https://doi.org/10.1093/ptj/pzaa166

Inouye, J. (2015). Practical Guide to Leading Indicators: Metrics, Case Studies & Strategies. National Safety Council. https://www.nsc.org/getmedia/a3f19e6b-6688-4474-84ed-54325c16155f/wp-practicalguidetoli.pdf

Interprofessional Education Collaborative. (2016). Core competencies for Interprofessional Collaborative Practice: 2016 update. https://hsc.unm.edu/ipe/resources/ipec-2016-core-competencies.pdf

Isham, A., Mair, S., & Jackson, T. (2020). Wellbeing and productivity: a review of the literature (CUSP Working Paper No.22). Guildford: University of Survey. http://www.cusp.ac.uk/powering-productivity

Jaegers, L. A., Ahmad, S. O., Scheetz, G., Bixler, E., Nadimpalli, S., Barnidge, E., Katz, I. M., Vaughn, M. G., & Matthieu, M. M. (2020). Total Worker Health® needs assessment to identify workplace mental health interventions in rural and urban jails. *American Journal of Occupational Therapy, 74*(3), 7403205020p7403205021-7403205020p7403205012. https://doi.org/10.5014/ajot.2019.036400

Jirathananuwat, A. & Pongpirul, K. (2017). Promoting physical activity in the workplace: A systematic meta-review. *Journal of occupational health, 59*(5), 385-393.

Karimi, A., Abbasi, M., Zokaei, M., & Falahati, M. (2021). Development of leading indicators for the assessment of occupational health performance using Reason's Swiss cheese model. *Journal of Education and Health Promotion, 10*, 158. https://doi.org/10.4103/jehp.jehp_1326_20

Kent, K., Goetzel, R. Z., Roemer, E. C., Prasad, A., & Freundlich, N. (2016, Feb). Promoting Healthy Workplaces by Building Cultures of Health and Applying Strategic Communications. *Journal of Occupational and Environmental Medicine, 58*(2), 114-122. https://doi.org/10.1097/jom.0000000000000629

Kirsten, W. (2010). Making the link between health and productivity at the workplace—A global perspective. *Industrial Health, 48*(3), 251-255. https://doi.org/10.2486/indhealth.48.251

Landsbergis, P. A., Grzywacz, J. G., & LaMontagne, A. D. (2014, May). Work organization, job insecurity, and occupational health disparities. *American Journal of Industrial Medicine, 57*(5), 495-515. https://doi.org/10.1002/ajim.22126

Lee, M. P., Hudson, H., Richards, R., Chang, C. C., C. L., & L., S. A. (2016). Fundamentals of Total Worker Health® approaches: essential elements for advancing worker safety, health, and well-being. National Institute for Occupational Safety and Health. https://www.cdc.gov/niosh/docs/2017-112/pdfs/2017_112.pdf

Lin, P. Y., Wang, J. Y., Shih, D. P., Kuo, H. W., & Liang, W. M. (2019, July 3). The interaction effects of burnout and job support on peptic ulcer disease (PUD) among firefighters and policemen. *International Journal of Environmental Research and Public Health, 16*(13). https://doi.org/10.3390/ijerph16132369

Magnavita, N. (2018, Apr 2). Medical Surveillance, Continuous Health Promotion and a Participatory Intervention in a Small Company. *International Journal of Environmental Research and Public Health, 15*(4). https://doi.org/10.3390/ijerph15040662

Marras, W. S. (2006). *Fundamentals and assessment tools for occupational ergonomics*. CRC Press. https://doi.org/10.1201/9781420003635

Mattke, S., Liu, H., Caloyeras, J. P., Huang, C. Y., Van Busum, K. R., Khodyakov, D., & Shier, V. (2013). Workplace wellness programs study: Final report. RAND Corporation. https://www.rand.org/content/dam/rand/pubs/research_reports/RR200/RR254/RAND_RR254.pdf

McLellan, D., Moore, W., Nagler, E., & Sorensen, G. (2017). Implementing an Integrated Approach: Weaving Worker Health, Safety, and Well-being into the Fabric of Your Organization. Harvad T.H. Chan School of Public Health Center for Work, Health, and Well-being. http://centerforworkhealth.sph.harvard.edu/sites/default/files/10.12.17_Guidelines_Screen_post.pdf

McMenamin, P., Wickstrom, R., Blickenstaff, C., Bagley, J., Johnson, C., Jones, K., Newquist, D., & Paddock, J. (2021). Current concepts in occupational health: Role of physical therapists in occupational health. *Academy of Orthopaedic Physical Therapy, 33*(1), 43-48.

National Institute for Occupational Safety and Health. (2021a). Making the business case for Total Worker Health®. Centers for Disease Control and Prevention. https://www.cdc.gov/niosh/twh/business.html

National Institute for Occupational Safety and Health. (2021b). Planning, assessment, and evaluation tools. Centers for Disease Control and Prevention. https://www.cdc.gov/niosh/twh/tools.html

National Safety Council. (2018). Work injury costs. https://injuryfacts.nsc.org/work/costs/work-injury-costs/

Newman, L. S., Scott, J. G., Childress, A., Linnan, L., Newhall, W. J., McLellan, D. L., Campo, S., Freewynn, S., Hammer, L. B., Leff, M., Macy, G. (2020). Education and training to build capacity in Total Worker Health®: Proposed competencies for an emerging field. *Journal of occupational and environmental medicine, 62*(8):e384.

Nobrega, S., Kernan, L., Plaku-Alakbarova, B., Robertson, M., Warren, N., & Henning, R. (2017, Apr). Field tests of a participatory ergonomics toolkit for Total Worker Health®. *Applied Ergonomics, 60*, 366-379. https://doi.org/10.1016/j.apergo.2016.12.007

Occupational Safety and Health Administration. (2016). Recommended practices for safety and health programs. U.S. Department of Labor. https://www.osha.gov/sites/default/files/OSHA3885.pdf

Pelkowski, J. M., & Berger, M. C. (2004). The impact of health on employment, wages, and hours worked over the life cycle. *The Quarterly Review of Economics and Finance, 44*(1), 102-121. https://doi.org/10.1016/j.qref.2003.08.002

Peters, S. E., Grant, M. P., Rodgers, J., Manjourides, J., Okechukwu, C. A., & Dennerlein, J. T. (2018). A Cluster Randomized Controlled Trial of a Total Worker Health® Intervention on Commercial Construction Sites. *International Journal of Environmental Research and Public Health, 15*(11). https://doi.org/10.3390/ijerph15112354

Peters, S. E., Trieu, H. D., Manjourides, J., Katz, J. N., & Dennerlein, J. T. (2020, Jul 15). Designing a participatory Total Worker Health® Organizational Intervention for commercial construction subcontractors to improve worker safety, health, and well-being: The "ARM for Subs" trial. *International Journal of Environmental Research and Public Health 17*(14). https://doi.org/10.3390/ijerph17145093

Prall, J., & Ross, M. (2019). The management of work-related musculoskeletal injuries in an occupational health setting: the role of the physical therapist. *Journal of Exercise Rehabilitation, 15*(2), 193-199. https://doi.org/10.12965/jer.1836636.318

Presser, H. B. (2005). *Working in a 24/7 economy: Challenges for American families*. Russel Sage Foundation.

Proper, K. I., & van Oostrom, S. H. (2019). The effectiveness of workplace health promotion interventions on physical and mental health outcomes - a systematic review of reviews. *Scandinavian Journal of Work, Environment & Health, 45*(6), 546-559. https://doi.org/10.5271/sjweh.3833

Punnett, L., Cavallari, J. M., Henning, R. A., Nobrega, S., Dugan, A. G., & Cherniack, M. G. (2020). Defining 'integration' for Total Worker Health®: A new proposal. *Annals of Work Exposures and Health, 64*(3), 223-235. https://doi.org/10.1093/annweh/wxaa003

Reitz, S. M., Scaffa, M. E., & Dorsey, J. (2020, May/Jun). Occupational Therapy in the Promotion of Health and Well-Being. *American Journal of Occupational Therapy, 74*(3), 7403420010p7403420011-7403420010p7403420014. https://doi.org/10.5014/ajot.2020.743003

Rodriguez-Alvarez, A., & Rodriguez-Gutierrez, C. (2018). The impact of health on wages: evidence for Europe. *The European Journal of Health Economics, 19*(8), 1173-1187. https://doi.org/10.1007/s10198-018-0966-2

Schaller, J., & Stevens, A. H. (2015). Short-run effects of job loss on health conditions, health insurance, and health care utilization. *Journal of Health Economics, 43*, 190-203. https://doi.org/10.1016/j.jhealeco.2015.07.003

Schwatka, N. V., Dally, M., Shore, E., Dexter, L., Tenney, L., Brown, C. E., & Newman, L. S. (2021). Profiles of Total Worker Health® in United States small businesses. *BMC Public Health, 21*(1), 1010. https://doi.org/10.1186/s12889-021-11045-8

Sheehan, C., Donohue, R., Shea, T., Cooper, B., & Cieri, H. D. (2016). Leading and lagging indicators of occupational health and safety: The moderating role of safety leadership. *Accident, Analysis and Prevention, 92*, 130-138. https://doi.org/10.1016/j.aap.2016.03.018

Sorensen, G., McLellan, D. L., Sabbath, E. L., Dennerlein, J. T., Nagler, E. M., Hurtado, D. A., Pronk, N. P., & Wagner, G. R. (2016). Integrating worksite health protection and health promotion: A conceptual model for intervention and research. *Preventive Medicine, 91*, 188-196. https://doi.org/10.1016/j.ypmed.2016.08.005

Stansfeld, S., & Candy, B. (2006). Psychosocial work environment and mental health—A meta-analytic review. Scand*inavian Journal of Work, Environment & Health, 32*(6), 443-462. https://doi.org/10.5271/sjweh.1050

Statista. (2021). Monthly number of full-time employees in the United States from April 2020 to April 2021. https://www.statista.com/statistics/192361/unadjusted-monthly-number-of-full-time-employees-in-the-us/

Strömberg, C., Aboagye, E., Hagberg, J., Bergström, G., & Lohela-Karlsson, M. (2017, Sep). Estimating the effect and economic impact of absenteeism, presenteeism, and work environment-related problems on reductions in productivity from a managerial perspective. *Value in Health: The Journal of the International Society for Pharmacoeconomics and Outcomes Research, 20*(8), 1058-1064. https://doi.org/10.1016/j.jval.2017.05.008

U.S. Bureau of Labor Statistics. (2013). Using workplace safety and health data for injury prevention. U.S. Department of Labor. https://www.bls.gov/opub/mlr/2013/article/using-workplace-safety-data-for-prevention.htm

U.S. Bureau of Labor Statistics. (2021). Occupational requirements survey: Handbook of methods. United States Department of Labor. https://www.bls.gov/opub/hom/ors/pdf/ors.pdf

U.S. Equal Employment Opportunity Commission. (2008). The Americans with Disabilities Act Amendments Act of 2008. https://www.eeoc.gov/statutes/americans-disabilities-act-amendments-act-2008

University of Massachusetts Lowell. (n.d.). Generate solutions using the IDEAS Tool. https://www.uml.edu/Research/CPH-NEW/Healthy-Work-Participatory-Program/generate-solutions/default.aspx

van Eerd, D., Cole, D., Irvin, E., Mahood, Q., Keown, K., Theberge, N., Village, J., St Vincent, M., & Cullen, K. (2010, Oct). Process and implementation of participatory ergonomic interventions: a systematic review. *Ergonomics, 53*(10), 1153-1166. https://doi.org/10.1080/00140139.2010.513452

Waddell, G., & Burton, K. (2006). Is work good for your health and well-being? The Stationery Office. https://cardinal-management.co.uk/wp-content/uploads/2016/04/Burton-Waddell-is-work-good-for-you.pdf

Washington State Department of Labor & Industries. (2021). Washington State Occupational Health Indicators—Current Data (2010-present). https://www.lni.wa.gov/safety-health/safety-research/files/2021/80_17_2021_WA_Indicators_2021Apr.pdf

White, M. I., Dionne, C. E., Wärje, O., Koehoorn, M., Wagner, S. L., Schultz, I. Z., Koehn, C., Williams-Whitt, K., Harder, H. G., Pasca, R., Hsu, V., McGuire, L., Schulz, W., Kube, D., & Wright, M. D. (2016, Apr). Physical activity and exercise interventions in the workplace impacting work outcomes: A stakeholder-centered best evidence synthesis of systematic reviews. International *Journal of Occupational and Environmental Medicine 7*(2), 61-74. https://doi.org/10.15171/ijoem.2016.739

Williams-Whitt, K., White, M. I., Wagner, S. L., Schultz, I. Z., Koehn, C., Dionne, C. E., Koehoorn, M., Harder, H., Pasca, R., Warje, O., Hsu, V., McGuire, L., Schulz, W., Kube, D., Hook, A., & Wright, M. D. (2015, Apr). Job demand and control interventions: a stakeholder-centered best-evidence synthesis of systematic reviews on workplace disability. *International Journal of Occupational and Environmental Medicine, 6*(2), 61-78. https://doi.org/10.15171/ijoem.2015.553

World Health Organization. (1999). *The World Health Report 1999: Making a difference*. Author.

World Health Organization. (2001). *International classification of functioning, disability and health*. https://apps.who.int/iris/bitstream/handle/10665/42407/9241545429.pdf?sequence=1&isAllowed=y

CHAPTER 12

Promoting Occupational Health and Productivity

Older Adults

Andrea Gossett Zakrajsek, OTD, OTRL, FNAP; Sharon Holt, MHS, OTRL; and Kathleen Tithof, LMSW, LCSW, LICSW

Learning Objectives

At the end of this chapter, the reader will:

1. Describe productive occupations and activities in which community-dwelling older adults engage (ACOTE B.1.2)
2. Analyze the engagement in productive occupations among older adults and the impact on health, well-being, and quality of life (ACOTE B.3.4)
3. Identify barriers and supports to meaningful participation in productive activities at the individual, community, and population levels (ACOTE B.3.5, B.5.1)
4. Select approaches to interpersonal assessments and assessment methods that can be used to understand health and well-being issues of older adults' engagement in productive activities (ACOTE B.4.4)
5. Locate and appraise community-based services, resources, and programs that afford older adult engagement in productive activities (ACOTE B.4.26)
6. Investigate community-based interventions to promote meaningful engagement of older adults in productive occupations and activities (ACOTE B.4.10, B.4.27)
7. Identify professionals outside individual professions who can assist older adults' engagement in productive activities in the community (ACOTE B.4.25)

The ACOTE Standards used are those from 2018.

Key Words

Caregiving, Encore Career, Formal Education, Informal Education, Leisure, Leisure Exploration, Leisure Participation, Paid Work, Productive Activities, Productive Occupations, Unpaid Work

Pizzi, M. A., & Amir, M. (Eds.). *Interprofessional Perspectives for Community Practice: Promoting Health, Well-Being, and Quality of Life* (pp. 217-235).

Introduction

Fifteen percent of the U.S. population is aged 65 years or older and this number is expected to increase to 23.5% by the year 2060 (Administration on Aging, 2017; Roberts et al., 2018). Life expectancy is increasing, and older adults are seeking out meaningful opportunities for engagement, such as second careers, travel, volunteering, and participating in higher education learning opportunities. It is clear that engagement in productive activities, which may also be understood as occupations, have a positive impact on health and quality of life (QOL) of older adults (Marfeo & Ward, 2020; Stav et al., 2012). Yet, older adults may encounter social and physical barriers in their environments or experience physical or mental impairments that impact meaningful participation in occupations or activities. Community-based practitioners have an important role to play in affording opportunities and promoting well-being among older adults, communities, and populations to engage in productive activities to support health promotion and well-being in later life. This chapter will focus on the several productive activities among older adults living in the community. Within each area of productive activity, interventions and programs will be presented that are implemented by community-based practitioners. Case studies focusing on interprofessional care provide the reader with an opportunity to reflect and develop critical reasonings skills related to promoting healthy productive activity. Resources, assessments, programs, and interventions are provided to support community-based practice. Community-based practitioners are uniquely qualified to promote engagement in healthy activity that promotes optimal productivity, life satisfaction, well-being, and QOL for community-dwelling older adults at individual, community, and population levels (see Appendix A).

Promoting Engagement in Healthy Productive Activity in Late Life

There has been an increased interest in older adults engagement in productive occupations and activities in the last few decades from various professional perspectives, as interprofessional gerontology research has included a focus on successful and productive aging (Hinterlong et al., 2007; Rowe & Kahn, 1997) and global and national healthy aging initiatives have recognized the contribution of health behaviors and habits in health, well-being, and disease prevention (National Prevention Council, 2016; World Health Organization [WHO], 2015). In their seminal work on healthy aging, Rowe and Kahn (1997) define **productive activities** as "all activities, paid or unpaid, that create goods and services of value" (p. 47). Occupations are the "everyday activities that people do as individuals, in families, and within communities to occupy time and bring meaning and purpose to life. Occupations include activities and tasks that "... people need to, want to, and are expected to do" (American Occupational Therapy Association [AOTA], 2020b, p. 7). The field of occupational therapy recognizes that these **productive occupations** and activities can contribute to "the maintenance or advancement of society as well as to the individual's own survival or development" (Creek, 1997, p. 34). Furthermore, productive occupations encompass a variety of tasks and activities that can be unpaid or paid. Categorizing these productive occupations of older adults varies within the literature and is discussed within and outside the health care field. In a qualitative study that aimed to examine productive occupations of 70 adults over the age of 60 years, key occupations were identified as homemaker, volunteer, caregiver, paid employee, and student (Knight et al., 2007). In a secondary analysis of the American's Changing Lives Study, Hinterlong et al. (2007) included five productive roles of older adults: paid worker, irregular paid worker, unpaid worker, caregiver, and provider of informal social assistance. Furthermore, productive occupations may not result in financial gain and can encompass unpaid occupations and activities that are of value to self and others (Knight et al., 2007) and include occupations that encompass education, work, play and leisure, social participation, and various instrumental activities of daily living (IADLs), such as care of others, care of pets and animals, home establish and management, meal preparation, and religious and spiritual participation (AOTA, 2020b).

The literature on older adults has overwhelmingly described the link between meaningful engagement in activities and health and well-being among community-dwelling older adults (Clark et al., 2012; Park et al., 2021; Stav et al., 2012). Specifically, positive associations have been found between productive activity (such as paid work, unpaid work, gardening, shopping, meal preparation) and mortality, self-reported health, and less-functional impairment among older adults living in the community (Hinterlong et al., 2007; Stav et al., 2012). In a systematic review of occupational engagement and health outcomes among community-dwelling older adults, Stav et al. (2012) found that productive occupations, including work, volunteering, physical activity, leisure, and social and religious activities, have a positive impact on the health and QOL for this population. In addition, altruism, pleasure, meaningful use of time, health, personal environment, and financial gain have been found to be motivators for engagement in productive occupations and activities (Knight et al., 2007). This finding suggests that benefits of engagement in productive activities and occupations reach beyond health to QOL and well-being (see Appendix B).

These findings align with the gerontological theories of aging, in particular, the Continuity and Activity Theories of aging. Activity Theory suggests that engaging in mental and physical tasks, along with meaningful occupations, increases satisfaction and happiness of older adults (Havighurst, 1961; Menec, 2003). In this, social participation, and engagement in positive relationships, which accompanies these tasks will increase life longevity. In contrast, Continuity Theory purports that aging adults tend to maintain their activities and behaviors, personality, and relationships as they age (Atchley, 1989, 1999). Furthermore, Continuity Theory holds that older adults attempt to preserve internal and external structures by making adaptive choices to continue participation in experiences that tie them to their social world, including productive occupations and activities. It is within the grounding of these theoretical frameworks that the benefit of continued engagement of these previously held occupations as well as the development of new productive activities is beneficial to the health, well-being, and QOL of older adults.

Along with the recognition of these benefits, it is important to consider barriers to productive occupations and activities that exist at the individual, community, and population/societal levels. Individual level barriers to older adults' participation of work and nonwork productive activities include gender, age, marital status, self-reported driving, self-reported health, physical function, and mental health, as found by Marfeo and Ward (2020). Individual's performance patterns (habits, roles, and routines), volition, and performance capacity also impact engagement in productive occupations (Taylor, 2017). Community and environmental-level barriers can include resources and services available in one's community and accessibility of physical spaces and services to users (Taylor, 2017). Population and societal-level barriers can include ageism and other discriminatory behaviors that are associated with stigma as well as governmental and organizational policies and practices that exclude groups within older adult populations (Gonzales et al., 2015). Figure 12-1 depicts potential barriers that can impact participation in productive participation of older adults at multiple levels.

Health care professionals use an evaluation and intervention process to collect data to guide and deliver intervention and to also determine the impact and quality of the intervention. Aspects of an evaluation may include an environmental assessment, identification of physical, social, emotional strengths and barriers, the goals of the client and/or caregiver, and resources available. Evaluation and intervention are completed at an individual level, at the community or environmental level or to identify population needs. For instance, evaluations can include occupation, leisure or work-focused assessments, QOL and life satisfaction surveys, home and environmental evaluations and screenings, mental health screenings, and needs assessments to name a few. It is beyond the scope of this chapter to identify all of the possible assessments that are available for each health care discipline and for each potential community dwelling older adult individual, group/community or population. Table 12-1 describes some categories of assessments to consider evaluation of performance, supports, and barriers to engagement in being a productive older person.

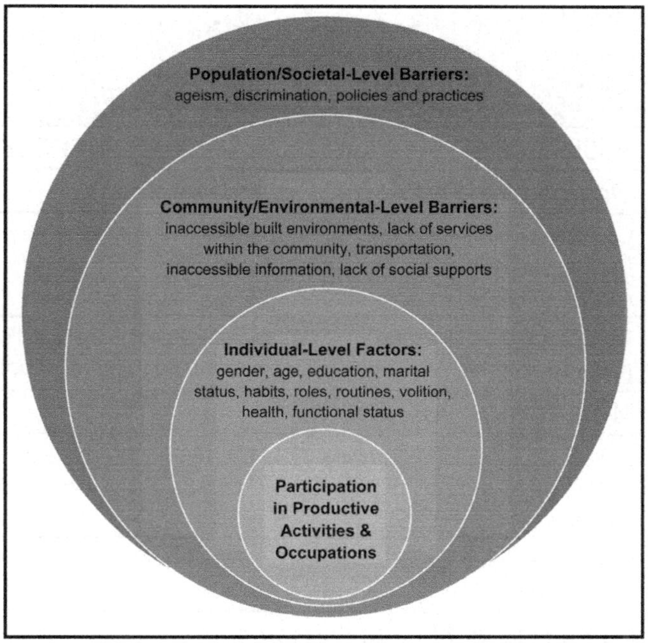

Figure 12-1. Individual, community/environmental, and population/societal level factors that present barriers to older adult participation in productive activities and occupations.

PAID WORK

Despite being past the age of typical retirement, around 67 years in the United States (Li, 2021), many community-dwelling elders continue to participate in work and volunteer occupations and activities (Stav et al., 2012). Furthermore, the U.S. Bureau of Labor Statistics projects that by 2024, 13 million people aged 65 years and older will still be working (approximately 8% of the working population, aged 16 and older), making up the fastest-growing segment of the workforce over that 10-year period (AARP, 2019). In one study using national study data following retirees longitudinally, the researcher found that about half of the retirees were partially retired, working part-time, or were "unretired," reversing their retirement decision and returning to paid employment (Maestas, 2010).

These various studies suggest that older adults do not necessarily desire to discontinue working in later life. Instead, older adults are returning to or continuing **paid work** for various reasons. Individual financial need is an obvious underlying reason for working in late life, as eligibility age for full Social Security benefits has increased, older adults do not have adequate savings for retirement, have a need for health insurance coverage, all while wages have been stagnant over the last decades, as well as economic recessions (Abraham & Houseman, 2020; Li, 2021). At a system level pertaining to financial need, the U.S. economy relies on older workers, especially the baby boomer generation, to fulfill worker roles (Gonzales et al., 2015). In addition, many older adults are participating in paid employment for nonfinancial reasons (Maestas, 2010). Research indicates that some of these reasons are choosing employment as a leisure pursuit, desire to

Table 12-1

Assessment Tools for Factors That Impact Productive Activities With Older Adults*

ASSESSMENT	FORMAT/PURPOSE	AVAILABILITY
Occupational Performance Interviews		
Canadian Occupational Performance Measure (COPM) (Law et al., 2019)	Outcome measure of a person's perception of satisfaction and performance in self-care, productivity, and leisure occupations	https://www.thecopm.ca/
Occupational Self-Assessment (OSA) (Baron et al., 2006)	Assessment of persons' perception of their own occupational competence on their occupational adaptation	https://moho-irm.uic.edu/
Work-Focused Assessments		
Work Environment Impact Scale (WEIS) (Moore-Corner et al., 1998)	Semi-structured interview addressing experiences and perceptions of a work environment	https://moho-irm.uic.edu/
Worker Role Interview (Bravemen et al., 2005)	Semi-structured interview addressing psychosocial and environmental factors that may be impacting return to work	https://moho-irm.uic.edu/
Caregiving and Health Assessments		
Adult Carer Quality of Life Questionnaire (AC-QoL) (Joseph et al., 2012)	Caregiver QOL assessment	https://doi.org/10.1108/1361 9321211270380
Geriatric Depression Scale (Marwijk et al., 1995; Parmelee et al., 1989)	Depression screen designed for older adults	https://www.sralab.org/rehabilitation-measures/geriatric-depression-scale
Perceived Social Support for Caregivers and Social Conflict Scales (Goodman, 1991)	Caregiver social support assessment	https://www.apa.org/pi/about/publications/caregivers/practice-settings/assessment/tools/perceived-support
Zarit Burden Interview (short and long forms) (Bédard et al., 2001; Zarit & Zarit, 1983)	Self-report measure designed to assess caregiver burden	https://www.apa.org/pi/about/publications/caregivers/practice-settings/assessment/tools/zarit
Outcome Measures Clearinghouse		
Health Measures Database that includes assessment clearinghouses: PROMIS, Neuro-QoL, ASCQ-Me, and NIH Toolbox.	National repository of patient reported outcome and QOL measures	https://www.healthmeasures.net/
Home and Community Environmental Assessments and Needs Assessments		
AARP - Livability Index and Livable Community Evaluation Guide	Assessment of neighborhoods and communities for the services, amenities and access	https://livabilityindex.aarp.org/ https://www.aarp.org/home-garden/livable-communities/info-2005/livable_communities__an_evaluation_guide.html
Community Health Assessment Toolkit	Resource for conducting a community health assessment and developing implementation strategies	https://www.healthycommunities.org/resources/community-health-assessment-toolkit
Community Integration Questionnaire (McColl et al., 2001)	Self-report survey of perceived communication integration in four dimensions	https://www.sralab.org/rehabilitation-measures/community-integration-measure

(continued)

Table 12-1 (continued)

Assessment Tools for Factors That Impact Productive Activities With Older Adults*

ASSESSMENT	FORMAT/PURPOSE	AVAILABILITY
Americans with Disabilities (ADA) Checklist	Developed by the New England ADA Center to assess access with the 2010 ADA Standards for Accessible Design	https://www.adachecklist.org
Safety Assessment for Function and Environment for Rehabilitation (SAFER); (SAFER-HOME v3) (Chiu et al., 2006)	Interview and observation-based rating scale to identify problems in community dwelling older adult living environments	https://www.cotainspires.ca/
Psychosocial Assessment		
EcoMap (Hartman, 1978)	Identifies the social and personal relationships of an individual within their environment	https://tinyurl.com/yc5drtu6 https://www.socialworkerstoolbox.com/ecomap-activity/
Self-Assessment Template (Lazarus, 1996; Pacheco, 2014)	Strengths based self-assessment designed to assess growth, value and mindset in the moment	http://socialworktech.com/2012/09/10/self-assessment/

*These are not all-encompassing but are included to provide a sample of options. You are encouraged to explore additional resources in your own community and work environment to support participation in productive occupations and activities.

stay physically and mentally active, and having opportunities to socially connect with others (Abraham & Houseman, 2020; Gonzales et al., 2015; Knight et al., 2007). In other words, older adults are promoting one's own occupational health and well-being by maintaining a sense of feeling fulfilled, having life satisfaction, and taking control of and optimizing one's own successful and productive aging.

While people are increasingly participating in paid work in later life, they may not necessarily be working in the same jobs or fields throughout their career. Marc Freedman (2007) introduced the term of **encore careers**, in which individuals in the second half of life continue work, often combining social impact, purpose, and income. In a small qualitative study, Murphy and Volpe (2014) found five factors motivating older adults to enter encore careers:

- Meaningful work
- Fun
- Novelty
- Work flexibility
- Work characteristics (e.g., autonomy, fewer physical demands, decreased travel requirements, less stress)

Furthermore, many older adults change jobs or industries as they have desires or needs to reduce hours due to other responsibilities or their own health issues, physical demands become too great in manual jobs or they lose jobs. System-level policies have a role in facilitating the worker role in late life. The U.S. Department of Labor (n.d.) Office of Disability Employment Policy offers reports, policies, and programs for support of older workers, such as the Return to Work Program, Job Accommodation Network, Senior Community Service Employment Program (SCSEP) and Age Discrimination in Employment Acts. Furthermore, in their 2020 analysis of older adults in the workforce, the Brookings public policy institution provides recommendations for workforce development policies that will improve the workforce services provided to older adults, such as having specialized staff at job resource centers who understand the needs of older adults, promoting self-employment of this populations, and developing program performance standards for older adults to eliminate disincentives for service provision (Abraham & Houseman, 2020).

It is also important to recognize possible widespread discrimination of older adults in the workplace. A survey study conducted by AARP suggested that over 60% of workers aged 45 years and older said they had experienced or observed age discrimination in the workplace (Terrell, 2018). Evidence of age discrimination has also been found during the application and processes of employment (Lahey, 2008; Neumark et al., 2019). Furthermore, work disparities based on gender, race, and ethnicity impact income, access to employment, and other practices in the workplace (Gonzales et al., 2015).

As older generations remain in or rejoin the workforce, community-based practitioners are well suited to address the individual needs of the person at the micro level as well as impact program development and delivery at the macro level to support engagement of older workers (Scaffa & Reitz, 2020). Oftentimes, professionals can be found in programs and services offered to older adults to engage in paid work. For example, the SCSEP is a community service and work-based job training program for older Americans. Authorized by the Older Americans Act, the program provides training for low-income, unemployed seniors. Participants also have access to employment assistance through American Job Centers. Another example is AARP's BACK TO WORK 50+. This is a program launched by AARP Foundation with the goal to increase the services and resources available to adult job candidates who are 50 or more years old nationally and in communities. The program also will facilitate their access to in-demand jobs .

Case Example 1

Robert is a 72-year-old male who lives in a mid-sized community near a large city. He lives alone, having lost his beloved wife to cancer last year. Robert enjoys being with his children and four grandchildren and tries to see them at least once every week. He also enjoys fishing and eating meals out with friends. Robert worked as a mechanic in the fire department and formally retired at 55 but continues to be a consultant, traveling around the state and teaching firefighters basic fire truck maintenance. To be effective in his job, he is required to climb in and around the fire trucks and do overhead maintenance. Robert has a past medical history of cardiac arrest with resultant Coronary Artery Bypass Graft X4 15 years ago and is currently experiencing increasing knee pain, which is impacting his ability to access the needed equipment and vehicles. He loves his job, feels his work is meaningful, and the income helps pay his bills, but he is identifying that the long hours and travel are becoming burdensome. He wants to continue working but is conflicted because of uncertainty about other options. During a recent follow-up visit to his doctor, and mentioning his concerns, his doctor recommended he meet with the care coordinator.

Reflective Questions

1. What questions might the care coordinator ask Robert? Are there further questions your profession may be interested in asking?
2. Which assessment tools can be utilized with Robert? Which assessment might provide *your* profession with the most pertinent information?
3. Considering supports and barriers at the individual, community, or population-level (Figure 12-1) what might impact Robert's ability and desire to continue working?
4. How might your profession assist Robert? Are there other professionals in the community who could also assist Robert?
5. Robert was provided information on a local state employment program and a pamphlet containing contact information for AARP. Look up the state employment resources in your area. What is the name of your local workforce development agency? What are the eligibility requirements? What might be available for Robert if he was living in your community?
6. In a situation in which you are working with an older adult on employment, as a community-based professional, what cultural considerations may there be?

Unpaid Work

Older adults engage in **unpaid work** as productive activities and occupations. In considering productive occupations, including activities that generate goods or services, unpaid work could include many IADLs. These are home management and maintenance, shopping, care of others, community mobility, and volunteering activities. Volunteering can be further differentiated as "formal" volunteering activities that parallel paid work in that these activities require specific tasks to be performed within timelines for a formal organization and "informal" volunteering activities that occur outside of an organization and include tasks such as helping family, neighbors, and friends. In a longitudinal study of characteristics and resources associated with volunteering among older adults in the community, having a higher education, reporting higher level of social capital, social functioning and physical functioning were significantly associated with formal volunteering (Cramm & Nieboer, 2014). This same study found that being younger, having a higher education, being married and male and reporting higher social capital, social functioning, and physical functioning were significantly associated with informal volunteering. Volunteering activities, whether formal or informal, decreased over time (Cramm & Nieboer, 2014). Conversely, Hinterlong et al. (2007) found that unpaid engagement among community dwelling older adults increases with age.

Individuals may volunteer in late life based upon individual characteristics (value of altruism, desire to help others, religiosity); resources (education, household income, physical or mental health); social factors such as social context (social environment, homeownership); social integration (social contacts people have); and social roles (marital and parental status; Dury et al., 2015). Personal benefits for older adults who volunteer are substantial (Gonzalez et al., 2015). In a critical review of 73 articles that described volunteering among older adult studies, benefits found to be associated with volunteering included: decreased symptoms of depression, higher levels and improvements in positive affect or happiness, increased self-reported health and QOL, improvements in social support and social networks, improvements in physical health and decreased functional limitations, and decreased mortality (Anderson et al., 2014). There are also many benefits of older adult volunteers to society. Older adults have skills and knowledge based upon their life experiences that are useful for volunteering. In addition, volunteers have an economic impact on the United States and global economy (Dury et al., 2015; Musick & Wilson, 2008).

Case Example 2

Charlotte is a 75-year-old female living with her husband Frank for the past 52 years. They reside in a two-story home in their small town of approximately 25,000 residents. Charlotte has been retired since age 65. Two of their three children live in the area along with five grandchildren. Every Sunday, Charlotte and Frank host a family dinner. They identify this weekly ritual as an important part of their lives to keep them connected to their family. Charlotte and Frank love to engage their grandchildren in helping to make Sunday dinner. They are also very active in helping their grandchildren with homework, playing games, and going to the park during the week. Charlotte loves to be active and participates in the "Silver Sneakers" program, paid for by her Medicare Advantage insurance, at the local YMCA with a group of her friends. She also enjoys traveling, attending concerts, reading, and socializing with friends on online social media platforms. Recently, Charlotte had a fall at home and broke a bone in her ankle. She spent 2 weeks in a local skilled nursing facility for rehabilitation and now is back home doing in-home rehabilitation. Due to new financial constraints and her decreased ability to engage in leisure interests, Charlotte has been experiencing symptoms of mild depression, which were discovered during a session with her home health care social worker.

Reflective Questions

1. Imagine you were working with a group of older adults in your community senior center who were interested in improving their leisure participation. What assessment tools could you utilize at the individual, community, or population level?
2. What community resources might be available if Charlotte were living in your community?
3. What might be potential barriers with accessing or utilizing these resources?
4. Who might be other disciplinary team members who are working with Charlotte in home health care? How might each discipline address Charlotte's depression and goal to re-engage in leisure pursuits?
5. In a situation in which you are working with an older adult, as a community-based professional, what cultural considerations may there be?

Participation in Caregiving

One productive occupation in which many older adults engage that can be unpaid or paid is family **caregiving**. According to the Family Caregiver Alliance ([FCA]; 2016), 34% of the over 43 million caregivers in the United States are aged 65 years or older. These caregivers may be unpaid, or informal caregivers, such as a spouse, partner, family member, friend, neighbor, or parent of an adult child with a disability. They may also be paid, or formal caregivers, providing services to others through private pay, government support such as Medicaid and veteran self-directed care programs, and long-term care insurance programs (U.S. Government Services and Administration, n.d.). Paid and unpaid older adult caregivers can assist with activities of daily living, medical care, and providing services such as shopping, food preparation, housekeeping, laundry, and transportation (FCA, 2016).

While the health of older adult caregivers has been associated with poorer physical and mental health and declines in physical activity participation (Queen et al., 2019), positive aspects of caregiving, such as positive association with the caregiving role, have been found to have a mediating effect on burden and satisfaction of caregivers (Fauziana et al., 2018). It is important to consider the intersectionality between caregiving and other productive occupations, such as working and leisure participation. Older adult caregivers may also be engaging in paid and unpaid work, leisure pursuits, and other occupations and activities. In fact, engagement in concurrent productive activities has been related to modest improvements in health and functional status in a national study of adults over the age of 60 years (Hinterlong et al., 2007). One study suggests that caregiving among older workers can be experienced as gratifying, as evidenced by the majority of study participants, but, at the same time, can evoke feelings of burden and stress (Grünwald et al., 2020). However, the same study finds that these caregivers who had access to resources, such as phased retirement and other employer and government support programs, experience caregiving as less burdensome and stressful.

Case Example 3

James, an 85-year-old man, lives in a rural town senior apartment complex with his wife Patricia, who has Alzheimer's disease. James and Patricia have lived in their community for 50 years and they have a very active social support system to assist with shopping and visiting with Patricia for a few hours each week. James ceased driving 2 years ago and now relies on the local senior taxi service for shopping and medical appointments for him and his wife. Sarah, their daughter, lives 20 minutes away. She comes once every week to help her dad with medical appointments and caregiving tasks, but James takes on the bulk of the responsibility for assisting Patricia each day. James was talking with the pastor at his church and expressed interest in talking with other caregivers for extra support. It is getting more difficult to care for Patricia each day and although he sees it as a last resort he feels it is time to learn about resources and living options for Patricia. The pastor, who had recently experienced a similar situation with his own father, provided James with information for the Country Alzheimer's Association.

Reflective Questions

1. Look up your nearest Alzheimer's association. What programs or resources do they offer? What resources or programs might be available for James and Patricia if they lived in *your* community?
2. How might living in a rural, urban, or suburban community impact accessing or utilizing these resources?
3. Working with loved ones who have dementia or Alzheimer's disease often requires a team approach. Who are some of the health professionals that might work with older adults with cognitive decline in the community? How could *your* profession assist James and Patricia to continue to engage in meaningful occupations?
4. In a situation in which you are working with a caregiver of an older adult, as a community-based professional, what cultural considerations may there be?

Participation in Education

Another role many older adults engage in is that of a student in education pursuits. The productive occupation of participation in education can occur in informal or formal educational systems. Informal education exists outside a structured curriculum in which older adult students engage collaboratively to explore, study, and participate in content and experiences that foster learning (Brown et al., 1989). Typically, this occurs within a social environment that is less controlled than in formal education, whereby students can learn from other individuals and scaffold learning from one another (Dewey, 1933). **Informal education** can have a clear objective for the learner with a broader plan, but this does not always occur. Examples of informal education in which older adults might engage include joining Bible study groups, attending hobbies and crafts classes, participating in forums or chats about topics of interest, attending lectures and seminars, and social media engagement.

Older learners may also participate in **formal education**, including higher education. Specifically, the landscape of university campuses is changing nationally and globally, as more and more "nontraditional" students (over the age of 25 years) are enrolled in post-secondary education. In fact, the National Center for Education Statistics reported 7.6 million nontraditional students were enrolled in higher education institutes (Hussar & Bailey, 2016). Older learners are seeking higher education opportunities for reasons such as career development, opportunities to interact with other learners of various ages and backgrounds, and, most commonly, to satisfy an intellectual curiosity and desire to learn (Kressley & Huebschmann, 2002). The infiltration of these nontraditional learners in institutions of higher education provide intrinsic benefit to the learner but also to the social milieu of college campuses the provision of intergenerational learning opportunities, older learners drawing on their past experiences to enhance in-class discussions, and the appreciation of complexity and richness that age brings university diversity (Ellis, 2013; Parks et al., 2013; Schaefer, 2009; Simon et al., 2020).

With the increase of age diversity in higher education, it has been recognized that the needs of older learners are different from younger, more traditional students who are typically aged 18 to 25 years. Many of these older learners have work and family responsibilities that they balance along with educational commitments (Rabourn et al., 2018; Silverstein et al., 2002). In addition, research has shown that older students experience barriers of engagement in formal higher education including: accessing student support program and services (Ellis, 2013; Silverstein et al., 2002; Simon et al., 2020), navigating physical spaces and virtual educational environments (Dauenhauer et al., 2016; Rabourn et al., 2018) and perceived deficits in technology proficiency, especially with the prevalence of online education (Brody et al., 2010; Rabourn et al., 2018). Finally, older learners may perceive themselves as "othered" on college and university campuses and less likely to engage in social aspects of educational life due to perceived stigma (Parks et al., 2013).

Age-inclusive initiatives, such as the Age Friendly University (AFU) global network, provide opportunities and resources for universities to explore and support diversity on campuses based upon age (Talmage et al., 2016). Paralleling other age-friendly initiatives, such as Age-Friendly Health Care Systems (Fulmer et al., 2018) and Age-Friendly Cities and Communities (WHO, n.d.) the AFU initiative was developed by Dublin City University, Arizona State University, and University of Strathclyde to better meet the needs of older adults. Ten principles were developed to foster age-friendliness of universities (Table 12-2).

Case Example 4

Gerry is a 60-year-old man who was recently laid off from his position of 25 years from a large industrial manufacturer, due to downsizing. Gerry was not ready to retire and although he applied for many positions he felt qualified for, he was unable to obtain employment. After much contemplation, Gerry decided that he would return to school to learn a new set of skills for the job market. Gerry is an Army veteran, having served two tours of duty in the 1980s. He obtained the rank of sergeant while in active duty and used his

Table 12-2

10 Principles of Age-Friendly University Global Initiative

AFU PILLAR	AFU PRINCIPLES
Educational Access and Lifelong Learning	1. To encourage the participation of older adults in all the core activities of the university, including educational and research programs. 2. To enhance access for older adults to the university's range of health and well-being programs and its arts and cultural activities.
Workforce & Personal Development	3. To promote personal and career development in the second half of life and to support those who wish to pursue second careers. 4. To recognize the range of educational needs of older adults (from those who were early school-leavers through to those who wish to pursue Master's or PhD qualifications). 5. To widen access to online educational opportunities for older adults to ensure a diversity of routes to participation.
Appreciation of Age Diversity and Intergenerational Exchange	6. To promote intergenerational learning to facilitate the reciprocal sharing of expertise between learners of all ages. 7. To increase the understanding of students of the longevity dividend and the increasing complexity and richness that aging brings to our society.
Research on Aging	8. To ensure that the university's research agenda is informed by the needs of an ageing society and to promote public discourse on how higher education can better respond to the varied interests and needs of older adults.
Campus-Community Connections	9. To engage actively with the university's own retired community. 10. To ensure regular dialogue with organizations representing the interests of the aging population.

Data source: Simon, A., Masinda, S., & Zakrajsek, A. (2020). *Age-friendly university environmental scan: Exploring "age-friendliness" with stakeholders at one regional comprehensive university.* Gerontology & Geriatrics Education. https://doi.org/10.1080/02701960.2020.1783259

skills of leading a team of soldiers effectively in his previous manufacturing leadership position. After speaking with a counselor at a local university, Gerry decided to apply to the nursing program as it was something that fit well with some of his experiences in the army and the job outlook was currently favorable. During the first week of class, Gerry felt out of place being the oldest person in his class. He also felt overwhelmed with the transition into his new role as a student.

Reflective Questions

1. Review a local college or university website. Are there any resources, professionals, or departments that might be available for Gerry to help him with his transitioning roles?
2. Considering supports and barriers at the individual, community, or population level (see Figure 12-1), what might impact Gerry's engagement in education? (Hint: supports and barriers could be social, physical, cultural, etc.)
3. Recently, the AFU where Gerry was taking classes was required to transition to online learning due to the COVID-19 pandemic. Gerry is now managing an online learning management system and Zoom conferencing for the first time. How might the university system support learners like Gerry?

Participation in Leisure or Recreational Activities

A final role of older adults is the pursuit and participation in leisure or recreational occupations and activities. This section focuses on definitions of the terms "leisure" and "recreation" from professional practice frameworks and will discuss the types of leisure and will also highlight research exploring emerging leisure activities of virtual reality and social media with the older adult population.

According to Merriam Webster dictionary, **leisure** is defined as "freedom provided by the cessation of activities, especially: time free from work or duties" and recreation is defined as, "refreshment of strength and spirits after work, also: a means of refreshment or diversion: hobby" (Merriam Webster Online Dictionary, n.d.). Health profession organizations further define leisure as an occupation in which people engage, distinguishing it from other occupations. The OTPF further differentiates between **leisure exploration**, "identifying interest, skills, opportunities, and leisure activities" (AOTA, 2020b, p. 250) and **leisure participation**, "planning and participating in leisure activities;... obtaining, using, and maintaining equipment and supplies" (AOTA, 2020b, p. 250) and recognizes the importance of balancing leisure activities with other occupations.

The profession of recreational therapy (RT) understands leisure and recreation as the core of the profession. The unique feature of RT that makes it different from other professions is the use of recreational modalities in the designed intervention strategies. RT is extremely individualized to each person by their past, present, and future interests and lifestyle. The recreational therapist has a unique perspective regarding the social, cognitive, physical, and leisure needs of the patient. Incorporating client's interests, and the client's family and/or community makes the therapy process meaningful and relevant. Recreational therapists weave the concept of healthy living into treatment to ensure not only improved functioning, but also to enhance independence and successful involvement in all aspects of life (American Therapeutic Recreation Association, 2013).

Furthermore, leisure can be broken down into three main times, as defined by Stebbins (2015): serious leisure, casual leisure and project-based leisure. "*Serious leisure* is the systematic pursuit of an amateur, hobbyist, or volunteer ... that is highly substantial, interesting, and fulfilling and where ... participants find a [leisure] career..." (Stebbins, 2015, p. 11). For example, serious leisure could include collecting stamps or maintaining a public wetland area. According to Stebbins, individuals undertaking serious leisure can be categorized as amateurs, volunteers, and or hobbyists. *Casual leisure* is defined as "...immediately, intrinsically rewarding; and it is a relatively short-lived, pleasurable activity requiring little or no special training to enjoy it" (Stebbins, 2015, p. 11). For example, watching TV or going for a swim are casual leisure activities. Finally, *project-based leisure* "Is a short-term, moderately complicated, either one-shot or occasional, though infrequent, creative undertaking carried out in free time" (Stebbins, 2015, p. 11). For example, working on writing a poem or building a garden feature are project-based leisure pursuits (see Appendix C).

For the well-being of older adults and enhancement of QOL, recreation or leisure plays a key role. Involvement in recreational activities satisfies a variety of needs for older adults, including increased health and fitness, opportunities for socializing, using talents and skills developed throughout their lifetime, and for learning new skills. The elder population is very diverse and has a large variety of interests, strengths, and abilities (Singh & Kiran, 2014). Older adults are increasingly searching out opportunities to remain physically active in retirement and participate in meaningful activities in their communities.

One leisure pursuit that older adults are increasingly participating in as social media participants. Mary Madden, former Senior Researcher at Pew Research Center, writes about *Older Adults and Social Media*, discussing the results of Pew Research Center's Internet & American Life Project (Madden, 2010). First, the research shows that social media users are much more likely to reconnect with people from their past, and these renewed connections can provide a powerful support network when people near retirement or embark on a new career. A second finding of this research indicates older adults are more likely to be living with a chronic disease and those living with these diseases are more likely to reach out for support online. And finally, research shows that social media bridges generational gaps. These social media spaces pool together users from very different parts of people's lives and provide the opportunity to share skills across generational divides (Madden, 2010).

There are many organizations that work with older adults that actively promote social media resources that are relevant to mature users. There are policy implications for supporting older adults and other individuals to have access and training to technology, such as the Federal Communications Commission's National Broadband Plan to invest in a digital literacy training program for older Americans (Federal Communications Commission, 2017). A program within this plan included training volunteers to teach digital skills to those who are least connected. With 86% of internet users ages 18 to 29 years using social networking sites and 60% doing so on a typical day, it is not hard to imagine that some of these young mentors would be eager to share their skills in profile management with older users (Madden, 2010).

Virtual reality is another opportunity for older adults' leisure participation. Virtual reality refers to an artificial reality that allows users to enter a 2D or 3D visual, auditory, and interactive virtual world through a computer interface while gaining experiences similar to those in the real world. Virtual reality, combined with sound, video, graphics, animation, text, and other technologies, involves high interaction and immediate responses, allowing users to have an "immersed" feeling. In one study that examined the meanings and values of virtual reality among older adults, elders, particularly those with disabilities, found it easier to get involved in virtual reality leisure activities than physical leisure activities (Cheng-Shih et al., 2018). The results of the study show that elderly respondents value virtual reality leisure activities that are fun, safe, and easy. Older adults also placed high value on feeling physically and mentally healthy, having firsthand experiences, and satisfied curiosity. Elderly respondents also hope that their chosen virtual reality leisure activities improve not only their relationships with others, but also their enjoyment, QOL, and sense of belonging (Cheng-Shih et al., 2018).

There are many retirement and senior communities across the nation that are embracing 3D virtual reality technology to assist older adults with activities such as virtual traveling and creating opportunities for shared experiences with older adult's families or friends. An example of this is AARP Innovation Lab's family-oriented virtual reality application, "Alcove" (AARP, 2020). This application offers a "virtual home filled with endless experiences to discover and explore...packed with casual games, world travel, media customization, relaxation and adventure" (AARP, 2020). This program bridges the physical distance between family members and empowers others to experience new things and places that they wouldn't normally be able to do because of cost, time, or mobility constraints. Virtual reality is not a new concept but with the community dwelling, older adult population it can be an exciting and wonderful opportunity of engagement in the productive occupation of leisure involvement (see Appendix D).

Case Example 5

Robert enjoys fishing and eating meals out with friends. He also enjoys spending time with his family and is very active with caring for and having fun with his grandchildren. Robert identifies that his knee pain is impacting his ability to engage in these occupations. He has also expressed a keen interest in trying new activities but is not sure what is available to him.

Reflective Questions

1. Identify five individual, community, and population resources in the community that you practice or live in that may be of interest to Robert or that could assist him with activity exploration.
2. Considering supports and barriers at the individual, community, or population level (see Figure 12-1), what might impact Robert's exploration and engagement in leisure activities?

Community-Based Program, Services, and Resources

Programs and services that can be offered by community-based practitioners have been identified in earlier specific sections. Table 12-3 provides names, descriptions, and links to services that foster engagement in productive occupations and activities. These provide useful resources for community-based practitioners to share with their clients. In addition, interprofessional teams collaborate within these programs to enhance the health and well-being of community dwelling older adults.

Engagement in meaningful and productive occupations and activities is critical to the health, well-being, and participation of older adults living in the community. However, access and engagement in productive occupations in late life can be impacted by individual, community, and population barriers. Community-based health professionals can address these barriers at the micro, meso, and macro levels providing services to older adults in community agencies, developing resources and programs to support active engagement in productive occupations, or advocating for laws and policies that afford opportunities to those in the second half of life. It is our hope that you use these resources, approaches, and findings to support your community-based practice.

Conclusion

Engagement in meaningful and productive occupations and activities is critical to the health, well-being, and participation of older adults living in the community. However, access and engagement in productive occupations in late life can be impacted by individual, community, and population barriers. Community-based health professionals can address these barriers at the micro, meso, and macro levels providing services to older adults in community agencies, developing resources and programs to support active engagement in productive occupations, or advocating for laws and policies that afford opportunities to those in the second half of life. It is our hope that you use these resources, approaches, and findings to support your community-based practice.

Table 12-3

Programs That Support Productive Participation*

PROGRAM/RESOURCES/ SERVICE	AIM OF PROGRAM/RESOURCE/SERVICE	LINK FOR MORE INFORMATION
Paid Work		
AARP Back to work 50+	Provides the training, coaching, and job seeking tools needed to compete with confidence for today's in-demand jobs	https://resourcenavigator.secure.force.com/WorkshopFinder/?intcmp=BTW-WORKSHOPS
Encore.org	Provides resources for encore career development	https://encore.org
The Senior Community Service Employment Program (SCSEP)	Provides training for low-income, unemployed seniors	https://www.careeronestop.org/LocalHelp/EmploymentAndTraining/find-older-worker-programs.aspx
Workforce Development	Provides resources for career exploration, training, and jobs and sponsored by the U.S. Department of Labor	https://www.careeronestop.org/
Unpaid Work		
AARP	Volunteer Databases	https://www.aarp.org/volunteer/
Volunteers of America	Volunteer Database	https://www.voa.org/
Volunteer Match	Volunteer Database	https://www.volunteermatch.org/
Caregiving		
AARP	Caregiver resources, information, and assistance	https://www.aarp.org
Alzheimer's Association	Caregiver resources, information, and assistance	https://www.alz.org
Eldercare	A public service of the U.S. Administration on Aging connecting you to services for older adults and their families	https://eldercare.acl.gov/
Family Caregiving Alliance	Caregiver resources, information, and assistance	https://www.caregiving.org
National Association of Area Agencies on Aging	Caregiver resources, information, and assistance	https://www.n4a.org/
PACE: Programs of All-Inclusive Care for the Elderly	Programs of All-Inclusive Care for the Elderly (PACE) is a Medicare and Medicaid program that helps people meet their health care needs in the community instead of going to a nursing home or other care facility	https://www.medicare.gov/plan-compare/#/pace?lang=en&year=2021
U.S. Department of Health and Human Services	Caregiver resources, information, and assistance	https://www.hhs.gov
Leisure and Recreation		
AARP	Various leisure topics and resources	https://www.aarp.org/
Local Senior Centers and/or Local Senior Apartment Complexes	Travel, organized activities, games, educational sessions, congregate meal sites, opportunities for leisure, and social activities	https://www.55places.com/blog/the-ultimate-hobby-guide-50-hobbies-for-seniors
National Recreation and Parks Association	Engagement in community, state and federal parks	https://www.nrpa.org
National Council on Aging	The Aging Mastery Program (AMP): an engaging education and behavior change incentive program for aging well	https://www.ncoa.org

(continued)

Table 12-3 (continued)

Programs That Support Productive Participation*

PROGRAM/RESOURCES/ SERVICE	AIM OF PROGRAM/RESOURCE/SERVICE	LINK FOR MORE INFORMATION
Older Adult Technology Services	Technology connection support program for older adults	https://oats.org/
Project GOAL	Organization that supports broadband and technology access for older adults	https://theprojectgoal.org/goal-at-the-silvers-summit/

*These are not all encompassing but are included to provide a sample of options. You are encouraged to explore additional resources in your own community and work environment to support participation in productive occupations and activities.

References

AARP. (2019). Who's working more? People age 65 and older. AARP Research, Work & Jobs. https://www.aarp.org/work/working-at-50-plus/info-2019/surging-older-workforce.html

AARP. (2020). Retirement communities embrace 3D virtual reality technology. Home and Family, https://www.aarp.org/home-family/personal-technology/info-2020/vr-social-connections.html

Abraham, K. G., & Houseman, S. N. (2020). Policies to improve workforce services for older Americans. Economic Studies at Brookings. https://www.brookings.edu/wp-content/uploads/2020/11/ES-11.19.20-Abraham-Houseman.pdf

Administration on Aging. (2017). Profile of older Americans. https://www.acl.gov/sites/default/files/Aging%20and%20Disability%20in%20America/2017OlderAmericans

American Occupational Therapy Association. (2017). AOTA's societal statement on health literacy. *American Journal of Occupational Therapy, 71*(Suppl. 2), 7112410065. https://doi.org/10.5014/ajot.2017.716S14

American Occupational Therapy Association (2020a). Occupational therapy in the promotion of health and well-being. *American Journal of Occupational Therapy, 74*, 7403420010. https://doi.org/10.5014/ajot.2020.743003

American Occupational Therapy Association. (2020b). Occupational therapy practice framework: Domain and process (4th ed.) *American Journal of Occupational Therapy, 74*(Suppl. 2), 7412410010. https://doi.org/10.5014/ajot.2020.74S2001

American Therapeutic Recreation Association. (2013). Standards for the practice of recreational therapy & self-assessment guide. ATRA Standards of Practice Committee. https://www.atra-online.com/page/SOP?&hhsearchterms=%22standards%22

Anderson, N. D., Damianakis, T., Kröger, E., Wagner, L. M., Dawson, D. R., Binns, M. A., ... & Cook, S. L. (2014). The benefits associated with volunteering among seniors: A critical review and recommendations for future research. *Psychological Bulletin, 140*(6), 1505.

Atchley, R. C. (1989). A continuity theory of normal aging. *The Gerontologist, 29*, 189-190.

Atchley, R. C. (1999). *Continuity and adaptation in aging: Creating positive experiences*. Johns Hopkins University Press.

Baron, B., Kielhofner, G., Iyenger, A., Goldhammer, V. & Wolenski, J. (2006). *Occupational self-assessment (OSA): User manual* (Version 2.2.). Model of Human Occupation Clearinghouse.

Bédard, M., Molloy, D.W., Squire, L, Dubois, S., Lever, J. A., & O'Donnell, M. (2001). The Zarit Burden Interview: A new short version and screening version. *Gerontologist, 41*(5), 652-657. https://doi.org/10.1093/geront/41.5.652.

Braveman, B., Robson, M., Velozo, C., Kielhofner, G., Fisher, F., Forsyth, K., & Kerschbaum, J. (2005). *Worker role interview (WRI) user manual* (Version 10.0.). Model of Human Occupation Clearinghouse.

Brody, T., Chan, A., & Caputi, P. (2010). Comparison of older and younger adults' attitudes towards and abilities with computers: Implications for training and learning. *British Journal of Educational Technology, 41*(3), 473-485. https://doi.org/10.1111/j.1467-8535.2008.00914.x

Brown, J. S., Collins, A., & Duguid, P. (1989). Situated cognition and the culture of learning. *Educational Researcher, 18*(1), 32-42.

Centers for Disease Control and Prevention. (2011). Healthy aging at a glance. http://stacks.cdc.gov/view/cdc/22022

Centers for Disease Control and Prevention. (2021). Health literacy. https://www.cdc.gov/healthliteracy/index.html

Cheng-Shih, L., Mei-Yuan, J., & Tsu-Ming, Y. (2018). The elderly perceived meanings and values of virtual reality leisure activities: A means-end chain approach. *International Journal of Environmental Research and Public Health, 15*, 663. https://doi.org/10.3390/ijerph15040663

Chiu, T., Oliver, R., Ascott, P., Choo., L. C., Davis, T., Gaya, A., . . . Letts, L. (2006). *Safety assessment of functional and the environment for rehabilitation-health outcome measurement and evaluation (SAFER-HOME) version 3 manual.* COTA Health.

Clark et al. (2012). Effectiveness of a lifestyle intervention in promoting the well-being of independently living older people: Results of the Well Elderly 2 randomised controlled trial. *Journal of Epidemiological Community Health, 66*, 782-790. https://doi.org/10.1136/jech.2009.099754

Cramm, J. M., & Nieboer, A. P. (2014). Behavioral characteristics, resources and volunteering among older adults (aged >= 70 years) in the community: a longitudinal study. *Geriatrics & Gerontology International*, 1-9. https://doi.org/10.1111/ggi.12404

Creek, J. (1997). The truth is no longer out there. *British Journal of Occupational Therapy, 60*(2), 50-52. https://doi.org/10.1177/030802269706000202

Dauenhauer, J., Steitz, D. W., & Cochran, L. J. (2016). Fostering a new model of multigenerational learning: Older adult perspectives, community partners, and higher education. *Educational Gerontology, 42*(7), 483-496. https://doi.org/10.1080/03601277.2016.1157419

Dewey, J. (1933). *How we think*. D.C. Heath.

Dury, S., De Donder, L., De Witte, N., Buffel, T., Jacquet, W., & Verté, D. (2015). To volunteer or not: The influence of individual characteristics, resources, and social factors on the likelihood of volunteering by older adults. *Nonprofit and Voluntary Sector Quarterly, 44*(6), 1107-1128. https://doi.org/10.1177/0899764014556773

Ellis, B. (2013). Older undergraduate students bringing years of experience to university studies: Highlights, challenges, and contributions. *Australian Journal of Adult Learning, 53*(3), 351-374.

Family Caregiver Alliance. (2016). Caregiver statistics: Demographics. https://www.caregiver.org/resource/caregiver-statistics-demographics/#

Fauziana, R., Sambasivam, R., Vaingankar, J. A., Abdin, E., Ong, H. L., Tan, M.-E., Chong, S. A., & Subramaniam, M. (2018). Positive caregiving characteristics as a mediator of caregiving burden and satisfaction with life in caregivers of older adults. *Journal of Geriatric Psychiatry and Neurology, 31*(6), 329-335. https://doi.org/10.1177/0891988718802111

Federal Communications Commission. (2017). Strategies for recommendations for promoting digital inclusion. Consumer and Governmental Affairs Bureau. https://www.fcc.gov/document/advancing-broadband-availability-through-digital-literacy-training

Freedman, M. (2007). *Encore: Finding work that matters in the second half of life*. Public Affairs.

Fulmer, T., Mate, K.S., & Berman, A. (2018). The Age-Friendly Health System Imperative. *Journal of the American Geriatrics Society, 66*: 22-24. https://doi.org/10.1111/jgs.15076

Goodman, C. C. (1991). Perceived social support for caregiving measuring the benefit of selfhelp/support group participation. *Journal of Gerontological Social Work, 16*(3-4), 63-175.

Gonzales, E., Matz-Costa, C., & Morrow-Howell, N. (2015). Increasing opportunities for the productive engagement of older adults: A response to population aging. *Gerontologist, 55*(2), 252-261. https://doi.org/11.1093/geront/gnu176

Grünwald, O., Damman, O., & Henkens, K. (2020). Providing informal care next to paid care: Explaining care-giving gratification, burden, and stress among older workers. *Aging & Society*, 1-19. https://doi:10.1017/S0144686X20000215

Hartman, A. (1978). Diagrammatic assessment of family relationships. *Social Casework, 59*, 465-476.

Havighurst, R. J. (1961). Successful aging. *The Gerontologist, 1*, 8-13.

Hinterlong, J. E., Morrow-Howell, N., & Prozario, P. A. (2007). Productive engagement in late life physical and mental health: Finding from a nationally representative panel study. *Research on Aging, 20*, 348-370. https://doi.org/10.1177/0164027507300806

Hussar, W. J., & Bailey, T. M. (2016). Projections of education statistics to 2023 (NCES 2015-073). U.S. Department of Education, National Center for Education Statistics. U.S. Government Printing Office.

Jackson, D. N., Trivedi, N., & Baur, C. (2021) Re-prioritizing digital health and health literacy in Healthy People 2030 to affect health equity. *Health Communication, 36*(10), 1155-1162, DOI: 10.1080/10410236.2020.1748828

Joseph, S., Becker, S., Elwick, H., & Silburn, R. (2012). Adult carers quality of life questionnaire (AC-QoL): Development of an evidence-based tool. *Mental Health Review Journal, 17*(2), 57-69. https://doi.org/10.1108/13619321211270380

Kressley, K. M., & Huebschmann, M. (2002). The 21st century campus: Gerontological perspectives. *Educational Gerontology, 28*, 835-851.

Knight, J., Ball, V., Corr, S., Turner, A., Lowis, M., & Ekberg, M. (2007). An empirical study to identify older adults' engagement in productivity occupations. *Journal of Occupational Science, 14*, 145-153.

Lahey, J. N. (2008). Age, women, and hiring: An experimental study. *The Journal of Human Resources, 43*, 30-56. https://doi.org/10.3368/jhr.43.1.30

Law, M., Baptiste, S., Carswell, A., McColl, M. A., Polatajko, H., & Pollock, N. (2019). *Canadian occupational performance measure* (5th ed.—revised). COPM Inc.

Lazarus, A. (1996). *Behavior therapy & beyond*. Jason Aronson, Inc.

Li, Z. (2021). The Social Security retirement age. Congressional Research Service. https://fas.org/sgp/crs/misc/R44670.pdf

Madden, M. (2010). Older adults and social media. Pew Research Center. https://www.pewresearch.org/internet/2010/08/27/older-adults-and-social-media/

Maestas, N. (2010). Back to work: Expectations and realizations of work after retirement. *Journal of Human Resources, 45*(3), 718-748. https://doi.org/10.1353/jhr.210.0011

Marfeo, E. E., & Ward, C. (2020). Older adults productive activity participation using the National Health and Aging Trends Study. *Gerontology & Geriatrics Medicine, 6*, 1-6. https://doi.org/10.1177/233372/4209/0657

Marwijk, H. W., Wallace, P., de Bock, G. H., Hermans, J., Kaptein, A. A., & Mulder, J. D. (1995). Evaluation of the feasibility, reliability and diagnostic value of shortened versions of the Geriatric Depression Scale. *British Journal of General Practice, 45*, 195-199.

McColl, M. A., Davies, D., Carlson, P., Johnston, J., & Minnes, P. (2001). The community integration measure: development and preliminary validation. *Archives of Physical Medicine and Rehabilitation, 82*, 429-434.

Menec, V. J. (2003). The relation between everyday activities and successful aging: A 6-year longitudinal study. *The Journals of Gerontology, 54B*, S74-S82.

Merriam Webster Online Dictionary. (n.d.) https://www.merriam-webster.com/

Miller, W. R., & Rollnick, S. (2012). *Motivational interviewing: Preparing people for change* (3rd Edition). Guilford Press.

Moore-Corner, R., Kielhofner, G., & Olsen, L. (1998). *A user's guide to Work Environment Impact Scale (WEIS), version 2.0.* Model of Human Occupation Clearinghouse..

Murphy, W. M. & Volpe, E. H. (2014). Encore careers: Motivating factors for career exit and rebirth. In A. M. Broadbridge and S. L. Fielden (Eds.), *Handbook of gendered careers in management* (pp. 425-444). Edward Elgar.

Musick, M. A., & Wilson, J. (2008). *Volunteers: A social profile.* Indiana University Press.

National Institutes of Health. (2021). Health literacy. https://www.nih.gov/institutes-nih/nih-office-director/office-communications-public-liaison/clear-communication/health-literacy

National Prevention Council. (2016). Healthy aging in action. Department of Health and Human Services, Office of the Surgeon General.

Neumark, D., Burn, I. & Button, P. (2019). Is it harder for older workers to find jobs? New and improved evidence from a field experiment. *Journal of Political Economy, 127*(2), 922-970. https://doi.org/10.1086/701029

Pacheco, I. (2014). Self-assessment. http://socialworktech.com/2012/09/10/self-assessment/.

Park, S., Lee, H. J., Jeon, B.-J., Yoo, E.-Y., Kim, J.-B., & Park, J.-H. (2021). Effects of occupational balance on subjective health, quality of life, and health-related variables in community-dwelling older adults: A structural equation modeling approach. *PLoS ONE, 16*(2), e0246887. https://doi.org/10.1371/journal.pone.0246887

Parks, R., Evans, B., & Getch, Y. (2013). Motivations and enculturation of older students returning to university. *New Horizons in Adult Education & Human Resource Development, 25*(3), 62-75.

Parmelee, P., Lawton, M., & Katz, I. (1989). Psychometric properties of the Geriatric Depression Scale among the institutionalized aged. *Psychological Assessment, 1*(4), 331-338.

Queen, T. L., Butner, J., Berg, C. A., & Smith, J. (2019). Activity engagement among older adult spousal caregivers, *The Journals of Gerontology: Series B, 74*(7), 1278-1282. https://doi-org.ezproxy.emich.edu/10.1093/geronb/gbx106

Rabourn, K. E., BrckaLorenz, A., & Shoup, R. (2018). Reimagining student engagement: How nontraditional adult learners engage in traditional postsecondary environments. *The Journal of Continuing Higher Education, 66*(1), 22-33. https://doi.org/10.1080/07377363.2018.1415635

Roberts, A. W., Ogunwole, S. U., Blakeslee, L., & Rabe, M. A. (2018). The population 65 years and older in the United States: 2016. American Community Survey Reports, ACS-38, U.S. Census Bureau.

Rowe, J. W., & Kahn, R. L. (1997). Successful aging. *The Gerontologist, 37*, 433-440.

Scaffa, M. E., & Reitz, S. M. (2020). Work and career transitions. In M. E. Scaffa & S. M. Reitz (Eds.), *Occupational therapy in community and population health practice* (3rd ed., pp. 303-317). F. A. Davis Company.

Schaefer, J. L. (2009). Voices of older baby boomer students: Supporting their transitions back to college. *Educational Gerontology, 36*, 67-90.

Self-Management Resource Center (n.d.). https://www.selfmanagementresource.com/

Silverstein, N. M., Choi, L. H., & Bulot, J. J. (2002). Older learners on campus. *Geriatrics Education, 22*(1), 13-30.

Simon, A., Masinda, S., & Zakrajsek, A. (2020). Age-friendly university environmental scan: Exploring "age-friendliness" with stakeholders at one regional comprehensive university. *Gerontology & Geriatrics Education*. https://doi.org/10.1080/02701960.2020.1783259

Singh, B., & Kiran, U. V. (2014) Recreational activities for senior citizens. *Journal of Humanities and Social Science, 19*(4), 24-30. https://doi.org/10.9790/0837-19472430

Stav, W. B., Hellenen, T., Lane, J., & Arbesman, M. (2012). Systematic review of occupational engagement and health outcomes among community-dwelling older adults. *American Journal of Occupational Therapy, 66*, 301-301. http://dx.doi.org/10.5014/ajot.2012.003707

Stebbins, R. (2015). *Serious leisure—A perspective for out time*. Transaction Publishers.

Talmage, C. A., Mark, R., Slowey, M., & Knopf, R. C. (2016). Age friendly universities and engagement with older adults: Moving form principles to practice. *International Journal of Lifelong Education, 35*(5), 537-554.

Taylor, R. R. (Ed.). (2017). *Kielhofner's model of human occupation: Theory and application* (3rd ed.). Wolters Kruwer.

Terrell, K. (2018). Age Discrimination common in workplace, survey says. AARP. https://www.aarp.org/work/working-at-50-plus/info-2018/age-discrimination-common-at-work.html

Tuijt, R., Tan, A., Armstrong, M., Pigott, J., Read, J., Davies, N., ... & Schrag, A (2020). Self-management components as experienced by people with Parkinson's Disease and their carers: A systematic review and synthesis of the qualitative literature. Parkinson's Disease. https://doi.org/10.1155/2020/8857385

U.S. Department of Health and Human Services. (2018). Healthy People 2030 framework. https://www.healthypeople.gov/2020/About-Healthy-People/Development-Healthy-People-2030/Framework

U.S., Department of Labor (n.d.). Older workers. https://www.dol.gov/agencies/odep/program-areas/individuals/older-workers

U.S. Government Services and Administration. (n.d.) https://www.usa.gov/#tpcs

World Health Organization. (n.d.). WHO global network for age-friendly cities and communities. https://www.who.int/ageing/projects/age_friendly_cities_network/en/

World Health Organization. (2015). World report on aging and health. WHO Press. http://apps.who.int/iris/bitstream/handle/10665/186463/9789240694811_eng.pdf;jsessionid=0BBD7582A1693DA5128B0A93425A845F?sequence=1

Zarit, S. H. & Zarit, J. M. (1983). Cognitive impairment. In P. M. Lewinsohn & L. Teri (Eds.), *Clinical geropsychology* (pp. 38-81). Pergamon Press.

Appendix A: Enhancing Individual Capacity to Promote Change in Engagement in Productive Occupations Through Motivational Interviewing

Motivational interviewing (MI) is a useful tool for community-based practitioners to use in supporting motivation to change in individuals who are seeking to enhance health, well-being, and participation in productive activities and occupations. Initially developed by William Miller and Stephen Rollnick as a counseling approach focused on changing addictive behaviors, MI has evolved and been adopted by health professionals from various disciplines as an intervention to foster people's ability to find their own motivation to change. The process of MI includes four key steps as described by Miller and Rollnick (2012): 1) Engaging, 2) Focusing, 3) Evoking, and 4) Planning.

FOUR STEPS OF MOTIVATIONAL INTERVIEWING PROCESS

Motivational Interviewing Step	*Aim*	*Examples of Questioning*
1. Engaging	Establish a helpful connection and working relationship	• I'm glad you are here. What is your goal for our conversation today? • What issues are important to you? • How do you hope that I might be able to help you?
2. Focusing	Develop and maintain a specific direction in the conversation about change	• What are the biggest problems you would like to address? What do you think is getting in the way? • You've mentioned a few items (name them). Where would you like to start?
3. Evoking	Use the focus on a particular change and harness the client's own ideas/feelings about why and how they might do it	• What ideas do you have for how you could_____? • How might you like things to be different (5 years from now)? • How does _____interfere with the things you like to do? • What needs to happen?
4. Planning	Develop a commitment to change and formulate a specific plan of action	• What would be a reasonable next step toward change for you? • Where does all this leave you? • So, what do you think you will do? • I wonder what you might decide to do.

Adapted from Miller, W. R., & Rollnick, S. (2012). *Motivational interviewing: Preparing people for change* (3rd ed.). Guilford Press.

Furthermore, the facilitator of a MI should keep in mind the following facilitation strategies while facilitating the steps of the conversation: asking open-ended questions, affirming one's desire and ability to change, applying reflective listening, and summarizing with the intention to identify action steps. As community-based practitioners serve older adults who have goals that focus on changing participation in productive occupations and activities, the MI process can be a very useful approach.

Reference

Miller, W. R. & Rollnick, S. (2012). *Motivational interviewing: Preparing people for change* (3rd ed.). Guilford Press.

Appendix B: Health Literacy to Support Participation in Productive Occupations of Older Adults

Health care professionals and organizations have an obligation to the persons, communities, and populations they serve to provide information that is easily understandable to inform decisions for health and well-being. This obligation reflects the practice of health literacy, or the ability to easily obtain and understand basic health information needed to make informed health decisions and includes an emphasis on making health information accessible at the personal, organizational, and digital levels (AOTA, 2017; CDC, 2021; Jackson et al., 2021). Healthy People 2030 has identified health literacy as a part of one of their five major goals to "eliminate health disparities, achieve health equity, and attain health literacy to improve the health and well-being of all" (U.S. Department of Health and Human Services [DHHS], 2018, para. 11).

Specific professions of community-based practitioners have explicitly indicated a commitment to health literacy as part of practice. For example, the profession of occupational therapy has identified health literacy as an ethical consideration when working with individuals, groups, and populations and as part of a larger role in health management and maintenance (AOTA, 2020a). Furthermore, the AOTA developed a societal statement on health literacy, promoting the positive impact health literacy has on occupational participation and well-being and the profession's commitment to facilitating health literacy among the people, groups, and communities they serve (AOTA, 2017).

However, it is the personal responsibility for practitioners to commit to health literacy, in communicating health information in an accessible and effective manner. The Center for Disease Control and Prevention and the National Institutes of Health have available training opportunities, community resources, research, and toolkits for health professionals and health care teams to learn, identify, and apply health literacy principles (CDC, 2021; National Institutes of Health, 2021). Addressing health literacy in community dwelling older adults can promote informed decision making to support healthy participation and engagement in meaningful and productive occupations.

References

American Occupational Therapy Association. (2017). AOTA's societal statement on health literacy. *American Journal of Occupational Therapy, 71*(Suppl. 2), 7112410065. https://doi.org/10.5014/ajot.2017.716S14

American Occupational Therapy Association. (2020a). Occupational therapy in the promotion of health and well-being. *American Journal of Occupational Therapy, 74*, 7403420010. https://doi.org/10.5014/ajot.2020.743003

Centers for Disease Control and Prevention. (2021). *Health literacy basics*. https://www.cdc.gov/healthliteracy/basics.html

National Institutes of Health. (2021). Health literacy. https://www.nih.gov/institutes-nih/nih-office-director/office-communications-public-liaison/clear-communication/health-literacy

U.S. Department of Health and Human Services. (2018). Healthy People 2030 framework. https://www.healthypeople.gov/2020/About-Healthy-People/Development-Healthy-People-2030/Framework

Appendix C: Health Management to Support Participation in Productive Occupations of Older Adults

Older adults, over the age of 65 years, make up the largest proportion of the population and these numbers are expected to grow (Administration on Aging, 2017). This population is disproportionately affected by chronic diseases, such as heart disease, diabetes, stroke, and arthritis. In fact, 80% of the older adult population has at least one chronic condition (CDC, 2011). Self-management of chronic diseases has been a focus of community-based interprofessional practice in order to enable participation in meaningful productive occupations. Evidence-based self-management programs, such as the Chronic Disease Self-Management Program, which was developed and tested at the Stanford University Patient Education Center, offer community-based practitioners (Self-Management Resource Center, n.d.). Key components of self-management approaches include: 1) medication management, 2) physical exercise, 3) self-monitoring, 4) psychological strategies, 5) maintaining independence, 6) social engagement, and 7) knowledge and information (Tuijt et al., 2020). The Self-Management Resource Center (https://www.selfmanagementresource.com/; Self-Management Resource Center, n.d.) provides resources, training, and programs. By managing health, older adults have the more physical resources to participate in productive occupations, such as paid and unpaid work, leisure, and education.

References

Administration on Aging. (2017). *Profile of older Americans.* https://www.acl.gov/sites/default/files/Aging%20and%20Disability%20in%20America/2017OlderAmericans

Centers for Disease Control and Prevention. (2011). *Healthy aging at a glance.* http://stacks.cdc.gov/view/cdc/22022

Self-Management Resource Center. (n.d.). https://www.selfmanagementresource.com/

Tuijt, R., Tan, A., Armstrong, M., Pigott, J., Read, J., Davies, N., … & Schrag, A (2020). Self-management components as experienced by people with Parkinson's Disease and their carers: A systematic review and synthesis of the qualitative literature. *Parkinson's Disease.* https://doi.org/10.1155/2020/8857385

Appendix D: Case Study to Further Examine Barriers, Health Management, and Health Literacy

Cha, an 80-year-old Hmong widowed woman, lives with her oldest son and his family of six in a city with a population of approximately 70,000 residents. She immigrated from Laos with her husband and two oldest children in the 1960s. In Laos she had lived in a rural farming village. Cha has no formal education, has never worked outside of her home, and speaks and understands limited English. Cha cannot read English or Hmong and can only print her name in English. Cha has a history of untreated hypertension and diabetes and now has to start dialysis at the local dialysis center due to end-stage renal disease.

Reflective Questions

1. Considering supports and barriers at the individual, community, or population level (see Figure 12-1), what might impact Cha's engagement in productive occupations?
2. What professionals in the community and dialysis center may be able to assist Cha?
3. What ways might you make health information understandable to Cha so she can make informed decisions?
4. In a situation in which you are working with an older adult, as a community-based professional, what cultural considerations may there be when considering health management?

Part V

PROMOTING MENTAL AND EMOTIONAL HEALTH

CHAPTER 13

Promoting Mental and Emotional Health
Children and Youth

Tina Champagne, OT, OTD, OTR, FAOTA and Catherine Cavaliere, PhD, OTR/L

Learning Objectives

At the end of this chapter, the reader will:

1. At the end of this chapter the reader will understand how community and family health impacts the mental health of children and adolescents (ACOTE B.3.1)
2. At the end of this chapter the reader will understand the protective and risk factors that impact child and adolescent mental health (ACOTE B.3.2)
3. At the end of this chapter the reader will understand the application of a public health model to community, family, child, and adolescent mental health (ACOTE B.4.27)
4. At the end of this chapter the reader will be able to understand some of the interprofessional contributions that support community, family, child, and adolescent mental health (ACOTE B.4.23)

The ACOTE Standards used are those from 2018.

Key Words

Adverse Childhood Experiences, Attachment, Attunement, Co-Regulation, Determinants of Health, Health, Health Disparities, Health Equity, Mental Health Prevention, Mental Health Promotion, Occupational Justice, Public Health Model, Resilience, Secure Base, Self-Regulation, Socioecological Contexts, Stress Response, Suicidal Ideation, Suicide, Toxic Stress, Trauma

Pizzi, M. A., & Amir, M. (Eds.). *Interprofessional Perspectives for Community Practice: Promoting Health, Well-Being, and Quality of Life* (pp. 239-262).

Case Study

Karl is a 9-year-old boy living with his grandparents who have custody of he and his sister Ivy. Both Karl and Ivy are receiving care in different residential programs. This is due to having had trauma histories in early childhood. They continue to struggle with safety, self-regulation, coping with loss, and functionally participating in daily routines and occupations. Karl's mother used substances while she was pregnant and both she and his father had mental health and substance abuse challenges. Both children were taken into protective custody until the grandparents were able to get custody back. Karl and Ivy's mother passed away when they were 8 and their father is in jail serving a 10-year sentence on substance abuse–related matters. The grandparents are of a low socioeconomic status. Karl and Ivy have and continue to experience trauma, loss, and other adverse childhood experiences during their early and formative developmental years. This case vignette will be elaborated on and referred to at different points throughout this chapter, demonstrating how some of the concepts and interventions explored are relevant to child, adolescent, and family mental health and well-being.

Introduction

The World Health Organization (WHO) defines **health** as, "a state of complete physical, mental and social well-being and not merely the absence of disease or infirmity" (WHO, 2017). Across the life span, mental health is an integral part of one's overall health status. The vision of the Healthy People 2030 (n.d.) framework is a society in which all people can achieve their full potential for health and well-being across the life span. This reference to all persons includes children and youth, with and without disabilities. Healthy People 2030's overarching goals are to:

- Attain healthy, thriving lives and well-being free of preventable disease, disability, injury, and premature death.
- Eliminate health disparities, achieve health equity, and attain health literacy to improve the health and well-being of all.
- Create social, physical, and economic environments that promote attaining the full potential for health and well-being for all.
- Promote healthy development, healthy behaviors, and well-being across all life stages.
- Engage leadership, key constituents, and the public across multiple sectors to take action and design policies that improve the health and well-being of all (Office of Disease Prevention and Health Promotion, n.d.).

Health equity refers to the right of all people, communities, and populations to equality in health, including mental/emotional health (Brennan Ramirez et al., 2008). **Health disparities** are differences in both the incidence and prevalence of health conditions and/or health status between groups of people. Health disparities often occur among people or populations that are vulnerable and/or marginalized, as with some of the following: differences in gender, sexual orientation, race/ethnicity, socioeconomic status, disability status, geographic (socioecological) setting, community or location, or any combination of these factors (Braveman et al., 2015). **Socioecological contexts** include the individual (age, genetics, health, education, income, social and emotional strengths, etc.), relationships (those within one's closest social circle), communities (neighborhoods, schools, workplaces, online communities), and societal factors (discrimination, historical trauma, media portrayal of social issues, widespread epidemics, etc.).

The conditions within the socioecological contexts can also impact health disparities, such as the communities and places where children and adolescents live, play, go to school, volunteer or work, and obtain health care services. For instance, health and school-related outcomes have been linked to the lack of stable and quality housing, thereby are included as **determinants of health** for youth (Cohen & Wardrip, 2011). Health determinants are the personal, social, economic, and environmental factors that influence health status. (Healthy People 2020, n.d). Unhealthy living conditions can have long-term negative health influences as well (e.g., exposure to lead, chronic dampness and mold, tobacco smoke, and pests), and housing mobility and instability can lead to negative consequences in children's academic performance. Access to health care and early intervention services, healthy nutrition, education, volunteer, employment and economic opportunities, and social supports are critical to health outcomes, including mental health of children and youth. For example, caretakers earning minimum wage do not have the ability to consistently purchase healthy foods that often cost more money. In addition, they may not live in areas with grocery stores that carry healthy and affordable options. Poor nutrition can adversely affect the mental health and development of infants, children, and adolescents (O'Neil et al., 2014).

Infant, child, and adolescent health status varies by race and ethnicity, family income, access to health insurance (Larson & Halfon, 2010), as does high-quality health care (Long et al., 2012). The cognitive, emotional, and physical development of infants and children is influenced by the health, nutrition, and mental health status and behaviors of their mothers during pregnancy and early childhood (Larson & Halfon, 2010). Access to resources to meet one's daily health and safety-related needs, such as the promotion of maternity care and related practices such as the promotion of breastfeeding (USDHHS, 2011), and having access to sleep environments that are safe, has a direct influence on maternal health status, health-related behaviors, and ultimately the health of future generations (Hoelscher et al., 2010). The *Roadmap to Reducing Child Poverty* (RRCP) outlines the links between child poverty, health, and wellness, and compares a variety of child and family assistance programs (National

Academies of Sciences, Engineering, and Medicine, 2019). Further, the research reviewed in the RRCP reveals evidence that low economic resources negatively impact a child's ability to develop (including potential mental health challenges) and achieve success into adulthood.

Related to the Healthy People 2030 vision and to health equity is the concept of **occupational justice (OJ)**. OJ refers to a type of justice that recognizes rights to inclusive participation in everyday meaningful activities (occupations) for all persons in society, regardless of age, ability, gender, social class, or other differences (Wilcock & Townsend, 2014). Participation in meaningful roles, routines, and occupations contributes to people's health and well-being and is essential to the development of identity and perceptions of competence and value (American Occupational Therapy Association [AOTA], 2014). The Participatory Occupational Justice Framework (POJF) describes structural factors and contextual factors that support or restrict occupational outcomes and occupational rights. Structural factors include underlying determinants such as economic conditions and federal policies as well as local and federal programs to support health, employment, and educational programs. Contextual factors include individual factors that within varying contexts can impact occupational outcomes (justice or injustice), these can include age, gender, sexual orientation, and ability/disability (Whiteford & Townsend, 2011). Issues related to OJ can have a significant impact on the mental health and well-being of children, youth, and families in that the lack of opportunities afforded to families (i.e., limited access to quality health care and education, employment opportunities, and a safe living environment), directly impacts the mental health and development of infants, children, and youth. For instance, Romero and Lee (2008) found that children from low-income families are more likely to be exposed to stressors that may threaten their cognitive and emotional development. Risk factors, including living in poverty, having a teenage parent, living in a single-parent household, low levels of parental education, unemployment, food insecurity, and poor parental health are associated with higher levels of absenteeism from school, leading to poor academic performance, and an increased risk of dropping out of school (Romero & Lee, 2008), which can have long-term negative impacts on mental health and OJ.

Human trafficking is another example of occupational injustice as well as trauma. Human trafficking encompasses exploitation that can include sexual activities, labor practices, domestic servitude, forced marriage, debt bondage, organ removal and trafficking, child soldiers, and any type of slavery practices (International Labour Organization [ILO], 2012). Victims and survivors of trafficking undergo occupational deprivation that can limit engagement in activities of daily living, formal education, social participation, and meaningful occupational pursuits (Bryant et al., 2021). This deprivation, compounded by lack of medical, mental health, and dental care, often results in considerable developmental delays (DDs), sensory-related deficiencies, and extensive biopsychosocial impairments.

Determinants of Child and Adolescent Mental Health

Determinants of health as defined above are the many different factors that impact the health of individuals, families, communities, and populations and are very much related to, and often referred to as, protective factors and risk factors (Office of Disease Prevention and Health Promotion., n.d.).

Protective and Risk Factors

Protective factors reduce the chance of mental health problems developing. Risk factors increase the chances that mental health problems will develop. See Table 13-1 for examples of mental health protective and risk factors in children and adolescents. Protective factors support occupational justice in that they provide a set of multitiered circumstances that allow an individual to engage in self-identified activities that are meaningful, and support health and well-being. It is well accepted that families, children, and youth possessing a diverse set of protective factors experience more positive outcomes. Further, children reared in safe and nurturing families and neighborhoods, with minimal instances of maltreatment or other adverse childhood experiences, are more likely to have better health outcomes as adults (Felitti et al., 1998; Anda et al., 2010). By coming together to explore and better understand the complex interactions between structural and contextual factors that impact communities, families, and child health, health professionals can work together to reduce health disparities and improve the conditions that promote health equity, occupational justice, and protective factors.

Stress and Toxic Stress

Stress and trauma are common experiences of children and adolescents, and therefore, also impact child and adolescent mental health. In fact, over the last several decades, there has been a significant increase in the interdisciplinary health science research on the prevalence and impact of stress, adversity, and trauma as contributing factors to health outcomes among individuals, communities, and populations (Carr et al., 2013). **Stress** is a term used to describe the neurophysiological response that occurs when a person experiences a challenge or some type of demand (Selye, 1956). The **stress response** is the term used to describe the

Table 13-1

Factors Associated With Positive Development and Prevention of Mental Health Problems Over Time

	INDIVIDUAL	FAMILY	SCHOOL AND COMMUNITY
Infancy and early childhood	• Secure attachment • Emotional regulation • Appropriate conduct • Making friends • Understanding self and others' emotions	• Adequate prenatal and postnatal health care • Nurturing relationship with caregiver (reliable, responsive, affectionate) • Support for the development of new skills	• Availability of high-quality childcare • Support for early learning • Access to supplemental services, such as screening for vision/hearing • Low ratio of caregivers
Middle childhood	• Academic achievement • Appropriate behavior • Positive peer relationships • Resilience (ability to adapt to life stressors) • Empathy • Satisfying friendships	• Emotionally responsive interactions with children • Consistent discipline • Language-based rather than physically based discipline • Parental resources, including positive personal efficacy and adaptive coping	• High academic standards and strong leadership • Teacher support • Effective classroom management • Positive family–school relations • School policies and practices to reduce bullying
Adolescence	• Physical health • Intellectual development • Psychological and emotional development • Social development • Connectiveness to peers, family, and community	• Physical and psychological safety • Appropriate structures (limits, rules, predictability) • Supportive relationships • Opportunities to belong • Positive social norms (expectations, values) • Opportunities for skill building • Integration to family, school, and community	• Physical and psychological safety • Appropriate structure (limits, rules, predictability) • Supportive relationships • Opportunities to belong • Positive social norms (expectations, values) • Opportunities for skill building • Integration to family, school, and community
Early adulthood	• Explore identity in love, work, and worldview (e.g., values) to obtain a broad range of life experiences and move toward making commitments around which to structure adult life • Subjective sense of adult status in self-sufficiency, making independent decisions, becoming financially independent • Future orientation and achievement motivation	• Behavioral and emotional autonomy • Balance of autonomy and relatedness to family	• Opportunities for exploration in school and work • Connectiveness to adults outside of family

Reproduced with permission from O'Connell, M. E., Boar, T., & Warner, K. E. (Eds.). (2009). Using a developmental framework to guide prevention and promotion. In *Preventing mental, emotional, and behavioral disorders among young people: Progress and possibilities* (pp. 78-80). National Academies Press.

neurophysiological processes occurring within the human body when experiencing stress at any age. In recent years, it has been emphasized that stress is not always health damaging. When stress is at a moderate level, not prolonged, and helpful in nature it is often referred to as eustress. For instance, stress is important to support attention to task, the ability to perform, meet deadlines, and can, therefore, be used for optimization of function at times (Crum et al.,

2020). **Toxic stress** occurs when a child or adolescent encounters frequent, prolonged, and/or intense stress that they are unable to control or diminish.

Trauma

Trauma is an experience that overwhelms the ability to cope with what is happening and to integrate the experience (American Psychiatric Association [APA], 2013). The more severe the overwhelm in the face of little or no support, the more severe the impact in most cases. Both stress and trauma can be acute (single event or situation that is short in duration), chronic (multiple trauma experiences over time), or complex (cumulative, often starting in childhood and continuing over longer timeframes). When stress becomes chronic or complex it can cause health problems such as high blood pressure, high blood sugar levels, difficulty fighting off infection, inflammation, depression, anxiety (Felitti et al., 1998; Anda et al., 2010). Many aspects of infant, child, and adolescent development may be seriously impacted by chronic, complex, or toxic stress, adversity and trauma, particularly when these experiences occur before the age of 5, in which crucial and highly sensitive periods of development occur. The magnitude of the cumulative effects of traumatic experiences in children and adolescents cannot be underestimated. According to the APA (2013), to say that an individual has experienced trauma requires that they have experienced "actual or threatened death, serious injury, or sexual violence" (p. 271). According to the Substance Abuse and Mental Health Services Administration (SAMHSA, 2020a), however, traumatic events in an individual's life may include:

- Neglect and psychological, physical, or sexual abuse
- Natural disasters, terrorism, and community and school violence
- Witnessing or experiencing intimate partner violence
- Commercial sexual exploitation
- Serious accidents, life-threatening illness, or sudden or violent loss of a loved one
- Refugee and war experiences
- Military family-related stressors, such as parental deployment, loss, or injury (SAMHSA, 2020a, p. 1)

While the different trauma-related diagnoses (APA, 2013) are not part of the focus of this chapter, it is important to note that the understanding of what constitutes trauma, traumatic events, and the similarities and differences when experienced at different or multiple points across one's life span, has been of significant study in recent years. This initiative has enriched our understanding of what constitutes stress and/or trauma and how it impacts human beings across the life span.

All types of trauma can impact family, child, and adolescent development and health; however, chronic and complex trauma can have very serious and widespread effects. When trauma occurs in utero and/or during the first 5 years, the nervous system is forming and is particularly vulnerable (Perry, 2009; van der Kolk, 2014). In fact, the APA (2013) created additional criterion under the diagnosis of post-traumatic stress disorder (PTSD), which speaks to the impact of trauma when experienced before the age of 6 years, due to the sensitive periods of development that occur up until that age. Thus, it is not uncommon to see a variety of developmental challenges emerge (e.g., emotion dysregulation, hypersensitivities, fine motor, muscle tone, and/or challenges with body coordination, dyspraxia; Perry, 2009; van der Kolk, 2014). We also know that chronic stress and/or trauma experienced by a mother during pregnancy may negatively impact the developing fetus (Smith et al., 2016). This does not discount the impact of trauma at other times across the childhood and adolescent years, rather it demonstrates how certain developmental challenges may occur as a result given that different types of sensitive periods occur at different age ranges. Further, it is now well documented that when experienced during childhood and adolescence, stress, and trauma may negatively influence overall health as well as family and school participation, social and community participation, and other child and adolescent roles, routines, and occupations. Signs of traumatic stress in young children at different stages of development may include some of the following:

- **Preschool age**: Difficulty eating or sleeping, crying a lot, nightmares, fearful of being separated from caregivers (unless caregiver is source of stress/trauma)
- **Elementary age**: Difficulty eating or sleeping, school refusal, anxiety, feelings of guilt or shame, difficulty with attention and/or concentration, aggression
- **Middle school**: Feelings of depression, feeling alone or that they don't belong, difficulty with eating or sleeping, self-injurious behaviors, experimenting with smoking or substances, becoming sexually active, and increased anxiety, anger, and aggression (SAMHSA, 2020b)

As we learn more about stress and trauma in children with DDs such as autism spectrum disorder (ASD), we are beginning to understand that children with disabilities may be more prone neurologically and physiologically to experiencing stress and toxic stress (Stack & Lucyshyn, 2018). In addition, children with DDs have communication challenges, are socially more naïve, and can experience social isolation making them more susceptible to adverse experiences that may go unidentified. Behaviors associated with some children with ASD, such as self-injury, and sensory processing challenges are also common to individuals who have experienced trauma, thereby making discrimination between ASD and the side effects of trauma clinically challenging (Brenner et al., 2017). Further, families of children with DDs experience high levels of familial stress (Stack & Lucyshyn, 2018). Thus, children with disabilities may be more prone to trauma-related symptomology.

Adolescence is the time in development where the child is transitioning toward and into adulthood—physically, cognitively, socially, and emotionally maturing. Adolescent health is significantly impacted by the early and foundational developmental periods of childhood, which includes the health determinants over time (Viner et al., 2012). In addition, similar to the early childhood period, the adolescent years also bring critical periods of development. The adolescent period, ages 9 to 25 years, is characterized by intense physical, physiologic, social/emotional, psychosocial, and cognitive growth. It is during this time that adolescents develop a sense of self and a sense of belonging in the world. Peer relationships and belonging to a social group become highly important. During this time, adolescents develop their moral and spiritual compass. This period of intense psychosocial, emotional, moral, and spiritual growth presents a set of challenges that, if not met with nurturance and support at varying levels, can lead to mental health challenges. Some examples of mental health, occupational challenges, and health risk behaviors that may begin to emerge during adolescence include (but are not limited to):

- Academic challenges
- Self-injurious behaviors
- Mental health symptoms/diagnoses (e.g., depression, anxiety)
- Suicidal ideation/suicide
- Homicidal ideation/homicide
- Smoking and/or substance use/abuse
- Motor vehicle accidents
- Nutrition and weight conditions
- Homelessness
- Sexually transmitted infections/diseases
- Teen/unintended pregnancies
- Challenges related to sexual identity and coming out (LGBTQ)
- Violence and victimization related to bullying and/or hazing

Since adolescents are in such a significant transitional period of development, across so many areas (e.g., biological, social, educational), adolescents are particularly sensitive to the pressures of this time of life (growing into becoming more independent) and to social experiences. With peer groups taking an increasingly more prominent role in the lives of teens, in addition to their families and communities, these social/relational experiences are critical influencers. School, community, and media further influence impressionable youth during this phase of development. Many events signifying rites of passage from childhood toward adulthood include but are not limited to, learning to drive, going to prom/dances, dating, playing competitive sports, volunteering or working, and more independence from family as the emphasis shifts on participating more socially with one's peer group(s). Some examples of programs and policies that support adolescent health include:

- School-based health care, including social/emotional support
- Clubs, sports, and other health supporting extracurricular activities
- Smoking and substance abuse prevention programs
- Violence prevention in schools and communities
- Anti-bullying initiatives
- Vocational programs
- Driver's education programs
- Teen pregnancy and sexually transmitted disease prevention

At the community and population level, stress, toxic stress and trauma can result from some of the following: homelessness, unsafe living environments, lack of access to health and other resources, lack of access to an equitable education, fear, and oppression. Collective trauma affects communities of people throughout generations and is often significantly correlated with challenges with health equity and occupational justice. As professionals, we must be aware of the impact that these factors can have on communities, families, and children and consciously take action to promote the health and well-being of all persons.

Adversity and Resiliency

Adverse childhood experiences are those that are traumatic or potentially traumatic in nature and experienced during ages 0 to 17 years (Felitti et al., 1998). A seminal study known as the **Adverse Childhood Experiences** (ACEs) study revealed many important facts related to the impact of ACEs on mental/emotional health as well as other health outcomes (Felitti et al., 1998; Anda et al., 2010). The ACEs defined in this study included the following categories: *abuse* (physical, sexual, or verbal, and physical or emotional neglect) and *household challenges* (having a household or family member with depression, mental illness, substance abuse, or has made a suicide attempt, or one that is incarcerated, witnessing domestic violence, and parental separation, divorce, or loss). Having an ACE score of 4 or more (i.e., 4 out of these 10 experiences) puts and individual at high risk for chronic physical and mental health conditions as an adult (e.g., asthma, heart disease, autoimmune disorders, disrupted neurodevelopment, health risk behaviors, trauma-related symptoms and mental health challenges, difficulty reaching one's full potential, and early death). Initially, the ACE study was focused on factors related to obesity that inadvertently discovered other very important information on the health outcomes of people who had experienced ACEs. It was found that ACEs are very common experiences with approximately two-thirds of adults reporting at least one. Such experiences have been linked to not only mental/emotional health challenges in adulthood but also to chronic diseases such as heart disease, cancer, and other physical health problems.

Table 13-2

Risk and Protective Factors Associated With Positive Mental Health

	POSITIVE FACTORS	RISK FACTORS
Individual	• Positive sense of self • Good physical health • Effective social skills • Close relationship to family • Good coping skills	• Low self-esteem • Chronic illness or physical disability • Poor social skills • Insecure attachment to family • Poor coping skills
Social	• Caring and supportive parents • Positive early attachment • Sense of belonging • Supportive relationships • Participation in the community	• Social isolation • Abuse, neglect, and/or violence • Peer rejection • Separation and loss
Systems	• Safe living environment • Economic security • Positive educational experience • Access to health and other supports	• Neighborhood violence and crime • Poverty • Unemployment • Homelessness • School failure • Lack of health and other supports

Adapted with permission from Barry, M. M., & Jenkins, R. (2007). *Implementing mental health promotion*. Churchill Livingston/Elsevier.

This study helped to broaden the scope of what was viewed as extreme stress vs. traumatic, which again is a very subjective experience. This study also significantly expanded the understanding of the tremendous impact that ACEs has on health and well-being across the life span.

Significant trauma in early childhood is exemplified by the case study of Karl and Ivy. They report having always been hungry, witnessing their parents fight and physically harm each other. Their mother used substances while pregnant and received minimal prenatal care during each pregnancy. Both parents had mental health challenges and struggled to care for themselves and their children. It is noteworthy that both parents experienced ACEs as they grew up as well; this demonstrates the intergenerational nature that ACEs and trauma can have. The Department of Social Services removed both children from the home when Karl was 5 and Ivy was 6 years old. They have both experienced extreme early childhood trauma, neglect, and have many ACEs. Both entered into the foster care system until the grandparents were able to adopt them.

Resilience is the capacity to overcome hardships experienced across the life span (King et al., 2018). Some refer to it as the ability to "bounce back" after facing adversity, including trauma. The more protective factors that a family or individual possess the more resilient they may be when faced with life stressors. Protective factors help to combat the neurophysiological cascade of changes that goes into play when facing stress, trauma, adversity and injustices thereby, supporting health and wellness even when these issues do occur. Protective factors include some of the following: stable, competent, and supportive caregiving that includes positive parenting approaches, parental resilience, developmental competencies (i.e., social, emotional, self-regulation, problem-solving skills), having a sense of purpose (through identity, cultural, spiritual means), supports such as activities and social connections that contribute to health and personal growth (i.e., team or community-based activities, social clubs) are just some examples. See Table 13-2 for developmental factors associated with supporting positive mental health (Bazyk & Arbesman, 2013, p. 8).

Social-Emotional Development and Attachment

Children's social-emotional development provides them the capacity to experience, manage, and express both positive and negative emotions, develop satisfying relationships with other children and adults, and actively explore their environment and learn (Pontoppidan et al., 2017). Early childhood (birth to 3 years) is an especially important period for social and emotional development. At the core of social-emotional development is the attuned caregiver relationship. **Attunement** refers to the ability to "tune into" and respond to the sensory, emotional, and relational needs and experiences of another person, ultimately resulting in a deeper connection. This interpersonal and relational connection, also referred to as **attachment**, refers to the relational bond between the primary caregiver(s) and child, which includes the ability to attune to each other, and to develop and maintain a loving relationship over time (Bowlby, 1968). Much of the health outcomes of children and adolescents is dependent largely on the attachment relationship or bond between the infant/child and primary caregiver(s). Research has demonstrated the importance of the attuned caregiver attachment relationship in the developmental throughout childhood and into adulthood. Children who are separated from their parents at a young age, particularly under the age of 3 years, are at significantly higher risk of physical, mental, and developmental disorders in childhood and into adulthood (Paksarian et al., 2015; Liu et al., 2010). Parent and child separation has become an increasing issue globally. Migration (people leaving rural areas to find jobs in urban areas) has resulted in a growing number of "left-behind children" (LBC) when their parents migrate to find work, particularly in low- or middle-income countries. Shi et al. (2021) found that the rate of social-emotional problems among children who are left behind in rural China is 36.8%.

Studies have also shown an association between caregivers' depressive symptoms and the emergence of social-emotional problems, speculated to be due to decreased responsivity in the parenting relationship, lower levels of daily stimulation and acceptance, and other variables often found in struggling home environments (Tan et al., 2020). Further, elevated and chronic symptoms of negative affect, can impede a mother's recognition or tolerance of the needs of her baby, which may, in turn, negatively impact the infant's social-emotional development (Gentile, 2017; Kingston et al., 2012). Elevated maternal negative affect during pregnancy, has also been linked to increased risk for psychopathology in the child including anxiety, depression, attention deficit hyperactivity disorder (ADHD), and schizophrenia (Monk et al., 2019). Thus, the developmental capacity, to attune and attach in a healthy, relational manner with one's primary caregiver(s), is foundational to the development of a positive sense of self, the ability to connect with others, self-regulate and co-regulate—this capacity in whole is referred to as a **secure base** (Bowlby, 1968). The secure base is a significant influence on all aspects of child development. Further, the secure base is responsible for the development of self- and co-regulation skills, which are the building blocks to social-emotional development, can be considered foundational to mental health and well-being in children and support the future mental health and wellness.

Self-regulation may be considered the ability to achieve and maintain a state of homeostasis in the face of ongoing changes, needs, and challenges by adapting to the environment, daily routine, and relational and activity demands at hand. This includes neurophysiological regulation, emotional regulation, behavioral regulation, and sensory and cognitive regulation. In infancy, self-regulation is developing across all of these areas with a particular emphasis on neurophysiological, in that the infant's nervous system is still developing and attempting to adapt to life outside of the womb. The caregiver is the primary conduit of regulation for the infant in that he/she/they meets the infants relational and basic needs, which otherwise would not be sufficiently met, such as the need for food, loving care, and comfort (Bowlby, 1968). As the infant develops, cognitive, sensory, relational, and behavioral flexibility and adaptability (that is supported by an increasingly more flexible neurophysiological state) develops, which helps the infant learn to manage emotions and behaviors (Ayres, 1979; Blaustein & Kinniburgh, 2018; Perry, 2009). Thus, building the capacity for self-regulation is very much influenced by the early and attuned caregiver relationship, leading also to the ability for **co-regulation**. Co-regulation is an interpersonal process that supports the ability to simultaneously regulate with another person and adapt behavior accordingly. The ability to co-regulate is a skill that develops over time that is foundational to developing the ability to acquire and maintain relational connections, to attune to others, and to feel a sense of safety within close relationships, thereby supporting optimal growth and maturation (Blaustein & Kinniburgh, 2018). Further, this developmental process provides the foundation for future social-emotional regulation and healthy relationship building. The aforementioned attachment, regulation, and co-regulation skills are considered the primary pillars of positive mental health in children and adolescents (Blaustein & Kinniburgh, 2018; Bowlby, 1968).

Executive functioning, sensory processing, and integration skills also play a role in one's ability to self-regulate and connect with others and may be impacted by challenges in developing a secure base or to other developmental and genetic challenges. Research demonstrates that better self-regulation in preschool-aged children predicts a multitude of short- and long-term outcomes, such as school readiness, academic achievement throughout primary school, adolescent and adult educational attainment, feelings of higher self-worth, an increased ability to cope with stress, less substance use and less law breaking, even among at-risk youth (Moffitt et al., 2011). Research also demonstrates that emotion regulation skills are also fundamental to both school readiness, academic participation, and achievement throughout childhood and adolescence (Hoffmann et al., 2020). Thus, the importance of developing self-regulation and emotion regulation capacities in early childhood cannot be disconnected from the attachment relationship or overlooked as a critical protective factor in promoting child, adolescent, family, and community mental health. Mental health promotion must include an emphasis on supporting caregiver-child attachment, attunement to support other critical developmental and functional capacities supporting child and family health, wellness, and occupational participation.

While there are many other determinants of health that impact the mental health of children and adolescents, the attachment relationship is one of the most critical. While all parents are human and therefore make mistakes, what has been referred to as "good enough" parenting is what constitutes an attachment relationship that is optimal to overall health. Thus, supporting the development of a strong

Table 13-3
Case-In-Point: Seven Cs for Building Resilience
COMMUNITY-BASED MENTAL HEALTH SERVICES: SEVEN STRATEGIES
YouthBuild is a well-established nonprofit organization whose mission is to create a world where all young people are seen for their potential and power to transform themselves and their communities. YouthBuild has long worked with young people in underserved and indigenous communities in 18 countries. The cornerstones of their work are to catalyze youth agency; enable youth access to information, learning, social capital, and peer-to-peer healing; and create assets to address inequities in education and economic opportunity systems. YouthBuild assumes youth as primary stakeholders and important facilitators of community building. YouthBuild programs build capacities that support healthy communities across the globe.

attachment relationship, in addition to the prevention of trauma and adverse childhood experiences as much as possible, is critical during these sensitive developmental periods and to relationship-building capacities.

Reflective Question

Consider the case of Karl and Ivy. Having early childhood caregiver relationships that were traumatic and chaotic created the perception that adult caregivers cannot be trusted or relied upon for nurturance, care, or safety. How might the lack of safety, early attunement, and co-regulation impact their ability to manage their emotions and behaviors?

Additionally, the diverse cultural contexts of co-regulation and attachment must be understood and honored when working with families and children. These cultural contexts include communities or groups of people with commonalities that may make them more vulnerable or not (race, sexual orientation, socioeconomic status). According to Buhler-Wasserman and Hibel (2021), caregiver-child interactions exist within a complex, dynamic, and fast-paced, complex world where caregiving occurs simultaneously while having to respond to many other responsibilities and pressures (e.g., rearing multiple children, personal needs, other social, community, financial/employment, political) and other demands. Further, there is the intergenerational transmission of cultural norms, and a variety of different behaviors, core assumptions, morals, and values that influence the way caregivers respond as parents (Buhler-Wasserman & Hibel, 2021). Being culturally responsive to the norms and behaviors of parents from diverse backgrounds allows to better understand and support their bonding relationship and co-regulation patterns with their children, thus helping to build healthy families and communities in a way that uses cultural sensitivity and cultural humility (see Table 13-2).

In addition to protective factors and developmental factors listed in Tables 13-1 and 13-2, the following seven core areas (seven Cs of building resilience) have been shown to foster attachment, development, health, and resilience in children and youth:

1. **Connection**: Building healthy attachments with primary caregivers and family members as relationships with friends, people in school, in the community, at work, and other areas of social life.
2. **Coping**: Supporting the exploration and use of strategies that support self-regulation and emotional intelligence.
3. **Confidence**: Supporting the development of strengths, abilities, talents and the belief in one's abilities.
4. **Competence**: Supporting the identification and growth of one's skills and talents.
5. **Contribution**: Identify and support engagement in opportunities for contributing to other's health and well-being.
6. **Character**: Support the ability to understand the differences between right and wrong, develop strong moral values that contribute to one's self-identity.
7. **Control**: Supporting problem solving and decision-making capacities that foster a sense of self-control (Ginsburg & Jablow, 2020, p. 21).

A primary prevention approach to the adverse consequences of toxic stress and adversity includes routine guidance and resources that strengthen the seven Cs, and provide social supports, which are the ability to learn and utilize positive parenting techniques that support the child's social, emotional, and relational skills (Garner et al., 2012). Increasingly, pediatricians are adopting practices that help to identify toxic stress and adversity in order to help children and families obtain the resources and supports needed to ultimately promote development and health across the life span (Garner et al., 2012). One example of a primary prevention and mental health promotion program that supports children and families is YouthBuild, which is discussed in Table 13-3.

Case Study

It is clear that Karl and Ivy's parents had mental health and substance abuse challenges. Consider how this may have come to pass. It is known that they also come from families where domestic abuse, mental health, and substance abuse challenges occurred as well. During that time, mental illness was highly stigmatized, and therefore, help was not accessed in the same way that it is today. Much less was understood about trauma, mental illness, and its intergenerational nature. While mental illness continues to be stigmatizing today, much progress has been made. This family case vignette demonstrates the impact of trauma, loss, mental illness, socioeconomic factors, and ACEs on an intergenerational scale—when not addressed. Having adopted the two children later in life, the paternal grandparents now serve as the primary caregiver supports, and the youth are back in their family system in a safer way although with caregivers that still support in developing optimal parenting skills. While placement with their grandparents is health supportive in many ways, a significant amount of community support continues to be required to help the family unit with establishing safe, healthy family boundaries and attachment relationships, resources, and care. Currently, both children have significant difficulty forming trusting relationships, with self-injurious behaviors, and engaging safely and functionally in a variety of roles, routines, and occupations of childhood. Currently, both youths reside in residential programs in order to help the family to connect, trust, and engage in family and daily life relationships and occupations safely. The youth have individual counseling as well as family therapy as part of the residential programming. The grandparents have agreed to participate in the Nurturing Health Parenting sessions offered through the residential program by interdisciplinary residential staff. Occupational therapy practitioners also support child and family engagement in preferred activities and occupations, such as leisure and social activities, active and safe participation during activities of daily living, home visits, and therapeutic groups.

Mental Health Disorders and Mental Illness

It is estimated that between 10% to 20% of children and adolescents worldwide experience mental health disorders, yet these are often minimized and not realized as one of the leading causes of health-related disability in children and adolescents (Kieling et al., 2011). It is also evident that trauma can cause severe mental health challenges and severe mental illness and substance abuse issues (Mauritz et al., 2013; Zarse et al., 2019). While traumatic experience is not necessarily the cause of serious mental illness (SMI) 100% of the time, it is widely recognized that trauma impacts mental health and can lead to mental illness in some situations (Mihelicova et al., 2017). Additionally, it is also reported that most people with mental illness also have trauma histories and/or adverse childhood experiences to some degree, whether it occurs before or after onset of SMI. This is why it is so important to realize the interconnection in order to address these challenges from a public health approach (Mihelicova et al., 2017). The better health professionals understand the origins of problems, the better they are able to address, within their scope of practice, the concomitant mental health challenges and other issues impacting meaningful participation in life.

Although there is a great deal of debate as to whether or not it is appropriate to label individuals with diagnoses, the current practice continues to view mental health and emotional challenges on a continuum. In addition, mainstream psychiatry continues to use the Diagnostic and Statistical Manual of Mental Disorders-5th edition (DSM-5) as its leading reference in identifying and labeling mental health-related illness (APA, 2013). Bazyk and Arbesman (2013) refer to mental health challenges of children and youth as mental illness and mental health that is on a continuum from mild to the most severe, using the following terms:

Mental illness and mental health disorders: diagnosable mental health conditions that are typically diagnosable (APA, 2013)

Mental health problems: mental health challenges that are typically more mild, common in nature, and shorter in duration than per those that become approached as diagnosable mental health conditions (e.g., symptoms of acute stress, anxiety, feeling depressed).While it is not the purpose of this chapter to explore mental health diagnoses in depth, the following list demonstrates the overarching categories of mental health disorders identified in the DSM-5 that are relevant to children and/or adolescents:

- Schizophrenia Spectrum and Other Psychotic Disorders
- Bipolar and Related Disorders
- Depressive Disorders
- Anxiety Disorders
- Obsessive-Compulsive and Related Disorders
- Trauma- and Stressor-Related Disorders
- Dissociative Disorders
- Somatic Symptom and Related Disorders
- Feeding and Eating Disorders
- Elimination Disorders
- Sleep-Wake Disorders
- Sexual Dysfunctions
- Gender Dysphoria
- Disruptive, Impulse-Control, and Conduct Disorders
- Substance-Related and Addictive Disorders
- Neurodevelopmental Disorders
- Intellectual Disability
- Language Disorder

- Autism Spectrum Disorder
- Specific Learning Disorder
- Developmental Coordination Disorder
- Other Conditions That May Be of Clinical Focus

Please note that while some of the aforementioned diagnoses tend to be more prevalent in adult populations (e.g., Schizophrenia), there is still evidence of emergence in childhood at times. The attachment disorders are largely contained within the trauma and stressor-related disorder category, with the exception of separation anxiety disorder, which remains in the anxiety disorder section (APA, 2013). There are other mental health behaviors and challenges in children and adolescents that are serious but not necessarily part of this diagnostic list, such as self-injury, fire starting, bullying, hazing, suicidal and homicidal thoughts and/or attempts, and sexualized or sexually exploitative behaviors.

Suicidality

The CDC reports that for individuals between the ages of 10 and 24 years, suicide has become the second leading cause of death, and that those between the ages of 10 and 14 are within the age range for the fastest-growing suicide rates (CDC, 2020). According to Thompson et al. (2019):

> suicide prevention and treatment for youth must be developmentally appropriate, attend to critical social determinants of health, assess the presence of adverse childhood events (ACEs) and trauma, incorporate parental or guardian support, and address consent considerations. (p. 1)

Suicide refers to death that occurs as a direct result of a person harming themselves with the intent to die. **Suicidal ideation** is the term used to describe suicidal thoughts that are passive (wish or desire to be dead) or active (specific thoughts and/or plans related to suicide) and both may lead to a suicide attempt (Kaslow, 2014). To best support youth that are at risk for suicide, interprofessional staff, schools, and communities must be educated and offer the supports and resources necessary to identify and target this growing issue. Parents, caregivers, and those in positions where they work closely with children must be skilled in the assessment and management of suicidality in children and adolescents and have the ability to swiftly provide the necessary supports. Suicide risk assessment, collaboratively developing corresponding safety plans, and processes for ongoing reassessment are strategies for those working with youth who are able to provide suicide prevention measures. Suicide risk assessment includes but is not limited to identifying barriers to mental health and safety, the frequency, duration, and intensity of suicidal thoughts and the potential for obtaining or presence of weapons such as firearms or other lethal means (medications, environmental) in the home, neighborhood, and wider community. Developing and implementing critical care pathways, frameworks, and curriculums targeting suicidality are examples of ways to target suicide prevention and mental health promotion for individuals, organizations, communities, and populations.

Risk factors for suicidality in children and youth often include some of the following (Kaslow, 2014):

- Intrapersonal: Feelings of hopeless, helplessness, guilt, shame, worthlessness; recent or serious loss; mental health symptoms; alcohol/substance use or abuse; and previous suicide attempt(s)
- Societal/Situational: Lack of support; sense of isolation; family history of suicide; child abuse or neglect; witnessing family violence; bullying/being bullied; recent or serious loss (divorce, death of a loved one, separation, loss of previously enjoyed sports, hobbies, clubs)
- Cultural/Environmental: Stigma associated with asking for help; barriers to accessing services; access to lethal methods; cultural or religious beliefs related to mental health, gender, and/or sexual identity, or other symptoms or beliefs; lack of support

Suicide prevention is supported by prevention and intervention strategies. Protective factors include some of the following: a strong support system and close relationships; community supports; nonviolent conflict resolution, problem solving, stress management, self-regulation and coping skills; and limited access to lethal means (Kaslow, 2014). Refer to Table 13-4 for examples of assessment tools often used with children and adolescents related to suicidality, trauma, and mental health (Professional Reasoning Box A).

A public health approach to mental health promotion requires a broad spectrum of areas of emphasis given the extent of the varied challenges at hand. When taking a population approach to addressing major public health concerns, much of the impact to individuals can be greatly minimized, and at times fully addressed, as a result. The following section describes a public health approach to mental health promotion and prevention.

A Public Health Approach to Mental Health Promotion and Prevention

In 2001, the WHO proposed a public health model, specific to mental health promotion. This public health model was expanded upon to specifically to address children's mental health promotion, prevention, and intervention (Bazyk, 2011). The addition of an occupational justice focus helps to provide a guiding framework for promotion and prevention efforts. Interprofessional efforts within this approach can lead to the building of effective, holistic, and sustainable

Table 13-4

Assessments: Child and Adolescent Mental Health*

AREAS OF ASSESSMENT	ASSESSMENT TOOL EXAMPLES
Attachment	• Dyadic Parent-Child Interaction Coding System, 4th Edition (Eyberg et al., 2013) • Parent-Child Relationship Inventory (Gerard, 1994)
Health, wellness, and quality of life	• Child Health Questionnaire (CHQ; Waters et al., 2001) • Youth Quality of Life Instrument – Research Version (YQOL-R; Topolski et al., 2001)
Mood and mental health	• Beck Anxiety Inventory (Beck & Steer, 1993) • Columbia Depression Scale (Shaffer et al., 2000) • Conners Comprehensive Behavior Rating Scales (Conners, 2008) • Vanderbilt ADHD Rating Scale (Wolraich et al., 1998)
Participation and performance	• CAPE/PAC: Children's Assessment of Participation and Enjoyment (CAPE) and Preferences for Activities of Children (PAC; King et al., 2004) • Canadian Occupational Performance Measure (Law et al., 2005) • School Function Assessment (Coster et al., 1998)
Substance use/abuse	• CRAFFT (Knight et al., 2002) • Screening to Brief Intervention Scales (S2BI; Levy et al., 2014)
Suicidality	• Columbia Suicide Severity Rating Scales (C-SSRS; Posner et al., 2011) • Suicide Assessment Scale (SUAS; Nimeus et al., 2000)
Trauma and adversity	• Child Trauma Screening Questionnaire (Kenardy et al., 2006) • Trauma Symptom Checklist for Young Children (Briere, 1996)

*List is not all inclusive.

Professional Reasoning Box A

Tommy is an 11-year-old boy with ADHD. In addition to academic challenges, Tommy is often involved in arguments on the playground and in the cafeteria. He has frequent outbursts in the classroom when there is a change in schedule or "things do not go his way." He does not have any close friends and recently has experienced bullying on social media as a result of his frequent emotional outbursts. Since the start of the bullying, he refuses to take the bus to school and began wetting the bed. Two weeks ago, Tommy climbed out of his bedroom window onto the roof threatening to jump. After a brief hospitalization, Tommy is back at home but refuses to go back to school. Identify two interprofessional interventions that can support Tommy and his family to prevent suicidality and support safe re-integration into the school environment.

programs. A **public health model** is often used to demonstrate the scope of an issue and is used to research and identify varieties of ways to address it. The three major levels of the public health model used in mental health (Bazyk & Arbesman, 2013) include:

1. **Universal**: Services are focused on a whole population and are often offered to a whole group or population rather than via individual services.
2. **Targeted** or **selected services**: Services provided to youth and/or families for mental/emotional health promotion and/or to prevention of mental health challenges from developing.
3. **Intensive individualized services**: Intensive individualized services or programs provided to decrease the impact of the mental/emotional health challenges youth and/or families on an individual basis. Typically, this service type is provided to youth and families that already have mental health challenges and/or diagnoses and is not within the scope of this chapter.

Public Health and Mental Health Promotion and Prevention

Mental health promotion can be defined as intervening to *optimize* positive mental health by addressing determinants of positive mental health before a specific mental health problem has been identified, with the ultimate goal of improving the positive mental health of the population

Professional Reasoning Box B

Related to primary prevention, consider being a professional working at a middle school in an underserved community. Identify one interprofessional mental health promotion initiative that you could develop or implement to support the positive mental health of the youth in the school. Specify the role of at least two professionals working as part of this initiative.

Table 13-5

Case-In-Point: Community Based-Services to Support Positive Mental Health in Families and Youth

BERGEN FAMILY CENTER
The Bergen Family Center (BFC) is an example of community-based programming located in New Jersey that supports the mental health of families, children, and youth by providing services to enhance family's ability to function independently in the community. Central to their mission is a commitment to help eliminate disparities caused by systemic inequities and unconscious bias and to promote equity and justice in the community (https://bergenfamilycenter.org). BFC provides an array of programs and services to support family and child and youth mental health.

(Youth.gov, n.d.). Mental health promotion in children and youth includes efforts to enhance individuals' abilities to achieve developmentally appropriate tasks referred to as developmental competence (Arbesman et al., 2013). It is through mastery of these competencies that children develop a positive sense of self that supports successful achievement of future competencies. See Tables 13-1 and 13-2 for factors associated with positive mental health development (Bazyk & Arbesman, 2013, p. 8).

Mental health prevention can be defined as intervening to minimize mental health problems by addressing determinants of mental health problems before a specific mental health problem has been identified in the individual, group, or population of focus with the ultimate goal of reducing the number of future mental health problems in the population (Youth.gov, n.d.). Mental health promotion and prevention are primary intervention types when employing a public health approach at the universal and targeted levels. Efforts toward promotion and prevention at the community, family, and individual levels should focus on strengthening protective factors and building capacities to support child and adolescent mental health as well as continued risk factors (Professional Reasoning Box B). These interventions may include some of the following:

- Support for underserved communities (i.e., childcare; job coaching; parenting coaching; head start)
- Support for parents (i.e., parent coaching; respite for new parents; paid family leave)
- Support for children (i.e., skill-building programs such as social emotional learning programs; school readiness programs; anti-bullying programs)
- Support for families, children, and youth with disabilities (i.e., inclusive environments and programming)
- Support for adolescence (i.e., mentorship programs in communities and schools; leisure exploration programs; leadership training programs)
- Ecological changes in schools and communities to support positive mental health (i.e., sensory friendly classrooms; cultural- and gender-informed and -responsive schools)
- Support for vulnerable or at-risk groups including families and children in underserved communities, parents and/or children with disabilities, those with a history of ACEs (i.e., Head Start programs, trauma-informed and -responsive schools and community agencies)
- The Bergen Family Center (BFC) is one example of a community-based provider that uses an interprofessional team in a manner that integrates a public health approach to supporting the positive mental health of families. Table 13-5 demonstrates some of the work of BFC in their efforts to support positive mental health as part of community-based services.

Screening and Assessment

From a public health approach, since families make up communities, mental health promotion and prevention efforts with families, children, and youth starts with assessing the needs of communities and populations. Issel and Wells (2018) identify the following best practices in planning and evaluation models related to community mental health:

1. Communicating with the targeted group, other team members, and stakeholders
2. Identifying community problems and issues

3. Establishing priorities, objectives, and resources
4. Designing, implementing, and evaluating program activities

With regards to family, child, and youth mental health, this process involves identifying and communicating with key stakeholders including families, youth, agencies, organizations, and professionals to identify needs and trends within their communities. Communicating and partnering with families, children, and youth in the places where they live, work, and learn such as schools, day care centers, and community centers is essential. The primary voice and choice should be that of the youth and family. Cultural competency and cultural humility are essential when working with all populations, including children and adolescent populations.

When working with individuals, communities, or populations, providing evidence informed intervention first requires screening(s) or assessment(s). The type of screening(s) or assessment(s) used depends specifically on what the youth and family, community, or population's needs are. For instance, early intervention services are often recommended when parents and/or the child's pediatrician has concerns about any aspect of a young child's development (0 to 3 years of age), which includes mental/emotional health. Some outpatient behavioral health settings also provide services to very young children and their primary caregiver(s). When there are mental health symptoms involved, a mental health clinician, psychologist, or psychiatrist may be enlisted to help with an assessment to discern whether mental health symptoms or an actual mental health diagnosis, and potentially therapy and medications may be warranted (APA, 2013). There are also assessment tools that may be used to explore attachment, to identify whether different types of trauma or abuse have been experienced, whether substance abuse, self-harm, or suicidality is of concern, or whether anger, anxiety, depression, dissociation, or other mental health symptoms are being experienced and to what degree. Occupational therapists can assess a child's sensory issues, which may contribute to one's positive or negative mental health. See Table 13-4 for some examples of assessment tools used when working with children and adolescents (list is not all-inclusive).

Other variables that may impact the type of assessment used, and whether a formal or informal approach is employed, is the level of acuity (severity of symptoms, challenges, behaviors, safety), level of care (i.e., acute, community-based), and care/educational setting (i.e., school [pre-school, elementary, high school], outpatient setting, inpatient behavioral health unit, juvenile justice setting, substance abuse program, community-based support group).

When taking a universal or targeted public health approach, understanding the types of programs that communities and schools currently have in place to address the overall health and wellness of their members is an important part of program development. Assessment should include identifying opportunities to strengthen already existing programs as well as identifying gaps in programming. For instance, the ACE study has helped to launch trauma-informed screening and assessment practices that are now used across mental health settings but also in pediatric annual visits and as part of many primary care practices (Anda et al., 2010; Felitti et al., 1998). Thus, the ACE study has provided critical information about the impact of adverse childhood experiences that has led to the creation of a prevention practice implemented across many communities and levels of care with the goal of ACEs identification, prevention, and health promotion. The ACE scale asks 10 questions related to childhood adversity, and the higher the ACE score (particularly when having 4 or more ACEs) the higher the probability of negative mental and physical health outcomes unless intervention is provided (Anda et al., 2010; Felitti et al., 1998). Some examples of resources that provide additional information related to child/adolescent mental health prevention, promotion and intervention include:

- AOTA Practice Guidelines for Mental Health Promotion, Prevention, and Intervention for Children and Youth (Bazyk & Arbesman, 2013)
- The National Child Traumatic Stress Network: https://www.nctsn.org/
- SAMHSA's programs targeting equity and the quality and service delivery of behavioral health services across the United States: https://www.samhsa.gov/programs
- U.S. Health and Human Services Resilience Resources: https://www.acf.hhs.gov/trauma-toolkit/resilience

Related to the case study, when Karl and Ivy each entered into residential care, each met with an interprofessional mental health care team who worked with them and their caregivers (as appropriate to therapeutic boundaries) to complete the assessment and screening processes to collaboratively determine what the therapeutic needs, goals, and interventions would be from a strengths-based and client-driven perspective. The grandparents were also central to this process, looking at their history, strengths, needs, and concerns in order to best support the family unit via family therapy and community support recommendations and utilization.

Reflective Question

Why is it important to include Karl, Ivy, and the grandparents in a collaborative manner that is central to the assessment and intervention process?

Intervention

As mentioned earlier, the attachment relationship is critical to a host of developmental capacities, abilities, and overall child and adolescent health (Blaustein & Kinniburgh, 2018; Bowlby, 1968; Perry, 2009). It was previously thought that self-regulation was a capacity built solely through teaching regulation skills, but it is through the attachment relationship that infants and children first develop self-regulation (Blaustein & Kinniburg, 2018; Bowlby, 1968; Perry, 2009). Building this capacity in families and communities is needed at the societal, family, and individual levels to support healthy communities. This is especially important in marginalized and vulnerable communities that experience disadvantage, adversity, and oppression of any kind.

Given that there are many individuals that do not have the attachment opportunities supportive of optimal mental health and wellness, it is important to identify areas in need of support in order to help child, family, and community mental health and wellness. There are several key skills that are essential to building self-regulation, social, and emotional skills that are needed for family and child mental health, which include but are not limited to the following:

- Self-awareness
  - Sensory awareness
  - Emotional awareness, regulation, and management
  - Social awareness
  - Self-management
- Relationship building
  - Empathy
- Mindfulness
- Growth mindset

For children, adolescents, and families that have experienced (or continue to experience) trauma and/or adversity or have other mental health challenges, it is important to help them create a sense of safety, and in some situations a literal "safe space." Supporting the development of positive social relationships and those that help the youth develop or further expand upon capacities for self- and co-regulation is critical. Consistency of rituals, routines, support, and ongoing reassurance can help to build a variety of developmental skills, and a positive sense of coherence and self-identity. Infusing a strengths-based, developmental perspective into solutions and strategies is only one of the key ways that helps children and adolescents that have experienced adversity. In addition, the focus on building healthy and strong social-emotional skills has shifted from a cognitive behavioral focus to supporting the mind-body connection. Yoga, massage, sensory integration and processing, and mindfulness activities are examples of interventions widely used by interdisciplinary professionals to support social-emotional skill building and stress reduction, thereby supporting positive mental health.

It is well understood that a holistic approach that intentionally targets the mind and body is becoming viewed as best and promising practices with youth with trauma, adverse childhood experiences and attachment difficulties (Blaustein & Kinniburg, 2018; May-Benson & Tisdale, 2019; Perry, 2009). Further, sensory processing and integration challenges are also evident in some children, adolescents, and adults with trauma histories (van der Kolk, 2005, 2014; Perry, 2009). For instance, sensorimotor challenges (coordination, postural control, praxis), sensory modulation challenges (i.e., over responsivity and under responsivity) have been evidenced in those with symptoms of post-traumatic stress (Engel-Yeger et al., 2013; Perry, 2009; Yochman & Pat-Horenczyk, 2020). Thus, sensory- and body-based approaches are being increasingly used as part of mainstream mental health assessment and treatment interventions with individuals with mental health, trauma, and attachment challenges.

One example of a program that can be used for mental health promotion, prevention, and intervention, when modified and individualized for the age ranges and settings where it is used, is the Sensory Modulation Program (SMP) (Champagne, 2011). The SMP may be implemented as part of a home, programmatic, school system's, or organization's routine (i.e., residential, juvenile justice). The SMP outlines the many different aspects of the sensory modulation-related, therapeutic components that may be used to support self-awareness, self-regulation, organizational and coping skills, social-emotional, and relational skills. The SMP includes the following:

- Therapeutic use of self (assessment through intervention that include exploring sensory processing and integration as part of the overall assessment and intervention process)
- Sensory activities and modalities: identification and use of those that are most helpful and when use may be for prevention and/or crisis intervention purposes
- Sensory diet: an intentional, strategic routine that incorporates the youth's coping and sensory supportive strategies that have been identified as most helpful for use for health promotion, prevention, and crisis intervention purposes
- Environmental enhancements, spaces, and support
- Caregiver participation, education, and support

The SMP is typically used when an individual or family has difficulty with trauma, dissociation, self-regulation, sensory integration and processing, and/or other mental health challenges. Individual and programmatic applications of the SMP are provided in Table 13-6. The SMP is also used for health and wellness promotion, in addition to stress and anxiety reduction, management, and prevention among youth, parents, and staff. One example is the creation of a sensory modulation-informed therapeutic space in a hospital or school setting.

The first step with people of all ages with trauma and mental health challenges is to help them establish a sense of safety and stabilization. Likely due to the trauma and ACEs that Karl and Ivy both experienced, each had self-regulation, sensory integration, social, and emotional challenges. Both youths had difficulty with feeling overwhelmed emotionally, socially, and had severe tactile and auditory over-responsivity (hyper-sensitivity to touch and sound) impacting the ability to participate in self-care activities, therapeutic groups, and enjoyable activities with caregivers. The SMP was part of what was utilized with each youth during residential services

Table 13-6

The Sensory Modulation Program: Individual and Programmatic Applications

SENSORY MODULATION PROGRAM	CLIENT/INDIVIDUAL APPLICATION	PROGRAMMATIC APPLICATION
Therapeutic use of self	Clinician/staff work with the client using a trauma-informed and sensory supportive approach to all assessment, goal-setting, and intervention planning (i.e., assessment process includes sensory modulation).	Staff are trained in verbal and nonverbal communication skills that are trauma-informed and sensory supportive.
Sensory-based activities	Support the client in identifying and planning for the use of sensory supportive strategies that help the client meet their goals.	Activities provided by the program are sensory supportive in nature (groups and/or individual sessions).
Sensory-based modalities	Support the client in identifying and planning for the use of sensory supportive modalities (i.e., weighted blanket, other therapeutic tools/ equipment).	Modalities provided by the program are sensory supportive in nature. • Group and/or individual use
Sensory diet (routine)	Collaborative creation and modification an individualized daily routine with sensory supports built in (strategically) for prevention purposes. Also, an individualized plan for strategies to use for de-escalation and crisis intervention purposes.	Creation and ongoing modification of the program's daily routine to help meet the goals of the clients receiving services for prevention, de-escalation, crisis intervention, and stress management goals.
Environmental modifications and enhancements	Help the client create spaces that support sensory needs (corner of their bedroom, an outdoor area/space, etc.).	Program management and staff co-create specific spaces/rooms and overall program modifications to the physical environment that are trauma informed and sensory supportive. Gather and utilize client feedback over time.
Caregiver education	Provide client and caregiver(s) education and resources to support the successful use of therapeutic, sensory-supportive routines, and strategies.	Staff education/training; create resources and methods for education and resources; identification for clients, caregiver(s), and families.

Data source: Champagne, T. (2011). *Sensory modulation and environment: Essential elements of occupation*. Pearson.

in order to support their ability to stabilize and feel safe. Each had a sensory diet (strategic routine with individualized sensory, relational and organizational supports used throughout the day, strategies for when feeling overwhelmed and unsafe, and extra staff support for recognizing and addressing tactile and auditory challenges proactively. Some examples include obtaining clothing that is comfortable, reminding them to use the quiet/nurturing space developed in their room to decrease noise and other forms of overwhelming stimulation as needed, and determining sensory supportive tools that are helpful and creating their own sensory kits. Each youth also met with an occupational therapy practitioner to address occupational participation needs and goals at school and to monitor how these sensory-based and other strategies supported occupational goals.

The Zones of Regulation (Kuypers, 2011) is another example of a program that supports the promotion of social-emotional and self-regulation skills in children and adolescents. The zones use visual color-coded cues to help children identify their current emotional state and the effect this has on those around them. It highlights the mind-body connection and encourages mindful awareness of body states as clues to regulation. The zones can be used in classrooms and in the home. The Zones of Regulation can be used as part of, or in conjunction with, the Sensory Modulation Program. There are a variety of other programs that support both self-regulation and social and emotional development from infancy through adulthood. All of the programs listed below are interprofessional in nature and require keen collaboration among professionals, parents, and the children themselves to foster integration of skills:

- Social Thinking and Me (https://www.socialthinking.com)
- 7 Mindsets (https://7mindsets.com)
- Interoception Curriculum (https://www.kelly-mahler.com)
- Habitudes (https://growingleaders.com)

While social-emotional skill building is vital to all children, it is especially critical in children that have experienced or are experiencing any adversity. While this is not an exhaustive list, post-traumatic skill development also includes prosocial skills training to help children learn to care not only for themselves but also for others, fostering organizational and problem-solving skills, the ability to maintain attention and concentration, the ability to identify when support is needed, and to seek appropriate forms of support. Since trauma is often most impactful because of one's perception (whether aware of it or not) of or actual loss of power or control, children and adolescents often need to work on learning to develop trust in different contexts and relationships. Through building trusting relationships youth are also able to learn that it is common for relationships to have struggles and opportunities for repair—and that they can be repaired. In this way, youth see adults modeling the use of their power by showing respect and treating others with care, kindness, compassion, and dignity. Further, a host of sensory- and body-oriented therapies, play therapies and interventions that foster creative and expressive arts, and animal-assisted therapies have and continue to emerge as both evidence informed and promising practices for children and adolescents across individualized and targeted intervention types (Champagne, 2011; Mims & Waddell, 2016; Perry, 2009; van der Kolk, 2014).

Additionally, children and adolescents that engage in regular physical activity and receive a healthy nutritional diet demonstrate enhanced neurophysiological development (even with those whose nervous systems have been negatively impacted by trauma and adversity), less depression, and increased school performance (Edwards & Pratt, 2016). Karl and Ivy resided in a group residence where therapeutic interventions such as expressive arts, pet therapy, sensory-based approaches, and play therapy were a central part of interventions offered. Engagement and participation in these important interventions can yield positive mental health benefits and support well-being (Professional Reasoning Box C).

Please see Table 13-7 for examples of evidence-based clinical and therapeutic models and/or programs used by interprofessional teams, largely for intensive intervention purposes with children and adolescents that have experienced stress, adversity, developmental trauma, and attachment-related challenges.

The cycle of building capacities for self-regulation and healthy social and emotional skills can be viewed from an individual, family, and community health perspective. Supporting skill development in early childhood, and in a culturally supportive manner, can lead to improved mental health outcomes as children transition to adulthood. This also supports and promotes the mental health of the family. Thus, child and youth mental health is intimately intertwined with family and community mental health using a public health approach.

Targeted and Universal Interventions: Community Programming

In addition to the examples provided throughout the chapter there are many other targeted and universal, evidence-based approaches employing interprofessional perspectives to working with children and adolescents to foster positive social and emotional development, health, wellness, and resilience, including the following:

- **Every Moment Counts** (EMC; Bazyk, 2010) is an example of a mental health promotion-oriented program for children and adolescents that is often provided within school and after-school programs, although application in other program types is expanding. Strategies are embedded in everyday school and after-school experiences, with the primary focus on enjoyment within the context of childhood occupations, such as school participation. EMC provides tools and intervention approaches that may be implemented by interprofessional staff that have had training.
- **RULER** (Recognizing, Understanding, Labeling, Expressing, Regulating) **Approach** was created by the Yale Center for Emotional Intelligence (Hoffman et al., 2020). The theory of emotional intelligence is central to this whole school approach, which emphasizes the coordinated efforts of all stakeholders, such as administrators, educators, therapists, counselors, and other school personnel, as well as parents and the students themselves, in supporting the mental, emotional, and social health. One key feature of the RULER approach is that all stakeholders participate in the program to allow for more emotionally intelligent and more regulated adults, which can then better support student mental and emotional health. The RULER approach supports the exploration of strategies and tools that can be used as ways to integrate emotion regulation skill-building and practice as part of curriculum design, direct teaching practices, and the daily routine.
- **The CATCH Program**: The CATCH (Coordinated Approach to Child Health) Program is an intentional and coordinated, school-based, evidence-based approach that uses a school-based intervention to teach and integrate regular opportunities for healthy eating/nutrition and engagement in regular movement and physical activity to support student health (Hoelscher et al., 2010; Office of Disease Prevention and Health Promotion, n.d.). The CATCH program is considered a leading program used in both the United States and Canada that has demonstrated evidence of improving the health-promoting behaviors of students in the areas of active engagement in physical activity and in making healthier food choices.

Professional Reasoning Box C

POLYVAGAL THEORY AND MENTAL HEALTH AND WELL-BEING

Mental health cannot be discussed without acknowledging the importance of the feeling of safety and its impact on mental health and well-being. The contribution of the **Polyvagal theory** (PVT; Porges, 2011) to this discussion is immense and has evolved from theoretical to practical and is being used as guiding lens to inform practice among many professions. PVT proposes that the **vagal system**, as controlled via the vagus nerve and mediated by the parasympathetic nervous system, is our "social engagement system," allowing our nervous system to detect cues of safety, which allows us to engage with others from that safe place (Porges, 2011).

Paramount to PVT is the concept of **neuroception**. Neuroception is our sense of safety and danger mediated by the autonomic nervous system (ANS; Porges, 2011). When we feel safe the ANS creates conditions within our bodies, such as a regulated and responsive heart rate, as well as regulated and responsive breathing. However, when we sense danger the ANS sets off a neurophysiological cascade of processes that are intended to protect us, such as increased heart rate and respiration needed to flee.

BRANCHES OF THE VAGUS NERVE

The **ventral branch** of the vagus nerve is the most recently evolved in relationship to human development. Its connections are primarily above the diaphragm, including the head and neck region. These innervations include eye lids, facial muscles, middle ear muscles, neck muscles, and laryngeal and pharyngeal muscles, which together allow for social engagement and connectedness to others.

The **dorsal branch** is the older of the two branches and supports survival. Its connections are below the diaphragm and include the gut, heart, and lungs. The activation of the dorsal branch supports the slowing down of bodily functions in the presence to danger, which serves to protect from harm resulting in immobilization.

- Sympathetic arousal or **fight or flight**, is a mobilized state of protection and survival. Meaning that a person is mobilized by fear or danger and ready to fight or flee. This activation can become chronic among those with trauma histories.

STATES OF REGULATION

VENTRAL VAGAL STATE

When in a state of ventral vagal regulation, we can connect and attune to others, form attachments, co-regulate, and self-regulate. This state is central to the human experience, however, can only be fully accessed and used in the presence of feelings of safety and thus, is a reciprocal fluid experience.

DORSAL VAGAL STATE

The dorsal branch is thought to mediate life-threatening protection and survival. When experiencing a prolonged dorsal vagal response, when in a prolonged fearful or perceived dangerous situation, shut down may occur. This includes hypo-arousal, flat affect, low voice volume, and limited eye contact. When in this protective hypo-aroused state, it is difficult to access safe and social cues that provide a sense of safety, thus difficult to shift out of this state into a ventral vagal state of connection. When in a chronic state of immobilization (dorsal vagal) or mobilization (fight or flight), our ability to detect safety becomes diminished or skewed. Thus, even when safety cues are present, a person may not be able to access those cues.

SYMPATHETIC STATE

A mobilized state (i.e., fight or flight) is characterized behaviorally as being "on edge," hypervigilant, can't sit still, anxious, having a limited attention span, and fleeting eye contact. When in this state, we are consciously and subconsciously searching for auditory, visual, and other sensory-based cues of danger vs. safety. In this hypervigilant state, stimuli-eliciting concerns, such as a high-pitched sounds, are prioritized. Therefore, those that are not supportive of the ability to discern one's degree of safety are not attended to or able to support regulation.

(continued)

- **Psychological First Aid** (PFA) and **Skills for Psychological Recovery** (SPR) are promising practices for disaster response, that focuses on mental health and recovery. Both PFA and SPR were primarily developed by the National Center for PTSD and the National Child Traumatic Stress Network (n.d.). PFA and SPR interventions are meant to be used with survivors or witnesses that have been exposed to disaster or terrorism. First responders and others that provide disaster relief and related services are often trained in these approaches.
- **Communities Advancing Resilience Toolkit** (CART): CART includes a theory-based and field-tested assessment survey that helps to evaluate a community's resilience and individual's relationships with their community, specifically exploring the following areas: connection and caring, transformative potential, disaster management, and information and communication. CART also provides tools to help identify the strengths and needs within a community in order to identify areas for intervention and increased supports (Pfefferbaum et al., 2011).

Professional Reasoning Box C (continued)

STATE SHIFTS

The ability to flexibly shift between states facilitates the ability to meet environmental, task, and relational demands behaviorally as well as physiologically. This neurophysiological flexibility supports the ability to behaviorally respond and adapt to the ever-changing environment and also supports self-regulated behavior.

The vagal brake (Porges, 2011) describes the role of the vagus nerve in increasing vagal tone in order to influence the neurophysiological process necessary to shift between states as through neuroceptive processing. The vagal brake is activated when we are called to attention *without threat* and when we need to become mobilized in the case of danger. For example, the vagal brake is initiated when answering a question in class as the neurophysiological shifts needed for attention and engagement are required. The brake is also initiated when faced with danger, such as having to move out of the way of a speeding car. This flexible ability to smoothly move in and out of states in response to stress or eustress, as well as to recover from stressors, can be considered an indication of resilience (Carnevali et al., 2018).

Stress, and trauma of all kinds, can significantly limit our ability to both access and give safe and social cues. This lack of feeling safe can impact communities, populations, and families over time and can often be experienced on a subconscious level. Understanding the dynamic impact of self-regulation on well-being using a polyvagal lens can provide insight to inform practices from a public health perspective.

Identify the ways that PVT might inform youth mental health promotion and prevention efforts for underserved populations including those with disabilities?

The aforementioned community programs and tools demonstrate some examples of those that are specific to mental health promotion, prevention, and intervention with child and adolescent populations across varied contexts (e.g., schools, communities, health care settings).

Two examples of comprehensive parenting programs that can be offered by interprofessional staff include:

- **Nurturing Parenting Programs** target all families at risk for abuse and neglect with children ages birth to 18 years. The programs feature activities used to foster positive parenting skills with nurturing behaviors, promoting healthy physical and emotional development, while teaching appropriate role and developmental expectations. Lessons can be delivered in the home, in a group setting, or in the combination of home and group settings (Family Developing Resources, 2021).
- **Triple P** (Positive Parenting Program) employs a parent-driven approach to providing practical strategies and tools to help make parenting more safe, enjoyable, more predictable, and loving for youth and parents (Triplep-parenting.com, n.d.).

Conclusion

Family, child, and youth mental health is inseparable from community mental health. Supporting the mental health of our children and youth is critical to building healthy communities and conversely, building healthy communities is critical to the mental health of our children and youth. Family, school, and community efforts are integral to positive family, child, and youth outcomes. Utilizing public health and occupational justice approaches helps to support the promotion of positive mental health through equity and choice for diverse communities and populations. Interprofessional collaborations to support the positive and healthy development of youth from infancy through adulthood is essential to building and maintaining mentally healthy communities. As professionals working in communities, we must be aware of the reciprocal impact that community health has on child, adolescent, and family mental health and take action to promote the health and well-being of all persons.

Table 13-7

Intensive Intervention Models and Programs

MODEL/PROGRAM	PURPOSE	RESOURCE
The Circle of Security (Powell et al., 2013)	A model and training program for parents, caregivers, teachers, and others focused on helping caregivers reflect upon children's attachment needs in order to promote a secure attachment with a child.	https://www.circleofsecurityinternational.com
Theraplay (Booth & Jernberg, 2010)	Theraplay is a training program for caregivers and professionals providing practitioner guidance to co-create playful and caring child-adult interactions fostering joyful, shared experiences supporting attunement.	https://theraplay.org/
Developmental Individual Relationship (DIR)/ Floortime Model (Greenspan & Wieder, 2006)	DIR provides a framework for understanding social-emotional development and how each person perceives and interacts with the world differently. The model highlights the power of relationships and emotional connections to fuel development. It is most often utilized with children with educational, social-emotional, mental health, and/or developmental challenges.	https://www.icdl.com/home
Neurosequential Model of Therapeutics (NMT) (Perry, 2009)	The NMT is an approach to intervention that integrates core principles of neurodevelopment and trauma to inform assessment and intervention practices when working with children, families, and communities.	https://www.neurosequential.com/
Safe Place (May-Benson & Tisdale, 2019)	Safe Place is a multidisciplinary approach to treating children with complex trauma and sensory processing disorder. It encompasses concepts from sensory integration, attachment, and complex developmental trauma theories.	https://thespiralfoundation.org/courses/safe-place-a-multi-disciplinary-approach-to-treating-children-with-complex-trauma-and-sensory-processing-disorder-a-training-program/
The Attachment, Regulation and Competence (ARC) Model (Blaustein & Kinniburgh, 2018)	The Attachment, Regulation and Competency (ARC) Framework is an intervention guide for caregiver systems working with children and adolescents that have experienced complex trauma (i.e., parents, caregivers, teachers, and other professionals).	https://arcframework.org/what-is-arc/
Somatic Experiencing (Levine, 2005)	The Somatic Experiencing, developed by Peter Levine, PhD, is a body-oriented approach to the healing of trauma and other stress-related by helping to release traumatic shock and restores connection to one's body and to others.	https://www.somaticexperiencing.com
Dialectical Behavior Therapy (DBT) (Linehan, 1993)	Dialectical behavior therapy is intended to teach people how to live in the moment, develop healthy ways to cope with stress, regulate their emotions, and improve their relationships with others. It is used broadly with persons that have mental health conditions including those who have experienced trauma.	https://behavioraltech.org
Trauma-Focused Cognitive Behavior Therapy (TF-CBT) (Cohen & Wardrip, 2011)	TF-CBT is an evidence-based, structured, short-term treatment model that helps improve a range of trauma-related outcomes in 8 to 25 sessions with the child/adolescent and caregiver.	https://tfcbt.org/

Other Website Resources

- 7 Mindsets: https://7mindsets.com
- Adverse Childhood Experiences Study at CDC: https://www.cdc.gov/violenceprevention/aces/index.html?CDC_AA_refVal=https%3A%2F%2F
- Building Bridges Initiative: http://buildingbridges4youth.org
- Children and Family Futures: https://www.cffutures.org/
- Child Trauma Academy: http://childtrauma.org
- Child Welfare Information Gateway: https://www.childwelfare.gov/
- Developmental Individual Relationship/Floortime Model: https://www.icdl.com
- Every Moment Counts: http://www.everymomentcounts.org

- Habitudes: https://growingleaders.com
- Interoception Curriculum: https://www.kelly-mahler.com
- National Center for Education in Maternal and Child Health: https://www.ncemch.org/about.php
- National Center for Safe Children: https://healthysafechildren.org
- National Center for Substance Abuse and Child Welfare: https://ncsacw.acf.hhs.gov/
- National Children's Advocacy Center: https://www.nationalcac.org/
- National Child Traumatic Stress Network: https://learn.nctsn.org/
- Nurturing Parenting Program: https://www.nurturingparenting.com
- OT Innovations: www.ot-innovations.com
- Social Thinking and Me: https://www.socialthinking.com
- Triple P Parenting Program: https://www.triplep-parenting.com/us/triple-p/
- Zero Suicide: https://zerosuicide.edc.org/
- Zero to Three: https://www.zerotothree.org/
- Zones of Regulation: https://zonesofregulation.com

References

American Occupational Therapy Association. (2014). Occupational therapy practice framework: Domain and process (3rd ed.). *American Journal of Occupational Therapy, 68*, S1-S48. https://doi.org/10.5014/ajot.2014.682006

American Psychiatric Association. (2013). *Diagnostic and statistical manual of mental health disorders* (5th ed.). https://doi.org/10.1176/appi.books.9780890425596

Anda, R. F., Butchart, A., Felitti, V., & Brown, D. (2010). Building a framework for global surveillance of the public health implications of adverse childhood experiences. *American Journal of Preventive Medicine, 39*(1), 93-98.

Arbesman, M., Bazyk, S., & Nochajski, S. (2013). Systematic review of occupational therapy and mental health promotion, prevention and intervention for children and youth. *American Journal of Occupational Therapy, 67*(6), 120-130.

Ayres, A. J. (1979). Sensory Integration and the Child. Los Angeles, California: Western Psychological Services.

Bazyk, S. (2010). Promotion of positive mental health in children and youth with developmental disabilities. *OT Practice, 15*(7), CE1-CE8.

Bazyk, S. (2011). *Mental health promotion, prevention and intervention with children and youth.* AOTA Press.

Bazyk, S. & Arbesman, M. (2013). *Occupational therapy practice guidelines for mental health promotion, prevention and intervention for children and youth.* AOTA Press.

Beck, A. T. & Steer, R. A. (1993). *Beck Anxiety Inventory manual.* Psychological Corporation.

Blaustein, M., & Kinniburgh, K. (2018). *Treating traumatic stress in children and adolescents: How to foster resilience through attachment, self-regulation, and competency* (2nd ed.). Guilford Press.

Booth, P., & Jernberg, J. (2010). *Theraplay: Helping parents and children build better relationships through play.* Wiley.

Bowlby, J. (1968). *Attachment and loss* (Vol. 1). Attachment. Basic Books.

Braveman, P. A., Heck, K., Egerter, S., et al. (2015). The role of socioeconomic factors in black–white disparities in preterm birth. *American Journal of Public Health, 105*(4), 694-702.

Brennan Ramirez, L. K., Baker, E. A., & Metzler, M. (2008). *Promoting health equity: A resource to help communities address social determinants of health.* Department of Health and Human Services, Centers for Disease Control and Prevention.

Brenner, J., Pan, Z., Mazefsky, C., Smith, K. A., & Gabriels, R. (2017). Behavioral symptoms of reported abuse in children and adolescents with autism spectrum disorder in inpatient settings. *Journal of Autism and Developmental Disorders, 48*, 3727-3735. https://doi.org/10.1007/s1080 3-017-3183-4

Briere, J. (1996). *Trauma Symptom Checklist for Children (TSCC): Professional manual.* Psychological Assessment Resources.

Bryant, A. S., Worjoloh, A., Caughey, A. B., et al. (2021). Racial/ethnic disparities in obstetric outcomes and care: Prevalence and determinants. *American Journal of Obstetrical Gynecology, 202*(4), 335-343.

Buhler-Wasserman, A. C., & Hibel, L. C. (2021). Studying caregiver-infant co-regulation in dynamic, diverse cultural contexts: A call to action. *Infant Behavior and Development, 64*. https://doi.org/10.1016/j.infbeh.2021.101586

Carnevali, L., Koenig, J., Sgoifo, A., & Ottaviani, C. (2018). Autonomic and brain morphological predictors of stress resilience. *Frontiers of Neuroscience, 22*(12). https://doi.org/10.3389/fnins.2018.00228

Carr, C., Martins, C., Stingel, A. M., Braga, V., & Juruena, M. (2013). The role of early life tress in adult psychiatric disorders, *The Journal of Nervous and Mental Disease, 201*(12), 1007-1020. https://doi.org/10.1097/NMD.0000000000000049

Centers for Disease Control and Prevention, National Center for Injury Prevention and Control (2020). Web-Based Injury Statistics Query and Reporting System (WISQARS). http://www.cdc.gov/injury/wisqars

Champagne, T. (2011). *Sensory modulation and environment: Essential elements of occupation.* Pearson.

Cohen, R., & Wardrip, K. (2011). *Should I stay or Should I go? Exploring the effects of housing instability and mobility on children.* Center for Housing Policy.

Conners, C. K. (2008). Conners (3rd ed.). Multi-Health Systems.

Coster, W., Deeney, T., Haltiwagner, J. T., & Haley, S. M. (1998). *School function assessment.* Psychological Corporation/Therapy Skill Builders.

Crum, A. J., Jamieson, J. P., & Akinola, M. (2020). Optimizing stress: An integrated intervention for regulating stress responses. *Emotion, 20*(1), 120-125. https://doi.org/10.1037/emo0000670

Edwards, O. W., & Pratt, H. (2016). Family meal participation as a corollary of positive youth development: Opportunities for counseling services. *International Journal for the Advancement of Counselling, 38*, 89-96.

Engel-Yeger, Z. B., Palgy-Levin, D., & Lev-Wiesel, R. (2013). The sensory profile of people with post-traumatic stress symptoms. *Occupational Therapy in Mental Health, 29*, 266-278.

Eyberg, S. M., Nelson, M. M., Ginn, N. C., Bhuiyan, N., & Boggs, S. R. (2013). *Dyadic parent-child interaction coding system: Comprehensive manual for research and training* (4th ed.). PCIT International.

Family Developing Resources. (2021). Nurturing parenting program. https://www.nurturingparenting.com/

Felitti, V., Anda, R., Nordenberg, D., Williamson, D., Spitz, A., Edwards, V., Koss, M., & Marks, J. (1998). Relationship of childhood abuse and household dysfunction to many of the leading causes of death in adults. The Adverse Childhood Experiences Study. *American Journal of Preventative Medicine, 14*(4), 245-258.

Garner, A., Shonkoff, J., Siegel, B., Dobbins, M., Earls, M., McGuinn, L., Pascoe, J., & Wood, D. (2012). Early childhood adversity, toxic stress, and the role of the pediatrician: Translating developmental science into lifelong health. *Pediatrics, 129*, e224-e231. https://doi.org/10.1542/peds.2011-2662

Gentile, S. (2017). Untreated depression during pregnancy: Short- and long-term effects in offspring. A systematic review. *Neuroscience 342*, 154-166.

Gerard, A. B. (1994). *Parent-Child Relationship Inventory (PCRI) manual*. WPS.

Ginsburg, K., & Jablow, M. (2020). *Building resilience in children and teens: Giving kids roots and wings* (4th ed.). American Academy of Pediatrics.

Greenspan, S. & Wieder, L. (2006). *Engaging autism: Using the floortime approach to help children relate, communicate and think.* Perseus Books.

Healthy People 2020. (n.d.). Adolescent health. https://www.healthypeople.gov/2020/topics-objectives/topic/Adolescent-Health

Healthy People 2030. (n.d.) School-based intervention teaches about healthy eating and physical activity. https://www.healthypeople.gov/2020/healthy-people-in-action/story/school-based-intervention-teaches-about-healthy-eating-and-physical-activity

Hoelscher, D. M., Springer, A. E., Ranjit, N., et al. (2010). Reductions in child obesity among disadvantaged school children with community involvement: The Travis County CATCH Trial. *Obesity, 18*(1), S36-S44.

Hoffmann, J. D., Brackett, M. A., Bailey, C. S., & Willner, C. J. (2020). Teaching emotion regulation in schools: Translating research into practice with the RULER approach to social and emotional learning. *Emotion, 20*(1), 101-109. https://doi.org/10.1037/emo0000649

International Labour Organization. (2012). ILO global estimate of forced labour: Results and methodology. http://www.ilo.org/wcmsp5/groups/public/ed_norm/ declaration/documents/publication/wcms_182004.pdf

Issel, L. M., & Wells, R. (2018). *Health program planning and evaluation: A practical systematic approach for community health* (4th ed.). Jones and Bartlett.

Kaslow, N. (2014). Suicidal behavior in children and adolescents. https://www.apa.org/about/governance/president/suicidal-behavior-adolescents.pdf

Kenardy, J. A., Spence, S. H., & Macleod, A. C. (2006). Screening for posttraumatic stress disorder in children after accidental injury. *Pediatrics, 118*(3), 1002-1009.

Kieling, C., Baker-Henningham, H., Belfer, M., Conti, G., Ertem, I., Omigbodun, O., Augusto Rohde, L., Srinath, S., Ulkuer, N., & Rahman, A. (2011). Child and adolescent mental health worldwide: Evidence for action. *The Lancet, 378*, 1515-1525. https://doi.org/10.1016/S0140-6736(11)60827-1

King, G., Law, M., King, S., Hurley P., Hanna, S., Kertoy, M., et al. (2004). *Children's Assessment of Participation and Enjoyment (CAPE) and Preferences for Activities of Children (PAC).* Harcourt Assessment.

King, G., Seko, Y., Chiarello, L. A., Thompson, L. (2018). Building blocks of resiliency: a transactional framework to guide research, service design, and practice in pediatric rehabilitation. *Disability and Rehabilitation, 42*(7), 1-10. doi: 10.1080/09638288.2018.1515266

Kingston, D., Tough, S., & Whitfield, H. (2012). Prenatal and postpartum maternal psychological distress and infant development: A systematic review. *Child Psychiatry Human Development, 43*, 683-714. https://doi.org/10.1007/s10578-012-0291-4.

Knight, J. R., Sherritt, L., Shrier, L. A., Harris, S. K., & Chang, G. (2002). Validity of the CRAFFT substance abuse screening test among adolescent clinic patients. *Archives of Pediatric Adolescent Medicine, 156*(6), 607-614.

Kuypers, L. (2011). *The zones of regulation.* Social Thinking Publishing.

Larson, K., & Halfon, N. (2010). Family income gradients in the health and health care access of U.S. children. *Maternal Child Health Journal, 14*(3), 332-342.

Law, M., Baptiste, S., Carswell, A., McColl, C., & Dillon, A. R. (2005). *The Canadian Occupational Performance Measure* (4th ed.). Canadian Association of Occupational Therapy.

Levine, P. (2005). *Healing trauma: A pioneering program for restoring the wisdom of your body*. Sounds True.

Levy, S., Weiss, R., Sherritt, L., Ziemnik, R., Spalding, A., Van Hook, S., & Shrier, L. A. (2014). An electronic screen for triaging adolescent substance use by risk levels. *JAMA Pediatrics, 168*(9), 822-828.

Linehan, M. (1993). *Skills training manual for treating borderline personality disorder*. Guilford Press.

Liu, Z., Li, X., & Ge, X. (2010). Left too early: The effects of age at separation from parents on Chinese rural children's symptoms of anxiety and depression. *American Journal of Public Health, 99*(11), 2049-2054.

Long, W., Bauchner, H., Sege, R., Cabral, H., & Garg A. (2012). The value of the medical home for children without special health care needs. *Pediatrics, 129*(1), 87-98.

May-Benson, T., & Tisdale, A. (2019). Validation of a sensory-based trauma informed intervention program using qualitative video analysis. *American Journal of Occupational Therapy, 73*, 7311520393. https://doi.org/10.5014/ajot.2019.73S1-PO2034

Mauritz, M. W., Goossens, P., Draijer, N., & van Achterberg, T. (2013) Prevalence of interpersonal trauma exposure and trauma-related disorders in severe mental illness, *European Journal of Psychotraumatology, 4*(1). https://doi.org/10.3402/ejpt.v4i0.19985

Mihelicova, M., Brown, M., & Shuman, V. (2017). Trauma-informed care for individuals with serious mental illness: An avenue for community psychology's involvement in community mental health. *Community Psychology, 61*, 141-152.

Mims, D., & Waddell, R. (2016). Animal assisted therapy and trauma Survivors. *Journal of Evidence Informed Social Work, 13*(5), 452-457.

Moffitt, T. E., Arseneault, L., Belsky, D., Dickson, N., Hancox, R. J., Harrington, H. L., Houts, R., Poulton, R., Roberts, B. W., Ross, S., Sears, M. R., Thomson, W. M., & Caspi, A. (2011). A gradient of childhood self-control predicts health, wealth, and public safety. *Proceedings of the National Academy of Sciences of the USA,108*, 2693-2698.

Monk, C., Lugo-Candelas, C., & Trumpff, C. (2019). Prenatal developmental origins of future psychopathology: Mechanisms and pathways. *Annual Review of Clinical Psychology, 15*, 317-344.

National Academies of Sciences, Engineering and Medicine (2019). *A roadmap to reducing child poverty*. The National Academies Press. https://doi.org/10.17226/25246

National Child Traumatic Stress Network. (n.d.). Psychological First Aid. https://www.nctsn.org/treatments-and-practices/psychological-first-aid-and skills-psychological-recovery/about-pfa

Nimeus, A., Alsen, M., & Traskman-Bendz, L. (2000). The suicide assessment scale: An instrument assessing suicide risk of suicide attempters. *European Psychiatry: The Journal of the Association of European Psychiatrists, 15*, 416-423. https://doi.org/10.1016/S0924-9338(00)00512-5

Office of Disease Prevention and Health Promotion. (n.d.). Social determinants of health. Healthy People 2030. U.S. Department of Health and Human Services. https://health.gov/healthypeople/objectives-and-data/social-determinants-health

O'Neil, A., Quirk, S. E., Housden, S., Brennan, S. L., Williams, L. J., Pasco, J. A., Berk, M., & Jacka, F. N. (2014). Relationship between diet and mental health in children and adolescents: A systematic review. *American Journal of Public Health 104*, e31_e42. https://doi.org/10.2105/AJPH.2014.302110

Paksarian, D., Eaton, W. W., Mortensen, P. B., Merikangas, K. R., & Pedersen, C. B. (2015). A population-based study of the risk of schizophrenia and bipolar disorder associated with parent-child separation during development. *Psychological Medicine, 45*(13), 2825-2837.

Perry, B. D. (2009). Examining child maltreatment through a neurodevelopmental lens: Clinical applications of the neurosequential model of therapeutics. Journal of Loss and Trauma, 14, 240-255.

Pfefferbaum, R. L., Pfefferbaum, B., & Van Horn, R. L. (2011). *Communities Advancing Resilience Toolkit (CART) survey*. Terrorism and Disaster Center at the University of Oklahoma Health Sciences Center.

Pontoppidan, M., Niss, N. K., Pejtersen, J. H., Julian, M. M., & Vaever, M. S. (2017). Parent report measures of infant and toddler social-emotional development: A systematic review. *Family Practice, 34*(2), 127-137.

Porges, S. (2011). *The polyvagal theory*. W.W. Norton and Company, Inc.

Posner, K., Brown, G. K., Stanley, B., Brent, D. A., Yershova, K. V., Oquendo, M. A., Currier, G. W., Melvin, G. A., Greenhill, L., Shen, S., & Mann, J. J. (2011). The Columbia-Suicide Severity Rating Scale: Initial validity and internal consistency findings from three multisite studies with adolescents and adults. *American Journal of Psychiatry 168*(12), 1266-1277.

Powell, B., Cooper, G., Hoffman, K., & Marvin, B. (2013). *The circle of security intervention: Enhancing attachment in early parent-child relationships*. Guilford Press.

Romero, M., & Lee, Y. (2008). The influence of maternal and family risk on chronic absenteeism in early schooling. National Center for Children in Poverty. http://www.nccp.org/publications/pdf/text_792.pdf

Selye, H. (1956). The Stress of Life. McGraw-Hill Book Company.

Shaffer, D., Fisher, P., Lucas, C. P., Dulcan, M. K., & Schwab-Stone, M. E. (2000). NIMH Diagnostic Interview Schedule for Children Version IV (NIMH DISC-IV): Description, differences from previous versions, and reliability of some common diagnoses. *Journal of the American Academy of Child & Adolescent Psychiatry, 39*(1), 28-38.

Shi, H., Wang, Y., Li, M., Tan, C., Zhao, C., Huang, X., Dou, Y., Duan, X., Du, Y., Wu, T., Wang, X., & Zhang, J. (2021). Impact of parent-child separation on children's social-emotional development: a cross-sectional study of left-behind children in poor rural areas of China. *BMC public health, 21*(1), 823. https://doi.org/10.1186/s12889-021-10831-8

Smith, M. V., Gotman, N., & Yonkers, K. A. (2016). Early childhood adversity and pregnancy outcomes. *Maternal Child Health Journal, 20*, 790-798. https://doi.org/10.1007/s10995-015-1909-5

Stack, A., & Lucyshyn, J. (2018). Autism spectrum disorder and the experience of traumatic events: Review of the current literature to inform modifications to a treatment model for children with autism. *Journal of Autism and Developmental Disorders, 49*, 1613-1625. https://doi.org/10.1007/s10803-018-3854-9

Substance Abuse and Mental Health Services Administration. (2020a). Recognizing and treating childhood traumatic stress. https://www.samhsa.gov/child-trauma/recognizing-and-treating-child-traumatic-stress#signs

Substance Abuse and Mental Health Services Administration. (2020b). Understanding child trauma. https://www.samhsa.gov/child-trauma/understanding-child-trauma

Tan, C., Zhao, C., & Dou, Y., et al. (2020). Caregivers' depressive symptoms and social–emotional development of left-behind children under 3 years old in poor rural China: The mediating role of home environment. *Childdren and Youth Services Review, 16*, 105-109.

Thompson, M. P., Kingree, J. B., & Lamis, D. (2019). Associations of adverse childhood experiences and suicidal behaviors in adulthood in a US nationally representative sample. *Child: Care, Health, and Development, 45*(1), 121-128.

Topolski, T. D., Patrick, D. L., Edwards, T. C., Huebner, C. E., Connell, F. A., & Mount, K. K. (2001). Quality of life and health risk behaviors among adolescents. *Journal of Adolescent Health, 29*(6), 426-435.

Triple P International. (n.d.). Triple P - Positive Parenting Program. Retrieved August 5, 2021, from https://www.triplep-parenting.com/us/triple-p/?cdsid=um0dq2d28h9smu1nsv6vam733b

U.S. Department of Health and Human Services. (2011). Office of the Surgeon General. The Surgeon General's Call to Action to Support Breastfeeding. Rockville, MD: Office of the Surgeon General.

van der Kolk, B. (2005). Clinical implications of neuroscience research and PTSD. *Annals New York Academy of Science, 1071*, 277-293.

van der Kolk, B. (2014). *The body keeps the score: Mind, brain, and body in the healing of trauma*. Penguin Group LLC.

Viner R. M., Ozer E. M., Denny S., Marmot M., Resnick M., Fatusi A., & Currie C. (2012). Adolescence and the social determinants of health. *Lancet, 379*(9826), 1641-1652. https://doi.org/10.1016/S0140-6736(12)60149-4.

Waters, E. B., Salmon, L. A., Wake, M., Wright, M., & Hesketh, K. D. (2001). The health and well-being of adolescents: A school-based population study of the self-report Child Health Questionnaire. *The Journal of Adolescent Health, 29*(2), 140-149.

Whiteford, G., & Townsend, E. (2011). Participatory Occupational Justice Framework (POJF): Enabling occupational participation and inclusion. In F. Kronenberg, N. Pollard, & D. Sakellariou (Eds.), *Occupational therapy without borders: Volume 2: Towards an ecology of occupation-based practices* (pp. 65-84). Elsevier Churchill Livingstone.

Wilcock, A. A., & Townsend, E. (2014). Occupational justice. In B. A. Boyt Shell, G. Gillen, & M. E. Scaffa (Eds.), *Willard and Spackman's occupational therapy* (pp. 541-552). Lippincott, Williams, & Wilkins

Wolraich, M. L., Feurer, I. D., Hannah, J. N., Baumgaertel, A., & Pinnock, T. Y. (1998). Obtaining systematic teacher reports of disruptive behavior disorders utilizing DSM-IV. *Journal of Abnormal Child Psychology, 26*(2), 141-152.

World Health Organization. (2001). *International Classification of Functioning, Disability and Health*. Author.

World Health Organization. (2017). *Determinants of health*. https://www.who.int/news-room/q-a-detail/determinants-of-health

Yochman, A., & Pat-Horenczyk, R. (2020). Sensory modulation in children exposed to continuous traumatic stress. *Journal of Child & Adolescent Trauma, 13*, 93-102.

Youth.gov. (n.d.). Mental Health Promotion and Prevention. Other Youth Topics. https://youth.gov/youth-topics/youth-mental-health/mental-health-promotion-prevention

Zarse, E., Neff, M., Yoder, R., Hulvershorn, L., Chambers, J., & Chambers, R. A. (2019). The adverse childhood experiences questionnaire: Two decades of research on childhood trauma as a primary cause of adult mental illness, addiction, and medical diseases. *Cogent Medicine, 6*(1). https://doi.org/10.1080/2331205X.2019.1581447

CHAPTER 14

Promoting Mental and Emotional Health
Adults

Christine Urish, PhD, OTR/L, BCMH, FAOTA, CCAP and
Michael A. Pizzi, PhD, OTR/L, FAOTA

Learning Objectives

At the end of this chapter, the reader will:

1. Identify assessments that can be utilized to address client wellness and foster interdisciplinary collaboration related to delivery of therapeutic intervention (ACOTE B.4.25)
2. Identify areas of meaningful activity as related to mental health promotion for adults (ACOTE B.4.3)
3. Identify strategies to foster change within clients who struggle or appear reluctant or experience difficulty with the change process (ACOTE B.4.1)
4. Understand the concept of flourishing and how this relates to the dimensions of wellness (ACOTE B.3.4)

The ACOTE Standards used are those from 2018.

Key Words

Dimensions of Wellness, Eudaimonic Well-Being, Health Behaviors, Hedonic Well-Being, Intentional Relationship Model, LEAP Approach, Motivational Interviewing, Ottawa Charter for Health Promotion, Recovery Model, Risk and Protective Factors, Two Continua Model

Case Study

Ray is a 43-year-old widower. His wife died 5 years ago due to colon cancer. Her cancer was undetected until it was stage 4 and from diagnosis to death was 8 months. Since her death, Ray has struggled with his physical, social, and emotional health. During this time Ray has experienced several failed romantic relationships. Currently he is being seen by a physical therapist due to low back pain. Ray is self-employed as an entrepreneurial consultant. He has a bachelor's degree in music performance, but his most significant skill

Pizzi, M. A., & Amir, M. (Eds.). *Interprofessional Perspectives for Community Practice: Promoting Health, Well-Being, and Quality of Life* (pp. 263-282).

set is social media marketing and interpersonal/community networking.

Ray has two children—David is a senior in high school and Lauren is a high school freshman. The family has struggled collectively with a variety of challenges since the death of Ray's wife. Ray easily acknowledges his challenges physically with low back pain and sleep apnea; however, he appears in denial of his overall state of emotional health. Ray is morbidly obese and has experienced increased anxiety and depression since the death of his wife. He is on medication for his depression and anxiety and recently sustained a shoulder injury during a move into a smaller living space.

Ray's primary care physician has referred him to a mental health counselor, who is a social worker at a local health care system. He has begun counseling sessions twice per month and has made progress with his anxiety; however, he continues to struggle with depression, which has impacted completion of activities of daily living, instrumental activities of daily living, social participation, and leisure engagement. Ray struggles with grief related to the loss of his wife. Further, Ray and his late wife had a clear division of labor related to home management and care of the children. Ray was the primary breadwinner working outside the home and his wife managed everything else. Although his children help in the home, Ray feels responsible for everything, which causes increased stress and anxiety.

Ray's physician referred him to physical therapy to address his lower back pain. The physical therapist identified that an occupational therapist would be beneficial to address limitations in areas of self-care, health maintenance, and sleep hygiene. Social work, occupational therapy, and physical therapy services are being provided at a local hospital outpatient clinic. Ray's children are receiving grief counseling services through the National Alliance for Children's Grief, and they have participated in Camp Kessem for the past 3 years to continue to process their feelings related to the loss of their mother. Ray recognizes his depression, anxiety, and grief are negatively impacting his life and well-being. His weight has been a long-standing challenge as well. He was able to gain approval from his insurance to have gastric sleeve surgery; however, all disciplines have shared with Ray that this is not a final solution. Ray attends therapy sessions with occupational therapists, physical therapists, and social workers, and he continues to struggle enacting individualized goals and home programs outside of the formal prescribed therapy sessions. The three disciplines are struggling with limited progress toward goals and are considering discharge, despite their awareness of his ongoing need for services. They worry about Ray's eating behaviors and seeming unwillingness to change after the gastric sleeve procedure.

Reflective Questions

1. How can occupational therapy, physical therapy, and social work collaborate to assure all the client's identified concerns are being met in the most efficient manner and work effective in an interprofessional fashion?
2. From an occupational therapy, physical therapy, and social work perspective what will each discipline address as goals to assure the client is at the center of the health care team?
3. How can the occupational therapy, physical therapy, and social work health care team facilitate active engagement on the part of the client in addressing health promotion goals, when there is little carry over and limited engagement in the established home program from the client?
4. What are the mental health challenges experienced by Ray and how would an interprofessional mental health team assess and intervene?

Introduction

Health is not the absence of disease or illness, but rather is composed of individual elements that allow individuals to engage in productive, satisfying lives (Centers for Disease Control and Prevention [CDC], 2018). A state of health enables social, economic, and individual development essential to well-being. The Ottawa Charter for Health Promotion (World Health Organization [WHO], 1986) goes much further and states:

> Health is created and lived by people within the settings of their everyday life; where they learn, work, play, and love. Health is created by caring for oneself and others, by being able to make decisions and have control over one's life circumstances and by ensuring that the society one lives in creates conditions that allow the attainment of health by all its members. Caring, holism, and ecology are essential issues in developing strategies for health promotion and wellness. (p. 1)

Within this definition, there are many concepts that relate directly to promoting mental health and well-being. Self-care (caring for oneself and taking care of one's own needs) also includes advocating for oneself, being self-directed, and having self-determination while having control over one's life circumstances relates to maintaining one's mental health and supporting overall health.

The WHO further defines mental health promotion as "a state of well-being in which the individual realizes his or her own abilities, can cope with the normal stresses of life, can work productively and fruitfully, and is able to contribute to his or her own community" (2018, para. 3).

Crucial to promoting positive mental health is the concept of "ensuring that the society one lives in creates conditions that allow the attainment of health by all its members" (WHO, 1986, p. 1). Interprofessional teams working with individuals, communities, or populations have the obligation and privilege to create those opportunities to reduce barriers to mental health in order for full participation, engagement, and positive coping in daily life to be realized. Positive mental health fosters the ability of individuals to cope with life challenges, be engaged in work, and offer contributions to the community (SAMHSA, 2020). Mental health promotion can assist an individual in critically examining individualized strategies to increase personal control to improve overall health (CDC, 2018).

Mental Health and Mental Illness

While mental illness in many societies is common, one in five adults in the United States experience mental illness annually (National Alliance on Mental Illness, n.d.). Unipolar depression is the most common illness that can lead to disengagement in life activity, and according to the WHO, can become the leading illness burden in developed and underdeveloped countries (WHO, 2008). The effects of mental illness, particularly depression, are keenly felt in families and communities, and individuals with depression, which is often accompanied by anxiety, are 40% more likely to experience cardiovascular and metabolic diseases (National Alliance on Mental Illness [NAMI], 2021a).

Promoting positive mental health and creating conditions for such within the context of one's life (e.g., families, schools, communities) can act as protective factors against mental illness. Sturgeon (2007), citing the WHO, states that "mental health promotion includes strategies to promote the mental well-being of those who are not at risk, those who are at increased risk and those who are suffering or recovering from mental health problems" (p. 37). Mental health promotion, a state of well-being as characterized earlier, helps to diminish any symptomatology of mental illness to a great degree and protects against the loss of positive mental health. Use of a public health approach can complement treatment (Keyes, 2007). While treatment targets those with mental illness, and use of a risk reduction approach can work with those at risk for mental illness, "mental health promotion targets those with good mental health and those with less than optimal mental health…." (Keyes, 2014, p. 180). Thus, it is vital that health professionals explore the risk and protective factors that impact the mental health of individuals, families, communities, and populations, whether mentally well or unwell, and examine how best to support and promote positive mental health through proper assessment and intervention using a public health approach.

Protective and Risk Factors for Mental Health

Each person has a unique set of factors in their lives that can either put them more at risk for or protect them from mental health issues. These factors do not exist in isolation and are often cumulative. Risk and protective factors also exist in multiple contexts, meaning mitigating one or two risk factors in the home does not mean the problem is solved at school or work (SAMHSA, n.d.). **Risk factors** are those health determinants such as poverty, injustice, familial issues, societal barriers, and poor community living conditions that place a person at risk for poor mental health (Rashbrook, 2019). **Protective factors** are those that shield one from poor mental health, or at least can reduce mental health issues for one to better cope with life circumstances (Rashbrook, 2019). Protective factors can include positive family relationships, resilience (being able to adapt and cope well with life circumstances), having a sense of belonging, and economic security (Rashbrook, 2019). Others include integration of ethnic minorities, empowerment, social participation, social services, and social support and community networks (Commission on Social Determinants of Health, 2004). See Table 14-1 for a more complete list of risk and protective factors for mental health that is inclusive of those risk and protective factors of childhood that impact mental health.

Knowing these risk and protective factors assist the interprofessional team with proper assessment and interventions. During the intake process for any health professional, part of a person's profile needs to include a checklist of risk and protective factors. For example, if one presents with depression, knowing risk factors such as family disruption, lower socioeconomic status, abuse, or feelings of isolation and alienation and protective factors such as having positive self-esteem and self-worth, social support, and self-determination would help the team work from a strength-based (protective factor) approach to further strengthen and promote positive mental health and well-being.

Table 14-1

Risk and Protective Factors

STAGE OF DEVELOPMENT	INDIVIDUAL RISK AND PROTECTIVE FACTORS	FAMILY RISK AND PROTECTIVE FACTORS	SCHOOL OR COMMUNITY RISK AND PROTECTIVE FACTORS
Early childhood	*Risk Factors*		
	• Difficult temperament • Insecure attachment • Hostile to peers, socially inhibited • Irritability • Fearfulness • Head injury • Motor, language, and cognitive impairments • Early aggressive behavior	• Parental drug/alcohol use • Cold and unresponsive mother behavior • Marital conflict • Negative events • Parental drug/alcohol use • Family dysfunction • Parental loss	• Poor academic performance in early grades • Specific traumatic experiences • Negative events • Lack of control or mastery experiences • Urban setting • Poverty
	Protective Factors		
	• Self-regulation • Secure attachment • Mastery of communication and language skills • Ability to make friends and get along with others	• Reliable support and discipline from caregivers • Responsiveness • Protection from harm and fear • Opportunities to resolve conflict • Adequate socioeconomic resources for the family	• Support for early learning • Access to supplemental services such as feeding, and screening for vision and hearing • Stable secure attachment to child care provider • Low ratio of caregivers to children • Regulatory systems that support high quality of care
Middle childhood	*Risk Factors*		
	• Negative self-image • Apathy • Anxiety • Dysthymia • Insecure attachment • Poor social skills: impulsive, aggressive, passive, and withdrawn • Poor social problem-solving skills • Shyness • Poor impulse control • Sensation-seeking • Lack of behavioral self-control • Impulsivity	• Parental depression • Poor parenting, rejection, lack of parental warmth • Child abuse/maltreatment • Loss • Marital conflict or divorce • Family dysfunction • Parents with anxiety disorder or anxious childrearing practices • Parental overcontrol and intrusiveness	• Peer rejection • Stressful life events • Poor grades/achievements • Poverty • Stressful community events such as violence • Witnessing community violence • Social trauma • Negative events • Lack of control or mastery experiences

(continued)

Table 14-1 (continued)

Risk and Protective Factors

STAGE OF DEVELOPMENT	INDIVIDUAL RISK AND PROTECTIVE FACTORS	FAMILY RISK AND PROTECTIVE FACTORS	SCHOOL OR COMMUNITY RISK AND PROTECTIVE FACTORS
Middle childhood	*Protective Factors*		
	• Mastery of academic skills (math, reading, writing) • Following rules for behavior at home, school, and public places • Ability to make friends • Good peer relationships	• Consistent discipline • Language-based rather than physically based discipline • Extended family support	• Healthy peer groups • School engagement • Positive teacher expectations • Effective classroom management • Positive partnering between school and family • School policies and practices to reduce bullying • High academic standards
Adolescence	*Risk Factors*		
	• Low self-esteem, perceived incompetence, negative explanatory, and inferential style • Anxiety • Low-level depressive symptoms and dysthymia • Insecure attachment • Poor social skills: communication and problem-solving skills • Extreme need for approval and social support	• Parent with anxiety • Parental/marital conflict • Family conflict (interactions between parents and children and among children) • Parental drug/alcohol use • Parental unemployment • Poor attachment with parents • Family member with psychiatric illness • Poor parental supervision • Parental depression • Sexual abuse	• Peer rejection • Poor academic achievement • Community-level stressful or traumatic events • School-level stressful or traumatic events • Community violence • School violence • Poverty • Low commitment to school • Not college bound • Aggression toward peers
	Protective Factors		
	• Positive physical development • Academic achievement/intellectual development • High self-esteem • Emotional self-regulation • Good coping skills and problem-solving skills • Engagement and connections in two or more of the following contexts: school, with peers, in athletics, employment, religion, culture	• Family provides structure, limits, rules, monitoring, and predictability • Supportive relationships with family members • Clear expectations for behavior and values	• Presence of mentors and support for development of skills and interests • Opportunities for engagement within school and community • Positive norms • Clear expectations for behavior • Physical and psychological safety

(continued)

Table 14-1 (continued)

Risk and Protective Factors

STAGE OF DEVELOPMENT	INDIVIDUAL RISK AND PROTECTIVE FACTORS	FAMILY RISK AND PROTECTIVE FACTORS	SCHOOL OR COMMUNITY RISK AND PROTECTIVE FACTORS
Early adulthood (18 to 25 years)	*Risk Factors*		
	• Early-onset depression and anxiety • Need for extensive social support • Childhood history of untreated anxiety disorders • Childhood history of poor physical health • Childhood history of sleep and eating problems • Poor physical health • Lack of commitment to conventional adult roles • Antisocial behavior • Head injury	• Parental depression • Spousal conflict • Single parenthood • Leaving home • Family dysfunction • Social isolation	• Decrease in social support accompanying entry into a new social context • Negative life events • Attending college • Substance-using peers • Social adversity
	Protective Factors		
	• Identity exploration in love, work, and world view • Subjective sense of adult status • Subjective sense of self-sufficiency, making independent decisions, becoming financially independent • Future orientation • Achievement	• Balance of autonomy and relatedness to family • Behavioral and emotional autonomy	• Opportunities for exploration in work and school • Connectedness to adults outside of family

Adapted from the U.S. Department of Health and Human Services. (n.d.) *Risk and protective factors*. https://iod.unh.edu/sites/default/files/media/2021-11/c3-handout-2-hhs-risk-and-proetctive-factors.pdf

Therapeutic Approaches to Promote Positive Mental Health

The foundation of the client/health care practitioner relationship is the effective use of a therapeutic approach. Practitioners may possess clinical skills within their individual disciplines; however, if the client does not feel seen, heard, and valued, the therapeutic relationship could be off to a challenging start. It is imperative that health care practitioners examine their own therapeutic approach when meeting with a client to address health and well-being needs in order to foster well-being and quality of life (QOL).

An approach by Amador (2012) focuses on **listening, empathizing, agreeing and partnering (LEAP)** and can be utilized by any health care discipline. The focus of this approach is to provide a judgment-free, genuine understanding from the client point of view, especially clients who deny there is a health care need and feel they do not need "help." Amador designed the approach to be utilized with individuals diagnosed with schizophrenia who have limited insight into their lack of reality-based thinking; however, it can be used with many other populations.

The health care practitioner engages with the client, first by **listening** intently to what the client has to say and observing client behavior, considering unspoken communications, in order to determine what areas need to be further discussed and addressed. For example, in the case of Ray, the client has experienced many changes in his life within the past 5 years; however, at this time he appears to be focusing on the gastric sleeve procedure as the intervention that will "completely change" his entire life related to his well-being. It is not apparent to Ray that he has difficulty with limited motivation to complete required daily tasks, engaging in parenting responsibilities, and follow through with agreed-upon goals outside of scheduled therapy sessions. Careful listening to the client perspective to address his limited insight into current challenges or denial of problems is vital. Health care practitioners cannot assume they understand the client's situation from a chart review or participation in team meeting.

Empathizing is the next step of the LEAP approach. This includes meeting the client where they are mentally and emotionally and empathizing with their current entire situation. Empathy helps to strengthen the therapeutic relationship by conveying that the practitioner understands the issues being discussed. The health care practitioner should utilize empathy in exploration of actions and strategies that have the potential to improve overall well-being. Using empathy with Ray regarding his health and wellness challenges over the past 5 years and addressing next steps for desired changes toward health and wellness demonstrates the health care practitioners' regard and esteem toward the client.

Agreement is the next step according to Amador (2012). Health care practitioners agree that the gastric sleeve procedure will have an impact; however, there are other areas that will need to continue to be addressed in a comprehensive fashion to achieve the overall health and wellness/well-being goals. Rather than the health care practitioner making a statement such as "well that's only one part to be addressed," one should acknowledge Ray's perceptions of the situation, help him appraise that situation, and develop an agreement about what can be done to develop positive alliances to move toward change. Throughout the practitioner/client relationship, the practitioner will discover several areas of agreement with the client, which continues to build on listening and empathy.

Partnering is the last strategy presented by Amador (2012). Partnering is when the health care practitioner actively engages the client as an equal partner in planning and implementing the desired change in thoughts, feelings, or behavior. From an interprofessional perspective, health care practitioners need to actively engage and partner with one another to address identified goals, supporting one another to comprehensively address all dimensions of well-being for the client. Although the client may present with many challenges, that same client also possesses many strengths. The interprofessional health care practitioner can partner with the client in their self-examination of strengths and how those strengths can be utilized to identify client-centered goals. Clients may struggle with challenging situations and want to rely on the interprofessional health care team to "fix" a situation. Partnering with the client values the client's involvement in the therapeutic process and desire to work collaboratively to address areas of concern utilizing a strengths-based approach (use of personal strengths).

For example, in the case of Ray, his social and financial dimension areas of wellness are strengths. The interprofessional health care team can partner with Ray on how these strength areas can be utilized effectively to address ongoing challenges in mental health promotion and to address the guiding principles of recovery according to the Substance Abuse and Mental Health Services Administration (SAMHSA; 2012).

The Intentional Relationship Model

Utilizing the intentional relationship model (Taylor, 2020) while engaging in interprofessional approaches can also assist in fostering a positive therapeutic relationship. This model can be utilized by any discipline and considers the client's individual context and behavior, prior to choosing a communication mode to utilize when interacting with the client. There are six therapeutic modes. Please refer to Table 14-2 for information regarding each mode and related definition.

Based upon the practitioner's choice of mode, and the client response to the practitioner, the interaction is examined by the practitioner to determine if the mode was effective (Taylor, 2020). If the practitioner does not feel the mode was effective, they may choose to utilize a different mode. Different therapeutic modes are beneficial for different client interactions, contexts, and challenges that may present during the assessment, intervention, and the discharge planning processes. The use of a variety of therapeutic modes can be directly related to the concept of recovery (SAMHSA, 2012). One of the guiding principles in recovery is person driven. Use of "advocating mode" or "problem-solving mode" could foster increased control on the part of the client and increase movement toward wellness and recovery. The use of "encouraging mode" could foster a sense of respect within the client. Health care practitioners are challenged to examine the therapeutic modes utilized and examine the relationship of mode use to guiding principles of recovery.

The importance of the six therapeutic modes is to examine the client's response to the therapeutic process and consider which mode could assist the client toward independence and goal attainment. In the case of Ray, when discussing challenges related to overall well-being, the interprofessional health care team may utilize empathizing and instructing (Taylor, 2020). When discussing plans for a home program to be utilized from one session to the next, the interprofessional health care practitioner may utilize problem solving to assist Ray in overcoming any challenges that may arise related to initiation and engagement in identified home program to be enacted between sessions.

In addition to therapeutic modes utilized by individual health care practitioners, Taylor designed various assessments that practitioners can utilize to gain insight into their

Table 14-2

Intentional Relationship Therapeutic Modes

MODE	DEFINITION
Advocating	Providing client knowledge of necessary services or resources. Increasing client knowledge of rights.
Collaborating	Releasing therapeutic control to foster client independence. Engaging client through following their lead.
Encouraging	The use of positive communication to encourage continued movement toward identified desired behaviors or goals. Instillation of hope, praise, motivational communication.
Empathizing	Utilization of active listening and communication that demonstrate intent and effort to clearly understand client experience and individual perspective.
Instructing	Utilizing teaching approaches to guide, educate, explain, and demonstrate.
Problem solving	Fostering client ability to identify and develop options for action. The use of Socratic questioning can be utilized.
Adapted from Taylor, R. (2020). *The Intentional Relationship Model: Occupational therapy and the use of self.* F.A. Davis.	

Table 14-3

Motivational Interviewing Processes

PROCESS	PROCESS DESCRIPTION
Engaging	Engaging is foundational for MI. Developing a productive working relationship requires careful listening, which promotes engagement with the client. This helps practitioners to understand and accurately reflect the person's experience and perspective. Affirming client strengths and supporting autonomy is essential.
Focusing	In order to help a client change health behaviors, it is crucial to help clients focus on that need for change. An agenda is negotiated between client and practitioners that agree on a shared purpose, which gives the clinician permission to move into a directional conversation about change.
Evoking	Evoking means to elicit the client's ideas and motivations for health behavior change, whereby the clinician gently explores and helps the person explore these concepts. Clients may be ambivalent; however, that is deemed normal and part of the process. Careful listening to the client discussion about change helps move the process along.
Planning	Planning explores strategies for change, the client commitment to change, and includes the client's insights, motivations, strengths, and their own ideas for how to make changes. This process should occur when the client is ready and poised to make change.
Adapted from *Understanding motivational interviewing.* (n.d.). https://motivationalinterviewing.org/understanding-motivational-interviewing	

own individual effectiveness within therapy. Health care practitioners can ask their client for feedback on therapeutic interaction by using the *Clinical Assessment of Modes: Communicating with Your Therapist* and across disciplines, health care practitioners can observe and provide feedback to one another utilizing the *Clinical Assessment of Modes—Observer Assessment.* These tools are available free of charge from the University of Illinois, IRM Assessment website (2021). It is important to engage in ongoing self-reflection and examination of therapeutic effectiveness as an individual practitioner, as well as a member of an interprofessional treatment team.

Motivational interviewing (MI) strategies can be utilized in conjunction with the LEAP approach. Practitioners need to be competent in the skills and techniques of motivational interviewing. Four processes essential to utilization of MI include engaging, focusing, evoking, and planning (SAMHSA, 2021). MI strategies are helpful in assisting the client in developing strategies toward change (SAMHSA, 2021). Please refer to Table 14-3 for information regarding the processes within MI.

Through the exchange of information using the processes described, there are basic core skills identified in MI that when practiced and utilized by the health care practitioner can yield positive transformative change for individuals in order to help them flourish in their daily lives and community living. See Table 14-4 for information related to the core skills of motivational interviewing.

Health practitioners need to be open to accepting feedback from one another, working as a team, and strengthening interprofessional communication. In addition, the client must be included as an active participant in the ongoing assessment of progress or change within the therapeutic environment, no matter the approach. Communication is

Table 14-4

Core Skills of Motivational Interviewing

CORE SKILLS	SKILLS DESCRIPTION
Open questions	Closed questions are generally yes/no, while open questions draw out and explore the person's experiences, perspectives, and ideas. These help to guide the client to reflect on how change may be meaningful or possible. Practitioners first explore what the person already knows and then seeks permission to offer what the practitioner knows and understands and then explores the person's response.
Affirmation	Affirming the very being of a person is a key component for client-centered care. Practitioners affirm the client strengths, efforts, and past successes to support the development of self-efficacy and to help to build the person's hope and confidence in their ability to change.
Reflections	Repeating, rephrasing, or offering a deeper guess about what the person is trying to communicate is helping one to reflect on what is being felt, heard, and said in the process. Listening is crucial for health practitioners. This is a foundational skill of MI.
Summarizing	Health practitioners summarize what has been said and heard, ensuring shared understanding and reinforces key points made by the client. Summarizing can then lead to planning for health behavior change.
Attending to the language of change	Crucial to the MI process is for health practitioners to pay careful attention to language being used that identifies supports and barriers for health behavior change, and encouraging a movement toward change.

Adapted from *Understanding motivational interviewing.* (n.d.) https://motivationalinterviewing.org/understanding-motivational-interviewing

essential for client and health care practitioner success to improve client overall health and well-being (Professional Reasoning Box A).

Positive Psychology and Well-Being

There are many identified factors that contribute to well-being. Well-being is measured by the extent that one flourishes, according to Seligman (2011). Przybylko et al. (2021) cites Seligmans' definition of **flourishing** as a "multi-dimensional construct that integrates the presence of positive emotions (hedonic well-being) with high levels of psychological functioning (eudemonic well-being)" (p. 1). **Hedonic well-being** focuses on happiness that can be attained by avoiding pain and attaining pleasure (Kahneman et al., 1999). It is subjective, has a cognitive component of appraising one's life satisfaction, and focuses on positive emotions, such as happiness. **Eudaimonic well-being** relates to meaning and striving toward excellence in functioning (e.g., positive coping, handling emotions, being mentally well, being purposeful in life; Di Fabio & Palazzeschi, 2015; Keyes, 2014).

The goal of positive psychology is to help people (and communities) flourish. Different than focusing on mental health problems or challenges, the focus of positive psychology is a strengths-based, subjective approach optimizing one's happiness, life satisfaction, and well-being among other factors. However, Seligman has altered this approach to focus more on well-being and flourishing, noting that life satisfaction measures one's rating of their satisfaction only at that singular moment of assessment, which could be mood dependent while happiness was dependent only on positive emotion, engagement, and meaning. Seligman adapted his original construct of positive psychology and added relationships and accomplishment that, together with positive emotion, meaning and engagement, help people flourish.

Flourishing rests upon five pillars identified by Seligman: positive emotion, engagement, relationships, meaning, and accomplishment (PERMA; Table 14-5).

As health care practitioners, we value health, well-being, and meaningful engagement. These are quintessential elements to consider for clients' mental health. Health care practitioners and interprofessional mental health teams are encouraged to critically examine their professional values and engage in focused promotion of health in each and every client interaction, rather than being deficit-focused in total (Duque, 2004). It is that singular approach that strengthens abilities to take control of one's life, be attentive to self-care, and helps one to flourish.

In focusing on pillars of flourishing as identified by Seligman (2011), interprofessional health care teams can incorporate these pillars in assessment, intervention planning, implementation, community engagement, and discharge. For example, the practitioner could ask the client to identify one thing they are grateful for at the beginning or end of a session. This would be utilizing the pillar of positive emotion as well as the therapeutic mode of encouraging and empathizing. This could be carried over to a home program developed by client and the interprofessional team. When the client feels discouraged, identifying progress and gratitude toward attained changes could serve as a motivator for continued progress. The use of the pillar of engagement can be accomplished in collaborating with the client to identify

Professional Reasoning Box A

Health care professionals are often challenged with clients who may desire "change" within their life but struggle to enact change from session to session or experience difficulty with follow through of home programs designed to foster behavioral change. Amador (2012) proposes using the LEAP Approach. Models such as the Transtheoretical Model (Prochaska & DiClemente, 1982) offer strategies to examine behavioral change process, from pre-contemplation, contemplation, preparation, action, and maintenance of a behavior. MI has also proven to be an effective strategy that can be utilized across disciplines, often utilizing the TTM (SAMHSA, 2021). The intentional relationship model, which could be utilized by any discipline examines the client's behavior, with the therapist choosing a communication mode to assist in fostering movement toward the agreed-upon goal (Taylor, 2020).

How do each of these models differ from and are complementary to each other?

Table 14-5

Definitions of the Pillars of Flourishing

WELL-BEING PILLAR	DEFINITION
Positive emotion	Examination of positive emotion of the past, present, or future through gratitude, mindfulness, focus on hope, and optimism.
Engagement	Focused attention on a challenging task and the use of personal strengths in task engagement and accomplishment. Engagement can foster "flow" where the individual may engage in the task for the enjoyment of engaging, rather than the potential outcome. Engagement is the benefit obtained.
Relationships	Connections to others offer purpose and meaning. When individuals engage in supportive acts toward others, well-being is increased.
Meaning	Engagement in something larger than oneself. Some examples include organized religion, political activities, social causes, professional organizations.
Accomplishment	Pursuit of achievement, competence, success, mastery. Could include areas of work and leisure.

Adapted from Seligman, M. E. P. (2011). *Flourish*. Simon & Schuster.

activities they prefer engaging in and "lose track" of time (flow state) due to their enjoyment of the activity. For example, in the case of Ray, he is struggling with pain and following his home program established by the treatment team. Upon further exploration, it is discovered that Ray loves to swim and that he can be in the pool and swim countless laps and lose track of time. The exercise is good for his overall physical health, can be accomplished as a rehabilitative technique to treat his shoulder concern, and is something he enjoys, which would be considered engagement. When Ray finishes his swim, he experiences a sense of accomplishment, which fosters further motivation to encourage him to continue with positive behavior changes that will improve his mental well-being.

The WHO has identified that there is no health without mental health. Mental health promotion involves direct actions that support psychological well-being (WHO, 2018). "An environment that respects and protects basic civil, political, socioeconomic and cultural rights is fundamental to mental health. Without the security and freedom provided by these rights, it is difficult to maintain a high level of mental health" (WHO, 2018 para. 1). Practitioner advocacy can be one strategy to utilize to actively work toward positive societal change.

Models for Promoting Positive Mental Health

In order to promote optimal mental health, practitioners view of health behaviors is essential. **Health behaviors** are those actions one takes that can promote and enhance one's health, such as daily exercise and activity, healthy eating, and practicing mindfulness while negative health behaviors can include smoking, negative self-talk, and drinking to excess (Short & Mollborn, 2015). There are many models in health promotion that can be utilized as frameworks for health behavior change, which have been mentioned elsewhere in this textbook. For the purposes of this chapter, two models related to promoting positive mental health include the Two Continua Model and the Recovery Model.

The Two Continua Model is a psychological well-being model created using the major dimensions of wellness that include Autonomy, Environmental Mastery, Personal Growth, Positive Relations with Others, Purpose in Life, and Self-Acceptance (Ryff & Keyes, 1995; Westerhof & Keyes, 2010). These psychological dimensions, attributed to the seminal work of Ryff (1989) and Ryff and Keyes (1995) are further defined as the following:

1. Self-acceptance: A positive and acceptant attitude toward aspects of self in past and present
2. Purpose in life: Goals and beliefs that affirm a sense of direction and meaning in life
3. Autonomy: Self-direction as guided by one's own socially accepted internal standards
4. Positive relations with others: Having satisfying personal relationships in which empathy and intimacy are expressed
5. Environmental mastery: The capability to manage the complex environment according to one's own needs
6. Personal growth: The insight into one's own potential for self-development (Westerhof & Keyes, 2010, p. 112)

The Two Continua Model examines the continuum of mental health and mental illness, noting that there is a relationship between the two; however, one can have a mental illness but also be mentally well within their own illness status. Those with high mental illness symptoms may have high subjective well-being, defined as incomplete mental illness, or low subjective well-being, or complete mental illness. Conversely, those with low mental illness symptoms and high subjective well-being would be considered to have complete mental health. While individuals with low subjective well-being would have incomplete mental health (Ryff & Keyes, 1995; Westerhof & Keyes, 2010).

This model is also affiliated with the Mental Health Continuum—Short Form (MHC-SF; Keyes, 2009) assessment (further described in the assessment section of this chapter) and can be a model that can be used in mental health promotion, even for those with persistent mental illness. The Two Continua Model is an innovative and constructive way to approach mental health care, providing hope and optimism for all coping with mental health challenges of any kind.

Another model that focuses on mental health promotion and is applicable to all disciplines and populations is the Recovery Model. The Recovery Model is client-centered, holistic, and fast becoming the standard model for recovery for mental health and mental illness. Recovery is "a process of change through which individuals improve their health and wellness, live a self-directed life, and strive to reach their full potential" (SAMHSA, 2012, p. 3).

The Recovery Model was first utilized and developed for people with substance use disorder, and it is beginning to be used in various health professions for different populations. Pizzi (2015) applied the model to occupational therapy students post–Hurricane Sandy. This devastating weather event disrupted academic and professional lives in profound ways. The Recovery Model provides a foundation in which health professionals can create interventions focused on hope, optimism, and enabling self-determination to improve one's self-worth, self-esteem, and coping with life challenges. Table 14-6 outlines the 10 factors that comprise the Recovery Model.

The use of either, or both, of these models to enable positive mental health and have a positive impact on health behaviors, is essential for all practitioners. These models are just two examples that serve as a framework for assessment and interventions.

Assessment

After meeting the client and obtaining a life and medical history, the health care practitioner explores the additional information needed to effectively plan intervention. While the client may present with specific physical or psychiatric concerns, it is important to be comprehensive in addressing the client's health and well-being. A responsibility of the health care team is the selection of assessments that will provide information to assist in effective treatment planning.

Mental health is just one facet of an individual's overall picture of well-being. SAMHSA (2016) has identified eight dimensions of wellness that are interconnected and relate to an individual's overall state of health. The dimensions included are emotional, spiritual, intellectual, environmental, financial, physical, occupational, and social (SAMHSA, 2016). As these aspects are interconnected, it is important for health care practitioners to be mindful of the interrelationship of all dimensions of wellness and the interaction and interplay of various dimensions with one another.

The Wellness Inventory (Swarbrick, 2017) is one clinically useful survey considering wellness across the eight SAMHSA dimensions. This inventory is a self-reported questionnaire with 89 items that are rated by the client according to a Likert scale from 1 = never true for me, to 4 = always true for me. The assessment offers the client a way to consider how they are thinking about what they are doing and how they are feeling. Clients are encouraged to consider behaviors toward wellness in which they are currently engaged while completing the assessment. When utilizing the assessment, it is important to communicate to the client there are no "right" or "wrong" answers. The assessment is scored by adding the ratings for each item within each dimension. The assessment could be re-administered to ascertain change within individual dimensions. This assessment is available free of charge from https://alcoholstudies.rutgers.edu/wellness-in-recovery/inventory/.

The Pizzi Health and Wellness Assessment (PHWA) is another assessment for the health care practitioner to consider (Pizzi, 2001; Pizzi & Richards, 2017; Serwe et al., 2019). This valid and reliable assessment was designed to assist the client in increasing their awareness regarding the most significant health issues that impact participation in meaningful daily activity and helps to develop a client-centered plan for health behavior change. Among the six health areas is mental/emotional health. Participants rate their perceptions

Table 14-6

Definitions of Components of Recovery

COMPONENT	DEFINITION
Self-direction	One's goals are defined through one's own choices and realized through control over one's own life.
Individualized and client-centered	Each person is unique, and thus recovery is unique for each individual.
Empowerment	Recovery can be made more achievable by enabling self-direction.
Holistic	One must embrace all aspects of one's life to maximize well-being and health.
Nonlinear	The forward and backward movement of recovery must be honored.
Strengths-based	Identifying and working with one's own capacities enable one to move forward in recovery and use them to build new life roles.
Peer support	A sense of mutuality and belonging aids the process of recovery.
Respect	Respect includes self-acceptance, valuation of oneself, and self-worth and requires elimination of stigma and exclusion.
Responsibility	Recovery requires acceptance of responsibility for oneself and one's own self-direction and is a self-guided process.
Hope	The internalized sense that the future holds a better QOL for individuals by overcoming barriers facilitates the recovery process.

Adapted from Substance Abuse and Mental Health Services Administration. (2010). *Illness management and recovery.* https://store.samhsa.gov/product/Illness-Management-and-Recovery-Evidence-Based-Practices-EBP-KIT/SMA09-4462

of health on a Likert scale 0 to 10, then answer questions related to daily activity participation and that specific area of health. It is the first assessment directly linking daily activity participation with perceived health status. The assessment can be obtained by contacting the author at mpizzi58@gmail.com.

The Flourishing Scale was developed by Diener et al. (2010). The authors identified eight important items related to promoting positive mental health: purpose and meaning, positive relationships, engagement, social contribution, competence, self-respect, optimism, and social relationships. Each item utilizes a seven-point Likert scale, from "strongly disagree" to "strongly agree," providing a cumulative score of 56. The measure has good psychometric properties and is strongly associated with other psychological well-being scales. The measure is available at https://ggsc.berkeley.edu/images/uploads/The_Flourishing_Scale.pdf.

The MHC-SF (Keyes, 2009) is a 14-question mental health assessment exploring one's emotional, psychological, and social well-being. It looks at frequency with which respondents perceive their own mental health. Flourishing mental health is rated when one records "every day" or "almost every day" on the 14 questions, 3 signs of hedonic well-being, and 11 signs of positive functioning in the last month. Low levels are categorized as one with "languishing" mental health. The form is found at https://www150.statcan.gc.ca/n1/pub/82-003-x/2014009/article/14086-eng.htm and permission is universally granted with credit to the author. This assessment corresponds directly to the Two Continua Mental Health Model. Additional assessments for health care practitioner consideration are presented in Table 14-7.

The health care practitioner is guided to utilize the assessment that provides data that will best assist the client and practitioner in clearly and effectively plan collaborative intervention plans and goals. Whichever assessment is chosen to be utilized, results need to be communicated across disciplines so that all health care team members are operating from a similar perspective (Professional Reasoning Box B).

INTERVENTION

Activities that are purposeless can cause the client to feel a sense of powerlessness or increase a feeling of distress (SAMHSA, 2016), thus it is essential that health care professionals consider engaging clients in activities that have meaning and purpose to the client. Practitioners are encouraged to begin building activities with clients that foster wellness into their daily routine such as planning each morning for things, which will contribute to wellness. This can set the intention and make evident the goals identified as important or essential to the client.

Przybylko et al. (2021) reviewed two experimental studies and found interventions that were provided in an interprofessional manner in an online format, which incorporated concepts of positive psychology and lifestyle medicine that had an impact on increasing human flourishing. Interprofessional perspectives can be beneficial to clients in

Table 14-7

Well-Being Assessments

ASSESSMENT	AUTHORS	INFORMATION	AVAILABLE
Psychological Well-Being Scale (PWB)	Ryff (n.d.)	• 42- or 18-item self-report using a Likert scale reporting (1 strongly agree, 7 strongly disagree) • Six subscales: 1. Autonomy 2. Environmental Mastery 3. Personal Growth 4. Positive Relations with Others 5. Purpose in Life 6. Self-Acceptance • 42-item report has been reported to be more statistically sound	Open-access assessment 42-item report: https://docs.google.com/document/d/1pn2oZi3NiSuEJjtxl0hfaFpEa4Ea0v6YtrlWTAkVUIY/edit 18-item report: https://docs.google.com/document/d/10wj6zmPlGNZMvZXVrXDbMoG1ybkuezapJLXwy2xVAHY/edit
Life Balance Inventory (LBI)	Matuska (2009)	• 53 questions, self-reported to examine life balance and imbalance • Examines daily activity patterns to address: Health, Relationships, Activity Challenge, and Personal Identity	https://minerva.stkate.edu/lbi.nsf
Perceived Wellness Survey (PWS)	Adams et al. (1997)	• 36-item self-report survey addressing perceived wellness perceptions within the following dimensions of wellness: physical, spiritual, psychological, social, emotional, and intellectual	https://perceivedwellness.com/scoring/
Health Promoting Lifestyle II	Walker et al. (1995)	• 52-item questionnaire measuring self-reported behaviors including: health responsibility, physical activity, nutrition, spiritual growth, interpersonal relations, and stress management. Instrument is available in English and Spanish	https://www.unmc.edu/nursing/faculty/English_HPLPII.pdf

Professional Reasoning Box B

How can interprofessional health care teams become more efficient in completing client assessment and sharing outcomes that are obtained from each discipline? Electronic health or electronic medical records can offer some assistance; however, practitioners should strive for establishing regular communication times to discuss client progress toward goals, client response to intervention, and challenges that have presented within the clinical environment. Health care practitioners can benefit from being able to communicate progress each client has made, as well as challenges to obtain insight and perspective from other disciplines.

creating an individual wellness lifestyle that includes routines that support all dimensions of wellness. Finding the correct information, resources, and supports to assist the client in tracking their progress and utilizing resources to meet the client's individual needs is essential (SAMHSA, n.d.). As in the case of Ray, helping him develop a healthy routine of a short walk each day, making dietary changes, and meditating each morning to music he enjoys can lead to positive mental health and prepare him for each day using a positive frame of mind. Each of these activities may require building a routine within each of them, and slowly building them into a routine utilizing all of them.

SAMHSA (2016) has developed a workbook, *Creating a Healthier Life: A Step-By-Step Guide to Wellness*. The workbook addresses the eight dimensions of wellness. This resource is available free of charge: https://store.samhsa.gov/sites/default/files/d7/priv/sma16-4958.pdf. Within each dimension of wellness, specific characteristics of the dimension are discussed, and resources provided. The workbook offers the individual completing it an opportunity to identify specifically what they will do to improve each dimension as well as what type of support is needed for each area of change. This section of the document is of significance as health care practitioners can collaboratively discuss client-identified needs and plans as well as to find the resources and support they could individually or collectively provide (SAMHSA, 2016).

For example, in the dimension of social wellness, the characteristics included are Community, New People, and Social Time. Within these areas the document lists questions the interprofessional health care team can pose to the client, as well as applicable resources for each area (SAMHSA, 2016). Practitioners will critically appraise each dimension of wellness with the client and explore the client's readiness to change, ability to embrace the steps for change, and willingness to take the necessary actions for change in order to flourish. It is important that all health care practitioners provide intervention from a holistic perspective to best meet the needs of the client and engage in collaborative engagement with other disciplines. There are a variety of evidence-based interventions available for health care team consideration based upon client needs/goals identified during the assessment process. See Table 14-8 for an overview of other interventions.

One evidence-based intervention that could be undertaken across disciplines is supporting the client in the development of a Wellness Recovery Action Plan (WRAP; Copeland, 2014). The WRAP program could be implemented by practitioners in a variety of ways. Each discipline could address a different area of the WRAP or one discipline could address all areas with the other disciplines reinforcing the work of the others. The key concepts of the WRAP program focus on Hope, Personal Responsibility, Education, Self-Advocacy, and Support (Copeland, 2014). Please refer to Table 14-9 for definitions of WRAP key concepts.

The concepts identified within WRAP are closely tied to SAMHSA (2012) concepts of recovery and are related to PERMA pillars of Seligman (2011). Included elements within the WRAP program address strategies for building a healthy lifestyle including exercise, diet, light, sleep, health care, and community. Strategies that have been found to be beneficial include scheduling, diversionary and creative activities, journaling, engaging in reality checks, focusing, connecting with warm or hotlines as needed as well as specific strategies to improve one's self-esteem (Copeland, 2014).

The WRAP is also available in an electronic form, as an app, for both Android and iPhone platforms. The elements of the WRAP include Wellness Tools, Daily Maintenance Plan, Stressors, Early Warning Signs, When Things are Breaking Down, and Developing a Crisis Plan. The wellness toolbox is considered the cornerstone of the WRAP program. It is a toolbox of activities an individual can do to feel better, stay well, and improve their individual QOL (Copeland, 2014). Examples of activities that could be included in the wellness toolbox could include call/text a friend, take a walk, do a Zentangle, or write a poem. In creating the wellness toolbox, the practitioner should encourage the individual to be specific about what they want to include. Rather than saying "exercise," encourage the client to be specific. For example, take a 30-minute walk or ride the stationary bike for 20 minutes. Another example is when a client may identify "eat better" as an item they wish to include in the wellness toolbox, the practitioner should encourage the client to be specific, such as eating three meals every day containing protein, complex carbohydrates, and avoiding highly processed foods.

In the case of Ray, the occupational therapist worked on the Wellness Toolbox development with him, the physical therapist worked with him on the development of his Daily Maintenance List, and the social worker worked with him on the identification of stressors and his Crisis Plan. Each discipline documented their work in the electronic medical record, and other disciplines reviewed work that was conducted and could reinforce the work of the other discipline on a regular basis for Ray to continue to develop and utilize his WRAP.

The goal of the Wellness Toolbox is to identify things that the person needs and wants to do to help themselves feel better and enjoy life. The Wellness Toolbox can be completed over several sessions. It is a dynamic plan that can be added to over time. The SAMHSA eight dimensions of wellness can be included within the Wellness Toolbox that is created by the client. The WRAP is considered an evidence-based intervention according to SAMHSA and a variety of research has been conducted to demonstrate the effectiveness of this intervention (Copeland Center, 2021). A variety of research studies describing the use of WRAP and outcomes can be obtained online at the Copeland Center: https://copelandcenter.com/resources-0.

Community Programs

The mental health of a community is mutually dependent on the individual and population mental health of community members. In considering development or engagement of clients in community-based programming, it is important to build upon the strengths present within the local community to foster a sense of commitment and empowerment of community members. This is especially important for those who have been marginalized or disadvantaged (Barry, 2019). The benefits of community-based interventions are far reaching. Programs have the potential to reach a wide audience of individuals. Community-based interventions can support social norms and promote specific structures and environments across the community (Barry, 2019). Refer to Table 14-10 for an overview of community-based mental health promotion programs.

Table 14-8

Evidence-Based Interventions for Mental Health Promotion and Well-Being

EVIDENCE-BASED INTERVENTION PROGRAM	PROGRAM OVERVIEW
Take Charge! A Workbook to Enhance Well-Being with the Eight Dimensions of Wellness (Policy Research Associates, 2020) https://www.prainc.com/product/take-charge-workbook-enhance-well-eight-dimensions-wellness/	Workbook that could be utilized individually or within a group setting, which examines eight dimensions: emotional wellness, social wellness, environmental wellness, occupational wellness, spiritual wellness, physical wellness, financial wellness, and intellectual wellness. Each section within the workbook offers a podcast, overview of the individual dimension, strategies to address the area of wellness, and additional resources. The workbook offers the participant the opportunity to begin with any area of wellness and offers the opportunity to document thoughts and reflections regarding each area. Cost ranges from $8.75 to $10.00 (+ shipping) depending on the number of workbooks ordered.
Do Live Well (Krupa et al., 2009) http://dolivewell.ca/tools-resources/#sthash.riHlpv2U.dpbs	Framework that examines dimensions of experience, activity patterns, and wellness/health outcomes. The model examines the personal and social forces that may impact these areas. Do Live Well offers the opportunity to examine various concepts of the model through resources available on the Do Live Well website. A coping with COVID-19 manual is available for download free of charge. This resource could be utilized with adults and older adults to cope with other types of occupational disruption aside of the pandemic.
Illness Management & Recovery (SAMHSA, 2010) https://store.samhsa.gov/product/Illness-Management-and-Recovery-Evidence-Based-Practices-EBP-KIT/SMA09-4462	Program dedicated to consumer empowerment related to illness management, recovery goals. and decision making for treatment and well-being. Provided in a psychoeducational module format with eight topics: Recovery Strategies, Facts about Mental Illness, Stress-Vulnerability Model and Treatment, Developing Social Supports, Drug and Alcohol Use, Reducing Relapses, and Coping with Stress. Significant emphasis is placed upon client coping strategies and relapse prevention.
Wellness Self-Management (Salerno et al., 2011) https://truegeorge.files.wordpress.com/2017/05/wsm-final-workbook.pdf	Wellness self-management focuses on principles of recovery and is provided in a format similar to the SAMHSA Illness Management & Recovery program. The program can be completed by and individual or within a group setting. A manual with 57 different topics is available free of charge from Practice Innovations (n.d.) The program addresses the connection between physical and mental health as well as overcoming challenges in accessing wellness services.
Solutions for Wellness Physical Activity (Lilly, 2013a) Healthy Eating (Lilly, 2013b) https://education.lillymedical.com/en-us/patient-education-resources/well-being/resources	The program focuses on physical activity and healthy eating. The manualized program could be provided individually or in a group setting. Free workbooks are available in an archived format from the National Council for Behavioral Health. Physical activity workbook has 17 lessons ranging in topics from physical activity and wellness, balance, stress, flexibility and strengthening. The Healthy eating workbook has 22 lessons ranging in topics from choosing healthy eating and wellness, benefits and barriers to healthy eating, weight management, stress, and food consumption.
UIC Solutions Suite for Health & Recovery https://www.center4healthandsdc.org/solutions-suite.html	The UIC Solutions Suite for Health & Recovery offers tools, curricula, and implementation manuals for free and immediate use in mental health centers, peer-run programs, or one's own life. You can introduce the entire complement of products to foster improved health and recovery. Or you can choose the ones that will work best for your program or your life. The Suite is co-directed by Dr. Peggy Swarbrick, OTR/L. Its products are co-developed with the Collaborative Support Programs of New Jersey.
Teledoc Health (2024) https://mystrength.com/	Online self-help and wellness portal that offers resources for individuals who experience depression or anxiety and stress-related concerns. The program offers interactive tools to address coping skills, daily inspiration, strategies to enhance motivation, goal setting and action plans, and modules to offer information on well-being and strategies to improve mental health and well-being. This tool could be utilized by the client outside of the formal treatment time and the interdisciplinary health care practitioner could follow up to assess client behavior and progress.

(continued)

Table 14-8 (continued)

Evidence-Based Interventions for Mental Health Promotion and Well-Being

EVIDENCE-BASED INTERVENTION PROGRAM	PROGRAM OVERVIEW
Pathways to Recovery (Child et al., 2006)	Group intervention facilitate by peer and mental health clinician for 12 weeks. Topics include living situation, social support, career path, motivation, and goals for the future.
Mindfulness Based Stress Reduction (MBSR) https://palousemindfulness.com/index.html	Mindfulness-Based Stress Reduction is a psychoeducational training to foster resilience and improve well-being (Palouse Mindfulness, n.d.).

Table 14-9

Definitions of Key Concepts of Wellness Recovery Action Plan

KEY CONCEPT OF WRAP	DEFINITION
Hope	The ability to see option for health, well-being, and fulfillment of life goals.
Personal responsibility	Individual responsibility for well-being and ability to ask/seek help.
Education	Learning about self and strategies to support decision making in all life areas.
Self-advocacy	Ability to engage with others regarding individual needs, wants for well-being and recovery.
Support	Receiving support and offer support to others and positive impact on well-being.

Adapted from Copeland, M. E. (2014). *WRAP for life*. Peach Press.

Table 14-10

Community-Based Mental Health Promotion Programs

PROGRAM	PROGRAM OVERVIEW
Big Brothers/Big Sisters https://www.bbbs.org/	Assist youth in achievement of potential through establishment of positive adult relationship. Adults benefit from altruism of engaging with youth and community program involvement (Barry, 2019).
Act-Belong-Commit (from Australia) https://www.actbelongcommit.org.au/	This program emphasizes physical, spiritual, social, and mental activity to increase belonging within the community (Barry, 2019). This program has a positive mental health focus on doing something, doing something with someone, and doing something meaningful. Although a similar program does not exist in the United States, a health care practitioner could utilize "meetup" to assist community members in finding like-minded individuals to engage in community-based activities (https://www.meetup.com/). By strengthening engagement within community networks social support and social inclusion are increased (Barry, 2019).
Volunteer Match https://www.volunteermatch.org/	Volunteer Match is a website in which an individual can search for volunteer opportunities within their community. A positive relationship between mental well-being and self-rated health was reported in research reviewed by Barry (2019).

For example, the Blue Zones approach moves from individual behavioral change to impacting change in community health. This is accomplished through making changes in multiple levels such as changing city spaces (walking paths, bike trails, smoking policies, sidewalks) as well as facilitating change within social networks, restaurants, grocery stores, employers, faith organizations, habitat, and overall community engagement. The program focuses on making comprehensive change within the community environment to foster positive health and economic well-being for the community (Blue Zones, 2021).

In the case of Ray, he desires to become more involved within his community. While at the swimming pool doing his workout, he sees a flyer for a Blue Zones group challenge. The group will meet for 4 weeks to focus on the development of healthy habit formation. The focus of the sessions is to improve the places and spaces where he would spend his time in addition to expanding his social circle. The program flyer states that the outcome of participation can include decreased stress, increased energy, improved sleep, better relationships, and ability to identify and stay at one's ideal weight (Blue Zones, 2021). The program is being offered free of charge and Ray figures he has nothing to lose, so he signs up to participate. He shares with his health care professionals his participation in the program, and they encourage his ongoing engagement. He identified feeling more engaged, energetic, and discovered a new restaurant with the other group members. Ray has participated socially in other community activities (fun walk/run, community music concert) as a result of meeting new people within the group. The program provided Ray with a variety of positive mental health promotion outcomes.

Another community-based program found to be successful was the InShape program (Naslund et al., 2017). The program was designed for young adults with serious mental illness. Persons with mental illness are at risk of medication-related weight gain and can benefit from total lifestyle-focused interventions to foster wellness across all dimensions as identified by SAMHSA (n.d.). The focus of the program is to improve physical and social well-being. It includes meetings with a fitness trainer on a weekly basis, a gym membership, and nutrition education. A key element of this program was to explore how mental health symptoms could interfere with health and well-being and how physical strategies can overcome challenges presented by symptoms. The outcomes for the participants of the InShape program at 12 months were weight loss and change in fitness level (Nashlund et al., 2017). Participants also demonstrated increased activity level, increased satisfaction with physical fitness, increased confidence in social engagement, and decreases in blood pressure and depressive symptoms.

Besides physical activity, individuals who engage in creative activity reported higher levels of flourishing (Tamlin et al., 2018). Spending time each day engaged in creative goals was indicative of a person doing well and also fostered positive feelings. This could include engaging in monthly crafting sessions at a local library or community center or participating in the painting of a mural at a community living area. A variety of creative community activities are offered through local parks and recreation departments, community centers, religious organizations, and local libraries. This could be a consideration for interdisciplinary health care teams to examine how they could incorporate creative activity within their traditional interventions to promote mental health, well-being, and an improved QOL.

A publication by the World Mental Health Association and the WHO (2004) provides comprehensive case studies from countries around the globe addressing mental health promotion. Each case study provides an overview of the program with the method, program design, and program evaluation. A great deal of wisdom can be gained from a review of the case studies provided relative to community programs and program development so that healthcare practitioners do not "reinvent the wheel."

In addition to WRAP, the National Alliance on Mental Illness (NAMI; 2021b), Mental Health America (MHA, 2021), National Depression and Bipolar Support Alliance (DBSA, 2021), and the CDC (2018) have educational resource materials relevant to the promotion of mental health and well-being for clients. Community programming information is also available that can be utilized by health care teams. It is important to be consistent in evaluating evidence of the efficacy and clinical

When clients are engaged in community-based interventions, the stigma and negative connotations of programs targeted toward specific groups has the potential to be diminished. Community engagement empowers the client and contributes not only to the betterment of the client, but also has the potential to positively impact the community as well (Barry, 2019). As such, it is important to interprofessional team members to be aware of resources within the community and share information with each other to support client mental health.

The Importance of Interprofessional Teams

Health care practitioners are directed to consider programs that have evidence of effectiveness and include interprofessional involvement. Rather than providing intervention in a silo, health care practitioners need to actively collaborate with one another and the client to identify and strive toward client-centered goals.

At times practitioners are concerned about their own roles and responsibilities and concerned about crossing the boundary into the area of another discipline. The IPEC competencies (2016) clearly state the importance of understanding values and ethics of each respective discipline (competency 1), but also emphasize the importance of possessing knowledge of the roles/responsibilities of other disciplines (competency 2). Professionals are directed to engage in respectful interprofessional communication that promotes health and prevents disease in clients served (competency 3). Practitioners are also responsible to determine strategies to deliver services in a "safe, timely, efficient and equitable manner" (competency 4; 2016, p. 10). As such, practitioners need to consistently discuss progress toward identified goals across all disciplines and support one another at every opportunity. Clearly understanding the emphasis and focus of the other profession is essential to this success and is outlined in IPEC competency 1, which states "work with individuals of other professions to maintain a climate of mutual respect and shared values" (2016, p. 10). These competencies have been illustrated throughout this chapter, and it is vital that health care professionals (and students) understand their importance in practice.

Professional Reasoning Box C

Although various disciplines are often presented with a client who is struggling with a physical, emotional, or social challenge, the client may also present with specific individual strengths. All too often, practitioners focus on the deficits, rather than addressing the strengths that clients possess that helps them flourish. Health care practitioners are encouraged to actively collaborate with the client and one another to identify individual strengths that can be built upon to address challenges that the client presents to the therapeutic environment with. Being mindful of the IPEC competencies (2016) in addition to addressing the dimensions of wellness from SAMHSA (n.d.) and the well-being theory of Seligman (2011), practitioners will be more effective in designing and implementing comprehensive interventions to address deficits within the client, while building upon the strengths that exist for the client as well. Practitioners are encouraged to challenge themselves and one another to begin and end each clinical session not with the question "what's wrong with you?" but "what matters to you?" and work from an area of strengths related to fostering well-being within the client.

Clients are complex individuals, often receiving care from many different health care professionals. Working collaboratively and not in a silo is essential to making progress with the client. Wellness is not just positive physical health. It is multidimensional and needs to include strategies to also strengthen one's mental health. When a physical therapist is working on increasing core strength in a client such as Ray, the practitioner could be engaging in conversation addressing the client's spiritual well-being (focusing on what provides the client meaning and purpose). The occupational therapist may be working on addressing the spiritual dimension of the client's wellness by focusing on meaning and purpose in daily activities with which the client may be struggling. When practitioners effectively communicate with one another regarding goals and therapeutic approaches, ultimately each discipline is more effective as they are working to support the ultimate client outcome: improvement in function, independence, and overall health and well-being (Professional Reasoning Box C).

Conclusion

Although clients bring a complex constellation of concerns to the therapeutic setting, when practitioners work in an effective interprofessional and constructive manner—with the individual client, community, or population needs of primary importance—individual disciplines can feel mutual respect and positive benefit in supporting one another to assist clients in achieving identified goals. Working in an interprofessional collaborative fashion offers the client the opportunity for multiple viewpoints to facilitate best practice and assist in promoting positive mental health, well-being, and QOL.

References

Adams, T., Bezner, J., & Steinhardt, M. (1997). The conceptualization and measurement of perceived wellness: Integrating balance across and within dimensions. *American Journal of Health Promotion, 11*(3), 208-218.

Amador, X. (2012). *I'm not sick and i don't need help*. Vida Press.

Barry, M. M. (2019). Implementing community based mental health promotion strategies (pp. 195-229). In M. M Barry, A. M. Clarke, I. Petersen, & R. Jenkins (Eds). *Implementing mental health promotion* (2nd ed). Springer.

Blue Zones. (2021). Blue zones project. https://www.bluezones.com/services/blue-zones-project/#section-1

Centers for Disease Control and Prevention. (2018). Well-being concepts. https://www.cdc.gov/hrqol/wellbeing.htm

Child, B., Castleton, D. K., Cross, H. L., & Green, C. A. (2006). *Group facilitator's manual for peer and mental health counselors to accompany pathways to recovery: A strengths recovery self-help workbook*. Kaiser Permanente Center for Health Research. https://research.kpchr.org/Portals/0/Docs/project%20websites/Recovery%20Group%20project/FullFacilitatorsManualV38.pdf?ver=2016-01-07-111016-723

Commission on Social Determinants of Health (2008). Closing the gap in a generation: health equity through action on the social determinants of health. Final Report of the Commission on Social Determinants of Health. Geneva, World Health Organization. Available: https://iris.who.int/bitstream/handle/10665/43943/9789241563703_eng.pdf?sequence=1

Copeland Center (2021). Research. https://copelandcenter.com/resource-type/research

Copeland, M. E. (2014). *WRAP for life*. Peach Press.

Di Fabio, A., & Palazzeschi, L. (2015). Hedonic and eudaimonic well-being: The role of resilience beyond fluid intelligence and personality traits. *Frontiers in Psychology, 6*, 1367. https://doi.org/10.3389/fpsyg.2015.01367

Diener, E., Wirtz, D., Tov, W., Kim-Prieto, C., Choi, D. W., Oishi, S., & Biswas-Diener, R. (2010). New well-being measures: Short scales to assess flourishing and positive and negative feelings. *Social Indicators Research, 97*(2), 143-156.

Duque, R. L. (2004). Health promotion and the values of occupational therapy. *World Federation of Occupational Therapists Bulletin, 49*(1), 5-8. https://doi.org/10.1179/ otb.2004.49.1.002

Interprofessional Education Collaborative. (2016). *Core competencies for interprofessional collaborative practice: 2016 update.* Interprofessional Education Collaborative.

IRM Assessments. (2021). Self assessment of modes, clinical assessment of modes: communicating with your therapist, clinical assessment of modes, observer version. https://irm.ahs.uic.edu/irm-assessments-and-products/

Kahneman D., Diener E., Schwarz N. (Eds). (1999). *Well-Being: The Foundations of Hedonic Psychology*. Russell Sage Foundation.

Keyes, C. L. M. (2007). Promoting and protecting mental health as flourishing: A complementary strategy for improving national mental health. *American Psychologist, 62*, 95-108.

Keyes, C. L. M. (2009). Brief description of the mental health continuum short form (MHC-SF). https://www.aacu.org/sites/default/files/MHC-SFEnglish.pdf

Keyes, C. L. M. (2014). Mental health as a complete state: How the salutogenic perspective completes the picture. In G. F. Bauer & O. Håmmig (Eds.), *Bridging occupational, organizational and public health: A transdisciplinary approach* (pp. 179-192). Springer Science+Business Media Dordrecht. https://doi.org/10.1007/978-94-007-5640-3_11

Krupa, T., Moll, S., & Gewurtz, R. (2009). *Do live well.* http://dolivewell.ca/about-us/#sthash.IIgCmAtH.dpbs

Lilly, E. (2013a). Solutions for wellness: Physical activity. https://www.thenationalcouncil.org/wp-content/uploads/2015/06/12-Solutions-for-Wellness-Choosing-Wellness-Physical-Activity.pdf?daf=375ateTbd56

Lilly, E. (2013b). Solutions for wellness: Healthy eating. https://www.thenationalcouncil.org/wp-content/uploads/2015/06/12-Solutions-for-Wellness-Choosing-Wellness-Physical-Activity.pdf?daf=375ateTbd56

Matuska, K. (2009). Life balance inventory. http://minerva.stkate.edu/lbi.nsf

Mental Health America. (2021). Living mentally healthy. https://mhanational.org/live-b4stage4

Naslund, J. A., Aschbrenner, K. A., Scherer, E. A., Pratt, S. I., & Bartels, S. J. (2017). Health promotion for young adults with serious mental illness. *Psychiatric Services, 68*, 137-143. https://doi.org/10.1176/appi.ps.201600091

National Alliance on Mental Illness. (n.d.). Mental health conditions. https://nami.org/About-Mental-Illness/Mental-Health-Conditions

National Alliance on Mental Illness. (2021a). Mental health by the numbers. https://www.nami.org/mhstats

National Alliance on Mental Illness. (2021b). Mental health education. https://nami.org/Support-Education/Mental-Health-Education

National Depression and Bipolar Support Alliance. (2021). Wellness tracker. https://www.dbsalliance.org/wellness/wellness-toolbox/wellness-tracker/

Palouse Mindfulness. (n.d.). Mindfulness based stress reduction. https://palousemindfulness.com/index.html

Pizzi, M. (2001). The Pizzi Holistic Wellness Assessment. *Occupational Therapy in Health Care, 13*(3-4), 51-66. https://doi.org/10.1080/J003v13n03_06

Pizzi, M. (2015). Hurricane Sandy, disaster preparedness and the recovery model. *American Journal of Occupational Therapy, 69*, 6904250010. https://doi.org/10.5014/ajot.2015.015990

Pizzi, M. A., & Richards, L. G. (2017). Promoting health, well-being and quality of life in occupational therapy: A commitment to a paradigm shift for the next 100 years. *American Journal of Occupational Therapy, 71*(4), 7104170010p1-7104170010p5.

Policy Research Associates. (2020). *Take charge! A workbook to enhance well-being with the eight dimensions of wellness*. Author.

Practice Innovations. (n.d). Wellness self-management workbook. https://practiceinnovations.org/Portals/0/WSMLibrary/WSM_sample_wkbk_20091029.pdf?ver=2015-10-16-134652-513

Prochaska, J. O., & DiClemente, C. C. (1982). Transtheoretical therapy: Toward a more integrative model of change. *Psychotherapy: Theory, Research, and Practice, 19*, 276-288.

Przybylko, G., Morton. D. P., Morton, J. K., Renfrew, M. E. & Hinze, J. (2021): An interdisciplinary mental wellbeing intervention for increasing flourishing: Two experimental studies. *The Journal of Positive Psychology, 17*(4), 573-588. https://doi.org/10.1080/17439760.2021.1897868

Rashbrook, E. (2019). Health matters: Prevention - A life course approach. Available: https://ukhsa.blog.gov.uk/2019/05/23/health-matters-prevention-a-life-course-approach/

Ryff, C. D. (n.d). Psychological wellbeing scale. https://sparqtools.org/mobility-measure/psychological-wellbeing-scale/

Ryff, C. D. (1989). Happiness is everything, or is it? Explorations on the meaning of psychological well-being. *Journal of Personality and Social Psychology, 57*, 1069-1081, https://doi.org/10.1037/0022-3514.57.6.1069

Ryff, C. D., & Keyes, C. L. M. (1995). The structure of psychological well-being revisited. *Journal of Personality and Social Psychology, 69*(4), 719-727. https://doi.org/10.1037/0022-3514.69.4.719

Salerno, A., Margolies, P., Cleek, A., Pollock, P. Gopalan, G., & Jackson, C. (2011). Wellness self-management: An adaptation of the Illness Management and Recovery Practice in New York State. *Psychiatric Services, 62*(5), 456-458. https://doi.org/10.1176/appi.ps.62.5.456

Seligman, M. E. P. (2011). *Flourish*. Simon & Schuster.

Serwe, K., Walmsley, A., & Pizzi, M. A. (2019). Reliability and responsiveness of the Pizzi Health and Wellness Assessment. *Annals of International Occupational Therapy, 3*(1), 7-13.

Short, S. E., & Mollborn, S. (2015). Social determinants and health behaviors: Conceptual frames and empirical advances. *Current Opinions in Psychology, 5*, 78-84. https://doi.org/10.1016/j.copsyc.2015.05.002

Sturgeon, S. (2007). Promoting mental health as an essential aspect of health promotion. *Health Promotion International, 21*(Suppl. 1), 36-41. https://doi.org/10.1093/heapro/dal049

Substance Abuse and Mental Health Services Administration. (n.d.). Risk and protective factors. https://www.samhsa.gov/sites/default/files/20190718-samhsa-risk-protective-factors.pdf

Substance Abuse and Mental Health Services Administration. (2010). Illness Management and Recovery. https://store.samhsa.gov/product/Illness-Management-and-Recovery-Evidence-Based-Practices-EBP-KIT/SMA09-4462

Substance Abuse and Mental Health Services Administration. (2012). Working definition of recovery. https://store.samhsa.gov/sites/default/files/d7/priv/pep12-recdef.pdf

Substance Abuse and Mental Health Services Administration. (2016). Creating a healthier life: A step by step guide to wellness. https://store.samhsa.gov/sites/default/files/d7/priv/sma16-4958.pdf

Substance Abuse and Mental Health Services Administration (2020). What is mental health. Available: https://www.samhsa.gov/mental-health

Substance Abuse and Mental Health Services Administration. (2021). Using motivational interviewing in substance use disorder treatment. Advisory. https://store.samhsa.gov/sites/default/files/SAMHSA_Digital_Download/PEP20-02-02-014.pdf

Swarbrick, P. (2017). Wellness inventory. http://cspnj.org/wp-content/uploads/2019/08/Wellness_Inventory.pdf

Tamlin, S. C., DeYoung, C. G., & Silvia, P. J. (2018) Everyday creative activity as a path to flourishing. *The Journal of Positive Psychology, 13*(2), 181-189. https://doi.org/10.1080/17439760.2016.1257049

Taylor, R. (2020). *The Intentional Relationship Model: Occupational therapy and the use of self.* F. A. Davis.

Teledoc Health (2024). myStrength. Available: https://mystrength.com/mobile

Understanding Motivational Interviewing. (n.d.). https://motivationalinterviewing.org/understanding-motivational-interviewing

Walker, S. N., Sechrist, K., & Pender, N. (1995). Health promoting lifestyle profile II. https://www.unmc.edu/nursing/faculty/English_HPLPII.pdf

Westerhof, G. J., & Keyes, C. L. M. (2010). Mental illness and mental health: The two continua model across the lifespan. *Journal of Adult Development, 17*, 110-119. https://doi.org/10.1007/s10804-009-9082-y

World Health Organization. (1986). Ottawa Charter for Health Promotion. https://www.euro.who.int/__data/assets/pdf_file/0004/129532/Ottawa_Charter.pdf

World Health Organization. (2008). *The global burden of disease: 2004 update.* WHO Press.

World Health Organization. (2018). *Mental health: Strengthening our response.* https://www.who.int/news-room/fact-sheets/detail/mental-health-strengthening-our-response

CHAPTER 15

Promoting Mental and Emotional Health
Older Adults

Laurel D. Abbruzzese, PT, EdD, FNAP and Phyllis Simon, OTD, OTR/L, FNAP

Learning Objectives

At the end of this chapter, the reader will:

1. Describe the factors that impact mental and emotional health in older adults (ACOTE B.3.5)
2. Identify screening and assessment tools used in clinical practice to assess and screen for mental health and emotional well-being that affect the daily functioning and quality of life of older adults (ACOTE B.4.0, B.4.4; CAPTE 7D-19, I)
3. Identify evidence-based interventions that may positively impact mental health by increasing social connectedness, promote resilience, reduce loneliness, and/or reduce stress (ACOTE B.4.3, B.4.10; CAPTE 7D-24)
4. Describe some of the unique mental health concerns for older adults with marginalized identities (ACOTE B.1.3; CAPTE 7D-37)
5. Identify community resources and programs that can be used by the interprofessional team to foster emotional well-being in older adults (ACOTE B.4.26; CAPTE 7D-28)
6. Identify the roles of the interprofessional team members in addressing the mental health and well-being of older adults in the community (ACOTE B.4.25)

The ACOTE Standards used are those from 2018.

Key Words

Emotional Health, Interprofessional Collaboration, Loneliness, Mental Health, Resilience, Social Connectedness, Social Isolation, Stress, Well-Being

Pizzi, M. A., & Amir, M. (Eds.). *Interprofessional Perspectives for Community Practice: Promoting Health, Well-Being, and Quality of Life* (pp. 283-302).

Case Study: JP

JP was initially referred by her friend to SAGE (a senior center that provides services and advocacy for LGBT elders) for case management due to a decline in physical and mental health. She was subsequently referred to ELINC (Elder LGBT Interprofessional Collaborative Care Team) for further management and care. ELINC is a community-based interprofessional program whose team consists of a nurse practitioner, occupational therapist, physical therapist, social worker, psychiatrist, psychologist, and patient navigator. The team uses the GRACE Team Care Model (Agency for Healthcare Research and Quality [AHRQ], 2017), beginning with a two-person comprehensive in-home assessment performed by the nurse practitioner and social worker. JP also received in-home assessments by physical and occupational therapy prior to the development of a comprehensive collaborative care plan.

JP is an 88-year-old who identifies as a white, Jewish lesbian woman and uses the pronouns she/her/hers. Her medical history includes hypercholesterolemia, diabetes, urinary incontinence, tinnitus, s/p left shoulder fracture 2 years prior, transient ischemic attack, recurrent falls, history of smoking ("but doesn't inhale"). Past surgical history includes a right meniscus repair and cholecystectomy. Her medications include Losartan, Metformin, Crestor, Detrol, Baby Aspirin, Calcium, Singulair, Restoril, and Mobic.

JP is retired from the airline industry and is financially secure. Her 2-week marriage to a man was annulled at age 21 years. She was estranged from her parents when they refused to accept her sexual orientation. She has no children and limited family. Her cousin serves as her power of attorney. Her last partner died several years ago of alcoholism. Her "family of choice" includes a network of friends that has been dwindling over time.

JP lives in a one-bedroom apartment in an elevated building in a busy urban environment where she has lived for 40 years. The building is old, with multiple safety hazards and mobility challenges including poor lighting, uneven floors, narrow hallways, heavy doors, loose scattered rugs, a broken oven, and limited counter space. Her medications are kept in a box on the kitchen table, where she spends much of her time reading the newspaper and managing her calendar. The home is filled with art, a piano, and personal mementos. The neighborhood is active with a local pharmacy and restaurants; however, the sidewalks are uneven and difficult for her to navigate.

JP has limited left shoulder range of motion attributed to a past fracture. She presents with an unsteady gait (frequently reaching out to touch the walls and furniture as she navigates the apartment). She is also extremely cautious when walking in the community. She has a history of several falls, fears falling, and ambulates without an assistive device despite recommendations by a previous physical therapist. Her Timed Up and Go time revealed being a fall risk.

JP carries out her ADLs, phone use, medication management, and shopping independently. She reports being fearful in the tub with difficulty showering but declined recommendations for grab bars or shower chair to increase safety. She needed assistance with heavy cleaning and laundry, managing finances, meal preparation and cooking, and transportation. Despite poor nutritional management and poor adherence to her diabetic diet, she declined offers for enrolling in delivered meal services from Meals on Wheels or going to a local senior center for lunch. Due to functional limitations, fear of falling, and the cost of transportation, JP self-limited her community mobility. She stated, "I am not comfortable taking the bus or train anymore and taxis are so expensive." JP used to frequent the theater with friends, but currently has limited social interactions with friends and has not seen her usual social circle for several months.

REFLECTIVE QUESTIONS

1. What red flags and life stressors may put an older adult at an increased risk for poor mental health and well-being?
2. What additional life stressors should be considered for an LGBT older adult?
3. How might poor physical health impact an older adult's mental and emotional health?
4. What assessment strategies and tools would be valuable to the interprofessional team when evaluating mental health risks and emotional well-being of community-dwelling older adults?

Introduction

There is a growing recognition of the importance of interprofessional teams in promoting the well-being of older adults. **Well-being** is a subjective construct with multiple domains including physical, economic, social, emotional, and psychological aspects. Well-being is connected to life satisfaction, positive outlook, and health. The Centers for Disease Control and Prevention (CDC) defines well-being as "judging life positively and feeling good" (CDC, 2018b). High levels of well-being are associated with having basic needs met (food, shelter, income), positive social relationships, and good physical and mental health. Health care teams can optimize patient outcomes and community well-being through interprofessional collaboration, bringing together the strengths of different discipline perspectives. A shared priority for all members of the interprofessional collaborative care team will be to promote the mental and emotional health of individuals and communities.

According to the CDC, "**Mental health** includes our emotional, psychological, and social well-being. It affects how we think, feel, and act. It also helps determine how we handle stress, relate to others, and make healthy choices" (CDC, 2018b). **Emotional health** is a component of mental health that involves being in control of one's thoughts and feelings. In 2015, Galderisi et al. proposed a new definition of mental health:

> Mental health is a dynamic state of internal equilibrium which enables individuals to use their abilities in harmony with universal values of society. Basic cognitive and social skills; ability to recognize, express and modulate one's own emotions, as well as empathize with others; flexibility and ability to cope with adverse life events and function in social roles; and harmonious relationship between body and mind represent important components of mental health which contribute, to varying degrees, to the state of internal equilibrium. (2015, p. 408)

The Galderisi definition emphasizes harmony and coping abilities, acknowledging that good mental health does not require complete happiness and an absence of stress or adversity.

The World Health Organization (WHO) states that health, including mental health, is "not merely the absence of disease or infirmity" (n.d.a, "Special Initiative for Mental Health [2019-2023]-Universal Health Coverage for Mental Health," 2017, p. 1); however, the WHO Special Initiative for Mental Health (2019-2023) focuses on coverage for mental health conditions such as depression, anxiety, substance abuse, suicide risk, intellectual disabilities, and neurocognitive disorders like Alzheimer's disease. According to the WHO, depression and dementia are the most common mental and neurological disorders among adults over age 60 years, affecting 5% and 7% of the population respectively. In addition, 3.8% of older adults are diagnosed with anxiety disorders (WHO, 2017). While screening for common mental health disorders in older adults is an important part of promoting well-being, the interprofessional team can also promote mental and emotional health by attending to common risk factors and stressors. Good mental health is dynamic and requires flexibility and capacity to manage challenging times. Most importantly, mental health is more than the absence of mental illness; it refers to psychological and emotional well-being and the ability to effectively cope with life's stressors in a healthy way. An important ingredient in mental health promotion is ensuring that older adults are socially connected and feel a sense of belonging and engagement with others.

Social Connectedness, Social Isolation, and Loneliness in Older Adults

Humans are social beings. **Social connectedness** (having meaningful, quality social relationships) is essential for health and well-being (National Academies of Sciences, 2020). Social connectedness involves several interacting factors. The structure of the connections includes relationships such as romantic partners, friends, service providers, and caregivers. The number of these relationships can be quantified. For each of these relationships, the quality may be neutral, negative, or positive. Some relationships are strained by conflict and stress, and others may be nurturing and supportive. The function of the social connection overlaps with subjective feelings of belonging or feeling alone. The function of each social relationship will depend upon the way people perceive and experience the interactions. An individual may have many social contacts that are deficient in quality and still feel lonely. In contrast, an individual may have very few contacts, but the quality and perceived support is high and fulfilling, and the individual does not feel lonely. Thus, **loneliness** and **social isolation** are related but different constructs.

In the absence of social connectedness, an individual may experience both social isolation (a reduced quantity of social contacts) and loneliness (the perception of feeling alone and disconnected from others). Social isolation and loneliness are the structural and functional components of social connectedness, respectively (Holt-Lunstad, 2018; Figure 15-1). Both are risk factors that put individuals at risk of poor physical and mental health including depression, cognitive decline, and higher rates of mortality (Perissinotto et al., 2012). According to the American Psychological Association (APA), loneliness and social isolation may be a greater threat to public health than obesity (APA, 2017). Donovan and Blazer (2020) report on the bidirectional relationship between social isolation and loneliness and mental health disorders in older adults. The negative impact and consequences include higher rates of depression, anxiety, self-harm, suicidal ideation, and dementia need to be addressed by clinicians (Donovan & Blazer, 2020). To improve health outcomes and address these social determinants of health, the Institute of Medicine (IOM) recommends collecting measures of social connections and social isolation as core domains in the health record (IOM, 2014).

The high prevalence of social isolation and loneliness among older adults has been documented in numerous surveys (Anderson & Thayer, 2018). In 2018, the prevalence of loneliness and social isolation ranged between 22% and 35% of community-dwelling older adults (Anderson & Thayer, 2018). According to the 2018 Committee on the Health and Medical Dimensions of Social Isolation and Loneliness in Older Adults, formed by the National Academies of Sciences, Engineering, and Medicine, 24% of community-dwelling Americans aged 65 years and older were considered to be socially isolated, and 35% of adults aged 45 years and older and 43% of adults aged 60 and older reported feeling lonely (National Academies of Sciences, 2020, p. 1). While these numbers do not represent most older adults, aging adults are at increased risk of social isolation and loneliness because they are more likely to lose family members and

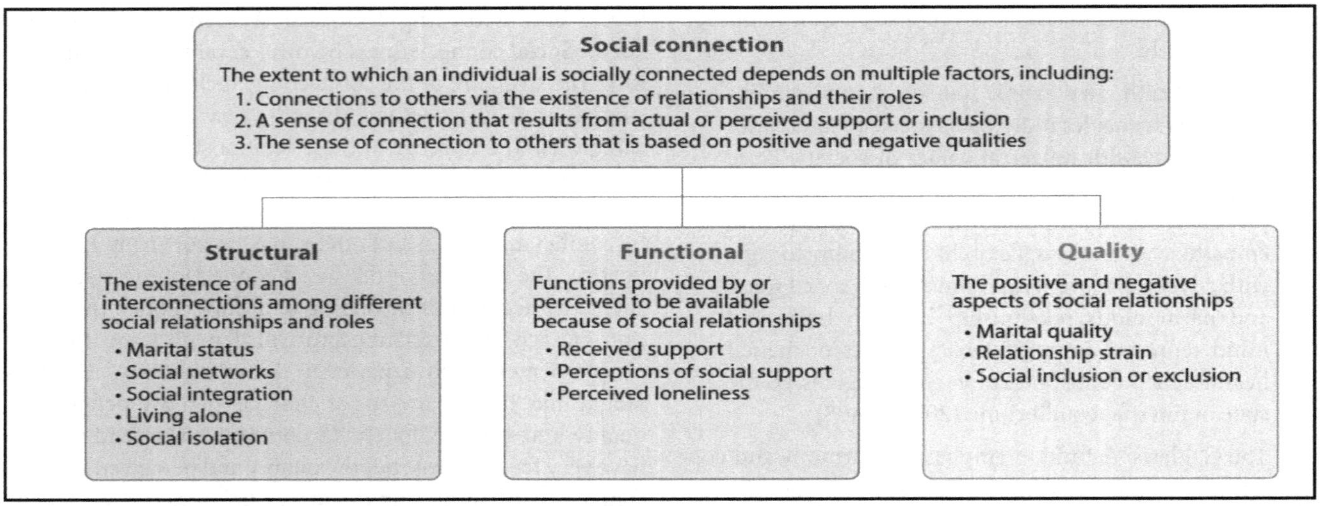

Figure 15-1. Social connection as a multifactoral construct, including structural, functional, and quality components. (Reproduced with permission from Holt-Lunstad, J. [2018]. Why social relationships are important for physical health: A systems approach to understanding and modifying risk and protection. *Annual Review of Psychology, 69*[1], 437-458. https://doi.org/10.1146/annurev-psych-122216-011902)

friends, experience chronic health conditions that limit mobility, have decreased community involvement (work, volunteerism), and to live alone.

Although social relationships may positively impact mental and emotional health, it is important to note that all social connections are not supportive and may instead be a source of stress. When the care being provided to an older adult includes verbal and nonverbal behaviors that cause distress and anguish, they constitute emotional or psychological abuse. Identifying and intervening in cases of caregiver burden may be a means of promoting mental and emotional health in older adults at risk of abuse (Committee on Family Caregiving for Older Adults, 2016).

An emerging body of literature has focused on the impact of COVID-19 on loneliness and mental health in older adults (Dahlberg, 2021; Lee et al., 2020; Wong et al., 2020). The COVID-19 pandemic posed heightened health risks for older members of society, who were understandably more fearful of becoming ill (Whitehead, 2020). In addition to the stress of personal illness and loved ones becoming infected or dying, the pandemic exacerbated social isolation and created new barriers to mental health services and community programs. The heaviest burden has been on older adults with marginalized identities (Garcia et al., 2020).

The WHO has identified social isolation and loneliness as a growing public health epidemic among older adults made worse by the COVID-19 epidemic. (WHO, 2021). In the 2021 WHO Advocacy Brief, "Social isolation and loneliness among older people," they highlight the numerous consequences of social isolation and loneliness (Figure 15-2), and recommend several strategies for reducing social isolation and loneliness in the aging population including: 1) structural changes, including policies and laws that combat ageism and inequitable access to services and digital resources; 2) fostering age-friendly communities, improved infrastructure, transportation and the built environment; and 3) targeted interventions for social engagement, social skills training, mindfulness, and cognitive behavior therapy, either face-to-face or through digital interventions (Figure 15-3; WHO, 2021). The interprofessional health care team is positioned to both evaluate and provide interventions for lonely and isolated older adults in community settings. Of particular concern are older adults from vulnerable and underserved populations. Practitioners may need to engage in targeted outreach efforts to meet the needs of marginalized groups with limited access to health services.

Physical and Mental Health

There is a myriad of evidence that has reported the connection and reciprocal relationship between mental and physical health in older adults (WHO, 2017). Evidence suggests both positive and negative impacts that each state has on older adults. Those in good physical health have been reported to have a lower prevalence of mental health disorders including depression, anxiety or dementia/neurocognitive disorders. Older adults with better physical health are more inclined to have better mental health (Ohrnberger et al., 2017). Physical activity has also been found to be a protective factor in preventing cognitive decline in older adults (Blondell et al., 2014; Smith et al., 2010; Sofi et al., 2011). Older adults who tend to be more active have less chronic conditions that allows for participation in chosen activities and more independent function.

Poor physical health has a negative impact on an older adult's mental health (Luo et al., 2014; Ohrnberger et al., 2017). Chronic conditions including cancer, cardiovascular disease, lung disease, and arthritis place older adults at higher risk of depression and anxiety (CDC, 2018a). These conditions can limit an individual's ability to perform daily routines or participate in physical activities and exercise. These situations can foster feelings of dependence, increased

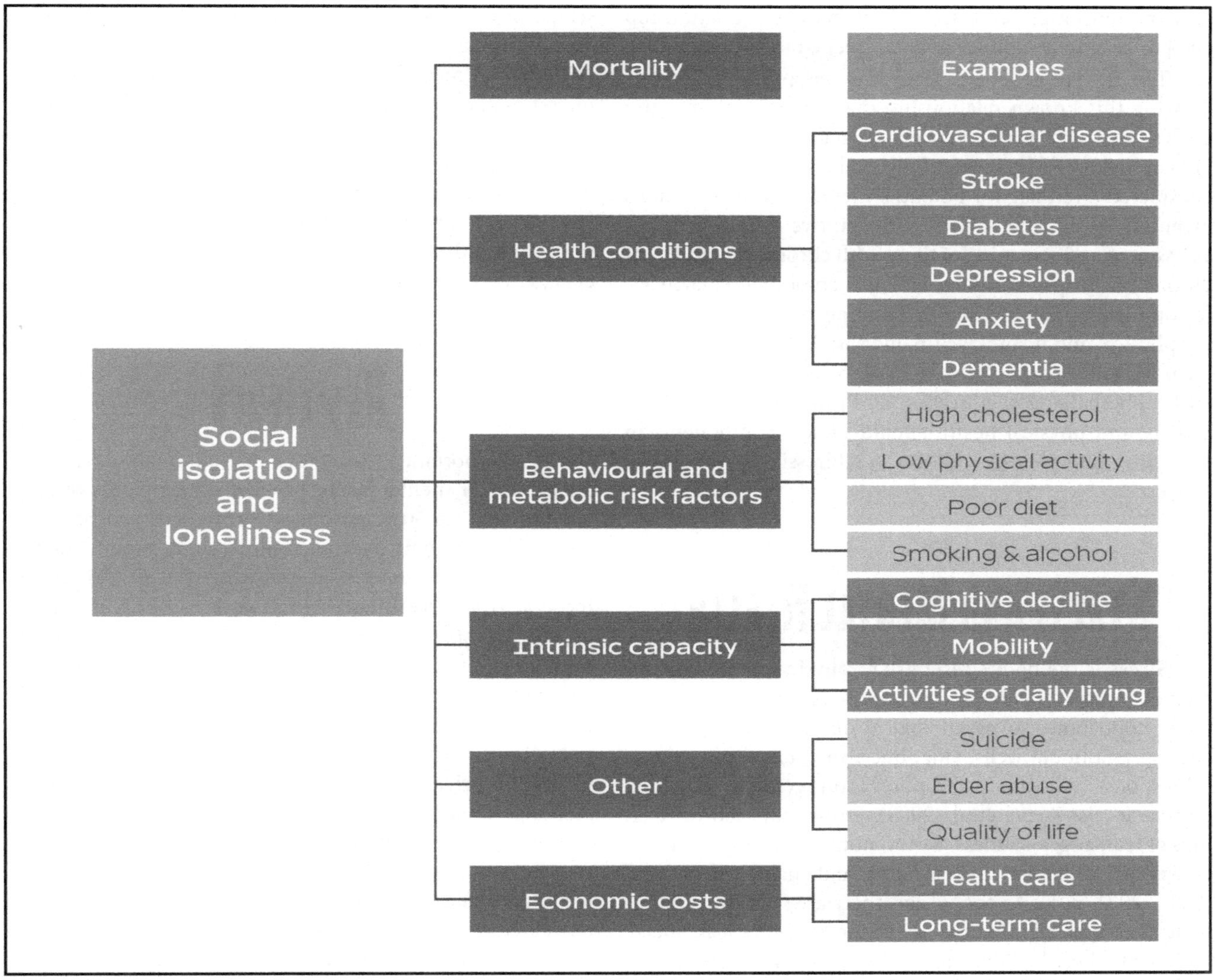

Figure 15-2. Consequences of social isolation and loneliness. (Reproduced with permission from World Health Organization [2021].)

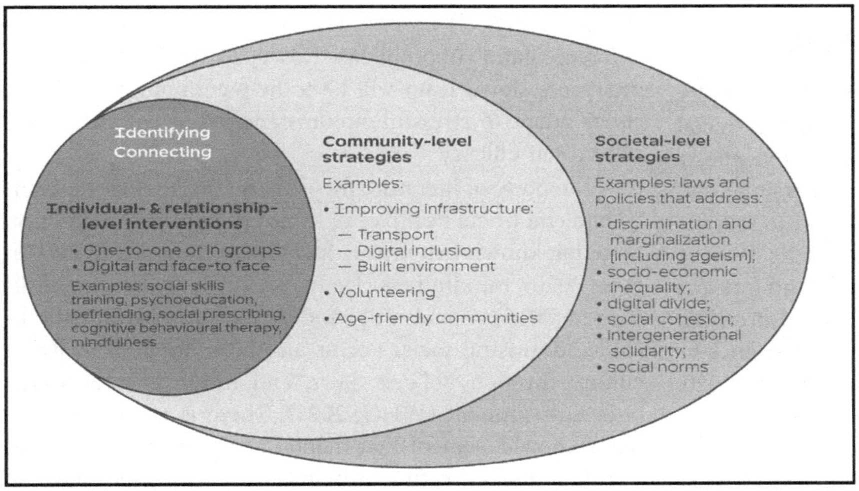

Figure 15-3. Interventions and strategies to reduce social isolation and loneliness. (Reproduced with permission from World Health Organization [2021].)

burden, and lower self-esteem. This cycle and relationship need to be closely monitored and screened for older adults.

The interprofessional team can be proactive in addressing this known relationship that can impact an older adult's functional performance and quality of life (QOL). A known history or presence of medical conditions should be considered a red flag for potential mental health conditions including depression, anxiety, or cognitive changes. Proper assessment and screening of those with chronic medical conditions can help identify mental and emotional challenges. Recommendations and interventions geared toward improving physical and mental well-being should be addressed and included in the team's care plan. For those with known mental health challenges, education and promotion of physical activity and physical health should be key components in the team's care plan in addition to addressing psychosocial concerns.

Stress and Mental Health

Stress is the body's response to physical, emotional, or mental pressure, and impacts health across the life span. Stress contributes to psychological distress, negatively impacting emotional well-being, but also elicits a physiological response (increased heart rate, blood pressure, and blood glucose levels; Kassel et al., 2003). Stress may lead to "feelings of fear, anger, sadness, worry, numbness, or frustration" as well as "difficulty concentrating and making decisions" (CDC, 2021, p. 1). As people age, there are numerous causes of stress, especially notable are changes in physical, social, and mental health. Table 15-1 cites many assessments to explore stress, QOL, and well-being among elders.

Marginalized Identities

In addition to the many stressors common among older adults, individuals from marginalized backgrounds (racial and sexual minorities) have endured the cumulative effects of a lifetime of systemic, structural, and interpersonal discrimination and victimization that can contribute to chronic stress and poor mental health (Cuevas et al., 2020; Wallace et al., 2016; Williams, 2018). "Older blacks, U.S. and foreign-born Hispanics report more chronic stress exposure than whites and are two to three times as likely to experience financial strain and housing-related stress" (Brown et al., 2020, p. 1). The experience of frequent microaggressions, harassment, and a lifetime of discrimination and marginalization has also been linked to poor mental health in LGBT older adults (Abbruzzese & Simon, 2018). The Minority Stress Theory (Meyer, 1995) highlights the deleterious and cumulative effects of bias and discrimination across the life span. Unfortunately, discriminatory practices related to race and sexual orientation or gender identity are layered on top of ageism, which leads to diminished QOL, including poor physical and mental health. Older adults with marginalized identities that experience ageism, racism, and sexism are more likely to experience isolation, loneliness, and depression (Velez et al., 2013). As we consider mental health promotion strategies that can be implemented at the community level, it is also important to address interventions that can improve health in high-risk subgroups (Fredriksen-Goldsen et al., 2017; Kim et al., 2017).

Resilience

It is important to recognize that although older adults are at risk for mental health problems, nearly 95% of older adults (over age 50 years) report being "satisfied" or "very satisfied" with their lives and most report prominent levels of mental and emotional well-being (CDC, 2018a). For those at risk, a **Resilience** Framework can be a useful approach to improving the mental and emotional well-being of older adults. "Resilience has been described in the mental health literature as the "capacity to maintain or regain well-being during or after adversity" (Whitson et al., 2016, p. 1). Resilience includes adaptive attitudes that enable individuals to thrive despite adverse events (Hardy et al., 2004). Although a variety of instruments have been developed to measure resilience, there remains a gap in the research for community-based interventions specifically targeting resilience, particularly among community-dwelling disabled and unwell elders. Psychological factors including dispositional optimism and expressive flexibility have been linked to resilience in the face of major stressors (Sardella et al., 2021). Interprofessional teams can promote healthy aging with a resilience framework by recognizing that older adults can constructively respond to environmental challenges (social and physiological), complementing a focus on identification and remediation of problems (Cosco, 2016). The focus of the interprofessional team will be to help community-dwelling elders adapt to stressful circumstances and cope with improved self-efficacy.

The body of literature focusing on improving the mental and emotional health of older adults currently focuses on targeting known risk factors including physical activity (An et al., 2020), mindfulness (Demarzo, 2018), and coping skills (Cosco, 2016). Community and systems-level strategies include addressing social norms and promoting an inclusive culture through policies, laws, and improvements to the built environment (WHO, 2021). There is an overwhelming acknowledgement that mental health is modifiable and can be improved with community-based interventions. An increased awareness of the importance of emotional well-being, prevention, and self-help programs for older adults could reduce stigma and facilitate access to important resources. According to the Life Course Model of Multimorbidity

Table 15-1

Screenings for Mental and Emotional Well-Being Constructs

SOCIAL CONNECTEDNESS/ LONELINESS/SOCIAL ISOLATION	QUALITY OF LIFE/ WELL BEING	STRESS/WORRY	RESILIENCE
• Social Connectedness Scale (Lee & Robbins, 1995) http://depts.washington.edu/uwcssc/sites/default/files//Social%20Connectedness%20Scale-Revised.pdf • UCLA Loneliness Scale (Russell, 1996) https://www.ncbi.nlm.nih.gov/pmc/articles/PMC2394670/ • Lubben Social Network Scale (Lubben, 1988) https://www.brandeis.edu/roybal/docs/LSNS_website_PDF.pdf • Multidimensional Scale of Perceived Social Support (Zimet et al., 1988) https://tnaap.org/wp-content/uploads/2022/06/MSPSS-Multidimensional-Scale-of-Perceived-Social-Support-pd.pdf • De Jong Gierveld Loneliness Scale (de Jong Gierveld & van Tilburg, 2006) https://www.nyc.gov/assets/dfta/downloads/pdf/about/dejong_gierveld_loneliness_scale.pdf	• Warwick-Edinburg Well-being Scale (Tennant et al., 2007) https://warwick.ac.uk/fac/sci/med/research/platform/wemwbs/ • PROMIS (Ader, 2007) https://www.healthmeasures.net/explore-measurement-systems/promis/intro-to-promis/list-of-adult-measures • Satisfaction with Life Scale (Diener, 1985) http://labs.psychology.illinois.edu/~ediener/SWLS.html • General Health Questionnaire (Vieweg & Hedlund, 1983) https://www.gl-assessment.co.uk/assessments/products/general-health-questionnaire/ • World Health Organization Quality of Life – Abbreviated Version (WHO-QOL-BREF; Harper & Power, 1998) https://www.who.int/tools/whoqol/whoqol-bref • DEMQOL-DEM QOL Proxy (Smith et al., 2006) https://www.bsms.ac.uk/research/neuroscience/cds/research/demqol.aspx	• Penn State Worry Questionnaire (Meyer et al., 1990) https://psychology-tools.com/test/penn-state-worry-questionnaire • Perceived Stress Scale (Jiang et al., 2017) https://www.mindgarden.com/documents/PerceivedStressScale.pdf	• The Connor Davidson Resilience Scale (CD-RISC; Connor & Davidson, 2003) http://www.connordavidson-resiliencescale.com • Brief Resilient Coping Scale (Sinclair & Wallston, 2004) https://emdrfoundation.org/toolkit/brcs.pdf • Resilience Scale (Wagnild & Young, 1993) https://www.resiliencecenter.com/products/resilience-scales-and-tools-for-research/theoriginal-resilience-scale/

Resilience, healthy aging can be achieved by developing resilience through individual, social, and environmental resources (Wister et al., 2016). Interprofessional teams can collaborate with community organizations and policy makers to support optimal aging by advocating for evidence-based mental health promotion models and interventions.

Before interprofessional teams can develop comprehensive intervention plans and implement community evidence-based strategies to address mental and emotional health, they need to assess risks and explore the many factors that contribute to mental and emotional health. Interprofessional team members then collaborate to address the barriers and challenges faced by older adults at the individual and community level.

Table 15-2

Screening Tools for Mental Health in Older Adults

DEPRESSION	ANXIETY	MENTAL STATUS AND COGNITIVE SCREENING TOOLS
• *Geriatric Depression Scale- (Short Form; Yesavage et al., 1982) https://geriatrictoolkit.missouri.edu/cog/GDS_SHORT_FORM.PDF • Patient Health Questionnaire (2) https://cde.drugabuse.gov/instrument/fc216f70-be8e-ac44-e040-bb89ad433387 • Hamilton Rating Scale for Depression (Hamilton, 1960) https://dcf.psychiatry.ufl.edu/files/2011/05/HAMILTON-DEPRESSION.pdf • Cornell Scale for Depression in Dementia (Alexopoulos et al., 1988) https://cgatoolkit.ca/Uploads/ContentDocuments/cornell_scale_depression.pdf • Beck Depression Inventory (Beck, 1961)	• *Geriatric Anxiety Inventory- Short Form (Pachana et al., 2007) http://gai.net.au/ • *Geriatric Anxiety Scale (Segal et al., 2010) https://gerocentral.org/wp-content/uploads/2013/03/Geriatric-Anxiety-Scale-v2.0_FINAL.pdf • *Adult Manifest Anxiety Scale – Elderly Version (Lowe & Reynolds, 2006) https://www.wpspublish.com/amas-adult-manifest-anxiety-scale • Goldberg Anxiety and Depression Scale (Goldberg et al., 1988)	• Mini-Mental Status Exam (Folstein et al., 1975) https://cgatoolkit.ca/Uploads/ContentDocuments/MMSE.pdf • *SLUMS (St Louis University Mental Status Exam; Tariq et al., 2006; Schwartz et al., 2019) https://www.slu.edu/medicine/internal-medicine/geriatric-medicine/aging-successfully/assessment-tools/mental-status-exam.php • Mini-Cog (Borson et al., 2003) https://mini-cog.com/ • MOCA (Montreal Cognitive Assessment; Nasreddine et al., 2005) https://www.mocatest.org/

*Designed for older adults.

Assessment of Mental and Emotional Health

The interprofessional team must gain an accurate assessment and profile of factors that contribute to emotional well-being and mental health. This is often part of a comprehensive geriatric assessment and is needed to intervene appropriately, make referrals, and provide resources. Varied tools and methods can be used to assess an older adult's mental and emotional health. Traditional (medical model) assessment tools include measures of depression, anxiety, and mental status and cognitive screening tools. Screening for mental illness is often prioritized by clinicians in a variety of practice settings and is typically part of a comprehensive geriatric assessment (Ellis et al., 2017). Table 15-2 includes traditional assessments and scales commonly used by the interprofessional team in clinical practice.

Any member of the interprofessional team may screen for depression, anxiety, or cognitive functioning. A quick screening item such as the PHQ-2, which is a two-item questionnaire asks about experiences of depressed mood and anhedonia over the past 2 weeks (Kroenke et al., 2003). Individuals with a positive screen should be followed up with a more comprehensive evaluation and/or referral to a mental health specialist to determine if they meet the criteria for a depressive disorder. For older adults showing symptoms of anxiety (restlessness, increased heart rate, rapid breathing, sweating), the Geriatric Anxiety Inventory (GAI) may be used to support a referral for anxiety using a tool validated in older adults that limits assessment of somatic symptoms that are also common in general medical conditions (Pachana et al., 2007).

In addition to screening for mental health disorders, the interprofessional team can measure mental and emotional health constructs including social connectedness, loneliness, social isolation, stress, resilience, self-efficacy, QOL, and well-being. A self-perceived degree of connectedness and social support is important to ascertain as this impacts one's overall well-being (Blazer, 2020). It is also important to gather information about the availability and quality of other sources that comprise one's support network. Measures such as the UCLA Loneliness Scale (Russell, 1996) and Social Connectedness Scale (Lee & Robbins, 1995) can be used to provide valuable information to the interprofessional team as an intervention plan is created and implemented (Lubben, 1988). Scales measuring stress and resilience can guide the interprofessional team toward strategies that promote adaptive coping and self-efficacy. While traditional assessment methods may explore these areas, these well-being constructs are often overlooked during the evaluation process in the medical model. Table 15-2 highlights measures that assess some of these mental health constructs associated with well-being.

Clinical Reasoning: Case of JP 1

Identification of depression, anxiety, or other mental health conditions is crucial to intervention planning for the interprofessional team. In JP's case, the PHQ-9 (Patient Health Questionnaire 9) score indicated moderate depression. The Saint Louis University Mental Status Exam (SLUMS) was administered due to complaints of forgetfulness and difficulty managing finances. Her score indicated a Mild Neurocognitive Disorder. The Social Connectedness Scale was administered to JP due to changes in her activity level and interaction with others as the result of her limited social participation and decline in physical status. Her score was consistent with her declining levels of social engagement.

Changes in JP's performance in daily activities and decline in physical and cognitive functioning are significant red flags and highlight her risk for poor mental and emotional health. Social isolation and loneliness with limited support networks are challenges faced by many older adults and has great impact on mental health. Life stressors including her financial concerns, changes in lifestyle post-retirement and the loss of her partner also places her at a high risk for poor mental health. Her identity as part of the LGBT community added additional stressors and has a unique set of barriers. Now in her later years, aging alone and without children, she has limited social supports, which is not uncommon for those in the LGBT older adult community.

The assessments thus far mentioned also highlight an important link between physical function and mental health. JP presented with several chronic conditions including diabetes and heart disease and was at risk for falls like one-third of all older adults. Changes and limitations in physical health pose significant challenges in JP's ability to perform the tasks, routines, and activities that she previously engaged in. These challenges served as barriers to social engagement and participation, which affected her mental and emotional well-being. Cognitive decline began to impact JP's ability to manage her own affairs, and at times concern for her safety and judgement had been expressed. Multiple stressors and losses likely produced a cumulative impact on her mental health and well-being. Identification of cognitive impairments is important as it impacts occupational performance, safety, and aging in place. Many factors influence an older adult's cognitive status including the presence of depression, altered blood values, underlying medical conditions, vison, and/or hearing impairments. The nurse practitioner or primary care provider (PCP) on the interprofessional team will typically take the lead on ordering any additional tests needed for the differential diagnoses.

The many circumstances surrounding JP's case underscore the importance of a comprehensive geriatric assessment and interprofessional care team to address the many factors contributing to her mental health and well-being. While JP faced similar challenges to her peers, including physical and cognitive decline, her identity as part of LGBT community posed additional obstacles. A cumulative impact of discrimination across her lifetime contributed to her reluctance to trust new providers and community resources. Ensuring that JP was connected to a culturally competent health care team was critical to her care plan. The ELINC team was an interprofessional collaborative care team committed to the culturally competent care of LGBT older adults.

The assessment process for older adults has multiple considerations. Practitioners should be mindful that not all assessments have been designed and validated for older adults. There may be differences between self-report and observational methods of evaluation. Practice setting, context, and even reimbursement may also drive assessment choices. Time allotted for the evaluation process varies in many clinical settings often being limited to a focus on physical and functional abilities and limitations. Practitioners need to consider the impact mental health has on physical and functional abilities. Role delineation and responsibilities among the interprofessional team is another consideration. Information pertaining to mental health concerns needs to be addressed and discussed by all members of the interprofessional team to establish a comprehensive intervention plan (Clinical Reasoning: Case of JP).

Interventions

There are a wide range of strategies that interprofessional teams may employ when developing an intervention plan to promote mental and emotional health in older adults. Intervention choices are impacted by the severity of the problem, economic costs, and resources, as well as personal preferences. Teams consider participant motivation (self-efficacy, outcomes, expectations), the likely health impact of the intervention (social connectedness, stress reduction, coping and resilience, mental health treatment) as well as the resources needed to implement a plan (health care providers, equipment, space, agency coordination). The pros and cons of delivery mode need to be considered (face-to-face, virtual, remote, hybrid). Ideally, interventions address multiple levels of capacity, including individual-level interventions, community-based interventions, and advocacy for policy and systems-level interventions (Madsen et al., 2019; WHO, n.d.a).

Individualized Mental Health Care

Mental health problems/disorders need to be respected and treated to the same extent as physical medical health problems/conditions. If a community-based screening program yields positive findings for a mental health problem such as depression, anxiety, or cognitive impairment, the interprofessional team serves a key role in connecting older adults with culturally competent, skilled providers for individual-level care.

Counseling services may be delivered by a range of providers including psychologists, clinical social workers, family nurse practitioners, and others. Additionally, occupational therapists, community mental health nurses, pastoral counselors, and mental health counselors also provide mental health services in a variety of settings. Pharmacological management of mental health conditions is typically addressed by a psychiatrist, or primary care provider (nurse practitioner, medical doctor). According to the WHO Special Initiative for Mental Health, the goal is to expand access to quality and affordable mental health care to at least 100 million more people between 2019 and 2023 (WHO, n.d.a). To support this initiative focused on individual care, there must be simultaneous efforts to scale-up services in community-based general health settings and specialist settings as well as improve mental health coverage polices.

Friendly Visiting Programs

Friendly visiting programs have been developed by several organizations to match isolated seniors with volunteers. Typically, volunteers are screened and trained, and commit to 1 year of visiting an older adult in their home on either a weekly or monthly basis with calls in-between. Examples of highly successful friendly visiting programs include DOROT, a nonprofit organization based in New York City, committed to alleviating social isolation among the elderly (DOROT, n.d.). SAGE, founded in 1979 and the first of its kind in the United States, matches volunteers from the community with LGBT older adults ("Friends at Home") to form relationships that are mutually rewarding and build community (SAGEnyc.org, n.d.a). The Council on Aging – Southern California benefits isolated older and disabled adults in California by addressing their basic, social, emotional, and environmental needs. In addition to addressing loneliness and cognition, these programs have provided a means of connecting isolated seniors to needed resources.

In the 2021 WHO Report on interventions to reduce social isolation and loneliness, "befriending" was among the examples listed for face-to-face or digital interventions (WHO, 2021), especially important for, as an example, an older adult with mobility impairments or fear of falling. In addition to reducing emotional stress, a strong, supportive personal connection may address barriers to other mental health interventions. Social ties also play a significant role in influencing health habits (U.S. Department of Health and Human Services, n.d.). Social support may help someone engage in healthier lifestyle behaviors like exercise or a healthier diet.

Group Activities

Numerous studies have investigated the benefits of participating in group activities on social connectedness, isolation, and loneliness (Findlay, 2003; Gardiner et al., 2016). Participation in group settings increases the number of social contacts, which addresses social isolation; however, engagement in group activities must be meaningful to combat feelings of loneliness. Programs that have a community development approach, are adaptable, and induce dynamic engagement will be among the most effective interventions for social isolation and loneliness (Gardiner et al., 2016).

Groups designed to promote connectedness typically either focus on an activity (e.g., gardening projects, painting, pottery, dance, music, drama, jewelry making, therapeutic writing, exercise, etc.) or a discussion topic (e.g., bible study, book club, aging topics, health topics). Skill development can also promote self-efficacy and resilience. In addition to developing a skill or learning about a particular topic, group members interact with each other, share individual experiences, and can offer each other emotional support. Feelings of "belonging to a group" can be enhanced when participation in a group activity persists over time.

For older adults with both physical and mental health challenges, augmenting individualized disease-management patient education with a referral to a group program could have the added benefit of promoting mental and emotional health. Group discussion topics that focus on health risks and chronic health conditions can be particularly beneficial to older adults that perceive health care professionals as not having enough time to answer all their questions (Agarwal & Brydges, 2018). There are numerous evidence-based programs focused on health conditions that offer both health education and social connectedness (e.g., Matter of Balance, the Chronic Disease Self-Management Program [CDSMP], Healthy Steps for Older Adults, Healthy Steps in Motion; NCOA, 2021).

Engaging vulnerable older adults in group activities may require targeted outreach and additional resources or training. Special attention should be given to older adults living alone, aging without a partner (divorced, widowed, single), with limited friend/family networks (Holt-Lunstad et al., 2017), reduced socioeconomic resources, and/or with marginalized identities (National Resource Center on LGBT Aging, 2020). If face-to-face options have too many barriers, virtual and online forms of engagement are a viable way to increase social connectedness (WHO, 2021; NCOA, 2021). Members of the interprofessional collaborative care team can help connect older adults to group programs and support training or implementation of evidence-based programs in community settings. Table 15-3 includes a list of evidence-based intervention options with mental health benefits that may be delivered in group settings.

According to the interventions and strategies to reduce social isolation and loneliness recommended by the WHO

Table 15-3

Evidence-Based Intervention Options With Mental Health Benefits

INTERVENTION	MENTAL HEALTH BENEFITS	PUBLIC RESOURCES	REFERENCES
Creative Arts			
Music	• Promotes a sense of well-being, belonging, and participation. • Taps into personal preferences and life history. • Reduces depression and confused mood.	https://www.arts.gov/state-and-regional-arts-organizations	Xu et al. (2017) Gold et al. (2019)
Dance	• Combines the benefits of physical activity with socialization and personal expression. • Integrates cognitive demands (learning steps and sequences) with motor execution. • Improves stress, anxiety, and depressive symptoms.	https://iadms.org/education-resources/dance-for-health/	Whitty et al. (2020) Barranco-Ruiz et al. (2020)
Arts on Prescription Program	• Improvements in mental well-being. • Participants report plans to continue artistic endeavors after the course ended.	https://www.hammond.com.au/healthcare-services/positive-ageing	Beauchet et al. (2020)
Mindfulness-Based Stress Reduction			
Standing, sitting and walking meditations, yoga, and body scanning activities	• Reduces depressive symptoms. • Enhances the resilience of Interprofessional teams.	https://www.apa.org/topics/mindfulness/meditation	Kabat-Zinn et al. (1985) Galante et al. (2021) Colgan et al. (2019)
Physical Activity and Exercise			
Physical activity	• Protective factor for cognitive decline and dementia. • Reduces anxiety. • Reduces depression risk. • Improves QOL. • There are not specific activity recommendations for brain health and cognitive function.	https://www.nia.nih.gov/health/exercise-physical-activity https://www.cdc.gov/physicalactivity/index.html https://tools.silversneakers.com/	Sofi et al. (2011) Smith et al. (2010) Mammen & Faulkner (2013)
High-intensity progressive resistive training	• Improves conflict resolution and selective attention. • Reduces depressive symptoms. • Delays onset of depression.		Nagamatsu et al. (2012) Singh et al. (2001)
Aerobic training	• Reduces depressive symptoms. • Delays onset of depression.		Bartholomew et al. (2005) Huang et al. (2015)
Aerobic training embedded within high-intensity interval training (HIIT)	• Improves memory.		Kovacevic et al. (2020)
Yoga	• Reduces depressive symptoms.	https://www.silversneakers.com/blog/yoga-for-seniors-which-class-best-for-you/	Patel et al. (2012)
Tai Chi	• Improves stress reduction. • Reduces anxiety. • Reduces depressive symptoms. • Improves mood.	https://taichihealth.com/tai-chi-fundamentals/ https://www.mayoclinic.org/tests-procedures/meditation/in-depth/meditation/art-20045858	Wang et al. (2013) Liu et al. (2015) Yohannes et al. (2010)

(2021), addressing social norms, discrimination, and marginalization (including ageism), and enacting polices that promote socioeconomic equality are societal-level strategies needed to support community-level interventions. Interprofessional Collaborative Practice Care (IPCP) team members can advocate for integrating assessment and program evaluation into novel program designs, to ensure group activities are effective at addressing targeted outcomes (Findlay, 2003). Agencies that provide group programs to older adults need to be mindful of the ways bias and discrimination can create barriers to needed services. Efforts to address the climate and develop culturally competent group facilitators will be a critical area of focus for group activity interventions (Abbruzzese & Simon, 2018).

Virtual Programs

Older adults with deteriorating physical status may benefit from virtual interventions when limited mobility or cumbersome transportation options create a barrier. While technology can be a resource for promoting social connectedness and delivering needed services, it can also serve as a potential barrier due to perceptions that technology is overly complex. The use of computers and smartphones to increase social connections, however, is growing rapidly among adults over age 50 years. According to a 2020 survey by the AARP, three quarters of all adults ages 50 and over engage with social media outlets like Facebook, Instagram, Youtube, and LinkedIn on a regular basis. An alternative to computers is the use of the telephones or video calls for reducing social isolation and loneliness in older people (Sundsli et al., 2014). For those who can overcome potential barriers of technology, virtual platforms can expand opportunities for connection. The Administration for Community Living offers seniors tips engaging virtually to combat loneliness and isolation (2021).

Online health communities have the potential to promote resilience in older adults (Kamalpour et al., 2021). In recent years, virtual programs have demonstrated improvements in cognitive function, depression, and anxiety levels in older adults with subjective cognitive decline (SCD) and appears to provide a feasible means of promoting activity remotely as an intervention for depression (Lambert et al., 2018). Interest and acceptance of online interventions is likely to grow. LEAVES (optimizing the mental health and resilience of older adults that have lost their spouse via blended, online therapy) is an online bereavement program that will support the prevention and treatment of prolonged grief. This program is designed to provide a virtual means of connecting with support and reducing stress.

There are virtual versions of many programs that were once delivered in person. For example, friendly visitor programs have been recreated in virtual spaces. Addressing Loneliness with Movement and Art (ALMA) is using technology to create intergenerational relationships between students and seniors in their 6-week student to senior program. The program is designed for independent living older adults and students. Students build personal friendships with seniors and explore meaningful topics and provide social emotional support (ALMA, n.d.). The Otago Exercise Program (OEP), primarily focused on reducing fall risk, has also been implemented in a virtual setting with success (Shubert et al., 2018). Although online interventions may be as effective as in-person programs, one of the problems cited in the virtual environment is increased attrition. Long-term adherence and in virtual settings may have unique drivers.

As with other interventions, the interprofessional collaborative practice team may need to focus on structural barriers to virtual interventions for mental and emotional health. Advocacy efforts are underway to increase broadband access to rural and under-resourced communities. Older adults on fixed incomes may not be able to afford the additional cost of an internet or cellular connection. Libraries and senior centers may offer computer access but would still be inaccessible to individuals with limited mobility or unreliable transportation. In some areas, low-cost internet may be an option (Senior Planet, 2021). Older adults also want policy makers to address reasonable concerns about privacy and vulnerability to scam artists in virtual spaces (Baig, 2021). Programs like "Older Adults Technology Services (OATS)" may help to connect older adults to valuable online resources (Senior Planet, 2021).

Physical Activity and Exercise

There are a myriad of activity and exercise evidence-based interventions that have been shown to have a positive impact on mental health (Biddle, 2016; Blondell et al., 2014). Most studies focus on delaying the onset of mental disease like dementia or depression. Some studies, however, also include improvement in symptoms like memory, executive function, and mood (Biddle, 2016; Blondell et al., 2014). Although the evidence for physical activity and exercise being beneficial for mental health is extensive, the methodology is varied. Interprofessional teams will be critical partners in connecting older adults to valuable community-based physical activity resources.

CDC guidelines for physical activity for older adults include being less sedentary, engaging in 150 to 300 minutes of moderate-intensity activity or 75 to 150 minutes of vigorous intensity activity per week and moderate intensity strength training at least twice per week (2021a). These activity recommendations are designed to promote bone health, muscle strength, functional mobility, healthy weight, as well as improved mood and cognition. Physical activity has been shown to positively impact mental and emotional health in numerous randomized controlled studies (Smith et al., 2010; Sofi et al., 2011). There are not, however, specific activity recommendations for brain health and cognitive function.

Physical activity "defined as the movement of skeletal muscles, resulting in energy expenditure exceeding the resting state" is a protective factor for cognitive decline and dementia (Blondell et al., 2014, p. 3). A meta-analysis of 21 prospective longitudinal studies, Blondell et al. (2014) concluded that higher levels of physical activity were associated with a 14% risk reduction for developing dementia. Previous systematic reviews have also concluded that physical activity is protective of cognitive decline (Smith et al., 2010; Sofi et al., 2011). A limitation for many of the studies reviewed is that physical activity is not consistently defined and is frequently assessed using self-report questionnaires. Details regarding frequency, type, and intensity of the physical activities are rarely provided.

In addition to providing protection against cognitive decline and dementia, physical activity has been shown to have additional brain health benefits including reduced anxiety, reduced depression risk, and improved QOL (Mammen & Faulkner, 2013). Individual studies focusing on older populations have revealed that both aerobic (Bartholomew et al., 2005; Huang et al., 2015) and resistive strength training (Singh et al., 2001) can reduce depressive symptoms in older adults and/or prevent the onset of depression. There are multiple systematic reviews demonstrating the effectiveness of tai chi as an antidepressant, including improved stress reduction, reduced anxiety, and reduced depressive symptoms (Liu et al., 2015; Wang et al., 2013); however, many of the studies are small and do not all specifically focus on older adults.

Healthy People 2030 has a stated objective to increase the percent of adults aged 65 years and over with reduced physical or cognitive function engaged in light, moderate, or vigorous leisure-time physical activities from 41.3% (2018) to 51% (n.d.) Exercise programs can be daunting to older adults that lack experience or knowledge. Although high-intensity exercise programs can be managed independently or in group settings led by lay personnel, older adults are sometimes reticent due to fears of musculoskeletal injury. For individuals with physical limitations and/or comorbidities impacting mobility, a physical or occupational therapist could provide personalized assistance with the exercise prescription and progression.

Group class–based activities like yoga or tai chi may be offered to older adults at a local gym, senior center, or through municipal programs. However, older adults on a fixed income may be worried about cost or transportation (Anderson & Mehegan, 2018). Our preliminary work on the facilitators and barriers to evidence-based programs among LGBT older adults suggests that instructor characteristics are especially important. In addition to being competent, the instructor needs to be likable and inclusive, particularly for marginalized populations (Abbruzzese et al., 2019). Internalized ageism may also be a major barrier to exercise and physical activity (WHO, n.d.b). Despite published guidelines, listing the many health benefits, older adults may see themselves as "too old" for exercise. Motivational interviewing may be a useful technique for promoting behavior change in individuals that are ambivalent about increasing activity levels (Brummel-Smith, 2015). Counseling and guidance from the Interprofessional team could help to ensure that older adults have the self-efficacy to seek out ways to be more active for mental health benefits and have safe plans for engaging in exercise and physical activity.

Nature-Based Social Prescribing

Leavell et al. (2019) have proposed "nature-based social prescribing" to improve social connectedness, mental well-being, and reduce stress. Activities may include park visits, walking clubs, gardening, forest bathing, bird watching, river walks, beach/coast walks, and trips to the Farmer's Market or Botanic Gardens. Recommending pet ownership, which has a positive effect on depressive symptoms and perceived well-being by reducing loneliness, stress, and anxiety, and promotes feelings of relaxation, may also promote connections with nature, and physical activity with purposeful daily walks outdoors (CDC, 2021). At the intrapersonal level, nature-based activities promote awe, enjoyment, purpose, belonging, competence, and autonomy. At the interpersonal level, they promote social involvement, shared learning, and relatedness. At the environmental level they offer access to nature, aesthetics, and place attachment. The interrelated elements of social connectedness, physical activity, cognitive attention, and stress reduction promote both improved physical health and mental well-being (Leavell et al., 2019). The intentional contact with nature is particularly important for individuals living in urban settings. The nature-based social prescriptions that have been investigated offer a low-cost, beneficial way to promote socially connected, active communities.

Mindfulness-Based Stress Reduction

Mindfulness-based stress reduction (MBSR), a meditation-based therapy developed by Kabat-Zinn in 1979, was originally designed for stress management, but has also been used to address mental illness, including depression and anxiety (Kabat-Zinn et al., 1985). Meditative activities address the thoughts, feelings, and behaviors that increase stress and negatively impact health. MBSR intervention techniques may include standing, sitting, and walking meditations, yoga, and body scanning activities, typically for 6 to 8 weeks, offered in community settings. The emerging evidence suggests that MBSR is a viable option for enhancing mental health in nonclinical settings (Galante et al., 2021) and the feasibility and possible benefits of MBSR in older adults is promising. In addition to implementing MBSR with older adult communities, Mindfulness-Based Wellness and Resilience (MBWR) interventions may enhance the resilience of interprofessional teams (Colgan et al., 2019).

Promoting Individual and Community Resilience

Promoting resilience in older adults and in communities requires multilevel engagement over time in social, unpredictable contexts. Older adults often have a deep connection to communities, thus efforts to enhance resilience should address community resources as well as personal and collective capacities through engagement in everyday circumstances (Madsen et al., 2019). The activities that have been identified as promoting resilience in communities are volunteering, collaborative decision making, collective action and participation, and community learning through collaborative action (Gibb, 2018; Madsen et al., 2019). At the personal level, individuals should be encouraged to volunteer in meaningful activities, and should be made aware of opportunities for them in their communities. At the community level, community facilities should be made affordable, grassroots advocacy and collaborative leadership is encouraged, equitable practices should be facilitated, and language and policies should be framed with a strengths-based approach to resilience (Madsen et al., 2019). Large-scale population efforts to provide older adults opportunities for engagement contributes to community well-being and mental health (Cosco et al., 2016).

The Village Model for aging in place is another great example of how communities can build both personal and collective capacities for resilience by coordinating services and supports within a local community. In the Village Model, participants provide functional, emotional, and social support to other members of the village. Neighbors help neighbors with nonmedical household tasks and work together to coordinate social, recreational, and educational programming (Village to Village Network [VtV], n.d.). Examples like the Beacon Hill Village in Massachusetts and Neighbor2Neighbor in Greenwich Village have been formed to empower older adults with the resources and support network to stay in their homes with confidence (VtV, n.d.). According to the according to the VtV, there are over 100 villages in the United States, and more being developed. One of their cited outcomes is having a positive impact on isolation, interdependence, health, and purpose of their members (VtV, n.d.).

Community-Based Programs

Community-based programs are a valuable resource for interprofessional teams concerned with the mental and emotional health of older adults. While interprofessional teams may consider referrals to health care providers with mental health expertise in traditional health care settings, these providers are also active in community programs designed to reach people outside of the medical model. Interprofessional teams in community programs can address day to day issues and concerns as they arise. Screening and routine monitoring are crucial and can more easily be performed in the community. Senior centers and community programs are staffed with providers including social workers, nurses, mental health workers, psychologists, and occupational and physical therapists who can address many attributes and facets of care to improve mental health and well-being (Anetzberger, 2019). Varied programming options offer flexibility and may be more amenable to an older adult from an access and financial perspective (Clinical Reasoning: Case of JP #2).

Community-based programs are most successful when a variety of environments/settings can be targeted (Healthy People 2030, n.d.). There are several community-based programs promoted by the CDC that specifically target mental/emotional well-being in older adults:

- **Lighten UP!** is an 8-week program consisting of 90-minute group session "designed to teach participants to identify and savor positive experiences across multiple domains of eudemonic well-being." This program has delivered robust improvements on Psychological Well-being Scale (PWB).

Clinical Reasoning: Case of JP 2

The ELINC team worked collaboratively to develop a multidimensional intervention plan to integrate and connect JP with community-based resources and care. Since JP had positive screens for both depression and mild cognitive impairment, she was referred for a follow-up with a behavioral health specialist. She had not had positive experiences in the past and did not feel that it would help her. Although JP was reluctant, it is important that older adults are connected to skilled providers. There are a range of skills-based therapeutic programs that have been shown to promote mental and emotional health in older adults including cognitive behavioral therapy, problem-solving therapy, reminiscence therapy, sleep and relaxation coaching, pain management therapy, bereavement therapy, and supportive therapy. Many of these evidence-based approaches are offered through the Institute on Aging (Institute on Aging, 2020). Practitioners that want to ensure that community partners are providing culturally competent care can refer to the National CLAS Standards, sponsored by the Office of Minority Health, U.S. Department of Health and Human Services.

In addition to referrals within the medical model, the interprofessional team helped connect JP to group programs offered in the SAGE Senior Center offered a robust calendar of events and a diverse menu of programs including Fall Prevention groups, Diabetes Self-Management groups, and exercise groups. JP did not like the idea of going to a senior center alone. She was also reluctant to follow through on the theater activity recommendations due to her impaired mobility. The team implemented home safety modifications and instructed JP in safe use of an assistive device and safe mobility. Although these interventions address physical limitations, her functional independence and safety was a barrier to social connectedness. JP made small adaptations in her home environment, including tacking down loose rugs, posting exercise sheets on the wall to prompt more consistent adherence, and wearing more supportive shoes. She also practiced using the cane for increased gait stability.

A major source of stress in JP's life was her social isolation and loneliness exacerbated by inaccessible and expensive transportation options. JP was unable to safely navigate public transportation. She would use private taxi services for medical appointments but was resistant to taking cabs/private transportation to engage in social/leisure activities due to limited finances. The team arranged transportation services (Access-A Ride) for ease and safety in the community.

Recommendations made by the interprofessional team also addressed underlying mental health concerns to help mediate JP's social isolation and loneliness. JP was also referred to the SAGE Friendly Visitor Program. The SAGE Friendly Visitor Program turned out to be the critical service that addressed JP's loneliness, stress of travelling alone, and support for other team recommendations like participation in SAGE community-based programs (SAGEnyc.org, n.d.b). Once connected to a friendly visitor, JP started participating in group activities at the SAGE senior center and resumed activities like attending the theater. Individuals with marginalized backgrounds often age alone, single, and without children. Like her aging peers, JP's social isolation combined with limited physical mobility may have been exacerbated by perceived lack of culturally responsive providers and sensitivity to JP's life story.

This intervention plan reflects the interprofessional perspectives of the team and the wide variety of community-based programs available to JP. JP was encouraged to attend an LGBT-friendly senior center to foster socialization, engagement, and participation in group-based physical activities. Community resources were provided for local theater and travel clubs based on her identified leisure interests. Promotion of home safety, physical activity, and strategies to decrease her sedentary behaviors were outlined. The individual/relationship-level friendly visitor service helped to connect JP to the recommended community resources. The combined interventions facilitated improved mental health and well-being in JP and highlights the benefits of culturally competent interprofessional collaboration.

- **IMPACT, the Improving Mood-Promoting Access to Collaborative Treatment** (IMPACT) collaborative care management program for late-life depression, is a 12-month program focused on brief psychotherapy for depression, and is supervised by a primary care provider and psychiatrist (https://aims.uw.edu/project/impact-improving-mood-promoting-access-to-collaborative-treatment/). Psychiatrists, primary care providers, and behavioral health care managers can receive free training in the IMPACT collaborative care model (https://www.psychiatry.org/psychiatrists/practice/professional-interests/integrated-care/get-trained).
- **PEARLS: Program to Encourage Active, Rewarding Lives for Seniors** includes 8 50-minute sessions delivered in the home over a 19-week period (CDC, 2018a). Older adults with minor depression or dysthymia are taught three depression management techniques including problem solving, social and physical activity planning, and participation planning for pleasant events. Participants are encouraged by counselors to utilize local community resources. Over 40 PEARLS programs have been implemented in the United States since 2008 (https://www.cdc.gov/prc/resources/tools/pearls.html). Members of the interprofessional team interested in implementing a PEARLS program can download the PEARLS Toolkit and participate in a 2-day training program.

Websites for Additional Mental Health Community Resources

- CDC Programs to Address Depression in Community Older Adults: https://www.cdc.gov/aging/pdf/mental_health_brief_2.pdf

- SAMHSA Older Adult and Mental Health Resources: https://www.samhsa.gov/resources-serving-older-adults
- World Health Organization: https://www.who.int/teams/social-determinants-of-health/demographic-change-and-healthy-ageing/social-isolation-and-loneliness
- The Treatment of Depression in Older Adults: Evidence Based Tool Kit: https://store.samhsa.gov/sites/default/files/d7/priv/sma11-4631-keyissues.pdf

Interprofessional Team

Geriatric care delivered by an interprofessional collaborative care team represents an optimal and comprehensive approach to the multidimensional needs of older adults. The multitude of factors impacting an older person's life including their physical and mental health, emotional well-being, and social and environmental challenges call for a coordinated team approach. The Interprofessional Education Collaborative identifies four core competencies for interprofessional collaborative care that include values and ethics for interprofessional practice, roles and responsibilities, interprofessional communication, and teams and teamwork (2016).

Unique contributions of multiple disciplines ensure that the needs of older adults are met. To address the mental and emotional health of older adults, an interprofessional team approach will provide varied perspectives and insights to address medical conditions, social support issues, physical, functional, and environmental barriers that are inter-related and all impact well-being and QOL.

There are an overwhelming number of community programs and resources designed to meet the mental and emotional needs of older adults. It is critical for clinicians to collaborate with team members and clients to identify needs and make needed referrals. The role of the clinician may be to share a resource, encourage and facilitate clients to engage and participate, monitor, and track needs and outcomes and most important support the older adult to facilitate well-being and improved QOL.

Conclusion

Older adults face a multitude of stressors, losses, and challenges in their later years that impacts their ability to function and cope. The different perspectives of the interprofessional team members provide a unique approach to address mental health and emotional well-being. Multiple members of the interprofessional team can promote health and well-being by promoting physical activity, connection to social support or needed services, medication management, and/or by increasing someone's functional independence. Different perspectives and approaches to address mental health concerns provide an avenue for a client-centered, comprehensive care and best practice. The interprofessional collaborative team approach begins with a multidimensional assessment process, followed by identification of interfering factors and challenges and finally development and implementation of a multidimensional intervention plan. Interventions occur at the individual, community, and societal level. Access to community resources and programs should be facilitated to enhance social connectedness, decrease stress and worry, increase physical activity, improve self-efficacy, and promote resilience. In some cases, this may mean addressing society-level policies that limit access and perpetuate discrimination. In other cases, it requires addressing individual barriers like mobility or befriending. Meaningful community engagement, which promotes flexibility, resilience, and adaptability, is key in helping older adults cope and facilitate satisfaction and QOL in their later years.

References

Abbruzzese, L. D., & Simon, P. (2018). Special concerns for the LGBT aging patient: What rehab professionals should know. *Current Geriatrics Reports, 7*(1), 26-36. https://doi.org/10.1007/s13670-018-0232-6

Abbruzzese, L. D., Simon, P., & Hall, P. (2019). *Facilitators and barriers to participation in evidence-based programs in urban senior centers serving LGBT older adults*. Unpublished manuscript.

Ader, D. N. (2007). Developing the patient-reported outcomes: Measurement Information System (PROMIS). *Medical Care, 45*(5). https://doi.org/10.1097/01.mlr.0000260537.45076.74

Administration for Community Living & Administration on Aging. (2021). Commit to connect. https://acl.gov/CommitToConnect

Agarwal, G., & Brydges, M. (2018). Effects of a community health promotion program on social factors in a vulnerable older adult population residing in social housing. *BMC Geriatrics, 18*(1). https://doi.org/10.1186/s12877-018-0764-9

Agency for Healthcare Research and Quality. (2017). GRACE Team Care. https://www.ahrq.gov/workingforquality/priorities-in-action/grace-team-care.html

Alexopoulos, G. S., Abrams, R. C., Young, R. C., & Shamoian, C. A. (1988). Cornell scale for depression in dementia. *Biological Psychiatry, 23*(3), 271-284. https://doi.org/10.1016/0006-3223(88)90038-8

ALMA. (n.d.). Student to senior. https://www.almamovement.org/sts

American Psychological Association. (2017, August 5). Social isolation, loneliness could be greater threat to public health than obesity. ScienceDaily. https://www.sciencedaily.com/releases/2017/08/170805165319.htm.

An, H.-Y., Chen, W., Wang, C.-W., Yang, H.-F., Huang, W.-T., & Fan, S.-Y. (2020). The relationships between physical activity and life satisfaction and happiness among young, middle-aged, and older adults. *International Journal of Environmental Research and Public Health, 17*(13), 4817. https://doi.org/10.3390/ijerph17134817

Anderson, G. O., & Mehegan, L. (2018). Sweating together: Exercise and social preferences among adults 18+. *AARP Research*. https://doi.org/10.26419/res.00229.001

Anderson, G. O., & Thayer, C. E (2018). Loneliness and social connections: A national survey of adults 45 and older. *AARP Research*. https://doi.org/10.26419/res.00246.001

Anetzberger, G. J. (2019). Community based services Chapter 29. In B. Bonder & V. D. Bello Haas (Eds.), *Functional performance in older adults* (pp. 437-451). F.A. Davis Company.

Baig, E. (2021). Older adults wary about their privacy online. https://www.aarp.org/home-family/personal-technology/info-2021/companies-address-online-privacy-concerns.html

Barranco-Ruiz, Y., Paz-Viteri, S., & Villa-González, E. (2020). Dance fitness classes improve the health-related quality of life in sedentary women. *International Journal of Environmental Research and Public Health, 17*(11), 3771. https://doi.org/10.3390/ijerph17113771

Bartholomew, J. B., Morrison, D., & Ciccolo, J. T. (2005). Effects of Acute Exercise on Mood and well-being in patients with major depressive disorder. *Medicine & Science in Sports & Exercise, 37*(12), 2032-2037. https://doi.org/10.1249/01.mss.0000178101.78322.dd

Beauchet, O., Cooper-Brown, L., Hayashi, Y., Galery, K., Vilcocq, C., & Bastien, T. (2020). Effects of "Thursdays at the Museum" at the Montreal Museum of Fine Arts on the mental and physical health of older community dwellers: the art-health randomized clinical trial protocol. *Trials, 21*(1). https://doi.org/10.1186/s13063-020-04625-3

Beck, A. T. (1961). An inventory for measuring depression. *Archives of General Psychiatry, 4*(6), 561. https://doi.org/10.1001/archpsyc.1961.01710120031004

Biddle, S. (2016). Physical activity and mental health: Evidence is growing. *World Psychiatry, 15*(2), 176-177. https://doi.org/10.1002/wps.20331

Blazer, D. (2020). Social isolation and loneliness in older adults—A mental health/public health challenge. *JAMA Psychiatry, 77*(10), 990. https://doi.org/10.1001/jamapsychiatry.2020.1054

Blondell S. J., Hammersley-Mather R., & Veerman J. L. (2014). Does physical activity prevent cognitive decline and dementia? A systematic review and meta-analysis of longitudinal studies. *BMC Public Health, 14*(1), 510. https://doi.org/10.1186/1471-2458-14-510

Borson, S., Scanlan, J. M., Chen, P., & Ganguli, M. (2003). The Mini-Cog as a screen for dementia: validation in a population-based sample. *Journal of the American Geriatrics Society, 51*(10), 1451-1454. https://doi.org/10.1046/j.1532-5415.2003.51465.x

Brummel-Smith, K. (2015). *Motivational interviewing for older adults*. Springer. https://link.springer.com/chapter/10.1007/978-3-319-16095-5_5.

Centers for Disease Control and Prevention. (2018a). Well-being concepts. https://cdc.gov/hrqol/wellbeing.htm.

Centers for Disease Control and Prevention. (2018b). PEARLS. Centers for Disease Control and Prevention. https://www.cdc.gov/prc/resources/tools/pearls.html.

Centers for Disease Control and Prevention. (2021). How much physical activity do older adults need? https://www.cdc.gov/physicalactivity/basics/older_adults/index.htm.

Colgan, D. D., Christopher, M., Bowen, S., Brems, C., Hunsinger, M., Tucker, B., & Dapolonia, E. (2019). Mindfulness-based wellness and resilience intervention among interdisciplinary primary care teams: A mixed-methods feasibility and acceptability trial. *Primary Health Care Research & Development, 20*. https://doi.org/10.1017/s1463423619000173

Committee on Family Caregiving for Older Adults. (2016). *Families caring for an aging America*. The National Academies Press. https://doi.org/10.17226/23606

Connor, K. M., & Davidson, J. R. T. (2003). Development of a new resilience scale: The Connor-Davidson Resilience Scale (CD-RISC). *Depression and Anxiety, 18*(2), 76-82. https://doi.org/10.1002/da.10113

Cosco, T. D., Kaushal, A., Richards, M., Kuh, D., & Stafford, M. (2016). Resilience measurement in later life: A systematic review and Psychometric Analysis. *Health and Quality of Life Outcomes, 14*(1). https://doi.org/10.1186/s12955-016-0418-6

Cuevas, A. G., Ong, A. D., Carvalho, K., Ho, T., Chan, S. W. C., Allen, J. D., Chen, R., Rodgers, J., Biba, U., & Williams, D. R. (2020). Discrimination and systemic inflammation: A critical review and synthesis. *Brain, behavior, and immunity, 89*, 465-479. https://doi.org/10.1016/j.bbi.2020.07.017

Dahlberg, L. (2021). Loneliness during the COVID-19 pandemic. *Aging & Mental Health, 25*(7), 1161-1164. https://doi.org/10.1080/13607863.2021.1875195

de Jong-Gierveld, J. & van Tilburg, T. G. (2006). A 6-item scale for overall, emotional, and social loneliness: Confirmatory tests on survey data. *Research on Aging, 28*(5), 582-598. https://doi.org/10.1177/0164027506289723

Demarzo, M. (2018). Effect of the Mindfulness-Based Health Promotion Program (MBHP) in the elderly: A RCT—Full Text View. https://clinicaltrials.gov/ct2/show/NCT03706807.

Diener, E., Emmons, R. A., Larsen, R. J., & Griffin, S. (1985). Satisfaction with Life Scale. *Journal of Personality Assessment, 49*(1), 71-75. https://doi.org/10.1207/s15327752jpa4901_13

Donovan, N. J., & Blazer, D. (2020). Social isolation and loneliness in older adults: Review and commentary of a National Academies Report. *The American Journal of Geriatric Psychiatry, 28*(12), 1233-1244. https://doi.org/10.1016/j.jagp.2020.08.005

DOROT. (n.d.). History. https://www.dorotusa.org/about/history

Ellis, G., Gardner, M., Tsiachristas, A., Langhorne, P., Burke, O., Harwood, R. H., Conroy, S. P., Kircher, T., Somme, D., Saltvedt, I., Wald, H., O'Neill, D., Robinson, D., & Shepperd, S. (2017). Comprehensive geriatric assessment for older adults admitted to hospital. *The Cochrane database of systematic reviews, 9*(9), CD006211. https://doi.org/10.1002/14651858.CD006211.pub3

Findlay, R. (2003). Interventions to reduce social isolation amongst older people: Where is the evidence? *Ageing and Society, 23*(5), 647-658. https://doi.org/10.1017/s0144686x03001296

Folstein, M. F., Folstein, S. E., & McHugh, P. R. (1975). "Mini-mental state." A practical method for grading the cognitive state of patients for the clinician. *Journal of Psychiatric Research, 12*(3), 189-198. https://doi.org/10.1016/0022-3956(75)90026-6

Fredriksen-Goldsen, K. I., Kim, H.-J., Bryan, A. E., Shiu, C., & Emlet, C. A. (2017). The cascading effects of marginalization and pathways of resilience in attaining good health among LGBT older adults. *The Gerontologist, 57*(Suppl. 1). https://doi.org/10.1093/geront/gnw170

Galante, J., Friedrich, C., Dawson, A. F., Modrego-Alarcón, M., Gebbing, P., Delgado-Suárez, I., … Jones, P. B. (2021). Mindfulness-based programmes for mental health promotion in adults in nonclinical settings: A systematic review and meta-analysis of randomised controlled trials. *PLOS Medicine, 18*(1). https://doi.org/10.1371/journal.pmed.1003481

Galderisi, S., Heinz, A., Kastrup, M., Beezhold, J., & Sartorius, N. (2015). Toward a new definition of mental health. *World Psychiatry, 14*(2), 231-233. https://doi.org/10.1002/wps.20231

Garcia, M. A., Homan, P. A., García, C., & Brown, T. H. (2020). The color of COVID-19: structural racism and the disproportionate impact of the pandemic on older Black and Latinx adults. *The Journals of Gerontology: Series B, 76*(3). https://doi.org/10.1093/geronb/gbaa114

Gardiner, C., Geldenhuys, G., & Gott, M. (2016). Interventions to reduce social isolation and loneliness among older people: an integrative review. *Health & Social Care in the Community, 26*(2), 147-157. https://doi.org/10.1111/hsc.12367

Gibb, H. (2018). Determinants of resilience for PEOPLE ageing in REMOTE places: A case study in northern Australia. *International Journal of Ageing and Later Life, 11*(2), 9-33. https://doi.org/10.3384/ijal.1652-8670.17-333

Gold, C., Eickholt, J., Assmus, J., Stige, B., Wake, J. D., Baker, F. A., … Geretsegger, M. (2019). Music Interventions for Dementia and Depression in Elderly care (MIDDEL): Protocol and statistical analysis plan for a multinational cluster-randomised trial. *BMJ Open, 9*(3). https://doi.org/10.1136/bmjopen-2018-023436

Goldberg, D., Bridges, K., Duncan-Jones, P., & Grayson, D. (1988). Detecting anxiety and depression in general medical settings. BMJ (Clinical research ed.), 297(6653), 897-899. https://doi.org/10.1136/bmj.297.6653.897

Hamilton, M. (1960). A rating scale for depression. *Journal of Neurology, Neurosurgery, and Psychiatry, 23*(1), 56-62. https://doi.org/10.1136/jnnp.23.1.56

Hardy, S. E., Concato, J., & Gill, T. M. (2004). Resilience of community-dwelling older persons. *Journal of the American Geriatrics Society, 52*(2), 257-262. https://doi.org/10.1111/j.1532-5415.2004.52065.x

Harper, A. & Power, M. (1998) Development of the World Health Organization WHOQOL-BREF Quality of Life *Assessment. Psychological Medicine, 28*(3), 551-558. https://doi.org/10.1017/s0033291798006667

Healthy People 2030. (n.d.). https://health.gov/healthypeople

Holt-Lunstad, J. (2018). Why social relationships are important for physical health: A systems approach to understanding and modifying risk and protection. *Annual Review of Psychology, 69*(1), 437-458. https://doi.org/10.1146/annurev-psych-122216-011902

Holt-Lunstad, J., Robles, T. F., & Sbarra, D. A. (2017). Advancing social connection as a public health priority in the United States. *American Psychologist, 72*(6), 517-530. https://doi.org/10.1037/amp0000103

Huang, T.-T., Liu, C.-B., Tsai, Y.-H., Chin, Y.-F., & Wong, C.-H. (2015). Physical fitness exercise versus cognitive behavior therapy on reducing the depressive symptoms among community-dwelling elderly adults: A randomized controlled trial. *International Journal of Nursing Studies, 52*(10), 1542-1552. https://doi.org/10.1016/j.ijnurstu.2015.05.013

Institute of Medicine. (2014). *Capturing social and behavioral domains and measures in electronic health records: Phase 2*. The National Academies Press. https://doi.org/10.17226/18951

Institute on Aging (2020, December 4) Top geriatric counseling services & in-home therapy for seniors in SF. https://www.ioaging.org/services/all-inclusive-health-care/psychological-services

Interprofessional Education Collaborative. (2016). *Core competencies for interprofessional collaborative practice: 2016 update*. Interprofessional Education Collaborative.

Jiang, J. M., Seng, E. K., Zimmerman, M. E., Sliwinski, M., Kim, M., & Lipton, R. B. (2017). Evaluation of the reliability, validity, and predictive validity of the subscales of the perceived stress scale in older adults. *Journal of Alzheimer's Disease, 59*(3), 987-996. https://doi.org/10.3233/JAD-170289

Kabat-Zinn, J., Lipworth, L., & Burney, R. (1985). The clinical use of mindfulness meditation for the self-regulation of chronic pain. *Journal of Behavioral Medicine, 8*(2), 163-190.

Kamalpour, M., Rezaei Aghdam, A., Watson, J., Tariq, A., Buys, L., Eden, R., & Rehan, S. (2021). Online health communities, contributions to caregivers and resilience of older adults. *Health & Social Care in the Community, 29*(2), 328-343. https://doi.org/10.1111/hsc.13247

Kassel, J. D., Stroud, L. R., & Paronis, C. A. (2003). Smoking, stress, and negative affect: Correlation, causation, and context across stages of smoking. *Psychological Bulletin, 129*(2), 270-304. https://doi.org/10.1037/0033-2909.129.2.270

Kim, H.-J., Fredriksen-Goldsen, K. I., Bryan, A. E., & Muraco, A. (2017). Social network types and mental health among LGBT older adults. *The Gerontologist, 57*(Suppl. 1). https://doi.org/10.1093/geront/gnw169

Kovacevic, A., Fenesi, B., Paolucci, E., & Heisz, J. J. (2020). The effects of aerobic exercise intensity on memory in older adults. *Applied Physiology, Nutrition, and Metabolism, 45*(6), 591-600. https://doi.org/10.1139/apnm-2019-0495

Kroenke, K., Spitzer, R. L., & Williams, J. B. (2003). The Patient Health Questionnaire-2. *Medical Care, 41*(11), 1284-1292.

Lambert, J. D., Greaves, C. J., Farrand, P., Price, L., Haase, A. M., & Taylor, A. H. (2018). Web based intervention using behavioral activation and physical activity for adults with depression (The eMotion Study): Pilot randomized controlled trial. *Journal of Medical Internet Research, 20*(7), e10112. https://doi.org/10.2196/10112

Leavell, M.A., Leiferman, J.A., Gascon, M., et al. (2019). Nature-based social prescribing in urban settings to improve social connectedness and mental well-being: A review. *Current Environmental Health Reports, 6*, 297-308. https://doi.org/10.1007/s40572-019-00251-7

Lee, K., Jeong, G. C., & Yim, J. (2020). Consideration of the psychological and mental health of the elderly during COVID-19: A theoretical review. *International Journal of Environmental Research and Public Health, 17*(21), 8098. https://doi.org/10.3390/ijerph17218098

Lee, R. M., & Robbins, S. B. (1995). Measuring belongingness: The social connectedness and the social assurance scales. *Journal of Counseling Psychology, 42*(2), 232-241. https://doi.org/10.1037/0022-0167.42.2.232

Liu, X., Clark, J., Siskind, D., Williams, G. M., Byrne, G., Yang, J. L., & Doi, S. A. (2015). A systematic review and meta-analysis of the effects of Qigong and Tai Chi for depressive symptoms. *Complementary Therapies in Medicine, 23*(4), 516-534. https://doi.org/10.1016/j.ctim.2015.05.001

Lowe, P. A., & Reynolds, C. R. (2006). Examination of the psychometric properties of the Adult Manifest Anxiety Scale-Elderly Version scores. *Educational and Psychological Measurement, 66*(1), 93-115. https://doi.org/10.1177/0013164405278563

Lubben, J. E. (1988). Assessing social networks among elderly populations. *Family & Community Health, 11*(3), 42-52. https://doi.org/10.1097/00003727-198811000-00008

Luo, M. S., Chui, E. W. T., & Li, L. W. (2020). The Longitudinal Associations between Physical Health and Mental Health among Older Adults. *Aging & mental health, 24*(12), 1990–1998. https://doi.org/10.1080/13607863.2019.1655706

Mammen, G., & Faulkner, G. (2013). Physical activity and the prevention of depression. *American Journal of Preventive Medicine, 45*(5), 649-657. https://doi.org/10.1016/j.amepre.2013.08.001

Madsen, W., Ambrens, M., & Ohl, M. (2019). Enhancing resilience in community-dwelling older adults: A rapid review of the evidence and implications for public health practitioners. *Frontiers in Public Health, 7*, 14. https://doi.org/10.3389/fpubh.2019.00014

Meyer, I. H. (1995). Minority stress and mental health in gay men. *Journal of Health and Social Behavior, 36*(1), 38-56. https://doi.org/10.2307/2137286

Meyer, T. J., Miller, M. L., Metzger, R. L., & Borkovec, T. D. (1990). Development and validation of the Penn State Worry Questionnaire. *Behaviour Research and Therapy, 28*(6), 487-495. https://doi.org/10.1016/0005-7967(90)90135-6

Nagamatsu, L. S., Handy, T. C., Hsu, C. L., Voss, M., & Liu-Ambrose, T. (2012). Resistance training promotes cognitive functioning brain plasticity in seniors with mild cognitive impairment. *Archives of Internal Medicine, 172*, 666-668. https://doi.org/10.1001/archinternmed.2012.379

Nasreddine, Z. S., Phillips, N. A., Bédirian V., Charbonneau, S., Whitehead, V., Collin, I., ... Chertkow, H. (2005). The Montreal Cognitive Assessment, MoCA: A brief screening tool for mild cognitive impairment. *Journal of the American Geriatrics Society, 53*(4), 695–699. https://doi.org/10.1111/j.1532-5415.2005.53221.x

National Academies of Sciences, Engineering and Medicine (2020). *Social isolation and loneliness in older adults: Opportunities for the health care system*. The National Academies Press. https://doi.org/10.17226/25663

National Council on Aging. (2021). Center for Healthy Aging Evidence-Based Programs. https://www.ncoa.org/article/evidence-based-program-healthy-steps-in-motion

National Resource Center on LGBT Aging. (2020). Inclusive services for LGBT older adults: A practical guide to creating welcoming agencies. https://www.lgbtagingcenter.org/resources/pdfs/Sage_GuidebookFINAL1.pdf

Ohrnberger, J., Fichera, E., & Sutton, M. (2017). The dynamics of physical and mental health in the older population. *The Journal of the Economics of Ageing, 9*, 52-62. https://doi.org/10.1016/j.jeoa.2016.07.002

Pachana, N. A., Byrne, G. J., Siddle, H., Koloski, N., Harley, E., & Arnold, E. (2007). Development and validation of the Geriatric Anxiety Inventory. *International Psychogeriatrics, 19*(1), 103. https://doi.org/10.1017/s1041610206003504

Patel, N. K., Newstead, A. H., & Ferrer, R. L. (2012). The effects of yoga on physical functioning and health related quality of life in older adults: a systematic review and meta-analysis. *Journal of Alternative and Complementary Medicine (New York, N.Y.), 18*(10), 902-917. https://doi.org/10.1089/acm.2011.0473

Perissinotto, C. M., Stijacic Cenzer, I., & Covinsky, K. E. (2012). Loneliness in older persons. *Archives of Internal Medicine, 172*(14). https://doi.org/10.1001/archinternmed.2012.1993

PROMIS. (n.d.). http://www.nihpromis.org/

Russell, D. W. (1996). UCLA Loneliness Scale (Version 3): Reliability, validity, and factor structure. *Journal of Personality Assessment, 66*(1), 20-40. https://doi.org/10.1207/s15327752jpa6601_2

SAGEnyc.org. (n.d.a). SAGE NYC. https://sagenyc.org/nyc/

SAGEnyc.org. (n.d.b). SAGE NYC. https://sagenyc.org/nyc/care/visitor.cfm

Sardella, A., Lenzo, V., Bonanno, G. A., Basile, G., & Quattropani, M. C. (2021). Expressive flexibility and dispositional optimism contribute to the elderly's resilience and health-related quality of life during the COVID-19 pandemic. *International Journal of Environmental Research and Public Health, 18*(4), 1698. https://doi.org/10.3390/ijerph18041698

Schwartz, S. K., Morris, R. D., & Penna, S. (2019). Psychometric properties of the Saint Louis University Mental Status Examination. *Applied Neuropsychology: Adult, 26*(2), 101-110. https://doi-org.ezproxy.cul.columbia.edu/10.1080/23279095.2017.1362407

Segal, D. L., June, A., Payne, M., Coolidge, F. L., & Yochim, B. (2010). Development and initial validation of a self-report assessment tool for anxiety among older adults: The Geriatric Anxiety Scale. *Journal of Anxiety Disorders, 24*, 709-714.

Senior Planet. (2021, August 25). Welcome to senior planet. https://seniorplanet.org/

Shubert, T. E., Chokshi, A., Mendes, V. M., Grier, S., Buchanan, H., Basnett, J., & Smith, M. L. (2018). Stand tall—A virtual translation of the otago exercise program. *Journal of Geriatric Physical Therapy, 43*(3), 120-127. https://doi.org/10.1519/jpt.0000000000000203

Sinclair, V. G., & Wallston, K. A. (2004). The development and psychometric evaluation of the Brief Resilient Coping Scale. *Assessment, 11*(1), 94-101 https://doi.org/10.1177/1073191103258144

Singh, N. A., Clements, K. M., & Singh, M. A. (2001). The efficacy of exercise as a long-term antidepressant in elderly subjects: A randomized, controlled trial. *Journal of Gerontology: Medical Sciences, 56A*, M497-M504. https://doi.org/10.1093/gerona/56.8.M497

Smith, P. J., Blumenthal, J. A., Hoffman, B. M., Cooper, H., Strauman, T. A., Welsh-Bohmer, K., ... Sherwood, A. (2010). Aerobic exercise and neurocognitive performance: A Meta-Analytic Review Of Randomized Controlled Trials. *Psychosomatic Medicine, 72*(3), 239-252. https://doi.org/10.1097/psy.0b013e3181d14633

Smith, S. C., Lamping, D. L., Banerjee, S., Harwood, R., Foley, B., Smith, P., ... Knapp, M. (2006). Development of a new measure of health-related quality of life for people with dementia: DEMQOL. *Psychological Medicine, 37*(05), 737. https://doi.org/10.1017/s0033291706009469

Sofi, F., Valecchi, D., Bacci, D., Abbate, R., Gensini, G. F., Casini, A., & Macchi, C. (2011). Physical activity and risk of cognitive decline: a meta-analysis of prospective studies. *Journal of Internal Medicine, 269*(1), 107-117. https://doi.org/10.1111/j.1365-2796.2010.02281.x

Sundsli, K., Söderhamn, U., Espnes, G. A., & Söderhamn, O. (2014). Self-care telephone talks as a health promotion intervention in urban home-living persons 75+ years of age: A randomized controlled study. *Clinical Interventions in Aging, 95*. https://doi.org/10.2147/cia.s55925

Tariq, S. H., Tumosa, N., Chibnall, J. T., Perry, M. H., 3rd, & Morley, J. E. (2006). Comparison of the Saint Louis University mental status examination and the Mini-Mental State Examination for detecting dementia and mild neurocognitive disorder—A pilot study. *The American Journal of Geriatric Psychiatry, 14*(11), 900-910. https://doi.org/10.1097/01.JGP.0000221510.33817.86

Tennant, R., Hiller, L., Fishwick, R., Platt, S., Joseph, S., Weich, S., ... Stewart-Brown, S. (2007). The Warwick-Edinburgh Mental Well-being Scale (WEMWBS): Development and UK validation. *Health and Quality of Life Outcomes, 5*(1), 63. https://doi.org/10.1186/1477-7525-5-63

U.S. Department of Health and Human Services. (n.d.). Social isolation, loneliness in older people pose health risks. National Institute on Aging. https://www.nia.nih.gov/news/social-isolation-loneliness-older-people-pose-health-risks.

Velez, B. L., Moradi, B., & Brewster, M. E. (2013). Testing the tenets of minority stress theory in workplace contexts. *Journal of Counseling Psychology, 60*(4), 532-542. https://doi.org/10.1037/a0033346

Vieweg, B. W., & Hedlund, J. L. (1983). The General Health Questionnaire (GHQ): A comprehensive review. *Journal of Operational Psychiatry, 14*(2), 74-81.

Wagnild, G., & Young, H. (1993). Development and psychometric evaluation of the Resilience Scale. *Journal of Nursing Measurement, 1*(2), 165-178.

Wallace, S., Nazroo, J., & Bécares, L. (2016). Cumulative effect of racial discrimination on the mental health of ethnic minorities in the United Kingdom. *American Journal of Public Health, 106*(7), 1294-1300. https://doi.org/10.2105/AJPH.2016.303121

Wang, F., Lee, E.-K. O., Wu, T., Benson, H., Fricchione, G., Wang, W., & Yeung, A. S. (2013). The Effects of Tai Chi on depression, anxiety, and psychological well-being: A systematic review and meta-analysis. *International Journal of Behavioral Medicine, 21*(4), 605-617. https://doi.org/10.1007/s12529-013-9351-9

Whitehead, B. R. (2020). COVID-19 as a stressor: Pandemic expectations, perceived stress, and negative affect in older adults. *The Journals of Gerontology: Series B, 76*(2). https://doi.org/10.1093/geronb/gbaa153

Whitty, E., Mansour, H., Aguirre, E., Palomo, M., Charlesworth, G., Ramjee, S., … Cooper, C. (2020). Efficacy of lifestyle and psychosocial interventions in reducing cognitive decline in older people: Systematic review. *Ageing Research Reviews, 62*, 101113. https://doi.org/10.1016/j.arr.2020.101113

Williams, D. R. (2018). Stress and the mental health of populations of color: Advancing our understanding of race-related stressors. *Journal of Health and Social Behavior, 59*(4), 466-485. https://doi.org/10.1177/0022146518814251

Wister, A. V., Coatta, K. L., Schuurman, N., Lear, S. A., Rosin, M., & MacKey, D. (2016). A lifecourse model of multimorbidity resilience: Theoretical and research developments. *The International Journal of Aging and Human Development, 82*(4), 290-313. https://doi.org/10.1177/0091415016641686

Wong, S. Y., Zhang, D., Sit, R. W., Yip, B. H., Chung, R. Y.-nork, Wong, C. K., … Mercer, S. W. (2020). Impact of COVID-19 on loneliness, mental health, and health service utilisation: a prospective cohort study of older adults with multimorbidity in primary care. *British Journal of General Practice, 70*(700). https://doi.org/10.3399/bjgp20x713021

World Health Organization. (n.d.a). Special initiative for mental health (2019-2023)—Universal health coverage for mental health. https://www.who.int/publications-detail-redirect/WHO-MSD-19.1

World Health Organization. (n.d.b). Ageism is a global challenge: UN. https://www.who.int/news/item/18-03-2021-ageism-is-a-global-challenge-un

World Health Organization. (2017). Mental health of older adults. World Health Organization. https://www.who.int/news-room/fact-sheets/detail/mental-health-of-older-adults

World Health Organization. (2021). New advocacy brief highlights serious consequences of social isolation and loneliness on the health of older people, calls for greater political priority to the issue. https://www.who.int/news/item/29-07-2021-new-advocacy-brief-highlights-serious-consequences-of-social-isolation-and-loneliness-on-the-health-of-older-people-calls-for-greater-political-priority-to-the-issue

Xu, B., Sui, Y., Zhu, C., Yang, X., Zhou, J., Li, L., … Wang, X. (2017). Music intervention on cognitive dysfunction in healthy older adults: A systematic review and meta-analysis. *Neurological Sciences, 38*(6), 983-992. https://doi.org/10.1007/s10072-017-2878-9

Yesavage, J. A., Brink, T. L., Rose, T. L., Lum, O., Huang, V., Adey, M., & Leirer, V. O. (1982). Development and validation of a geriatric depression screening scale: A preliminary report. *Journal of Psychiatric Research, 17*(1), 37-49. https://doi.org/10.1016/0022-3956(82)90033-4

Yohannes, A. M., & Caton, S. (2010). Management of depression in older people with osteoarthritis: A systematic review. *Aging & Mental Health, 14*(6), 637-651. https://doi.org/10.1080/13607860903483094

Zimet, G. D., Dahlem, N. W., Zimet, S. G., & Farley, G. K. (1988). The multidimensional scale of perceived social support. *Journal of Personality Assessment, 52*(1), 30-41. https://doi.org/10.1207/s15327752jpa5201_2

Zung, W. (1965). A self-rating depression scale. *Archives of General Psychiatry, 12*(1), 63. https://doi.org/10.1001/archpsyc.1965.01720310065008

PART VI

PROMOTING FAMILY HEALTH

16

CHAPTER

Promoting Family Health
Children and Youth

Kelle DeBoth Foust, PhD, OTR/L;
Madalynn Wendland, PT, DPT, ATP, Board-Certified Pediatric Clinical Specialist;
and John M. Schaefer, PhD, BCBA-D

Learning Objectives

At the end of this chapter, the reader will:

1. Understand the family culture in promoting health well-being for children and youth Understand the family culture in promoting health well-being for children and youth (ACOTE B.1.2, B.4.4, B.4.5; CAPTE 7D10, 7D11, 7D34; CEC 1.2)
2. Describing the reciprocal relationships within family networks that promote health (ACOTE B.4.23, CAPTE 7D8; CEC 2.2)
3. Identify barriers and facilitators for optimal participation and engagement in the community setting (ACOTE B.4.14, B.4.27; CAPTE D19, 7D31, 7D37; CEC 7.3)
4. Distinguish the roles and responsibilities among members of an interprofessional team (ACOTE B.4.23, B.4.25; CAPTE 7D7, 7D39; CEC 7.2)
5. To describe how Family Systems Theory applies to promoting health and well-being for families, and family needs for interprofessional assessment, intervention, and community support (ACOTE B.4.23; CAPTE 7D10, 7D16; CEC 2.2)
6. To apply theoretical, interprofessional intervention approaches for each family member (ACOTE B.4.23; CAPTE 7D19, 7D27, 7D34, 7D37)
7. To analyze the contributions of the interprofessional team on an individual, family, community, and policy/advocacy level (ACOTE B.4.23, B.4.25; PT 7D7, 7D14)

The ACOTE Standards used are those from 2018.

Pizzi, M. A., & Amir, M. (Eds.). *Interprofessional Perspectives for Community Practice: Promoting Health, Well-Being, and Quality of Life* (pp. 305-326).

Key Words

Family Systems Theory, Health Literacy, Inputs, Learned Helplessness, Least Restrictive Environment, Mental Health, Outputs, Passive Dependency, Resilience or Resiliency, Shared Decision-Making

The network of parents, caregivers, siblings, and other extended relatives or community members that constitute a child's "family" as the family defines and recognizes it has a significant impact on participation and overall health and well-being. Children's health, quality of life (QOL), and opportunities for meaningful occupational engagement are shaped by the perceptions, attitudes, and health of their caregivers and family. From habits and routines within the home setting, cultural and spiritual practices, available resources, collective physical, mental, and social health all have a reciprocal influence on family members' overall health.

Families that have children with disabilities often face greater barriers to participation, achieving health and wellness, and have a poorer QOL. Participation in a fulfilling home life, establishing meaningful relationships, and finding joy and meaning in shared experiences and activities in and outside of the home can be more challenging. Families that have a child with a disability often do not feel the same sense of belonging in different settings and environments that may not appear to welcome or be designed for children of varying levels of abilities, limiting perceived opportunities. Therefore, caregivers' perceptions about how and where the family is able to meaningfully engage in the community has a direct effect on their children's participation (Huang et al., 2018; Schaaf et al., 2011; Bar et al., 2016; Pfeiffer et al., 2017; Fletcher et al., 2019). Similarly, children with disabilities often have limited social interactions, relationships, and others available to engage in play with outside of their immediate family (Solish et al., 2010; Taheri et al., 2016). This limits social participation for both children and the adults within the family unit. One of the most important qualities for caregivers and children who have a disability is resilience. Caregivers are found to be more resilient when they understand and have knowledge about their child's condition, who find joy and fulfillment in their roles and have adequate social supports (Sagester & Mazzarella, 2020; Suzuki et al., 2015). Resilience often depends on family members' ability to cope with stressors and negative events and resilience also builds positive mental health traits (Marshall et al., 2003; Suzuki et al., 2015). Therefore, it is unsurprising that caregivers and families, especially those who face disability limitations, desire community spaces that support meaningful engagement between family members (DeBoth et al., 2021), and can help build resilience.

Family participation in activities and occupations occur across multiple settings—home, school, and in the community. In addition, families make points of contact with a variety of different health care professionals in each of these different settings. The interprofessional team of experts and service providers have a critical role in supporting not just the health of the child, but the QOL and well-being of the entire family. This chapter will explore ways to assess family health, different interprofessional approaches to intervention, and describe successful examples of community programs that are designed by interprofessional teams to support family community engagement (Case Study Box A).

Reflective Questions

1. What are family characteristics that contribute positively or negatively to well-being and QOL?
2. What are barriers families face to optimal participation and engagement in desired activities and occupations?
3. How can an interprofessional team best serve the needs of children with disabilities and their families?

Introduction

A Biopsychosocial Model of Disability

The World Health Organization (WHO) embraces a biopsychosocial model of disability that can be used to understand interactions between a child with a disability, their family, and how the personal factors of each of these unique individuals interact with the environment, either supporting or hindering participation in activities that are integral to overall health and wellness (WHO, 2007). The International Classification of Functioning, Disability and Health (ICF) uses this model to provide a standard language for describing health, including both social and medical models that incorporate biological, individual, and social perspectives. For a child with a disability, the ICF model considers dysfunction at the level of impairment (body), activity limitations (whole person), and participation restrictions (the whole person in a social context). One of the most important contexts for a child is that of the family, and therefore how a disability can influence activities and participation (Figure 16-1).

Other contextual factors that affect family health outcomes, including how people work, play and live, are considered the social determinants of health (SDOH). The five key areas include education, social and community context, health and health care, neighborhood and built environment, and economic stability (Figure 16-2, CDC, n.d.). Each

Case Study Box A

The Smith family includes a White mother and Black father, who have been married for 17 years. They have three children—Steven, 15 years of age, Adam, 13 years of age, and Susan, 11 years of age. Steven has a diagnosis of autism spectrum disorder, and presents with hypotonia, motor incoordination, dyspraxia, mild fine motor deficits, moderate sensory processing differences, poor visual perception, impaired handwriting skills, and a significant learning disability. On his most recent Evaluation Team Report (ETR) from his school district, he scored in the "Very Low" range for all subtests of the Beery-Buktenica Developmental Test of Visual Motor Integration (VMI), Sixth Edition, in the "Well Below Average" range for all sections of the Bruininks-Oseretsky Test of Motor Proficiency, Second Edition (BOT-2), and in the "Very Low" range (age equivalent <11 years, 0 months) on the Motor-Free Visual Perception Test – Third Edition (MVPT-3). Clinical observation and assessment of handwriting skills were also completed, finding significant difficulties with independent written expression, poor motor planning, and sensory processing, below average grip strength, and difficulties completing activities of daily living independently. Steven needs supports and supervision, at minimum given cues for organizing and completing tasks as well as safety, for all tasks within his primary performance settings. Steven has been homeschooled by his mother since kindergarten, and his primary social interactions are with family and the therapists he works with in a private outpatient clinic. He participates in a pragmatic language social group with other peers of a similar age, but has yet to establish long-term, meaningful friendships and demonstrates anxiety when interacting with new people. Steven receives weekly occupational therapy and speech therapy in addition to the social language group, and a child psychologist works with him and his family on a monthly basis.

Adam has a diagnosis of autism spectrum disorder, is nonverbal, has a mitochondrial disorder that results in significant fatigue, he has a history of seizures, and presents with significant maladaptive behaviors that interfere with participation across activity domains. He uses an augmentative communication device to communicate his basic wants and needs, primarily tangible or food items he desires. Adam also has a history of significant self-stimulating and self-injurious behaviors that interfere with his ability to engage in purposeful activities across settings. Adam has a very low IQ and cognitive capacity and is unable to participate in most standardized assessments. The Pediatric Evaluation of Disability Inventory (PEDI), although standardized up to age 7.5 years of age is appropriate for older children with more significant impairments, suggest that Adam functions in the "Well Below Average" range for functional skills (self-care, mobility, social function) and caregiver assistance (self-care, mobility, social function). Adam engages socially with familiar adults and family members. He does not engage regularly with other children outside his home and is also homeschooled. He has limited leisure interests, and due to fatigue often needs wheelchair assistance to get from one place to another. Adam receives weekly occupational therapy, speech therapy, and physical therapy, and also consults regularly with a behavior specialist to help manage his behaviors and his educational curriculum at home. The neurologist who manages his seizure medications also works in the outpatient clinic and sees Adam every other month.

Susan currently attends a private, Catholic school getting mostly Bs, and her primary extracurricular activity is taking piano lessons. She attempts to help out at home with her brothers, and often spends her afternoons at the private outpatient clinic where they receive many of their services.

Mr. Smith is an accountant and works for a local firm. He is 44 years old, spends evenings and weekends with his family, and since he was born in another state, he does not have other family members that live nearby. Mr. Smith has a few casual acquaintances from work but does not feel he has time to engage with them outside of the office. Mrs. Smith homeschools her two sons and has not worked outside the home since Steven was born. Her mother lives nearby and often comes to help and spend time with the children in the evenings and on the weekends. The Smith family lives in a large home in the suburbs, and they regularly attend a nearby Christian church where they enjoy support from the community. The Smiths attempt to venture out into the community, such as going to nearby parks, downtown museums, and special events of interest when they are able. Often they have to bring a wheelchair for Adam, and their outings are frequently rescheduled due to behavior problems, medical issues, or when Adam is too fatigued.

of these have implications for assessment, intervention, and forming collaborative interprofessional health care teams. To begin applying the ICF and SDOH frameworks to family health, it is important to first understand the composition of the family.

Family Systems Theory

When a team seeks to make decisions about a child's treatment, families should be a central part of the decision-making process. Incorporating families in decision making today requires a broad conception of how families are structured and how members of the family interact with each other and with the team (Rothbaum et al., 2002; Turnbull et al., 2015).

Bowen's **Family Systems Theory** (Bowen, 1966, 1978) challenges the traditional view of the narrowly defined nuclear family of two opposite-sex biological parents adhering to strict gender roles, married, and raising one to four children in the same house. Instead, Family System Theory allows for the membership of a family to be more varied and flexible and emphasizes the importance of the relationship of members to each other and to the whole unit (Rothbaum et al., 2002; Turnbull et al., 2015). Teams today should not

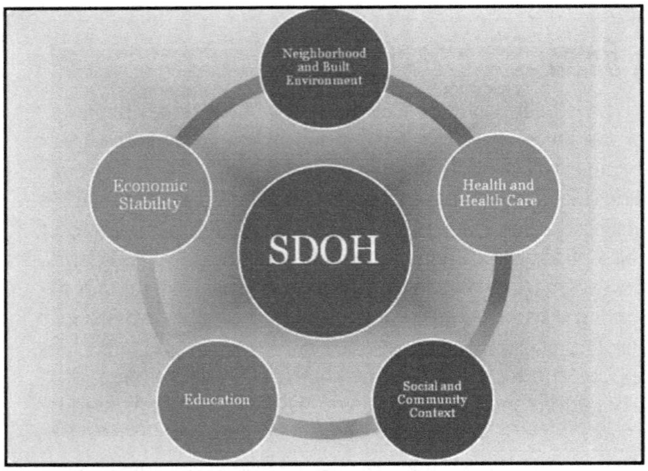

Figure 16-1. SDOH. (Reproduced with permission from Healthy People 2020. [n.d.]. https://www.healthypeople.gov/2020/topics-objectives/topic/social-determinants-of-health)

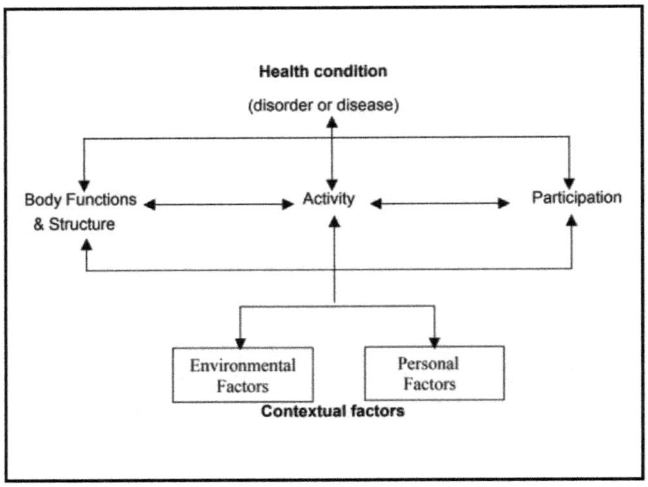

Figure 16-2. Five Key Areas. (Reproduced with permission from the World Health Organization. [2001]. International Classification of Functioning, Disability and Health. http://apps.who.int/iris/bitstream/10665/43737/1/9789241547321_eng.pdf)

expect to always be working directly with a biological mother who does not work outside the home only. That is one possible description of a caregiver or significant other that may be involved in decision making on behalf of a child in need of intervention. However, teams often may be working with multiple caregivers supporting a single child, including but not limited to extended family members and siblings acting as caregivers or guardians appointed by the state. All of these parties may have an important role in decision making.

Family System Theory describes the relation of the range of possible caregivers to the child the team is working with in terms of their role in the child's life. For example, Adam Smith lives with Mr. and Mrs. Smith, Adam's parents. At home Adam is regularly also supported by Steven and Susan who have a sibling relationship with Adam and also a parental relationship with Mr. and Mrs. Smith, and Adam's grandmother who frequently interacts with the family. Everyone in the house regularly engages Adam in play, leisure, and other activities of daily living. The first task of a collaborative team working with a new child is to get to know who are the key members of the family unit that will be supporting the child's engagement with therapy and be part of the decision-making process.

Once a team determines which key family members are involved in the decision-making process, it is necessary to understand what is impacting that family and how the family is impacting the child. All family units are impacted by what Family Systems Theory calls **inputs** that are factors that shape how the family interacts with others and the outside world. Some inputs are from individuals, for example, a strongly held religious belief by a family leader like a parent, might encourage the whole family unit to engage more in a faith community. Other inputs are external to the family and may offer unique challenges, such as poverty, incarceration, and so on. One input discussed in Family System Theory literature is particularly relevant here; exceptionality status of the family members can have a large impact on the whole unit. For example, if a family member has a physical disability, it can impact everything from the configuration of the home to the modes of transport available. If a family member has a cognitive impairment or developmental disability, it can impact educational choices and future outcomes like independent living and employment. Regardless, having at least one family member with an exceptionality tends to place additional demands on the family unit financial, logistically, and emotionally and tends to shape how all members of the unit interact.

On the opposite side of Family Systems Theory, all families also have **outputs**, or the specific products of the family unit interaction. For example, families often provide financial and emotional support to their children. Families often teach norms, self-concept, and perceptions of the dominant culture outside of the family. These outputs do not need to be generalized across all family members, and in fact, it is often not (Rothbaum et al., 2002; Turnbull et al., 2015). In the example of the family with a religiously observant parental figure, the input reflects what the family unit does as a group (i.e., attend religious services regularly) together, but the output can be individualized to each member. One child might independently engage and adhere to the parent's beliefs while another might react differently and move away from their parent's beliefs intentionally (Case Study Box B).

The last key element to Family Systems Theory that might be relevant to collaborating with a team, is called the "family life cycle." This idea holds that the membership of a family and the relationships of the members to each other change over time as members get added and removed (e.g., birth, marriage, death, estrangement) and as the family goes through predictable stages (e.g., centering around young children, centering around caring for elderly members). Teams should be open to and responsive to these changes in family structure.

A team adopting this broader view of how families operate and relate to each other is essential for family

Case Study Box B

QUESTION: CULTURAL INFLUENCES

How do you think the inputs and outputs of the Smith family's religious affiliation affects each of the family members? How would an interprofessional team of health care providers incorporate this into their overall approach?

Case Study Box C

QUESTION: CONSIDER FAMILY STRUCTURE

Consider how an interprofessional team of service providers may differ in composition and approach if the Smith family were Hispanic? Asian? If English was not their first language? How else might you reconsider the efforts of the interprofessional team if Steven Smith was homosexual? Or if Mrs. Smith was transgender? Identify additional services and resources that might be necessary to address any additional challenges or barriers posed by these familial factors.

decision-making process in areas such as prioritizing intervention, supports to offer, or long-term goals to target, which are impacted by family dynamics, culture, and beliefs. For example, for younger children transitioning into schools, families should be closely involved in the decision of how much their child will be included in general education environments and what supports are needed to be successful in those environments. For older children beginning to transition to adulthood, families should be deeply involved in how the team prepares the individual to live more independently. Some caretakers come from cultural backgrounds that often prioritize caring for adults with intellectual disability in the family home and stigmatizes paying for supported independent living. Other families have a strongly held belief that individuals with intellectual disabilities should be encouraged to live as independently as possible. Both of those attitudes might exist in the same family between parents, or between a parent of their other adult children who will one day be responsible for supporting the decision making of the individual with disabilities. Family System Theory does not indicate which voice is the most important in any scenario, it simply argues that there are multiple voices that teams need to be aware exist.

Although the case study presented in this chapter is one that is reflective of a more "traditional" family model, with married parents raising their own children in a middle class, suburban neighborhood, it is necessary to mention that this is not representative of all family dynamics or stressors that may exacerbate challenges managing disabilities within families. Grandparents, foster parents, or other relatives may assume primary caregiving responsibilities for a child with a disability. Those caregivers may be married, divorced, widowed, or of sexual orientation/gender identification other than heterosexual and binary. Considering these differences in addition to cultural, religious, ethnic, or other inherent family differences require that practitioners gain a holistic picture of the family unit, those who have influence and interactions with the family across settings, and consider these unique traits within the scope of addressing family health from an interprofessional perspective (Case Study Box C).

PASSIVE DEPENDENCY AND RESILIENCY

There are certain inputs and outputs of the family systems that can either hinder or support family functioning. Two such interrelated concepts this chapter will focus on are **passive dependency** and **resiliency**. Passive dependency, or what may have been more commonly referred to as learned helplessness, is common among families that have children with disabilities. Learned helplessness as described by Maier and Seligman (1976) suggests that when people encounter aversive stimuli, they may be conditioned to feel that those encounters are inescapable and therefore instead of attempting to escape, they essentially submit or give up. Historically, this term was used to describe children with mental retardation (currently known as intellectual disability) and is found to be a predictor of psychological disorders, in particular, depression (Reynolds & Miller, 1985; Weisz, 2013). More recently, studies have examined the notion of learned helplessness in relationship with perceived successes and self-efficacy (Filippello et al., 2015). If caregivers or other well-intended family members continuously do more than is necessary for a person with a disability to avoid learned helplessness and prevent their child from repetitive exposure to aversive stimuli, or failure, it limits the self-fulfillment of achievement (Mešl et al., 2012). This impairs the child's autonomy, decreases confidence in decision-making ability and feelings of self-worth, and deprives the individual of their ability self-determination, the drive for self-improvement thus dampening intrinsic motivation. As this concept has evolved, there is a current trend to refer to this idea as passive dependency. Competing medical and social models of disabilities suggest that parents may view their children as physically *limited* and restricted in activity participation, yet they may still be *able* to participate with the appropriate supports and accommodations which promotes a child well-being and overall QOL (Smith, 2013). Passive dependency suggests that children who learn to become dependent on their parents, caregivers, or others to fulfill their basic needs may not learn to be self-sufficient. While this may be rooted in protectionism over children that are more vulnerable, it also limits the ability of a child with a disability to have the same learning experiences necessary for achieving behavioral autonomy and independence (Cureton & Silvers, 2017). As described in the following sections, parent education is a critical component of the overall intervention process.

It is well documented that parents or caregivers of a child with a disability experience more stress than parents who do not have a child with a disability (Golfenshtein et al., 2016; Pastor-Cerezuela et al., 2021). The characteristics of the child and their diagnosis, in particular problem behaviors exhibited by the child, in addition to the level of understanding caregivers have about the disability, coping strategies and parenting supports are all key factors (Hsiao, 2018). Perceived barriers to participation and lack of reliable, robust social networks frequently pose significant challenges. In addition, caregivers of children with a disability have more internalizing factors such as depression and other negative psychological symptomatology that may be influenced by stigma, poor self-esteem, and lack of social supports (Cantwell et al., 2015; Papadopoulos et al., 2019). These family dynamics contribute to increased adversity, challenges, and barriers that families must adjust to, impacting overall QOL and well-being. How well families and individual family members cope with these challenges is often referred to as resiliency. *Resilience* (as a process) and *resiliency* (as a characteristic; Maurović et al., 2020) are concepts that have evolved with three components, or "waves": 1) individual qualities, assets, characteristics that help people overcome adversity; 2) reintegration of those characteristics and identification of assets that promote coping strategies over time; and 3) interprofessional creation of experiences and interventions for clients to help self-actualize such qualities (Richardson, 2002). Family resilience includes constructs of individual resilience as well as community resilience (Table 16-1).

Within this context, resilience is related to the exposure to risk and adversity, as well as how well a family can adjust to these conditions (Maurović et al., 2020), and how adaptive they are in a crisis situation. Resiliency is closely linked with parental stress (Pastor-Cerezuela et al., 2021), **mental health**, and QOL. The WHO defines mental health as "a state of well-being in which the individual realizes his or her own abilities, can cope with the normal stresses of life, can work productively and fruitfully, and is able to contribute to their community" (WHO, 2017). Having a child with a disability has a significant impact on the mental health of their caregivers (Whiting, 2014). Access to resources and socioeconomic status (SES) also have an impact on mental health, and the WHO considers SES to be a key modulator of both physical and mental health for families, suggesting a reciprocal relationship between poor mental health and social disparities (WHO, 2017). In fact, low levels of financial hardship and the accessibility of culturally relevant resources appear to significantly contribute to a family's overall resilience (McConnell et al., 2014; Case Study Box D).

Although the focus thus far has been on the impact of a child's disability on the family, it is also worth noting that the family structure can have significant impacts on the mental health of the child. When abuse, neglect, or trauma are present within the home, there is a significant increase in psychiatric hospitalization rates (Behere et al., 2017). Evaluating the unique intricacies of the familial context is important for understanding the relationships and prioritizing needs for family interventions.

Assessment

Three main areas need to be explored to promote family health: function, activity, and participation. Function here refers to internal factors, such as the impact of a child's health conditions on their physical abilities and impairments. However, when evaluating activity and participation, it is necessary to also consider external contextual variables related to the child's family's background, resources, and priorities. Understanding a family's norms, values, beliefs, and priorities for their child is essential to determining what activities are relevant and preferable. These factors also impact what level of participation expectation can contribute to a "just-right challenge" without settling unrealistic expectations and leading to frustration. Understanding more about a family's history and lived experience—especially in the context of their child's previous treatment—can help inform teams about how to best plan for success.

The interprofessional team assesses physical and cognitive demands of a child's activities and relative to their place in the family, after which they can start to make choices, in collaboration with the family, regarding activities that should be prioritized. Then the team evaluates to what degree the child engages with and participates in the activities during treatment sessions and with their family between treatment sessions. Most standardized participation measures look across environments and will capture what is happening at home, in the community, and in schools.

Activity participation needs to incorporate the child's preferences into the activities planned. This can be as simple as theming visual or auditory stimuli in the environment or providing manipulatives tailored to the child's interests. For example, if the goal is for the child to work on trunk stability while reaching across midline, reaching for a child's favorite toy can impact a child's motivation to participate or their tolerance for task demands.

Table 16-1

Proposed Indicators of Risk, Protective Factors, and Outcomes*

	RISK	PROTECTIVE FACTORS	GOOD OUTCOME
Individual level	• Vulnerability of the individual family member (traumatic events, illness, chronic exposure to negative social conditions, etc.)	• Intelligence • Capacity to identify and control emotions • Executive function • Established belief system (religious or other) • Self-efficacy & personal agency strategies • Problem-solving skills • Higher education or higher skill level • Easy temperament • Female sex • Positive views and strong sense of meaning in life • Spirituality	• Competency in achieving developmental tasks • Mental health • Subjective well-being
Family level	• Vulnerability of family (traumatic events, illness, chronic exposure to negative social conditions, etc.) • Family structure, size • Low socioeconomic status	• Family functioning (cohesion, flexibility, communication, problem solving, family roles, affective response, behavior control) • Family coherence • Family hardiness • Transcendence and spirituality • Stable and sufficient income • Appropriate housing	• Fulfilment of family functions (especially those that are threatened by the risk factors) • Satisfaction with family life • Gains from risk
Community level	• Community as source of risk • Vulnerability of the community (social injustice, high unemployment, vandalism, abandoned houses, run-down property, racial and ethnic conflicts, criminality, etc.)	• Informal support (friends and relatives) • Formal support (access to social services, quality educational and health system, etc.) • Social justice (equal opportunities) • Integreation in the community • Safe neighborhood • Opportunities for cultural and civic engagement • Strong community and cultural identity	• Social capital, social cohesion, social networking, collaboration

*Adjusted from Antonovsky & Sourani, 1988; Benzies & Mychasiuk, 2009; Khanlou & Wray, 2014; Liebenberg & Joubert, 2019; Masten & Coatsworth, 1998; Masten, 2001; Patterson, 2002b; Walsh, 2003; Openshaw, 2011; Oh & Chang, 2014.

Reproduced with permission from Maurović, I., Liebenberg, L., & Ferić, M. (2020). A review of family resilience: Understanding the concept and operationalization challenges to inform research and practice. *Child Care in Practice, 26*(4), 337-357.

Case Study Box D

QUESTIONS: RESILIENCY

The Smith family has many inter- and intrapersonal factors that make them vulnerable to increased risk exposure and stressors. Consider the following questions:

1. What are the primary stressors you perceive for each of the family members?
2. How could these stressors negatively impact well-being and QOL?
3. What familial factors exist that could potentially build resilience for the Smiths?

Although evaluation of the child is most frequently the focus of a team's assessment plan, it is also important to consider tools that can evaluate important aspects of the family including participation, QOL, resiliency, and health literacy. For example, the Activities Questionnaire (Solish et al., 2010) that includes background information about the child and parents grouped into several relevant subscales: Social Activities, Recreational Activities, Leisure Activities, and Friendship. The Family Resilience Assessment Scale accounts for factors of each family member (Gardiner et al., 2019; Sixbey, 2005). Resiliency is strongly related with QOL and is also linked with health literacy. Therefore, it is unsurprising that measures of these constructs are also often combined. Examples include the Parenting Resilience Elements and the Quality of Life Questionnaire (Widyawati et al., 2020), the Health Literacy and Resiliency Scale: Youth (HLRS-Y; Bradley-Klug et al., 2017), and the Construct of Resiliency in the Health Literacy and Resiliency Scale in combination with the Child and Youth Resiliency Measure (CYRM-28; Cambric, 2019). Historically, health literacy was considered a measure of oral literacy and reading comprehension. More recent definitions include contextual factors, how information is processed, comprehended, and utilized. Assessment tools that are more multifaceted and take into account interrelated constructs of health literacy are beginning to emerge (Altin et al., 2014). Countless tools exist that measure different aspects of health literacy, including objective, subjective, and mixed-measurement options. It is important to select an assessment tool that meets the team's need for evaluation while also considering cultural differences and composition of the family. For specific assessments addressing specific factors, please see Appendix A.

Interventions

Education

Parent, caregiver, or family education is an important component of the intervention process and is identified as one of the key SDOH areas. Parents and caregivers often experience grief and elevated levels of stress when receiving a child's diagnosis (Wayment & Brookshire, 2018). Health care practitioners can proactively support well-being by helping a family to understand the diagnosis and prognosis, identify resources, understand their rights and the rights of their children, and to recognize their potential feelings of loss. Psychoeducational intervention programs for caregivers have been found to be especially helpful giving parents' insights to their child's disability and identifying supports (Frantz et al., 2018) in addition to working on psychological acceptance of their child's condition (Weiss et al., 2012). Interprofessional teams are necessary to educate families on the medical diagnoses/conditions, comorbidities, and prognosis, and create intervention plans that address any and all areas of need. Expert practitioners can also refer families to support groups and help identify community resources and accessible spaces that can promote family engagement. Families may become overwhelmed attempting to coordinate these services on their own, highlighting the importance of a cohesive interprofessional team that helps bridge effective services.

Another important concept within client and family education is that of **shared decision making**. Shared decision making aligns with the biospsychosocial model putting clients holistically at the center of the health care team. This concept elucidates the idea that health care professionals should not make isolated, unilateral decisions for their clients. Instead, practitioners need to work together with the client and their family as the starting point for the decision-making process. This may require clients and their families to be educated in order to make the best, informed decisions about their health. Shared decision making can then be defined as the process by which clients reach an optimal decision (either at a health crossroads, or when multiple options are viable) where all involved team members share information and perspectives that help the client and their family guide the final decision and the plan to reach the agreed upon outcome (Barry & Edgman-Levitan, 2012). This approach should encourage education, conversation, respect for the client and family, and an equal partnership between all team members.

Case Study Box E

QUESTION: EDUCATION AND HEALTH LITERACY

Health literacy is an asset and skillset that is important for all members of a family. How might each member of the interprofessional team promote health literacy for the Smith family? In other words, what are important aspects of health literacy related to each field, and how can practitioners individually and jointly promote improved health literacy for this family?

Health Literacy

Related to education, health literacy can also impact a family's health and wellness. **Health literacy** is defined as "the degree to which individuals have the capacity to obtain, process, and understand basic health information and services needed to make appropriate health decisions" (Hernandez, 2009, p. 1; IOM, 2004) and is an important consideration for Healthy People 2030 (ODPHP, 2021). Health literacy, which may or may not be related to overall literacy, impacts the family's ability to make health-related decisions and is related to child outcomes as well as perceived barriers to health and well-being (Yin et al., 2012). Families need to be able to access information about their child's disability and health care options, but also be able to obtain and utilize information regarding family health such as identifying resources, health care providers, or other community opportunities that can improve QOL. In addition, it is important to consider how discrepant levels of health literacy between providers and family members create barriers to successful health management (Hollar & Rowland, 2015). Even well-informed interprofessional teams may not be well versed in identifying health literacy levels or trained in how to promote health literacy with their clients. Significant variability exists between health professional academic programs regarding the amount of exposure to health literary and clinical training implementing health literacy interventions (Harrington & Engelke, 2016; Rajah et al., 2018). Therefore, additional training is often needed for practitioners to accurately evaluate health literacy and provide effective interventions, and utilizing interprofessional education (i.e., educating teams of providers synchronously) can improve outcomes (Ulbrich et al., 2013). Health care providers should be critically aware of how they present information to family members and clients, including taking cultural, demographic, socioeconomic, educational, language and communication abilities, behaviors, and attitudes of the client and their family into consideration (Harrington & Engelke, 2016).

Health literacy and resiliency are inextricably linked (Bradley-Klug et al., 2017). Therefore, programs that can improve health literacy will naturally support increased family resiliency. Practitioners can help families identify, access, and utilize quality information about health from a variety of sources, including online search engines (Armstrong-Heimsoth et al., 2019). Mobile health applications provide new methods for delivering important information about health, accruing knowledge and resources, and can be a viable part of designing an intervention program (Case Study Box E). However, the use of mobile applications also requires that clients and families become competent in e-health literacy and can pose additional barriers such as equitable access to technology and concerns regarding privacy and security (Kim et al., 2019).

Mental Health Promotion

The WHO suggests that mental health promotion and interventions need to address health inequities during different stages of life and build social supports for families within communities to reduce long-term risk for stressors and adversity as well as to cope with those circumstances (WHO, 2017). Therefore, the specific focus on caregiver mental health and coping mechanisms for dealing with stress is critical for building family resiliency and overall QOL (Fairfax et al., 2019). It is also important to consider cultural influences, as caregivers from different backgrounds may differentially perceive events or circumstances as aversive. Reducing parental stress and enhancing well-being and self-efficacy can be accomplished using a combination of psychological interventions (such as Cognitive Behavioral Therapy), respite care, case management, parent-led support networks, and family-specific intervention programs. Individual parental intervention as well as group intervention have been found to be effective (Frantz et al., 2018). Improving parenting skills through behavioral parent interventions are also helpful for teaching caregivers to manage challenging behaviors associated with many pediatric disabilities such as autism spectrum disorders (Tarver et al., 2019). Other models such as Rational Emotive Family Health Therapy (Ede et al., 2020) teach caregivers to address their child's emotional and behavioral needs, including programs such as Predictive Parenting (Hallet et al., 2021), which have been effective for improving caregiver coping strategies. In addition, programs such as Strengthening Family Coping Resources (Kiser et al., 2010; Kiser et al., 2015) and techniques such as mindfulness-based interventions (Weitlauf et al., 2020) also improve outcomes. Evidence suggests that interventions assisting parents to manage their child's behavior and other diagnostic symptoms or characteristics are instrumental in reducing

Professional Reasoning Box A

Rishi is an adopted 12-year-old boy with who experienced significant childhood trauma. He came from a household where abuse was prominent, and he was removed from his parents' care at the age of 5 years. Rishi spent several years between foster homes and was adopted by his current family at age 9 years. In his adoptive family, Rishi is the oldest of four siblings in a family that live together in a modest suburban home. His mother is a physician at a local hospital and typically works four 12-hour shifts per week, and his father is an engineering faculty at a nearby university. Rishi attends public school, as do his three younger siblings. He receives occupational therapy, physical therapy, and speech therapy at school, and he has an aide that comes to the home during after school hours. Rishi continues to struggle with coping mechanisms, his parents are often unsure about his triggers and have difficulties helping him to manage and regulate his behaviors. Between managing his behaviors, the needs of his siblings, juggling work and family demands, they feel their QOL is poor. His occupational therapist identified a program "Rebuilding Resiliency" offered by an interprofessional team of occupational therapists and social workers at a local private practice. The program was an 8-week program designed for children who have experienced trauma and their caregivers. The program was designed around evidence-based practices and included sessions for Rishi in a group with similar peers and his parents in a group with other caregivers. Over the 8-week period Rishi engaged in activities that helped him identify and communicate his emotions, work on emotional regulation, identify coping strategies he could use for self-regulation, and apply positive coping strategies in different situations with peers. His parents completed coursework that helped them understand resiliency, how to build resiliency within families, identify coping strategies for caregivers (including mindfulness techniques) as well as strategies to offer their child, identifying community resources, and learning how to advocate for themselves and their child. Two months following the completion of this program, Rishi continues to utilize appropriate coping strategies and maladaptive behaviors have significantly decreased. His parents feel more confident in supporting Rishi, feel more knowledgeable about his needs, and they have started to venture out into new community settings increasing the family's participation and enhancing their QOL.

overall parental stress. Building social supports and coping strategies in caregivers to improve their own personal mental health and well-being, as well as to attend to the needs of their child with a disability, helps to establish protective factors for families who are vulnerable to chronic stress and increase resilience (Kiser et al., 2010; Professional Reasoning Box A).

Inadequate social supports for families who have a child with a disability can also become a barrier to community participation (Hartini, 2017; Simplican et al., 2015), and therefore impact QOL and well-being. Restraints on caregivers' time can prohibit seeking and maintaining social connections and building supportive social networks. Caregivers benefit from the ability to share lived experiences with other families dealing with similar issues, exchanging ideas, sharing resources and connections, helping to counterbalance many of the familial stressors. Creating opportunities for positive interactions between caregivers, other caregivers and the community can improve perceived sense of social supports and acceptance. Health care providers can be instrumental in helping to identify places in the community to facilitate these interactions, such as businesses offering "sensory-friendly" events or allowing alternative hours for children with special needs, locations that adhere to the spirit of universal design to promote equitable access, and connecting families to organizations that promote family wellness (DeBoth et al., 2021). Facilitating social connectedness and improving caregiver confidence supporting their child's disability can also help overcome participation barriers and each of these types of interventions contribute to the process of building resilience. To determine if interventions successfully improve resilience, three overall components have been proposed as indicators: 1) the successful fulfilment of family functions; 2) adequate balance between life satisfaction and risk exposure within the family; 3) gains from the process of building resilience within the family (Maurović et al., 2020).

Environmental Modifications and Participation

A relationship exists between SDOH and how families interact with, and therefore participate in, different environments. Social and community contexts and as well as the neighborhood and the built environment contribute to QOL. Successful participation in the community builds social capital, a sense of belonging, confidence in the ability to access and utilize the built environment and provides novel opportunities for growth and learning. Unsuccessful participation across different environments exacerbates perceived barriers and learned helplessness. Despite ADA requirements for community spaces to meet minimum accessibility demands, spaces often remain inaccessible or unwelcoming for families with children who have disabilities. Modifying the environment has been successful for improving community participation (Cermak et al., 2015; Kinnealey et al., 2012; Wood et al., 2019), and health care providers have a distinct role and ability to consult with organizations to ensure the spirit of ADA is applied for all disabilities, not simply physical disabilities (Umeda et al., 2017). Environmental considerations should include physical, social, and sensory-related features. Physical spaces created to accommodate wheelchairs or

Case Study Box F

QUESTION: FAMILY INTERVENTIONS

Consider the diverse needs of the Smith family. What interventions do you feel should be prioritized? Are there certain types of interventions that Mr. and Mrs. Smith could benefit from in particular? What members of the interprofessional team are the best fit for providing these interventions?

walkers may still utilize materials, sounds, or visual stimuli that are overstimulating and prohibitive for universal access. Pedestrian traffic patterns, crowd control, visual aids and cues, transportation, equipment and machinery present, and weather conditions are examples of many additional variables that can influence access and participation. For a family like the Smiths, fluctuating health conditions are only one hindrance to participation in community events. Having places to sit and rest, facilities that have space for full wheelchair access, acoustic panels to control noise, adequate shade or temperature control, appropriate lighting, and sensory break rooms or quiet spaces if behaviors are heightened, are examples of modifications that can help support increased participation. Health care providers trained in environmental assessment, such as occupational therapists, can take a lead role on an interprofessional team to help determine a family's needs and possible solutions (Case Study Box F).

In summary, an interprofessional team of health care providers can use their collective expertise to provide individual and group interventions that can impact and improve family health. Meeting the needs of caregivers to increase knowledge about their child's disability, available resources, building coping mechanisms and resiliency, promoting health literacy, and addressing environmental modifications represent some of the collective efforts that can make a significant impact on the lives of a child with a disability and their family.

Interprofessional Perspectives

Throughout this chapter, we have identified the need for an interprofessional approach to addressing family health. Beyond the notion that each profession can provide different assessments and intervention services integral to youth and family health, it is also important to recognize interprofessional team dynamics and how these interplay with the roles of caregivers and families.

Interprofessional teams working with children and their families may include any of the following: medical doctors, nurse practitioners, social workers, occupational therapists, physical therapists, speech-language pathologists, recreational therapists, psychologists, psychiatrists, art therapists, music therapists, in-home respite care providers, community organizations or agencies, and school personnel. Families may also have cultural connections with religious organizations, require interpreters, or have advocates. This exemplifies the diversity of the many professionals working closely with families, and therefore, the need to coordinate services is evident.

Many caregivers and families feel that there is a distinct lack of interprofessional collaborative practice (IPCP) between members of their care teams, and that they are not fully included or respected as equal team members (Cooper-Duffy & Eaker, 2017). This is in stark contrast to shared decision making and family-centered care that puts the client and family at the center of team-based models of interprofessional collaboration. Several groups have examined strategies to create effective teams. Cooper-Duffy and Eaker (2017) summarized and condensed these findings into the following critical team-building components: goal setting, roles and responsibilities, effective and efficient process, communication and interpersonal relationships, collaborative problem solving, and evaluation. These strategies mirror the five interprofessional competencies previously described in other chapters, namely values and ethics, roles and responsibilities, interprofessional communication, and team and teamwork (Interprofessional Education Collaborative [IPEC], 2016).

Goal setting should begin by understanding the outcomes that are most important for the child, the child's caregivers, and the child's family. Often, results from assessment tools are more reflective of skill deficits than how those skills affect family participation in various settings and contexts. The caregiver and family perspective is critical for designing intervention plans that meet the needs of the family and will therefore improve engagement, adherence, and satisfaction with outcomes. Strategies to include the family in goal setting are to explain the information you need from them, ask them about their desired outcomes, give families time to consider options before making decisions, listen to their problems and concerns, and respectfully share recommendations (Cooper-Duffy & Eaker, 2017). Members of the interprofessional team should each absorb these strategies, and help families understand priorities for interventions and resources that could best meet their needs. Goals should be collectively identified and agreed upon; in particular, if opportunities for carryover between professionals exists (e.g., incorporating speech-language pathology strategies into occupational therapy and physical therapy sessions).

During initial meetings with the client and family, practitioners should introduce the roles of each team member successful organization and productivity. It may be appropriate for older children to be fully participating members of the team, whereas younger children or those with more significant cognitive impairments may need to rely on their caregivers to best represent their needs. It may be beneficial to establish a team leader from the professional team who can help coordinate care and be the point of contact for the family. Finally, strategies to include caregivers and families more during role delineation include meeting with families to discuss their role, invite family members to share their expertise, acknowledge caregivers as experts and advocates for their children, encourage family members to share information, and each team member can explain how their role contributes to the expertise of the family (Cooper-Duffy & Eaker, 2017).

Effective and efficient process refers to the process by which the team will meet the stated goals and objectives. For this to be effective, the team requires a plan with steps, a sequence and strategies, identified resources, and management of the plan (Cooper-Duffy & Eaker, 2017). This is reflective of the IPEC competency "Team and Teamwork" that aims to plan, deliver, and evaluate patient care. Modifications of the plan may also be necessary in different settings to help achieve the goals. For example, if a child is working on self-feeding and swallowing with the occupational therapist and speech-language pathologist in a clinical setting, the practitioners would provide a modified feeding plan with previously mastered foods and food delivery in order to maintain skills at home. In order to incorporate the family in this process, it is recommended that the team ask the family about their habits and routines, provide the family information about how team meetings are conducted and with necessary information to prepare for meetings, and allow the family to add suggestions to the meeting agenda (Cooper-Duffy & Eaker, 2017).

Effective interprofessional teams work with families to develop effective and timely strategies for communicating important information, adopt a shared goal and vision to become more effective communicators, and emphasize open communication (D'Alimonte et al., 2019). Achieving these aims may require education and training for the practitioners and the family members. Additionally, recommended strategies for building communication with caregivers and family include using common language and reducing jargon, using active listening strategies and attending to positive nonverbal communication, acknowledging the family's requests, demonstrating a shared interest in and care for the child, using shared decision making, being aware of and offering potential resources, having an open dialogue to resolve problems and concerns, asking clarifying questions, being willing to look up information you do not already have, avoiding judgment, and speaking positively about the child as much as possible to counterbalance the many negative things families often hear (Cooper-Duffy & Eaker, 2017).

Caregivers often offer unique perspectives of how they anticipate potential solutions will be feasible or effective in their various family settings. The best, most creative, and innovative ideas will fall short of being successful if the family does not feel it is realistic or find value in its merit. Families can be more integrated into the problem-solving process by giving them visuals or outlines of the problem and its components, asking the family to identify challenges and barriers, and actively listening and welcoming proposed solutions from the family (Cooper-Duffy & Eaker, 2017).

Over time, the family may feel more connected to some team members more than others, and those members may be able to have a more honest and open conversation with the family about the team and its outcomes. Team members can also engage in self-reflection exercises to consider their roles and possible changes that could enhance the effectiveness of the overall team function (Blaiser & Nevins, 2017; Professional Reasoning Box B).

Policy

One additional area with which interprofessional teams can assist families is understanding and navigating relevant health care or other policies and their implications. Families need to gain knowledge about their rights, the rights of their child, what services they are entitled to and when, how to advocate for their child, and what community resources are available to support them. At the time a family officially enters the school system it may be their first encounter with the Individuals with Disabilities Education Act (IDEA, 2004) that guarantees free, appropriate public education to all eligible children. Under this act, students with disabilities are expected to be placed in the **least restrictive environment** (LRE) in order to provide equitable education and are integrated into classrooms with nondisabled peers. Determining LRE requires input and expertise from the interprofessional team. Caregivers may desire to hire an advocate who is versed in policy matters in order to help them better understand their rights and make informed decisions. Families may hire a legal advocate, and some areas offer pro bono advocates on a volunteer basis.

The world of health care and reimbursement mechanisms is also a dynamic, challenging web for families to traverse. Some health care services will be covered by insurance more than others. Families may obtain supplemental insurance to offset costs or be eligible for government assistance. The interprofessional team needs to be aware of a family's health care coverage and options especially before making recommendations or referrals for additional services. The team also needs to understand and share with the family information about what types of diagnoses, interventions, and services are covered and to what degree. When all of these components have been identified, the team can then work together to help establish intervention priorities. Although the family and child may need an array of services, more often than not finances will be limited and require discernment regarding prioritization and best practices (Case Study Box G).

Professional Reasoning Box B

Rosa is a speech-language pathologist working on an interprofessional team leading the care of a 6-year-old boy with autism named Marco who is nonverbal. He and his family are Hispanic, his parents' first language is Spanish, they also speak English fluently, and Marco seems to respond similarly to English and Spanish directions. The team has been working together for approximately 5 months, and Rosa procured an iPad and an augmentative communication program using picture symbols to provide Marco an independent means of communication. His parents requested that his communication device be set up in English, and Rosa provided training to the family on how to use the device. Marco's physical therapist, Collin, noticed one day that Marco was demonstrating increased self-injurious behaviors when encouraged to use his device during therapy. The therapist asked his parents if he has been using it at home, and they reported he has not and that a lot of vocabulary that they would like to use at home was not on the device. Collin relayed this information to Rosa and suggested that they call a team meeting. Rosa initially became defensive and told Collin she would address the problem with the family herself, but Collin reminded her that the team has agreed for open dialogue and free brainstorming, including the family, when new concerns arise for Marco.

During the team meeting, Collin asked Marco's parents to talk about their experiences with the device. They shared it was more frustrating than helpful at home, although they admitted he was using it proficiently in speech therapy and in his kindergarten classroom. Marco's social worker suggested that his parents make a list of the most common words and phrases they use at home in Spanish, and she would have them translated. Rosa considered this suggestion and then added that she would like to have the iPad training worksheet and instructions she provided them also translated into Spanish. When Rosa received the list from Marco's parents, she was surprised at some of the terms that the family used most often. Two weeks later, the team reconvened to determine if Marco was using his device more frequently at home and if his parents were more comfortable using it with him. His parents happily reported that he now had the pictures and vocabulary that are more meaningful to them, and that they are more comfortable using and modifying it to add content as well.

REFLECTIVE QUESTIONS

1. What components of interprofessional collaboration and practice made the resolution to this concern for Marco successful?
2. How might other disciplines have contributed to solving this problem?
3. How should the team continue moving forward to keep Marco and his family at the center of the team function across disciplines?

Case Study Box G

QUESTIONS: INTERPROFESSIONAL TEAM

Consider the number of potential providers that may be involved in the ongoing care for the Smith family. Who are the necessary core team members and what services will they provide? What settings will these be provided in? Who should take leadership roles, and what are best communication strategies to implement between the team and the family? What is the expertise of Mr. and Mrs. Smith you would most rely on? What policies might the team need to help the Smiths negotiate?

Community Programs

Many community programs and organizations recognize the need to support children with disabilities and their families inclusively into community activities, events, and spaces. Some of the more common venues are museums, parks and green spaces, and community-based organizations.

Museums

The Children's Museum of Cleveland (CMC; https://cmcleveland.org/) has made significant efforts over time to be more inclusive of the disability community. CMC recently renovated a historic mansion on "millionaire's row" in the city of Cleveland, Ohio. During the interim between the closing of the old museum and grand opening of the new facility, CMC participated in a joint effort with Cleveland State University (CSU) faculty to offer families a "sensory-friendly" museum exhibit experience on the university campus. Working with university occupational therapists, physical therapists, speech therapists, and special education teachers, CMC staff created activities and exhibits as part of an event designed for children with mobility and/or sensory impairments and their families. The CSU program PLAAY (Participation in Leisure Allowing Access for EverYone) on the Move (https://www.csuplaayonthemove.com/) hosts free events on a regular basis that utilize multidirectional, overground, hands-free harness systems and adapted ride-on cars to increase participation for children with disabilities. The presence of licensed therapists and health professional students at the events also offers parents an opportunity to learn, share, rest, and connect. As part of the multi-million-dollar CMC renovation project, consideration for children of all abilities was central to the design with regard for families and caregivers as well. Designers included resting and gathering places for caregivers, an elevator for easy transitions between floors, a sensory break room to help redirect heightened behaviors, and a large café space for snacks and small meal breaks. These components of environmental design are small, but meaningful and can have a dramatic effect on participation. CMC continues to partner with CSU to offer sensory-friendly times during off-hours to reduce noise and crowds for families who can benefit from reduced sensory stimulation.

Parks and Green Spaces

The Cleveland Metroparks system includes 18 reservations covering more than 24,000 acres, has over 300 miles of trails, eight golf courses, eight lakefront parks, and a nationally recognized zoo (Cleveland Metroparks, 2021; https://www.clevelandmetroparks.com/accessibility). Metroparks offers daily programming for individuals and families intended to be accessible for persons of all abilities, with optional accommodations that can be scheduled prior to events. Beach wheelchairs are available for the lakefront properties and SoloRider golf carts can be reserved to increase accessibility on the golf course. Most programs are free of charge and many of the parks offer fidget bags, assisted listening devices, sign language interpreters, and staff that are trained to adapt equipment to accommodate individual needs. Utilization of accessible parks and green spaces strengthens the relationships between children and caregivers, as well as between families and the community (Vaznonienė & Vaznonis, 2017). In youth, green spaces enhance well-being by encouraging personal development, increasing physical activity and functioning, improving emotional regulation, and may be associated with fewer internalizing symptoms, less screen time, and more physical activity (Reuben et al., 2020; Vaznonienė & Vaznonis, 2020). At the community level, green spaces provide social, economic, and environmental benefits, that improve the well-being of individuals and families and therefore QOL (Mensah et al., 2016). For families, the ability to participate in nature may also be a successful intervention for improving mental health (Reuben & Himschoot, 2021). Health care providers should be aware of the benefits of green spaces and parks and can seek out similar types of programming locally. In addition, community-based therapists can work with families to increase participation and structure therapeutic activities on-site when local parks and playgrounds are available. Finally, health care providers also have a calling to advocate for their clients and families to ensure that parks and green spaces are accessible so that children with disabilities and their families can receive the same benefits from these spaces as do others in their communities.

Community-Based Member Organizations

Two organizations in the Cleveland, Ohio area provide free and accessible opportunities for children with disabilities. Gigi's Playhouse (2021; https://gigisplayhouse.org/) has over 54 locations worldwide, including one in Cleveland, Ohio. Gigi's uses a playhouse model to provide free educational, therapeutic-based and career development programs for individuals with Down syndrome, their families, and the community. They strive to gain acceptance for children with Down syndrome as well as build a support network for their families. Gigi's Playhouse offers programs that promote skills development, tutoring services, social development and interactions, pragmatic skills, physical exercise, and career training programs. This organization is family centered and they have removed the major cost barrier by offering free services and programming to the community.

Another program, Youth Challenge (YC, 2021; https://www.youthchallengesports.com/), aims to bring youth with physical disabilities together with teenage volunteers and engage in play, adapted sporting activities, recreational opportunities, and social experiences. The teen volunteers are trained by professionals, and YC offers programs such as basketball, baseball, swimming, skiing, tennis, arts and crafts, music, sailing, bowling, nature programs, dancing, and field trips. The focus on engaging children with disabilities with typically developing teenage peers strengthens community participation and integration. Children also develop sports and leisure skills that can translate into other community settings, enhancing overall community engagement. YC does not charge families a fee for programming and offers free transportation as well for families in need.

Practitioners should be aware of community-based organizations and opportunities that are appropriate for their clients and families. Free or reduced-cost opportunities to enhance community participation, increase social networks, and gain new or strengthen skills are important factors that can enhance QOL. Each member of the interprofessional team may be aware of different community organizations and supports, some targeting the child, some focused on caregivers, and others focused on peers or siblings and promoting socialization. Practitioners can also offer families expertise on what adaptations, modifications, or supports would be necessary to promote full engagement of children and their families in different community programs (Professional Reasoning Box C and Case Study Box H).

Professional Reasoning Box C

Gianna is a 7-year-old girl with mixed-type quadriplegic cerebral palsy. Her legs are more affected than her upper body and are primarily spastic, and she typically uses a wheelchair for mobility. Her mother is a single mother, she is Black, and resides in a first-floor apartment with Gianna's grandmother. Gianna receives occupational, physical, and speech therapy in the home in addition to services provided by the school district. The family lives in an under-resourced urban neighborhood 5 minutes outside the downtown area. Recently Gianna's mother and grandmother expressed to the team that they wanted to see her engage in more community activities and increase social engagement with peers. The family is unable to take Gianna themselves, as her grandmother has limited mobility, is without a car or personal transportation, and her mother works two jobs outside the home. Between school and in-home therapy, and the extra time required for Gianna's self-care, opportunities for community engagement are limited. The interprofessional team of community service providers collaborated with the school team and determined that many of the skill development goals could continue to be addressed in the school setting, and the community team could revise some of their goals to incorporate community inclusion and more opportunities for peer interactions. A local organization offers a leisure and recreation program pairing children with disabilities with teenage volunteers to engage in recreational activities. The community team worked with the organization to ensure staff were trained to handle Gianna's unique needs, manage transfers in and out of her wheelchair, utilize her assistive communication devices, and support independent functioning as much as possible. The therapists each took one session a month to attend the events with Gianna and her teen companion. They observed, make additional recommendations, and provided training and tips as needed and reported back to the team. Within 3 months, Gianna was comfortable and enjoying time with her companion and was introduced to many new peers and activities through the organization's events.

REFLECTIVE QUESTION

1. What other options might the interprofessional team have explored? What do you think are the most positive outcomes for the family?

Case Study Box H

QUESTIONS: COMMUNITY PROGRAMMING

The Smith family enjoys being out in the community. Based on the examples of community programming provided, which do you feel would be beneficial for them? Based on your experiences in your own community, what other types of programs or resources could be a good fit for the Smiths? What barriers to participation in these programs do you think each could face, and what are potential ways an interprofessional team could work to solve them?

Conclusion

Family health and well-being is critical to the health and QOL of the larger community. It is important for practitioners to keep the client and their family at the center of the intervention process and maintain the integrity of shared decision making. Practitioners need to understand how to recognize familial factors that affect the family and child's well-being, how to identify barriers, how to improve participation for children with disabilities and their families at home and in the community, and how interprofessional team members can each contribute to these outcomes. Without addressing the needs of caregivers and other family members, many contextual factors affecting a child cannot be fully integrated into intervention planning. In addition, the SDOH that impact caregivers and the family unit are important considerations for intervention recommendations, tapping into available resources, and connecting children and families with opportunities within or surrounding their communities.

References

Altin, S. V., Finke, I., Kautz-Freimuth, S., & Stock, S. (2014). The evolution of health literacy assessment tools: a systematic review. *BMC Public Health, 14*(1), 1-13.

Armstrong-Heimsoth, A., Johnson, M. L., Carpenter, M., Thomas, T., & Sinnappan, A. (2019). Health management: Occupational therapy's key role in educating clients about reliable online health information. *The Open Journal of Occupational Therapy, 7*(4), 1-12.

Bar, M. A., Shelef, L., & Bart, O. (2016). Do participation and self-efficacy of mothers to children with ASD predict their children's participation? *Research in Autism Spectrum Disorders, 24*, 1-10.

Barry, M. J., & Edgman-Levitan, S. (2012). Shared decision making—The pinnacle patient-centered care. *New England Journal of Medicine, 366*(9), 780-781. https://doi.org/10.1056/NEJMp1109283

Bedell, G. (2009). Further validation of the Child and Adolescent Scale of Participation (CASP). *Developmental Neurorehabilitation, 12*, 342-351.

Bedell, G., & McDougall J. (2015). The Child and Adolescent Scale of Environment (CASE): Further validation with youth who have chronic conditions. *Developmental Neurorehabilitation, 18*(6), 375-382.

Behere, A. P., Basnet, P., & Campbell, P. (2017). Effects of family structure on mental health of children: A preliminary study. *Indian Journal of Psychological Medicine, 39*(4), 457-463.

Berg, M., Jahnsen, R., Frøslie, K. F., & Hussain, A. (2004). Reliability of the pediatric evaluation of disability inventory (PEDI). *Physical & Occupational Therapy in Pediatrics, 24*(3), 61-77.

Blaiser, K. M., & Nevins, M. E. (2017). Practitioner reflection that enhances interprofessional collaborative practices for serving children who are deaf/hard-of-hearing. *Perspectives of the ASHA Special Interest Groups, 2*(9), 3-9.

Bowen, M. (1966). The use of family theory in clinical practice. *Comprehensive Psychiatry, 7*, 345-374.

Bowen, M. (1978). *Family therapy in clinical practice*. Rowman & Littlefield.

Bradley-Klug, K., Shaffer-Hudkins, E., Lynn, C., Jeffries DeLoatche, K., & Montgomery, J. (2017). Initial development of the health literacy and resiliency scale: Youth version. *Journal of Communication in Healthcare, 10*(2), 100-107.

Cambric, M. N. (2019). Validating the Construct of Resiliency in the Health Literacy and Resiliency Scale (HLRS-Y) with the Child and Youth Resiliency Measure (CYRM-28). University of South Florida. ProQuest Dissertations Publishing, 13905118.

Cantwell, J., Muldoon, O., & Gallagher, S. (2015). The influence of self-esteem and social support on the relationship between stigma and depressive symptomology in parents caring for children with intellectual disabilities. *Journal of Intellectual Disability Research, 59*(10), 948-957.

Centers for Disease Control and Prevention. (n.d.) Ten essential public health services and how they can include addressing social determinants of health inequities. https://www.cdc.gov/publichealthgateway/publichealthservices/pdf/ten_essential_services_and_sdoh.pdf

Cermak, S. A., Stein Duker, L. I., Williams, M. E., Lane, C. J., Dawson, M. E., Borreson, A. E., & Polido, J. C. (2015). Feasibility of a sensory-adapted dental environment for children with autism. *American Journal of Occupational Therapy, 69*, 6903220020. https://doi.org/http://dx.doi. org/10.5014/ajot.2015.013714

Cleveland Metroparks Organization. (2021). Accessibility. https://www.clevelandmetroparks.com

Cooper-Duffy, K., & Eaker, K. (2017). Effective team practices: Interprofessional contributions to communication issues with a parent›s perspective. *American Journal of Speech-Language Pathology, 26*(2), 181-192.

Coster, W., Bedell, G., Law M., Alunkal Khetani, M., Teplicky, R., Liljenquist, K., Gleason, K., & Kao, Y. C., (2011). Psychometric evaluation of the Participation and Environment Measure for Children and Youth (PEM-CY). *Developmental Medicine & Child Neurology, 53*(11), 1030-1037.

Cureton, A., & Silvers, A. (2017) Respecting the dignity of children with disabilities in clinical practice. *HEC Forum, 29*, 257-276. https://doi.org/10.1007/s10730-017-9326-3

D'Alimonte, L., McLaney, E., & Di Prospero, L. (2019). Best practices on team communication: interprofessional practice in oncology. *Current opinion in supportive and palliative care, 13*(1), 69-74.

DeBoth, K., Wendland, M., Bilinovic, T., & Sanford, C. (2021). Caregiver perceptions of child participation in sensory friendly community events. *Journal of Occupational Therapy, Schools, & Early Intervention*, 1-16.

Ede, M. O., Anyanwu, J. I., Onuigbo, L. N., Ifelunni, C. O., Alabi-Oparaocha, F. C., Okenyi, E. C., ... & Victor-Aigbodion, V. (2020). Rational emotive family health therapy for reducing parenting stress in families of children with autism spectrum disorders: A group randomized control study. *Journal of Rational-Emotive & Cognitive-Behavior Therapy*, 1-29.

Fairfax, A., Brehaut, J., Colman, I., Sikora, L., Kazakova, A., Chakraborty, P., & Potter, B. K. (2019). A systematic review of the association between coping strategies and quality of life among caregivers of children with chronic illness and/or disability. *BMC Pediatrics, 19(*1). https://doi.org/10.1186/s12887-019-1587-3

Filippello, P., Sorrenti, L., Buzzai, C., & Costa, S. (2015). Perceived parental psychological control and learned helplessness: The role of school self-efficacy. *School Mental Health, 7*(4), 298-310.

Fisher, W. W., Piazza, C.C., Bowman, L.G., & Amari, A. (1996). Integrating caregiver report with a systematic choice assessment. *American Journal on Mental Retardation, 101*, 15-25.

Fletcher, T., Anderson-Seidens, J., Wagner, H., Linyard, M., & Nicolette, E. (2019). Caregivers' perceptions of barriers and supports for children with sensory processing disorders. *Australian Occupational Therapy Journal, 66*(5), 617-626.

Frantz, R., Hansen, S. G., & Machalicek, W. (2018). Interventions to promote well-being in parents of children with autism: A systematic review. *Review Journal of Autism and Developmental Disorders, 5*(1), 58-77.

Fuchs, W. W., Mundschenk, N. J., & Groark, B. (2017). A promising practice: School-Based mindfulness-based stress reduction for children with disabilities. *Journal of International Special Needs Education, 20*(2), 56-66.

Gardiner, E., Mâsse, L. C., & Iarocci, G. (2019). A psychometric study of the Family Resilience Assessment Scale among families of children with autism spectrum disorder. *Health and Quality of Life Outcomes, 17*(1), 1-10.

Gigi's Playhouse. (2021). Down syndrome achievement centers. https://gigisplayhouse.org/

Golfenshtein, N., Srulovici, E., & Medoff-Cooper, B. (2016). Investigating parenting stress across pediatric health conditions: A systematic review. *Comprehensive Child and Adolescent Nursing, 39*(1), 41-79.

Hallett, V., Mueller, J., Breese, L., Hollett, M., Beresford, B., Irvine, A., ... & Simonoff, E. (2021). Introducing 'Predictive Parenting': A feasibility study of a new group parenting intervention targeting emotional and behavioral difficulties in children with autism spectrum disorder. *Journal of Autism and Developmental Disorders, 51*, 323-333.

Harrington, M., & Engelke, M. K. (2016). Health literacy: Perceptions and experiences of pediatric nephrology interprofessional team members. *Nephrology Nursing Journal, 43*(1), 15.

Hartini, R. (2017). The increasing model of family's social support and child with disability's environment. *Journal Sampurasun: Interdisciplinary Studies for Cultural Heritage, 3*(2), 56-68.

Hernandez, A. (2009). *Roundtable on health literacy*. Board on Population Health and Public Health Practice, & Institute of Medicine.

Hollar, D. W., & Rowland, J. (2015). Promoting health literacy for people with disabilities and clinicians through a teamwork model. *Journal of Family Strengths, 15*(2), 5.

Hsiao, Y. J. (2018). Parental stress in families of children with disabilities. *Intervention in School and Clinic, 53*(4), 201-205.

Huang, H. H., Chen, Y. M., Huang, H. W., Shih, M. K., Hsieh, Y. H., & Chen, C. L. (2018). Modified ride-on cars and young children with disabilities: effects of combining mobility and social training. *Frontiers in Pediatrics, 5*, 299.

Individuals with Disabilities Education Act, 20 U.S.C. § 1400 (2004).

Institute of Medicine. (2004). *Health literacy: A prescription to end confusion*. Author.

Interprofessional Education Collaborative. (2016). *Core competencies for interprofessional collaborative practice*. Author.

Khetani, M. A., Graham, J. E., Davies, P. L., Law, M. C., & Simeonsson, R. J. (2015). Psychometric properties of the Young Children's Participation and Environment Measure (YC-PEM). *Archives Physical Medicine and Rehabilitation, 96*(2), 307-316.

Kim, H., Goldsmith, J. V., Sengupta, S., Mahmood, A., Powell, M. P., Bhatt, J., ... & Bhuyan, S. S. (2019). Mobile health application and e-health literacy: Opportunities and concerns for cancer patients and caregivers. *Journal of Cancer Education, 34*(1), 3-8.

King, G. A., Law, M., & King, S. (2006). Measuring children's participation in recreation and leisure activities: Construct validation of the CAPE and PAC. *Child: Care, Health, and Development, 33*, 28-39.

Kinnealey, M., Pfeiffer, B., Miller, J., Roan, C., Shoener, R., & Ellner, M. L. (2012). Effect of classroom modification on attention and engagement of students with autism or dyspraxia. *American Journal of Occupational Therapy, 66*(5), 511–519. doi:10.5014/ajot.2012.004010

Kiser, L. J., Backer, P. M., Winkles, J., & Medoff, D. (2015). Strengthening family coping resources (SFCR): Practice-based evidence for a promising trauma intervention. *Couple and Family Psychology: Research and Practice, 4*(1), 49.

Kiser, L. J., Donohue, A., Hodgkinson, S., Medoff, D., & Black, M. M. (2010). Strengthening family coping resources: The feasibility of a multifamily group intervention for families exposed to trauma. *Journal of Traumatic Stress, 23*(6), 802-806.

Maier, S. F., & Seligman, M. E. (1976). Learned helplessness: Theory and evidence. *Journal of Experimental Psychology, 105*(1), 3.

Marshall, E. S., Olsen, S. F., Mandleco, B. L., Dyches, T. T., Allred, K. W., & Sansom, N. (2003). "This is a spiritual experience": Perspectives of Latter-Day Saint families living with a child with disabilities. *Qualitative Health Research, 13*(1), 57-76.

Maurović, I., Liebenberg, L., & Ferić, M. (2020). A review of family resilience: Understanding the concept and operationalization challenges to inform research and practice. *Child Care in Practice, 26*(4), 337-357.

McConnell, D., Savage, A., & Breitkreuz, R. (2014). Resilience in families raising children with disabilities and behavior problems. *Research In Developmental Disabilities, 35*(4), 833-848.

Mensah, C. A., Andres, L., Perera, U., & Roji, A. (2016). Enhancing quality of life through the lens of green spaces: A systematic review approach. *International Journal of Wellbeing, 6*(1).

Mešl, N., Kodele, T., & Čačinovič Vogrinčič, G. (2012). The role of contemporary social work concepts in dealing with learned helplessness of children with learning difficulties. *Ljetopis Socijalnog Rada, 19*(2), 191-213.

Naeem Mohsin, M. (2011). Ecological inventory: An approach for assessment of children with intellectual disability. *International Journal of Early Childhood Special Education, 3*(2), 148-159.

Office of Disease Prevention and Health Promotion. (2021, June 23). Health literacy. HealthyPeople2020. https://www.healthypeople.gov/2020/topics-objectives/topic/social-determinants-health/interventions-resources/health-literacy

Papadopoulos, C., Lodder, A., Constantinou, G., & Randhawa, G. (2019). Systematic review of the relationship between autism stigma and informal caregiver mental health. *Journal of Autism and Developmental Disorders, 49*(4), 1665-1685.

Pastor-Cerezuela, G., Fernández-Andrés, M. I., Pérez-Molina, D., & Tijeras-Iborra, A. (2021). Parental stress and resilience in autism spectrum disorder and Down syndrome. *Journal of Family Issues, 42*(1), 3-26.

Pfeiffer, B., Coster, W., Snethen, G., Derstine, M., Piller, A., & Tucker, C. (2017). Caregivers' perspectives on the sensory environment and participation in daily activities of children with autism spectrum disorder. *American Journal of Occupational Therapy, 71*(4), 7104220020p1-7104220028p9.

Rajah, R., Ahmad Hassali, M. A., Jou, L. C., & Murugiah, M. K. (2018). The perspective of healthcare providers and patients on health literacy: A systematic review of the quantitative and qualitative studies. *Perspectives in Public Health, 138*(2), 122-132.

Reynolds, W. M., & Miller, K. L. (1985). Depression and learned helplessness in mentally retarded and nonmentally retarded adolescents: An initial investigation. *Applied Research in Mental Retardation, 6*(3), 295-306.

Reuben, A., & Himschoot, E. (2021). Nature as a mental health intervention: State of the science and programmatic possibilities for the conservation community. *Parks Stewardship Forum, 37*(2).

Reuben, A., Rutherford, G. W., James, J., & Razani, N. (2020). Association of neighborhood parks with child health in the United States. *Preventive Medicine, 141*, 106265.

Richardson, G. E. (2002). The metatheory of resilience and resiliency. *Journal of Clinical Psychology, 58*(3), 307-321.

Rothbaum, F., Rosen, K., Ujiie, T., & Uchida, N. (2002). Family systems theory, attachment theory, and culture. *Family Process, 41*(3), 328. https://doi.org/10.1111/j.1545-5300.2002.41305.x

Sagester, G., & Mazzarella, J. (2020). *Measuring and building resilience in children with developmental disabilities: A scoping review*. Manuscript in progress.

Schaaf, R. C., Toth-Cohen, S., Johnson, S. L., Outten, G., & Benevides, T. W. (2011). The everyday routines of families of children with autism: Examining the impact of sensory processing difficulties on the family. *Autism, 15*(3), 373-389.

Simplican, S. C., Leader, G., Kosciulek, J., & Leahy, M. (2015). Defining social inclusion of people with intellectual and developmental disabilities: An ecological model of social networks and community participation. *Research in Developmental Disabilities, 38*, 18-29.

Sixbey, M. (2005). Development of the family resilience assessment scale to identify family resilience constructs. PhD thesis. University of Florida.

Smith, S. (2013). Citizenship and disability: Incommensurable lives and well-being. *Critical Review of International Social and Political Philosophy, 16*(3), 403-420. http://dx.doi.org/10.1080/13698230.2013.795708

Solish, A., Perry, A., & Minnes, P. (2010). Participation of children with and without disabilities in social, recreational and leisure activities. *Journal of Applied Research in Intellectual Disabilities, 23*(3), 226-236.

Suzuki, K., Kobayashi, T., Moriyama, K., Kaga, M., Kiratani, M., Wantanabe, K., Yamashita, Y., & Inagaki, M. (2015). Development and evaluation of a parent resilience elements questionnaire (PREQ). *PLOS ONE, 10*(12).

Taheri, A., Perry, A., & Minnes, P. (2016). Examining the social participation of children and adolescents with intellectual disabilities and autism spectrum disorder in relation to peers. *Journal of Intellectual Disability Research, 60*(5), 435-443.

Tarver, J., Palmer, M., Webb, S., Scott, S., Slonims, V., Simonoff, E., & Charman, T. (2019). Child and parent outcomes following parent interventions for child emotional and behavioral problems in autism spectrum disorders: A systematic review and meta-analysis. *Autism, 23*(7), 1630-1644.

Turnbull, A. P., Turnbull, H. R., Erwin, E., Soodak, L. & Shogren, K. A. (2015). *Families, professionals, and exceptionality: A special partnership* (7th ed.). Merrill Publishing Company.

Ulbrich, S., Campbell, J., Dyer, C., Gregory, G., & Hudson, S. (2013). Interprofessional education on health literacy: Session development, implementation, and evaluation. *Annals of Behavioral Science and Medical Education, 19*(1), 3-7.

Umeda, C. J., Fogelberg, D. J., Jirikowic, T., Pitonyak, J. S., Mroz, T. M., & Ideishi, R. I. (2017). Expanding the implementation of the Americans with Disabilities Act for populations with intellectual and developmental disabilities: The role of organization-level occupational therapy consultation. *American Journal of Occupational Therapy, 71*(4), 7104090010p1-7104090010p6.

Vaznonienė, G., & Vaznonis, B. (2017). Social benefit of green spaces to local community. In: Rural Development 2017 [elektroninis išteklius]: Bioeconomy Challenges: Proceedings of the 8th International Scientific Conference, 23-24th November 2017, Aleksandras Stulginskis University. Akademija: Aleksandras Stulginskis University.

Vaznonienė, G., & Vaznonis, B. (2020). Strengthening youth wellbeing through green spaces: Case study of a small town. *Management Theory and Studies for Rural Business and Infrastructure Development, 42*(2), 178-192.

Wayment, H. A., & Brookshire, K. A. (2018). Mothers' reactions to their child's ASD diagnosis: Predictors that discriminate grief from distress. *Journal of Autism and Developmental Disorders, 48*(4), 1147-1158.

Weiss, J. A., Cappadocia, M. C., MacMullin, J. A., Viecili, M., & Lunsky, Y. (2012). The impact of child problem behaviors of children with ASD on parent mental health: The mediating role of acceptance and empowerment. *Autism, 16*(3), 261-274.

Weitlauf, A. S., Broderick, N., Stainbrook, J. A., Taylor, J. L., Herrington, C. G., Nicholson, A. G., ... & Warren, Z. E. (2020). Mindfulness-based stress reduction for parents implementing early intervention for autism: an RCT. *Pediatrics, 145*(Suppl. 1), S81-S92.

Weisz, J. R. (2013). Learned helplessness and the retarded child. In *Mental retardation* (pp. 36-49). Routledge.

Whiting, M. (2014). Children with disability and complex health needs: The impact on family life. *Nursing Children and Young People, 26*(3).

Widyawati, Y., Otten, R., Kleemans, T., & Scholte, R. H. J. (2020). Parental resilience and the quality of life of children with developmental disabilities in Indonesia. *International Journal of Disability, Development and Education*, 1-17.

Wood, E. B., Halverson, A., Harrison, G., & Rosenkranz, A. (2019). Creating a sensory-friendly pediatric emergency department. *Journal of Emergency Nursing, 45*(4), 415–424. doi:10.1016/j.jen.2018.12.002

World Health Organization. (2007). *International classification of functioning, disability and health: Children & youth version.* http://apps.who.int/iris/bitstream/handle/10665/43737/9789241547321_eng.pdf;jsessionid=8AF639DAE00F37F60D3FD93849B48C28?sequence=1

World Health Organization and Calouste Gulbenkian Foundation. (2017). Policy options on mental health: A WHO-Gulbenkian Mental Health Platform collaboration. Author.

Yin, H. S., Dreyer, B. P., Vivar, K. L., MacFarland, S., van Schaick, L., & Mendelsohn, A. L. (2012). Perceived barriers to care and attitudes towards shared decision-making among low socioeconomic status parents: Role of health literacy. *Academic Pediatrics, 12*(2), 117-124.

Young, N. L., Williams, J. I., Yoshida, K. K., & Wright, J. G. (2000). Measurement properties of the activities scale for kids. *Journal of Clinical Epidemiology, 53*(2), 125-137.

Youth Challenge. (2021). https://www.youthchallengesports.com/

Ziviani, J., Ottenbacher, K. J., & Shephard K. (2002). Concurrent validity of the Functional Independence Measure for Children (WeeFIM™) and the pediatric evaluation of disabilities inventory in children with developmental disabilities and acquired brain injuries. *Physical & Occupational Therapy in Pediatrics, 21*(3), 91-101.

Appendix A: Family Health: Children and Youth Assessment Instruments

Assessment	Authors/ Citation	Population	Development	Environment	Participation	Preferences	Resiliency	Quality of Life	Health Literacy
Pediatric Evaluation of Disability Inventory (PEDI)	Berg et al. (2004)	Children and youth	✓						
Functional Independence Measure for Children (WeeFIM)	Ziviani et al. (2002)	Children and youth	✓						
Activities Scale for Kids (ASK)	Young et al. (2000)	Children and youth		✓					
Child and Adolescent Scale of Environment (CASE)	Bedell & McDougall (2015)	Children and youth		✓					
Ecological inventory	Naeem Mohsin (2011)	Child and family		✓					
The Child and Adolescent Scale of Participation (CASP)	Bedell (2009)	Children and youth			✓				

(continued)

Assessment	Authors/ Citation	Population	Development	Environment	Participation	Preferences	Resiliency	Quality of Life	Health Literacy
The Participation and Environment Measure for Children and Youth (PEM-CY)	Coster et al. (2011)	Children and youth			✓				
Young Children's Participation and Environment Measure	Khetani et al. (2015)	Children and youth		✓	✓				
Children's Assessment of Participation (CAPE) with supplemental assessment, Preferences of Children (PAC)	King et al. (2006)	Children and youth			✓	✓			
Reinforcer Assessment for Individuals with Severe Disability (RAISD)	Fisher et al. (1996)	Children and youth				✓			
Activities Questionnaire	Solish et al. (2010)	Child and family			✓				
Family Resilience Assessment Scale	Gardiner et al. (2019); Sixbey (2005)	Child and family					✓		

(continued)

Assessment	Authors/ Citation	Population	Development	Environment	Participation	Preferences	Resiliency	Quality of Life	Health Literacy
Parenting Resilience Elements and the Quality of Life Questionnaire	Widyawati et al. (2020)	Child and family					✓	✓	
Health Literacy and Resiliency Scale: Youth	Bradley-Klug et al. (2017)	Child and family					✓		✓
Construct of Resiliency in the Health Literacy and Resiliency Scale (HLRS-Y)	Cambric (2019)	Child and family					✓		✓
Child and Youth Resiliency Measure (CYRM-28)	Cambric (2019)	Child and family					✓		

Reflective Questions

1. Why are we concerned about resiliency in families who have a child with a disability?

Resiliency is a measure of a family's ability to cope with adverse events in their lives. Resilient families have better overall outcomes, greater feelings of well-being, and a perceived better QOL. The health (physical, mental, and social) of each member of the family contributes to its overall resilience. Over time, appropriate coping strategies, activities that support positive mental health, interventions that support knowledge, skill-building, and increase participation will all build family resilience. Interprofessional health care teams have the ability to assess resilience, provide education, and other relevant interventions, filling needs and previously unidentified gaps, and track progress over time.

Using the ICF framework as a starting point, interprofessional team members can holistically evaluate the needs of the child while including critical information about the family and their environment. It is not simply enough to utilize developmental checklists, but rather each member of the team should consider what limitations each family member faces and assess how those limitations impact participation in the home, school, and community settings. Team members should also consider evaluation tools that extend beyond typical clinical assessments and incorporate related areas such as resiliency, participation, and health literacy. Each team member should consider how factors such as these could influence a successful intervention plan. For example, speech therapists might assess community participation as a complement to speech and pragmatic language to better understand how the child and family competently interact with others in the community. The occupational therapist might incorporate prescribed language supports into recommendations, such as environmental adaptations, that they make for the family to access different community spaces such as museums or community events. Completing an evaluation with this type of approach is optimal for supporting overall health and well-being of the child and their family.

2. How can an interprofessional team consider the needs of caregivers as part of the intervention process?

Frequently, interventions and intervention plans are focused on the child. However, the child is part of a dynamic family unit that should be considered holistically by the team. Family interventions may be an option, or providing resources for family members to find individual or group supports. This can be in the form of education, social supports, and networking, training, or identifying community resources that are accessible and would support increased participation for the family. Interprofessional teams should think beyond the typical view of clinical intervention, considering other family members, their roles and occupations, what the family's priorities are, and how the team can help support positive outcomes in the child's home and out in the community.

CHAPTER 17

Promoting Family Health
Adults

Erica K. Wentzel, OTD, OTR/L and Holly Putnam Bacasa, PT

Learning Objectives

At the end of this chapter, the reader will:

1. Define the first three stages of adulthood (ACOTE B.1.1)
2. Explain how the concept of family is unique to adults and families (ACOTE B.1.2)
3. Describe characteristics of the 21st century family (ACOTE B.1.2)
4. Explain how social determinants of health affect adult and family health (ACOTE B.1.3)
5. Compare adverse childhood experiences to positive childhood experiences and how they relate to health outcomes in adulthood (ACOTE B.1.3)
6. Discuss the reciprocal nature of health and wellness between family and community (ACOTE B.3.4)
7. Explain the family-centered care framework (ACOTE B.2.1)
8. Articulate the importance of interprofessional collaboration when working with adults and their families (ACOTE B.4.25; CAPTE 7D7)
9. Demonstrate an understanding of how to select and apply family-centered assessment tools that consider client needs and cultural and contextual factors (ACOTE B.4.5)
10. Demonstrate an understanding of how family-centered, place-based interventions can enhance a family's health, well-being, and quality of life (ACOTE B.4.10)

The ACOTE Standards used are those from 2018.

Pizzi, M. A., & Amir, M. (Eds.). *Interprofessional Perspectives for Community Practice: Promoting Health, Well-Being, and Quality of Life* (pp. 327-341).

Key Words

Community, Community Health Resilience, Context, Emerging Adulthood, Evidence-Based Practice, Family, Family-Centered Care, Family Dynamics, Health, Health Management, Household, Householder, Interprofessional Collaboration, Middle Adulthood, Motivational Interviewing, Occupations, Quality of Life, Resilience, Roles, Social Determinants of Health, Socioeconomic Status, Well-Being, Young Adulthood

Case Study

Rose is a 30-year-old woman and mother with an opioid use disorder (OUD), which the Centers for Disease Control and Prevention (CDC) define as "a problematic pattern of opioid use that causes significant impairment or distress. Opioid use disorder is a medical condition that can affect anyone—regardless of race, gender, income level, or social class" (CDC, 2020, para. 2). Rose admits to struggles with addiction to prescription opioid pain pills, which were first prescribed to her at 17 years of age after an anterior cruciate ligament (ACL) surgery. Rose was raised by a single mother, and she moved frequently from one apartment to another. She explains she was exposed to substance abuse early in her life, and she suffered from verbal, physical, and sexual abuse when she was growing up. When she began taking prescription opioid medication after her surgery, she discovered it took away both her physical pain and her emotional pain. She increased her dosage and was able to secure prescription pain relievers from friends after her prescription ran out. Rose's mother discovered her daughter's addiction a year later and found her help. At the age of 18 years, Rose began going to a methadone clinic, a treatment facility for people addicted to opioid drugs, where she began taking a daily dose of methadone, a medication used in medication-assisted treatment (MAT) to help people reduce or quit their use of heroin or other opiates. The treatments helped Rose make lifestyle changes, move away from her hometown, and stay clean for 7 years. After moving back to her hometown 3 years ago, Rose succumbed to addiction again. Rose substituted her previous opioid pain pills to now using heroin because it was cheaper and easier to get. Two years later, with threats from her mother, Rose returned to the methadone clinic for treatments with hopes of getting and staying clean. She stayed clean for 2 years but relapsed once again. During her relapse, Rose discovered she was pregnant and immediately stopped using heroin but continued taking methadone. Rose moved in with her mother and has continued to stay clean.

When Rose went to her first prenatal doctor appointment, she met with a social worker who encouraged her to participate in Healthy Beginnings Plus (HBP), a Pennsylvania state program that assists low-income, pregnant women in meeting their psychosocial and medical needs so they can have positive prenatal experiences. Participants in the program have a dedicated interprofessional care team that includes a doctor or certified nurse midwife, nurse care coordinator, social worker, lactation support, and a registered dietician. Rose was leery about social workers, and worried that she would lose custody of her baby, so she never enrolled.

Rose was maintained on the drug methadone, a medication approved by the Food and Drug Administration (FDA) to treat OUD, throughout her pregnancy. She has a 9-month-old daughter, Hope, who was born with neonatal abstinence syndrome (NAS), a group of problems that occur as the result of exposure to opioid drugs in the womb. Problems may include the following withdrawal symptoms: tremors, seizures, fussiness, fever, breathing problems, stuffy nose or sneezing, diarrhea, poor feeding skills, and trouble sleeping. Hope and her family received care from physicians, nurses, occupational therapists, physical therapists, and social workers during her 6-week admission stay to the neonatal intensive care unit (NICU).

Rose worried the hospital staff would be judgmental because she was a mother on methadone. She was all too aware of the stigma, or negative attitudes and discrimination, associated with addiction. Rose was relieved to discover a warm and supportive staff who had received training about OUD and NAS, and said she really appreciated how they treated her and her baby without judgment.

Rose lives with her mother and her maternal grandfather. She explained that their relationship has been strained since her teenage years but is getting better now that she is clean and has a baby. She has one good friend who also recently had a baby. Rose says Hope's father, whom she is no longer with, has been fading from the picture. Rose had to quit her job because she could not find affordable childcare for Hope. Rose's mom works several jobs, and her grandfather's health is failing so he is unable to care for a baby.

The same social worker Rose met at her first prenatal visit showed up at Rose's first postnatal doctor visit and provided more details about the HBP program. The social worker explained that the program was offering a free weekly group program for new mothers struggling with OUD who are in a **MAT** program, a holistic treatment approach that combines medication with counseling and behavioral therapies. A team, including a nurse navigator, social worker, and recovery specialist, provide the women with the tools they need to maintain recovery, keep their children safe, and promote healthy families. Rose was thrilled to discover she could bring her daughter, who would be watched and cared for by volunteers. Rose has not missed a week and says attending the community-based meetings has made a huge difference in her life. Rose said, "This is the first time in my life I have ever felt truly supported, or ever felt like I was even a part of a community. I have learned so much about myself, about my baby, about how to be a strong family. Hope has weekly early intervention services with an occupational therapist who comes into my home and coaches my mom, my grandpa, and me about what we can do to support Hope's development. I don't know where I would be without having these people from the community in my corner."

Reflective Questions

1. How might your personal feelings about maternal opioid addiction and NAS affect your thoughts and actions if you were to be assigned to work with this client?
2. What are the unique contributions your profession can make to the health care team working with Rose and Hope?
3. Thinking about all the members of the health care team mentioned in the case study, what are their roles in the context of this case study? Discuss any potential interprofessional overlap.

Introduction

In order to optimize family health outcomes, practitioners need to appreciate and integrate the diversity of the twenty-first-century family structure and culture into their practice. Adults, typically the leaders of families, play important roles in family health regardless of the family structure. As leaders, adult family members are responsible for promoting the health and well-being of their families, which ultimately impacts family health outcomes. "Health has a particular value for individuals because it is essential to an individual's well-being and ability to participate fully in the workforce and a democratic society" (Braveman et al., 2011, p. 149). The Healthy People Initiative, released by the U.S. Department of Health and Human Services (HHS), has set national objectives for health promotion and disease prevention each decade since 1980. One of the overarching goals of Healthy People 2030, which applies to families, is the promotion of "healthy development, healthy behaviors, and well-being across all life stages" (Office of Disease Prevention and Health Promotion [ODPHP], n.d.a). Research supports the belief that the health of an individual family member can affect overall family health and wellness, as well as the health of the community in which they live (Barnes et al., 2020). Furthermore, family health has the best opportunity to thrive when the communities that surround them are health conscious. It is important to empower adult family members so they can be active participants in promoting the health and well-being of their families.

Adults Defined

Adults have traditionally been defined as people between 18 and 65 years of age (Arnett et al., 2014); however, age-based norms have been changing (Silva, 2012) and vary across and within cultures (Arnett, 2016). Definitions of adulthood have shifted over the course of time.

Emerging adulthood is a newer term used to describe a period of development from the ages of either 18 to 25 years of age (Arnett & Mitra, 2018), 18 to 29 years of age, (Barlett et al., 2018) or 19 to 25 years of years (Krettenauer et al., 2016). Emerging adulthood is considered the stage of life that begins at the end of adolescence and ends at the start of young adulthood. According to Arnett (2015), emerging adulthood is represented by five characteristics: identity exploration, self-focus, instability, optimism and feeling of possibilities, and feeling in-between. Arnett (2000) describes individuals in the stage of emerging adulthood as people who no longer consider themselves to be adolescents, yet they do not consider themselves to be full-fledged adults (Professional Reasoning Box A).

Young adulthood is a term used to describe the period of development from the ages of 26 to 45 years of age (Krettenauer et al., 2016) and is the stage of adulthood that follows emerging adulthood. This is typically the stage of adulthood when individuals either marry for the first time or cohabitate with a significant other and establish themselves as part of a new family. In 2020, the U.S. Census Bureau (USCB) determined that the estimated median age to marry, 30.5 years for men and 28.1 years for women (USCB, 2020a), occurs during this stage of adulthood. The mean age for women to give birth and become first-time mothers also occurs in this stage of adulthood and was 26.3 years in 2014 (Mathews & Hamilton, 2016).

Middle adulthood is a term used to describe the period of development from the ages of 40 to 64 years of age (Lodi-Smith et al., 2017) or 46 to 65 years of age (Krettenauer et al., 2016). This is the stage of adulthood when family structures change, and transitions occur. This is often the time of grandparenthood and the time when family members become part of the sandwich generation, a term used to describe adults who are caring for both elderly parents and their own children.

Professional Reasoning Box A

Maria and Edward have been happily married for 30 years. They have three grown daughters, all of whom join them for a weekly Sunday dinner. The family of five recently started planning a camping trip that will include their daughters' significant others.

How do family relationships impact individual family members' health and well-being across the life course?

Professional Reasoning Box B

Justin and George recently adopted Justin's 3-year-old nephew, after Justin's sister died from a drug overdose. They live on the third floor of a subsidized apartment building with several adult extended family members. Justin, his nephew, and George are sharing a bedroom. The closest neighborhood park is six blocks away and the playground equipment is broken and unsafe.

How is family health affected by the community in which they live?

Families in the Twenty-First Century

Adults, as leaders of families, are important members of the interprofessional health care team. The team must recognize that the concept of family is unique to different individuals and to different families. Family relationships impact an individual's health and well-being across their life span. The twenty-first-century family is much more diverse than in the past, in both structure and process. The 2020 U.S. Census defines **family** as a "group of two or more people (one of whom is the householder) related by birth, marriage, or adoption and residing together; all such people (including related subfamily members) are considered as members of one family" (USCB, 2020b, para. 15). A **householder** refers to the "adult or adults in whose name the housing unit is owned or rented (maintained) or, if there is no such person, any adult member. The person designated as the householder is the "reference person" to whom the relationship of all other household members, if any, is recorded" (USCB, 2020b, para. 26)). A **family household** is a "household maintained by a householder who is in a family (as defined earlier), and includes any unrelated people (unrelated subfamily members and/or secondary individuals) who may be residing there" (USCB, 2020b, para. 17). Cohabitation, or living together in the same household as unmarried partners, has become an increasingly popular alternative to marriage. Health benefits can come from peers, not just partners or spouses. Close friendships can have positive influences on health and well-being (Chopik, 2017).

Family living arrangements are much more diverse now than in previous decades. Family diversity refers not just to structural differences (e.g., single-parent, two-parent, divorced), but also to racial, ethnic, socioeconomic, generational, cultural, spiritual, gender, and sexual orientation differences. Research supports the fact that family forms and family homes do look different today than in the past. Although two-parent households continue to be most common, the percentage dropped from 88% in 1960 to 69% in 2016 (USCB, 2019a). Other common living situations include a child living with a single mother (23%), a single father (4%), and neither parent (4%; Livingston, 2020). The percentage of married households that are interracial or interethnic grew across the United States from 7.4% in the year 2000 to 10.2% between the years 2012 and 2016 (USCB, 2019b). The number of cohabitating partners living in the United States increased significantly from 6 million to 17 million in the last two decades (USCB, 2020a). According to the U.S. Census, there are nearly 1 million U.S. households with same-sex partners, with 58% being married and 42% unmarried (USCB, 2020d). Another trend that continues to increase in the twenty-first century includes grandparents who are taking active roles in helping to raise their grandchildren.

In order to support families, there must be an understanding that families can function effectively regardless of differences in their structure and process. Family forms do not necessarily influence or predict health outcomes for family members. A study that compared different-sex couples who are married and cohabitating, single parents who are divorced or never married, and same-sex couples suggested that the physical health of a child related more to demographic and socioeconomic differences than to being a part of a specific family form (Cenegy et al., 2017). Being sensitive to family diversity and **family dynamics**, or the patterns of interactions among family members will allow for members of the interprofessional care team to build on a family's strengths to promote their health, well-being, and quality of life (QOL; Professional Reasoning Box B).

Role of Adults in Family Health

Regardless of family structure, adults may occupy many roles in the context of their families. These roles change throughout the life span, with the acquisition of new roles and the loss of old roles. The American Occupational Therapy Association (AOTA) defines **roles** in the *Occupational Therapy Practice Framework: Domain and Process, Fourth Edition* (*OTPF-4*) as follows:

> For persons: "Sets of behaviors expected by society and shaped by culture and context that may be further conceptualized and defined by the client."
>
> For groups and populations: "Sets of behaviors by the group or population expected by society and shaped by culture and context that may be further conceptualized and defined by the group or population." (AOTA, 2020, p. 82)

Roles of family members are revealed in occupations. Participation in daily occupations is fundamental for all individuals and has a positive effect on health and well-being. An **occupation** is defined as "everyday personalized activities that people do as individuals, in families, and with communities to occupy time and bring meaning and purpose to life" (AOTA, 2020, p. 79). Adult occupations include **instrumental activities of daily living** (IADLs), "activities that support daily life within the home and community" (AOTA, 2020, p. 30) such as taking care of others, child rearing, communication management, driving and community mobility, financial management, home establishment and management, meal preparation and cleanup, and shopping. Occupations also include rest and sleep, education, work, leisure, and social participation. An important adult occupation is **health management**, which includes "activities related to developing, managing, and maintaining health and wellness routines, including self-management, with the goal of improving or maintaining health to support participation in other occupations" (AOTA, 2020, p. 32).

Family roles are often based on individual family members' positions within the family. The establishment of clearly defined roles and role expectations promote healthy family functioning. Adult roles may include, but are not limited to, spouse, partner, friend, parent, caregiver, household manager, volunteer, and worker. Adults, as leaders of families, take on multiple roles including the role of primary decision makers. The decisions they make can determine whether or not stable, secure, and nurturing family environments and relationships are established. Adults are responsible for other family members' development and/or sustaining other members' physical and emotional health, well-being, and QOL. The establishment and identification of an adult health care leader role, or family health manager role, will help guide an interprofessional team of health care providers in offering appropriate supports that can promote family health.

Consider Rose in her new role as a mother and caregiver of a child born with NAS. She is the primary decision maker for her daughter, Hope. She is responsible for not only her own health and wellness but for her daughter's as well. She is also maintaining the role of daughter and granddaughter. Rose has taken on many new demands in her roles and occupations, in addition to losing the role of worker, having had to quit her job because she could not find affordable childcare for Hope. Multiple demands can lead to role overload and occupational overload, which can have a negative effect on health and well-being and can affect family relationships.

Family Relationships

Family relationships influence the health, well-being, and QOL of both the family and individual family members. As family relationships change over the life span, family dynamics change, which can impact the overall health and wellness of a family. The World Health Organization (WHO) defines **health** as "a state of complete physical, mental and social well-being and not merely the absence of disease or infirmity" (WHO, n.d., para. 1). **Well-being** is defined as a "general term encompassing the total universe of human life domains, including physical, mental, and social aspects, that make up what can be called a 'good life'" (AOTA, 2020, p. 84). **QOL** is the "dynamic appraisal of life satisfaction (perception of progress toward identifying goals), self-concept (beliefs and feelings about oneself), health and functioning (e.g., health status, self-care capabilities), and socioeconomic factors (e.g., vocation, education, income)" (AOTA, 2020, p. 82).

Healthy family relationships require reciprocity and reciprocal relationships are associated with health benefits. "Reciprocal relationships support people with empowering feelings, such as love, empathy and resemblance, and give them strength to be loyal. Reciprocal relationships strengthen one's overall well-being and give meaning to one's life" (Törrönen et al., 2017, p. 40). The quality of family relationships affects the health and well-being of family members. Family members are inextricably linked to each other, and the social connections and influences continue throughout all stages of life (Umberson et al., 2010). Happy marriages, for example, lead to better mental and physical health for adults (Umberson et al., 2010). Parenthood has its own health benefits. Adult children influence the social connections of their parents, throughout their life span, and often take on the role of caregivers for their aging parents (Umberson et al., 2010).

Strong relationships promote family resiliency. **Resilience** is defined as "the capacity of a dynamic system to adapt successfully to disturbances that threaten its function, viability, or development" (Masten, 2014, p. 10). The family is a dynamic system. Adults, who assume the roles of leaders and family health managers, are responsible for providing positive environments and relationships, which can

Professional Reasoning Box C

An occupational therapist, who is working with the family of a toddler diagnosed with cerebral palsy, is reviewing outcomes and strategies written on the Individualized Family Service Plan (IFSP) with the toddler's mother. The occupational therapist became defensive when the mother shared how happy she was that the physical therapist helped explain her toddler's sensory processing issues at yesterday's therapy visit. The occupational therapist felt as if sensory processing was her profession's turf.

How is this an example of an interprofessional collaboration blind spot, and what does this mean?

foster resilience and promote healthy outcomes for families. Healthy families make efforts to overcome life's adversities that requires resilience. Healthy families also recognize when they need assistance and accept help. Consider Rose's family relationships: Rose's mother, who assumed the role of health manager, sought out assistance and accepted help from community resources, which led to improved family health outcomes for her daughter. Rose followed the example set by her mother and took on the role of health manager for herself and her own daughter (Professional Reasoning Box C).

A relationship with one stable, supportive, and caring adult could promote positive health outcomes for a child (Center on the Developing Child at Harvard University, 2021). Research supports the fact that supportive adult relationships are important for all children, especially those who have experienced hardships, because they serve as a buffer from developmental delays and help children build resilience and recover from these hardships (National Scientific Council on the Developing Child, 2018). Consider how these relationships illustrate the cyclical nature of health and wellness. The relationships adult family members have with their children may influence their children's future adult health. Childhood experiences, both adverse and positive, can affect a child's future family health during adulthood.

Just as **adverse childhood experiences** (ACEs) are linked to negative health outcomes in adulthood (Chang et al., 2019), **positive childhood experiences** (PCEs) are associated with positive mental and relational health in adults (Bethell et al., 2019). ACEs are defined as "potentially traumatic events that occur in childhood (0 to 17 years)" (CDC, 2021, para. 1). These events may include experiencing or witnessing violence, abuse or neglect; experiencing a family member attempt or die by suicide; growing up in a household with substance abuse or mental health problems; exposure to instability as the result of parental separation or household members being in prison (CDC, 2021). PCEs are defined as "essential, interrelated experiences that engage the child, the parent, and the parent-child relationship in order to achieve the designated child health outcomes" (Sege & Harper Brown, 2017, p. 81). PCEs are organized into four broad categories:

> (a) being in nurturing, supportive relationships; (b) living, developing, playing, and learning in safe, stable, protective, and equitable environments; (c) having opportunities for constructive social engagement and to develop a sense of connectedness; (d) learning social and emotional competencies. (Sege & Harper Brown, 2017, p. 81)

Findings from a study by Bethell et al. (2019) suggest that exposure to PCEs may lead to positive mental and relational health in adulthood, even when they co-occur with ACEs. Furthermore, their findings support the idea that families can adapt to and overcome adversities and develop resilience when they experience positive environments and relationships, which ultimately leads to optimal health outcomes in adulthood (Bethell et al., 2019).

Role of Community in Family Health

A healthy family establishes links with the community in which they live, and these communities affect the health and well-being of individual family members and family units living there. A **community** is "a collection of populations that is changeable and diverse and includes various people, groups, networks, and organizations" (AOTA, 2020, p. 75). The health of a community can influence the health of a population. A population refers to an "aggregate of people with common attributes such as contexts, characteristics, or concerns including health risks" (AOTA, 2020, p. 81). The health of a community and its members is influenced more by lifestyle and environment than actual health care. Health care accounts for only 10% to 20% of health outcomes for a population. The other 80% to 90% is attributed to **social determinants of health** (SDOH) , or health-related behaviors, and socioeconomic and environmental factors (Hood et al., 2016). The health of family members, families, and communities is influenced by the environment in and around their community, a place where people live, work, grow, learn, and age.

Health is community driven. The health of a community influences the health and well-being of all family members (ODPHP, n.d.b). This cyclical nature of health and wellness between families, communities, and populations occurs across the life span. The health of families is essential to the health of communities, and of the population. Furthermore, the health of a community influences the health of families living in those communities. A foundational principle that guides decisions about the Healthy People 2030 Framework is that "the health and well-being of all people and communities is essential to a thriving, equitable society" (ODPHP, n.d.a, para. 4). The Healthy People Initiative was created as a national health promotion and disease prevention program. The initiative has been updated every decade since its inception in 1980. *Healthy People 2030* continues to promote public awareness of SDOH, as it is recognized that economic stability, education, health and health care, neighborhood and built environment, and social and community context have a major impact on a family member's health, well-being, and QOL (ODPHP, n.d.a).

Socioeconomic status (SES), the combination of an individual or family's social and economic status, has an influence on the physical health and well-being of families. Health can improve through lifestyle choices, such as participating in physical activity, increasing social interactions, and engaging in stress management skills (Wang & Geng, 2019). Families who fall into the range of lower SES may require more assistance in removing barriers that interfere with their ability to achieve and maintain healthy lifestyles. Barriers might include lack of transportation, low health literacy, and accessibility of safe housing, healthy food, quality education, and quality health care. Noted health disparities exist for families whose SES falls in the lower range (Dankwa-Mullan & Pérez-Stable, 2016). Providing stable housing to families with lower SES has been found to improve overall health outcomes and decrease health care costs (Taylor, 2018). It is important that all families have access to quality health care and have the opportunity to participate in community programs that promote healthy lifestyles.

Place-based approaches to support adults and their families focus on entire communities, and look to remove neighborhood barriers like poor housing, social isolation, limited services, and limited economic opportunities (Centre for Community Child Health, 2011). Place-based approaches can build healthier communities by keeping families and communities more engaged and connected to each other. Examples of healthy communities are those that have places for families to engage in healthy lifestyles. According to Dankwa-Mullan and Pérez-Stable (2016), "Place is characterized by structural resources such as schools, hospitals, recreational facilities, retail outlets, and housing. Healthier places have health-promoting environments such as parks, safe walking spaces, maintained homes, full-service food stores, and environmental protection" (p. 637). When a community can offer these places as resources for adults and their families, it can improve their health outcomes, and in turn, they may be more likely to offer something back to their community.

Resilience, discussed earlier in the chapter, refers to the way a dynamic system adapts successfully to adversity. A community, like a family, is a dynamic system. **Community Health Resilience** (CHR) is defined as "the ability of a community to use its assets to strengthen public health and health care systems and to improve the community's physical, behavioral, and social health to withstand, adapt to, and recover from adversity" (U.S. Department of Health and Human Services [USDHHS], 2015, para. 1). Resilient communities lead to healthy communities where adults and their families are supported, connected to each other, and have equal access to both quality health care and healthy living resources (USDHHS, 2015). Strong, healthy communities promote strong, healthy families. Consider Rose's community and how it contributed to her resilience. The same social worker who Rose met at her first prenatal visit revisited Rose at her first postnatal doctor visit to share information about community-based resources that would meet Rose's family's needs. This continuity of care increased Rose's trust with the social worker and gave her confidence to rebuild her life with the support she was being offered by her community. Rose was able to connect to other mothers struggling with OUD and receive free childcare while receiving the support she needed to achieve and maintain her health, well-being, and QOL.

Evidence-Based Practice in the Health Promotion of Families

Evidence-based practice (EBP) integrates research outcomes with health care practitioners' clinical expertise and clients' preferences, beliefs, and values (AOTA, n.d.a). Health care professionals use a variety of evidence-based theories (systems of ideas intended to explain something), models (representations of theories), and frameworks (tools to guide actions and support clinical reasoning during the assessment and intervention process) in practice.

A classification system that provides a standardized interprofessional language through a biopsychosocial framework for the description of health and health-related states, the *International Classification of Functioning, Disability and Health* (ICF), was developed by the WHO (2001). The ICF does not focus on an individual's disability. Instead, it considers how the individual or family can function and perform in society, regardless of a disability or health condition. The ICF can be used to promote family health by including family priorities and goals.

Instead of focusing on what the individual or family cannot do, the ICF looks at the strengths and potentials for that individual and family. The standardized language of the ICF promotes interprofessional communication and allows

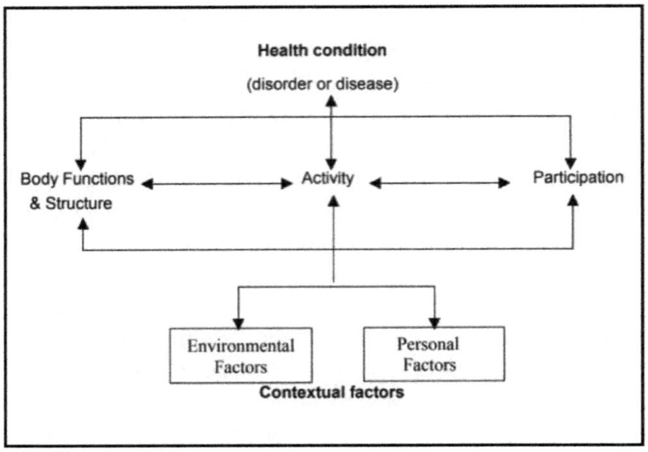

Figure 17-1. Interactions between the components of ICF. (Reproduced with permission from the World Health Organization. [2001]. International Classification of Functioning, Disability and Health. http://apps.who.int/iris/bitstream/10665/43737/1/9789241547321_eng.pdf)

for greater interprofessional collaboration in family assessments and interventions (WHO, 2001). The ICF diagram is a useful health promotion tool and can be used for both individual family members and entire families. It is separated into two parts; one part identifies function and disability such as body functions and body structures, activities, and participation. The second part identifies contextual factors such as environmental and personal constructs. Figure 17-1 illustrates the interactions between components of the ICF. According to the WHO (2001), the three dimensions of disability are impairments in body functions or body structures (e.g., vision loss, loss of the use of one's limb, depression); activity limitations (e.g., difficulty in the execution of a task like seeing or walking or driving or taking the bus), and participation restrictions in meaningful life situations (e.g., going on family hikes, going to work, cooking dinner for the family, providing care to family members). Contextual factors include environmental factors (e.g., the physical terrain, social attitudes, and social structures) and personal factors (e.g., age, coping styles, education, and employment; WHO, 2001).

The Family Systems Theory views the family as an emotional unit and suggests that individual family members are so interconnected, they are unable to separate themselves from this emotional unit (Bowen, 1993). Bowen contends that each family member plays a different role and follows certain rules, thus a change in one family member's functioning leads to reciprocal changes in the functioning of other family members. This theory focuses on what is happening in the family's present state instead of focusing on what happened in the past, and attention is placed on identifying and interrupting negative behavioral exchanges (Johnson & Ray, 2016). Consider Rose's family dynamics. In order for Rose to stay in recovery and continue to live with her mother, she must get and stay connected with healthy relationships at home and in the community, and she must embrace a healthier lifestyle.

An interprofessional team that uses the Family Resilience framework is invested in the well-being of at-risk adults and children and recognizes that life challenges affect the family unit (Walsh, 2016). Family resilience, a family's ability to withstand and bounce back from adversity, stronger and more resourceful than they were before, is at the core of this model (Walsh, 2016). Walsh emphasizes that a family-centered care approach is the key to reducing dysfunction and promoting resilience. Walsh (2016) explains:

> In facing adversity, the family approach and response are crucial for resilience. Key processes enable the family to rally in highly stressful times to reduce the risk of dysfunction and to support positive adaptation. Although some families are more vulnerable or have experienced severe trauma or persistent hardships, a family resilience perspective is grounded in a deep conviction in their potential for repair and growth. (p. 617)

The family resilience framework includes nine key processes organized into three domains of family functioning (Walsh, 2016). The three domains are family belief systems, organizational processes, and communication processes. Each domain includes three key interactive processes. The belief system domain includes making meaning of adversity; positive outlook; and transcendence and spirituality. The organizational processes domain includes flexibility; connectedness; and mobilization of social and economic resources. The communication process domain includes clarity; open emotional sharing; and collaborative problem solving (Walsh, 2016). Using this framework aids in identifying individual family strengths and values, which can ultimately help foster resilience when a family is faced with adversity (Walsh, 2016).

Consider Rose's situation. Rose has experienced stress and adversity throughout her life. One must endure stress or adversity before one can develop resilience, and before one can learn how to make positive adaptations (Windle, 2011). Applying the Family Resilience framework to practice can inform and guide the interprofessional team, during assessments and interventions, in order to promote optimal health outcomes for Rose and her family.

A **family-centered care** framework is an approach where all members of the family are engaged in health care decisions. It emphasizes a partnership approach to the decision making between the health care providers and the family (Institute for Patient and Family-Centered Care, n.d.). In families with children, it recognizes the adults (parents or caregivers) as the primary decision makers for the family. This approach to assessment and intervention helps to establish mutual trust and respect between health care professionals and the family. It considers how family members interact within the family unit and as a family unit within the community. An interprofessional care team must individualize services based on the unique needs of the family (regardless of race, ethnicity, and cultural background), must demonstrate flexibility in when and where services are provided, and be sensitive to the needs of each family member and family unit. A family-centered care approach recognizes this interdependence of family members, builds on the family's strengths, and promotes the health and well-being of the whole family. Consider Rose, who now lives at home with her mother, grandfather, and daughter. The interprofessional team involved in her care used a family-centered care approach. This approach included all members of the family, and provided services in clinics, in the community, and in Rose's home.

Assessment

Family-centered practice begins with evaluating a family's occupational participation in the context of their life. Evaluation and assessment provide members of the health care team with the valuable information they need to determine a family's health needs. Evaluation refers to "the comprehensive process of obtaining and interpreting the data necessary to understand the person, system, or situation. Evaluation requires synthesis of all data obtained, analytic interpretation of that data, reflective clinical reasoning, and consideration of occupational performance and contextual factors" (AOTA, 2020, p. 76).

Each initial client evaluation begins with the completion of an occupational profile, followed by an analysis of occupational performance. An occupational profile is a tool used by occupational therapists that summarizes a client's "occupational history and experiences, patterns of daily living, interests, values, needs, and relevant contexts" (AOTA, 2020, p. 80). Other professions may have narratives or past medical histories of people that inform them of who the person is in order to provide client-centered care. This profile helps a provider determine what it is the client wishes to do but has difficulty doing, as well as the strengths of the person to promote health and well-being. The information gathered in an occupational profile will assist providers in choosing appropriate assessment tools. It should be noted that, in a family-centered approach, the family is considered the client. Therefore, the occupational profile is suited to be used as a family-centered evaluation tool.

An assessment is "a specific tool, instrument, or systematic interaction ...used to understand a client's occupational profile, client factors, performance skills, performance patterns, and contextual and environmental factors, as well as activity demands that influence occupational performance" (AOTA, 2020, p. 74). According to the American Physical Therapy Association (APTA), "Physical therapist services include the use of assessments to identify the presence of risk factors, and cognitive and environmental barriers and opportunities that may be targets for health promotion activities" (p. 3). Social workers use assessments to address the needs of families. Social workers who practice in health care settings include the entire family in screenings and assessments in order to develop evidence-informed family care plans based on each family's unique needs (NASW, 2016).

Assessments must address more than just physical aspects of health. They must also address other dimensions that could be interfering with a client's health, well-being, or QOL. When completing a family assessment, regardless of the health care provider's discipline, it is important to move beyond an assessment form and engage family members in ongoing, individualized discussions that pertain to their unique situations.

Family-centered assessments determine the family's strengths, needs, interests, concerns, and priorities. Information gathered from family health assessments will generate information about family structure and function, both of which are needed to establish a family's health status and plan appropriate interventions. The use of comprehensive, standardized family assessments can be used as a guide for intervention planning. Although there is no single assessment tool that works for every family, there are many possible assessments that can be used to determine a family's strengths and needs.

According to the Comprehensive Family Assessment Guidelines, a Comprehensive Family Assessment is often used by social workers and it must be completed collaboratively with the family. A Comprehensive Family Assessment focuses

> not only the presenting issues at a specific time, but also the underlying causal factors for behaviors and conditions affecting children. A comprehensive family assessment also includes evaluation of contributing factors such as family history, domestic violence, substance abuse, mental health, chronic health problems, and poverty. In addition, the family's strengths and protective factors are assessed to identify resources that can support the family's ability to meet its needs and better protect the children. (National Child Welfare Resource Center for Family-Centered Practice, 2005, p. 5)

The Family Assessment Device (FAD) is a self-report measure of perceived family functioning. This assessment, which can be administered to family members age 12 years and older, is used to identify families who are experiencing problems, identify specific domains in which families are experiencing problems, and it can be used to assess changes after interventions (Family assessment device, 2018). The FAD is based on the McMaster Model of Family Functioning (MMFF), and it consists of six scales that assess the six dimensions of the MMFF. These dimensions include affective involvement, affective responsiveness, behavioral control, communication, problem solving, and roles. A seventh scale measures general family functioning. This assessment includes 60 statements about a family, and individuals are required to rate how well each statement describes their own family; higher scores indicate poor levels of family functioning (Child Welfare Information Gateway, n.d.).

QOL assessments measure family members' well-being and satisfaction with life. The WHO QOL (WHOQOL) assesses family members' QOL within the context of their family's culture, value systems, goals, standards, and priorities (WHO, n.d.). Two versions, the WHOQOL-100 and the WHOQOL-BREF are available and can be either self-administered or interview-administered for adolescents and adults. The WHOQOL-100 generates scores related to specific features of QOL (e.g., positive feelings, social support, financial resources), scores relating to larger domains (e.g., physical, psychological, social relationships) and a score related to overall health and QOL. The WHOQOL-BREF generates domain scores, but not specific individual scores. Both assessments can be used, at no cost, in a variety of cultural settings (WHO, n.d.).

Motivational interviewing is an approach to care where the therapist determines an individual's readiness to change, provides personalized health education to meet the individual's identified needs and learning styles, and empowers that individual to be a more active participant in the management of their health. Empowering adults and their families with the tools they need to successfully engage in meaningful occupations, improve family relationships, and decrease stress will lead to improved health, well-being, and QOL. Consider Rose and what seemed to help make her ready for change. When she became pregnant, she was willing to stop using drugs and was willing to accept support from her mother. When she had her baby, she was willing to trust and accept support from the social worker. Rose's readiness to change seemed to be linked to her pregnancy and the birth of her child.

Evidence-based health care professionals who wish to promote family health, well-being, and QOL must first identify appropriate assessments that identify family strengths and needs, thus equipping them with the information needed to create successful family-centered interventions that include preventive services and health promotion.

Intervention

Health care professionals use information gathered through evaluations and assessments to select interventions best suited to meet the unique needs and improve outcomes for clients. These interventions, plans based on results of the assessments, are created to promote the health and well-being of individual family members, entire families, and the communities in which they live. Interventions can be incorporated into the family's routine and can also provide new structure for the family while making adjustments for new roles and expectations, in order to promote the health and well-being of everyone in the family. In order to be effective, intervention approaches must focus on the family unit. It is important to recognize the family's strengths and resources, instead of focusing on the family's problems, when developing interventions. Just as family-centered practice begins with evaluating a family's occupational participation in the context of their life, interventions must also consider contextual factors. **Context** includes the environment and the people in that environment. "Parent and family contextual factors are often defined as characteristics of parents' social, psychological, or intellectual functioning as well as parental attitudes, behaviors and competencies and family dynamics and context" (Baker-Ericzén et al., 2010, p. 397).

A holistic approach to interventions, which includes all aspects of a person's life and lifestyle, is most useful for best practice and family-centered care. Health promotion is a prevention strategy that helps individual family members and families improve their overall health. Occupational therapists, physical therapists, social workers, along with many other disciplines, are well suited to offer health promotion services to adults and their families, and both disciplines espouse positions supporting their roles in health promotion. The AOTA's Fact Sheet states:

> The path to health and well-being is intricately linked to participating in daily occupations. Occupational therapy focuses on enabling clients to maximize their capacity to participate in life activities that are important and meaningful to them, to promote overall health and wellness. (AOTA, n.d.b)

The APTA states:

> Physical therapists play a unique role in society in prevention, wellness, fitness, health promotion, and management of disease and disability by serving as a dynamic bridge between health and health services delivery for individuals and populations. This means that although physical therapists are experts in rehabilitation and habilitation, they also have the expertise and the opportunity to help individuals and populations improve overall health and avoid preventable health conditions. (n.d.a)

The National Association of Social Workers (NASW) states:

> Social workers have a responsibility to advocate for the needs and interests of clients and client support systems. Social workers in health care settings serve as client advocates by promoting client access to health care, identifying and removing barriers to services delivery, and helping clients navigate between and among complex health and social services systems. Social workers also strive to promote clients' self-advocacy skills and to enhance the capacity of communities to support clients' biopsychosocial–spiritual quality of life. (2016, p. 29)

Interventions must build upon a family's internal interactions between family members and external interactions

Professional Reasoning Box D

WHY UNDERSTANDING THE ROLE OF THE ADULT IN FAMILY HEALTH IS IMPORTANT

- Adults, who serve as family health care managers, play an essential role in the promotion of family health,
- Family-centered care has been associated with better health care outcomes, well-being, and QOL,
- The promotion of community-based interventions and partnerships improves health at the community level,
- Establishing meaningful therapeutic relationships and partnering with adults, their families, and community organizations to promote health has the potential to improve family well-being, QOL, and reduce the overall cost of health care.

within its community (Hanson & Lynch, 2013). This approach to intervention, which considers a family's values, beliefs, spirituality, ways of life, and social environment allows a family to be more actively engaged in decision making and intervention services. This approach also leads to a more individualized and flexible delivery of family-centered intervention services (Hanson & Lynch, 2013). Health begins at home. Health behaviors are learned, developed, maintained, and changed at home; focusing on family systems, instead of individual family members, may lead to improved health outcomes in individuals, families, and communities (Garcia-Huidobro, 2015). Since family members are so interconnected, supportive family-centered interventions could lead to positive health outcomes for all members of a family.

Consider Rose's situation. Her addiction harms not only her health and well-being, but that of her family. Addressing her addiction requires implementation of effective intervention strategies that provide structure, setting her up for success for her new roles. Intervention strategies might include educating Rose and her family by promoting healthy lifestyle practices, helping Rose and her family develop strategies that will produce behavior changes to improve health, self-esteem, more independence, and collaborating with the community to identify and/or establish accessible resources for health and wellness. Professionals who work with individuals and families struggling with substance abuse or addiction must remain empathetic and nonjudgmental. Addiction affects both the body and the mind, so an interprofessional approach to treatment, one that views the individual and family from a holistic lens, is essential. Intervention strategies to promote a healthy lifestyle might include exercise therapy, massage, meditation, and mindfulness practice. Evidence supporting occupational therapy and physical therapy in the treatment of addiction has gained momentum within the last decade. "Occupational therapy is uniquely positioned to assist people who are struggling to recover from substance abuse, by helping them to reestablish the roles and identities most meaningful to them" (Opp, n.d.). The profession of physical therapy is also well-suited to become a member of an interprofessional addiction treatment team. Physical therapy is known to help individuals reduce pain and stress, but the profession's ability to engage clients in effective motivational interviewing, can lead to client's having an expectation of improvement (APTA, 2018). The NASW (2013) states:

> Social work practice is in a unique position to influence the delivery of services by addressing the acute and chronic needs of clients with SUDs, including co-occurring disorders and polysubstance patterns. By developing and applying evidence-informed approaches that incorporate established interventions and evolving techniques based on emerging research findings, social workers can markedly improve treatment services for clients and their families. (p. 6)

Interprofessional Perspectives

Interprofessional collaboration (IPC) , a practice that happens when health care providers from different professional backgrounds work together with individuals, families, and communities to deliver high quality of care, is essential in order to assist and empower adults and their families to assume control of their health, well-being, and QOL. Each member of the interprofessional health care team works together, contributing their unique practice skills, to promote health outcomes for all members of families. The ultimate goal of interprofessional collaboration is to collectively assist the client and family in making the lifestyle changes they need to, want to, and agree to make (Garcia-Huidobro, 2015).

According to the WHO, "collaborative practice in health-care occurs when multiple health workers from different professional backgrounds provide comprehensive services by working with patients, their families, carers and communities to deliver the highest quality of care across settings" (2010, p. 13). Families are best served by an interprofessional health care delivery model that supports this collaborative practice. Each member of the interprofessional team will have specialized disciplinary knowledge relevant to the health care situation, which will help guide collaborative, informed health care decisions during the assessment process. Holistic health and wellness assessments, which should focus not only on identifying problems but on identifying strengths, provide the interprofessional health care team with the information they need to provide culturally sensitive, evidenced-based interventions that promote health and wellness for families (Professional Reasoning Box D).

Interprofessional collaboration is thought to lead to improved patient outcomes and quality of care. The Interprofessional Education Collaborative (IPEC) focuses on the Triple Aim of improving population health, enhancing patient experiences, and reducing health care costs (IPEC, 2016). Health care professionals from two or more disciplines must collaborate and focus on four core competencies (IPEC, 2016, p. 10):

1. Work with individuals of other professions to maintain a climate of mutual respect and shared values
2. Use the knowledge of one's own role and those of other professions to appropriately assess and address the health care needs of the patients and populations served
3. Communicate with patients, families, communities, and other health professionals in a responsive and responsible manner that supports a team approach to the maintenance of health and the treatment of disease
4. Apply relationship-building values and principles of team dynamics to perform effectively in different team roles to plan and deliver patient-/population-centered care that is safe, timely, efficient, effective, and equitable

Barriers to IPC might include lack of awareness of one another's professional roles and areas of expertise, lack of information sharing, and lack of interprofessional training. Interprofessional blind spots and professional turf wars can arise without proper interprofessional education and training. Consider Rose's interprofessional health care team and how they collaborated successfully on these four core competencies to assess, intervene, and promote positive health outcomes for Rose and her family.

Community Programs

Community programs, also considered place-based interventions, are interventions that take place in communities or neighborhoods, and are meant to support adults and their families by improving life opportunities and promoting positive health outcomes. The goal of educational and community-based programs is to "increase the quality, availability, and effectiveness of educational and community-based programs designed to prevent disease and injury, improve health, and enhance quality of life" (ODPHP, 2021). Consider the community-based programs available to Rose. These family-centered programs were easily accessible and aimed to improve both Rose's health and the health of her family.

HBP is a Pennsylvania program that assists low-income, pregnant women who are eligible for Medical Assistance, a program that pays for health care services for eligible individuals (Pennsylvania Department of Human Services, n.d.). The aim of this program is to meet the unique, individualized medical and psychosocial needs of pregnant and parenting women, and ensure that women have a healthy pregnancy and that their babies have a good start in life. Rose was referred to the program offered through HBP, which is paid for by Medicaid and supports and empowers pregnant and parenting women who are in MAT. Rose was able to meet and develop trusting relationships with other moms and counselors during weekly meetings. Rose thrived in this environment, attributing her ability to stay in recovery to her participation in this program. The HBP care team relied on interprofessional collaboration between doctors or midwives, nurses, social workers, and counselors.

Pregnant and parenting women who have been identified as needing substance use interventions are referred to the RASE Project for Recovery Support Services. The vision of the RASE Project is "To provide innovative, quality services; reduce the stigma associated with Substance Use Disorder (SUD); and enhance the recovery process by weaving authenticity, dignity, passion and integrity throughout every aspect of the organization" (n.d., para. 1). Rose participated in this community-based program and was assigned a drug addiction counselor who completed an assessment, created a recovery plan, helped Rose in developing a positive support network and a set of skills needed to maintain recovery, and made referrals to appropriate health care providers. Rose credits her RASE counselor with helping her to maintain a healthy, drug-free lifestyle.

Rose and her daughter, Hope, who was exhibiting mild developmental delays, participated in an Early Intervention (EI) program, which provided state funded, family-centered support in the home. EI includes family-centered services and supports that are available to babies and young children with developmental delays and disabilities and their families (CDC, 2019). EI services may include speech therapy, physical therapy, and other services based on the needs of the child and family. These services provide families the skills they need to overcome challenges and promote positive health outcomes, well-being, and QOL for families.

Conclusion

Family health begins at home. Family relationships play a crucial role in shaping an individual family member's health and well-being across the life span. Adults, as leaders and managers of family health, are responsible for promoting and maintaining the health of themselves and their families. Family health is influenced by the individual family members as well as the communities in which they live. In this chapter, the authors described many ways to understand families in context. These included a discussion of the different stages of adulthood and the role adults play in family health. This was followed by a discussion about the twenty-first-century family and how the definition of family is unique to individual family members and families. In addition, several family-centered theories, models, and frameworks were explored as the foundation for family assessments and interventions. Finally, the authors discussed how family health has the potential to flourish in strong communities. Successful interprofessional collaboration of health care providers and community collaborators can promote positive lifestyle changes that will improve health, well-being, and QOL for families and communities.

Reflective Questions

1. What are the three stages of adulthood and what typically occurs during these stages?
2. What are social determinants of health and why is it important for members of the health care team to address them?
3. What are the four interprofessional core competencies?
4. How have twenty-first-century families changed and why is it important for health care providers to recognize, understand, and support the twenty-first-century family?
5. Why is the community important to the health of a family?

References

American Occupational Therapy Association. (n.d.a). https://www.aota.org/Practice/Health-Wellness/Evidence-Based.aspx

American Occupational Therapy Association. (n.d.b) Occupational therapy's role in health promotion. https://www.aota.org/~/media/Corporate/Files/AboutOT/Professionals/WhatIsOT/HW/Facts/FactSheet_HealthPromotion.pdf

American Occupational Therapy Association. (2020). *Occupational therapy practice framework; Domain and process* (4th ed.).

American Physical Therapy Association. (n.d.a) Physical therapists' role in prevention, wellness, fitness, health promotion, and management of disease and disability. https://www.apta.org/apta-and-you/leadership-and-governance/policies/pt-role-advocacy

American Physical Therapy Association. (n.d.b) Standards of practice for physical therapy. https://www.apta.org/siteassets/pdfs/policies/standards-of-practice-pt.pdf

American Physical Therapy Association. (2018, July 2). 2018 NEXT: Physical therapy can play a part in addiction treatment. https://www.apta.org/news/2018/07/02/2018-next-physical-therapy-can-play-a-part-in-addiction-treatment

Arnett, J. J. (2000). Emerging adulthood: A theory of development from the late teens through the twenties. *American Psychologist, 55*(5), 469-480. https://doi.org/10.1037/0003-066X.55.5.469

Arnett, J. J. (2015). Emerging Adulthood: *The winding road from the late teens through the twenties*. Oxford University Press.

Arnett, J. J. (2016). Life stage concepts across history and cultures: Proposal for a new field on indigenous life stages. *Human Development, 59*(5), 290-316. https://doi.org/10.1159/000453627

Arnett, J., & Mitra, D. (2018). Are the features of emerging adulthood developmentally distinctive? A comparison of ages 18–60 in the United States. *Emerging Adulthood, 8*(5), 412-419. https://doi.org/10.1177/2167696818810073

Arnett, J. J., Žukauskienė, R., & Sugimura, K. (2014). The new life stage of emerging adulthood at ages 18–29 years: Implications for mental health. *The Lancet Psychiatry, 1*(7), 569-576. https://doi.org/10.1016/s2215-0366(14)00080-7

Baker-Ericzén, M.J., Jenkins, M.M., & Brookman-Frazee, L. (2010). Clinician and parent perspectives on parent and family contextual factors that impact community mental health services for children with behavior problems. *Child Youth Care Forum, 39*, 397-419. https://doi.org/10.1007/s10566-010-9111-9

Barlett, C., Barlett, N., & Chalk, H. (2018). Transitioning through emerging adulthood and physical health implications. Emerging Adulthood, 8(4), 297-305. https://doi.org/10.1177/2167696818814642

Barnes, M., Hanson, C., Novilla, L., Magnusson, B., Crandall, A. & Bradford, G. (2020). Family-centered health promotion: Perspectives for engaging families and achieving better health outcomes. *INQUIRY: The Journal of Health Care Organization, Provision, and Financing, 57*, 4695802092353-46958020923537 https://doi.org/10.1177/0046958020923537

Bethell, C., Jones, J., Gombojav, N., Linkenbach, J., & Sege, R. (2019). Positive childhood experiences and adult mental and relational health in a statewide sample. *JAMA Pediatrics, 173*(11), e193007-e193007. https://doi.org/10.1001/jamapediatrics.2019.3007

Bowen, M. (1993). *Family therapy in clinical practice*. Jason Aronson.

Braveman, P., Kumanyika, S., Fielding, J., LaVeist, T., Borrell, L., Manderscheid, R., & Troutman, A. (2011). Health disparities and health equity: The issue is justice. *American Journal of Public Health, 101*(S1), S149-S155. https://doi.org/10.2105/ajph.2010.300062

Cenegy, L. F., Denney, J. T., & Kimbro, R. T. (2017). Family diversity and child health: Where do same-sex couple families fit? *Journal of Marriage and Family, 80*(1), 198-218. https://doi.org/10.1111/jomf.12437

Center on the Developing Child at Harvard University. (2021). Three principles to improve outcomes for children and families, 2021 update. http://www.developingchild.harvard.ed

Centers for Disease Control and Prevention. (2019, December 9). What is "early intervention" and is my child eligible? https://www.cdc.gov/ncbddd/actearly/parents/states.html

Centers for Disease Control and Prevention. (2020, October 22). Opioid overdose prevention saves lives. https://www.cdc.gov/drugoverdose/pubs/featured-topics/substance-abuse-prevention-awareness.html

Centers for Disease Control and Prevention. (2021, April 6). Preventing adverse childhood experiences. https://www.cdc.gov/violenceprevention/aces/fastfact.html

Centre for Community Child Health, The Royal Children's Hospital Melbourne. (2011). Place-based approaches to supporting children and families (Policy Brief 23). https://www.rch.org.au/uploadedFiles/Main/Content/ccch/Policy_Brief_23_-_place-based_approaches_final_web2.pdf

Chang, X., Jiang, X., Mkandarwire, T., & Shen, M. (2019). Associations between adverse childhood experiences and health outcomes in adults aged 18-59 years. *PLOS ONE, 14*(2), e0211850. https://doi.org/10.1371/journal.pone.0211850

Child Welfare Information Gateway. (n.d.). Comprehensive family assessment guidelines. https://www.childwelfare.gov/pubPDFs/family_assessment_23.pdf

Chopik, W. J. (2017), Associations among relational values, support, health, and well-being across the adult lifespan. *Personal Relationship, 24*, 408-422. https://doi.org/10.1111/pere.12187

Dankwa-Mullan, I., & Pérez-Stable, E. (2016). Addressing health disparities is a place-based issue. *American Journal of Public Health, 106*, 637-639. https://doi.org/10.2105/AJPH.2016.303077

Family Assessment Device. (2018). The National Child Traumatic Stress Network. https://www.nctsn.org/measures/family-assessment-device

Garcia-Huidobro, D. (2015). Family oriented care: Opportunities for health promotion and disease prevention. *Journal of Family Medicine and Disease Prevention, 1*(2). https://doi.org/10.23937/2469-5793/1510009

Hanson, M. J., & Lynch, E. W. (2013). *Understanding families: Supportive approaches to diversity, disability, and risk.* Brookes Publishing.

Hood, C., Henusso, K., Swain, G., & Catlin, B. (2016). County health rankings: Relationships between determinant factors and health outcomes. *American Journal of Preventive Medicine, 2*, 1290135. https://doi.org/10.1016/j.amepre.2015.08.024

Institute for Patient and Family-Centered Care. (n.d.) Patient- and family-centered care defined. https://www.ipfcc.org/bestpractices/sustainable-partnerships/background/pfcc-defined.html

Interprofessional Education Collaborative. (2016). Core competencies for interprofessional collaborative practice: 2016 update. https://hsc.unm.edu/ipe/resources/ipec-2016-core-competencies.pdf

Johnson, B., & Ray, W. (2016). Family Systems Theory. In *Encyclopedia of family studies* (pp. 1-5). John Wiley & Sons. https://doi.org/10.1002/9781119085621.wbefs130

Krettenauer, T., Murua, L., & Jia, F. (2016). Age-related differences in moral identity across adulthood. *Developmental Psychology, 52*(6), 972-984. https://doi.org/10.1037/dev0000127

Livingston, G. (2020, May 30). The changing profile of unmarried parents. Pew Research Center. https://www.pewresearch.org/social-trends/2018/04/25/the-changing-profile-of-unmarried-parents/

Lodi-Smith, J., Spain, S., Cologgi, K., & Roberts, B. (2017). Development of identity clarity and content in adulthood. *Journal of Personality and Social Psychology, 112*(5), 755-768. https://doi.org/10.1037/pspp0000091

Masten, A. S. (2014). Global perspectives on resilience in children and youth. *Child Development, 85*, 6-20. https://doi.org/10.1111/cdev.12205

Mathews, T. & Hamilton, B. (2016). Data Briefs—Number 232—January 2016. https://cdc.gov. https://www.cdc.gov/nchs/products/databriefs/db232.htm.

National Association of Social Workers. (2016). *NASW standards for social work practice in healthcare* Settings. Author.

National Association of Social Workers . (2013). *NASW standards for social work practice with clients with substance use disorders.* Author.

National Child Welfare Resource Center for Family-Centered Practice (2005). Comprehensive Family Assessment Guidelines. Children's Bureau. https://www.acf.hhs.gov/sites/default/files/documents/cb/family_assessment.pdf

National Scientific Council on the Developing Child. (2018). Center on the Developing Child at Harvard University. https://developingchild.harvard.edu/science/national-scientific-council-on-the-developing-child/

Office of Disease Prevention and Health Promotion. (n.d.a). Healthy People 2030 framework. Healthy People 2030. U.S. Department of Health and Human Services. https://health.gov/healthypeople/about/healthy-people-2030-framework

Office of Disease Prevention and Health Promotion. (n.d.b). Social determinants of health. Healthy People 2030. U.S. Department of Health and Human Services.https://health.gov/healthypeople/objectives-and-data/social-determinants-health

Office of Disease Prevention and Health Promotion. (2021, June 23). Educational and community-based programs. Healthy People 2020. https://www.healthypeople.gov/2020/topics-objectives/topic/educational-and-community-based-programs

Opp, A. (n.d.). *Recovery with purpose: Occupational therapy and drug and alcohol abuse.* American Occupational Therapy Association. https://www.aota.org/About-Occupational-Therapy/Professionals/MH/Articles/RecoveryWithPurpose.aspx

Pennsylvania Department of Human Services. (n.d.) Healthy Beginnings Plus. https://www.dhs.pa.gov/providers/Providers/Pages/Medical/Healthy-Beginnings.aspx

Rase Project, The. (n.d.). A recovery community organization. https://raseproject.org/

Sege, R. D., & Harper Browne, C. (2017). Responding to ACEs with HOPE: Health outcomes from positive experiences. *Academic Pediatrics, 17*(7), S79-S85. https://doi.org/10.1016/j.acap.2017.03.007

Silva, J. M. (2012). Constructing adulthood in an age of uncertainty. *American Sociological Review, 77*(4), 505-522. https://doi.org/10.1177/0003122412449014

Taylor, L. (2018, June 7), Housing and health: An overview of the literature. Health Affairs. https://www.healthaffairs.org/do/10.1377/hpb20180313.396577/full/

Törrönen, M., Munn-Giddings, C., & Tarkiainen, L. (2017). *Reciprocal relationships and well-being: Implications for social work and social policy.* Routledge.

Umberson D., Pudrovska T., & Reczek C (2010). Parenthood, childlessness, and well-being: A life course perspective. *Journal of Marriage and Family, 72*, 612-629. https://doi.org/10.1111/j.1741-3737.2010.00721.x

U.S. Census Bureau. (2019a). Majority of children live with two parents. https://www.census.gov/library/stories/2017/08/majority-of-children-live-with-two-parents.html

U.S. Census Bureau. (2019b). Race, ethnicity and marriage in the United States. https://www.census.gov/library/stories/2018/07/interracial-marriages.html

U.S. Census Bureau. (2020a). New estimates on America's families and living arrangements. https://www.census.gov/newsroom/press-releases/2020/estimates-families-living-arrangments.html

U.S. Census Bureau. (2020b). Subject definitions. https://www.census.gov/programs-surveys/cps/technical-documentation/subject-definitions.html#family

U.S. Census Bureau. (2020d). U.S. Census Bureau releases CPS estimates of same-sex households. https://www.census.gov/newsroom/press-releases/2019/same-sex-households.html

U.S. Department of Health and Human services. (2015, June 9). Community resilience. https://www.phe.gov/Preparedness/planning/abc/Pages/community-resilience.aspx

Walsh, F. (2016). Applying a family resilience framework in training, practice, and research: Mastering the art of the possible. *Family Process, 55*(4), 616-632. https://doi.org/10.1111/famp.12260

Wang, J., & Geng, L. (2019). Effects of socioeconomic status on physical and psychological health: Lifestyle as a mediator. International *Journal of Environmental Research and Public Health, 16*(2), 281. https://doi.org/10.3390/ijerph16020281

Windle, G. (2011). What is resilience? A review and concept analysis. *Reviews in Clinical Gerontology, 21*(2):152-169.

World Health Organization. (n.d.). The World Health Organization Quality of Life (WHOQOL). https://www.who.int/publications/i/item/WHO-HIS-HSI-Rev.2012.03

World Health Organization. (2001). *International classification of functioning, disability and health*. http://apps.who.int/iris/bitstream/10665/43737/1/9789241547321_eng.pdf.

World Health Organization. (2010). Framework for Action on Interprofessional Education and Collaborative Practice. https://apps.who.int/iris/handle/10665/70185

CHAPTER 18

Promoting Family Health
Older Adults

Andrea Gossett Zakrajsek, OTD, OTRL, FNAP
and Elizabeth Oates Schuster, MSW, PhD

Learning Objectives

At the end of this chapter, the reader will:

1. Describe social and cultural contexts and factors that influence families that include older individuals (ACOTE B.3.1, B.5.1)
2. Understand the unique needs presented by diverse populations and people within families and implications for interprofessional practice (ACOTE B.5.21)
3. Apply interdisciplinary theoretical concepts to the understanding of families with older adults and community-based practice (ACOTE B.3.1)
4. Appraise key issues that impact families with older adults, that include grandparents raising grandchildren, caregiving, and care transitions to community-based settings (ACOTE B.4.23, B.5.2)
5. Identify community-based programs and services that support older persons within family systems and relevant to interprofessional practice collaboration (ACOTE B.4.10, B.4.25, B.4.27)
6. Reflect upon the lived experiences of families that include older adults through interaction with a case study of a three-generational family. (ACOTE B.4.2)
7. Develop collaborative practices as health care professionals with older adults, families, and other health care professionals (ACOTE B.4.10, B.4.20, B.4.25, B.4.26)

The ACOTE Standards used are those from 2018.

Pizzi, M. A., & Amir, M. (Eds.). *Interprofessional Perspectives for Community Practice: Promoting Health, Well-Being, and Quality of Life* (pp. 343-360).

Key Words

Family, Family Life Cycle, Life Course Perspective, Grandparents Raising Grandchildren, Custodial Grandparents, Family Caregiving, Primary Caregivers, Secondary Caregivers, Caregiver Intensity, Care Transitions

Charlie Case: Part A

Charlie is a 72-year-old man who retired 10 years ago as a sales representative for a construction company that sold equipment to contractors. Charlie was diagnosed with irregular heartbeat, arrhythmia, when he was in his mid 60s. This condition resulted in the implant of a pacemaker that has helped him to function normally, although he does experience bouts of fatigue. During his early years of retirement, he enjoyed golfing with his former coworkers and participated in his church, serving food for events and greeting parishioners before services on Sundays. He was married in his 20s and has three adult children, two daughters and a son, and five grandchildren whom he describes as his "pride and joy." Eight years ago, Charlie's wife was diagnosed with breast cancer, and he became her primary caregiver as her health declined and she ultimately died. This loss deeply impacted him emotionally and he still misses his wife's companionship. His wife's death made it necessary for Charlie to learn how to do many household chores such as cooking, laundry, and shopping, and he still golfs occasionally. In recent years, Charlie has become very close to his daughters, who live in the same city. In addition, he has begun taking care of their children after school, eating dinner with them, and attending various events. His son lives in a different state but each year the two take an annual fishing trip to upstate Michigan.

DISCUSSION QUESTIONS

1. Describe the family life cycles that have taken place in Charlie's life with his family.
2. Identify meaningful occupations and activities in which Charlie engages. How has that changed over the past 10 years?
3. What are some of the key events that have impacted Charlie's life course?
4. Considering the five distinctive themes of the life course perspective (personal biography and social history; human agency and self-regulation; historical time and place; timing in lives; and linked lives) identify where two of the themes are occurring within the Charlie case.

Introduction

Older adults and their families often have complex, varied, and challenging issues and concerns that require an interprofessional and multifaceted approach to generating solutions at individual, community, and systems levels (Charlie Case: Part A). This chapter will describe relevant contributions from the interdisciplinary fields of gerontology and others that shape our understanding of older individuals within families, present current trends in the sociocultural influences on families with older adult members, promote and describe community-based programs and services that address concerns of families with older adults, and reflect upon the need for an interprofessional approach to address the needs of this population. The lived experience of a three-generational family will be woven throughout the chapter to provoke thoughts and ideas about older adults and families, formulate collaborative assessment and intervention strategies, and apply theory to practice.

Theoretical and Social Constructs Informing the Understanding of Families

To begin, it is important to understand the concept of **family**. Family theorists suggest that families are social groups that have key distinguishing characteristics. First, they exist for a considerably longer period of time than other social groups, such as co-workers and close friends, in that membership can be involuntary and oftentimes lifelong. Second, families are intergenerational, existing as a rare social group that spans large age differences. Third, they can contain both biological and affinal relationships between members (e.g., connected by marriage, adoptions, or other arrangements) and, fourth, these relationships link them to larger kinship groups (e.g., extended families; White et al., 2019).

It must also be recognized that family composition is impacted by societal and cultural influences. Current trends indicate that a number of factors, such as lower fertility, higher rates of childlessness, changes in traditional family structures, and increases in divorce and never-married status may result in smaller families (National Academies of Sciences, Engineering, and Medicine, 2016). Furthermore, a reduction in available caregivers through these population trends, in particular fewer adult children and spouses, presents a challenge to care of older adults who experience disability, impairment, and participation issues with age. Sociocultural influences, such as race, ethnicity, gender, LGBTQ status, socioeconomic status, immigrant, and culturally displaced families, greatly impact the choices and access to resources of families that include older adults (Dilworth-Anderson et al., 2004).

In addition, families are not a stagnant entity; rather, the **family life cycle** is reflective of developmental stages and shifts in the make-up of families over time. Carter and McGoldrick (1988) present six stages of the family life cycle, emphasizing that these stages are not chronologically determined but are reflective of stages of family systems:

1. Leaving home—single young adults (accepting emotional and financial responsibility for self)
2. Joining of families through marriage—new couple (commitment to new system)
3. Families with young children (accepting new members into the system)
4. Families with adolescents (increasing flexibility of family boundaries to include children's independence)
5. Launching children and moving on (accepting many exits and entrances into the family system)
6. Families in later life (accepting shifting of generational roles)

Disruptions within the family life cycle, access to services, and diminished choices among families with older adults all provide opportunities for program development and intervention by community-based practitioners to promote health and well-being.

Life Course Perspective

By what road did you arrive where you are?
Florida Scott-Maxwell (1968)

It is useful to consider the health and participation of older adults and their families within the gerontology **life course perspective**. This interdisciplinary perspective provides a context for understanding the life situations of clients who are served by community-based practitioners. The life course, which is understood as a perspective rather than a theory, involves an ongoing interpretive process and provides a lens through which to view and better understand the human experience. By viewing the lived experience through the life course lens there is a realization that no one exists in a vacuum. Instead, there are multiple interdependent and interlocking pathways and various life trajectories, such as family, education, and work pathways, which are interwoven into what may be described as a life tapestry (Elder, 1994). Trajectories tend to be long in scope and exist within the spheres of education, family, work, and leisure. Embedded within these trajectories are short-term transitions that happen gradually and are typically tied to the acquisition or relinquishment of roles (graduation, retirement). Events also occur along trajectories and are often abrupt and a one-time occurrence (such as a sudden death of a parent or winning the lottery). Transitions and events provide meaning and distinction within the trajectories (Elder, 1974, 1985; Elder & Johnson, 2003; Mortimer & Shanahan, 2003; Quadagno, 1999; Settersten, 2002). In understanding the life course perspective, it is useful to reflect on your own life course. Please see the Appendix A for questions to guide your personal reflection and application.

The life course perspective encompasses five distinctive themes: *personal biography and social history*; *human agency and self-regulation*; *historical time and place*; *timing in lives*; and *linked lives*. It is important to note that the themes may be applied to individuals, a family unit, a community, society, and to institutions such as schools and governments (Elder, 1994). In this discussion, the themes are being applied primarily to the individual's experience.

The interweave of *personal biographies and social histories* creates the life course tapestry, which involves textures, colors, hues, and the subtleties and forms patterns that become more clear and visible throughout the life developmental process of aging. Multiple aspects of life development contribute to these patterns including race, ethnicity, culture, gender, sexual orientation, social class, and birth cohort. These are all threads of the life course tapestry that are affected by previous cohorts and by the unfolding of history within an individual's lifetime (Elder, 1985; Moen et al., 1995).

Human agency and self-regulation refers to the act of decision making. These decisions are the building blocks of the life course and are influenced by the timing of decisions and by personal histories and experiences. Importantly, they are deeply impacted by the interpretation of the choices that have been made. When people are young, most of the big decisions in their lives are made for them (e.g., where a child lives and goes to school). As individuals move through the developmental process, they gain autonomy and the ability to make their own choices. In adulthood, the decisions that are made through human agency often affect not only the individual making those decisions but all of those whose lives are linked with that individual (Elder, 1994; Settersten, 2002, 2005).

The *historical events and conditions* of an individual's lifetime and of previous cohorts powerfully shape a person's own life course and worldview. The events of previous and current generations influence how persons interpret their

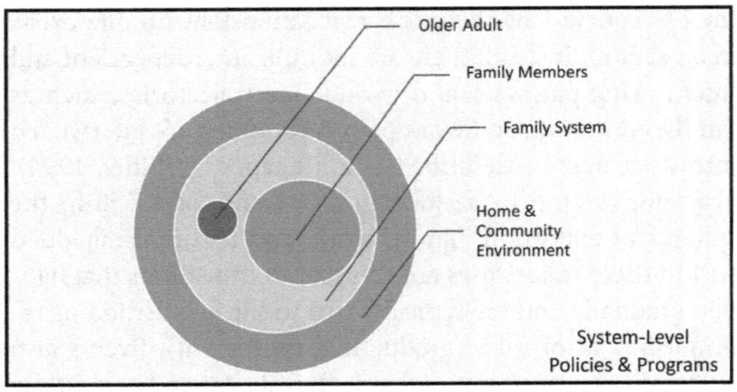

Figure 18-1. Considerations for assessment for older adults and families for community-based practice.

lives (Settersten, 2002, 2005). For example, if persons of various ages and backgrounds are asked to describe what it was like to live through the COVID-19 pandemic, a wide range of interpretations and what it meant to them personally would be expressed based on a number of factors including age, health, and well-being, and the availability and accessibility of support and resources, to name a few.

The *timing in lives* refers to biological and social transitions. Some typical biological time markers that may be socially and culturally embedded include the timing of puberty, childbirth, and menopause. Various events can disrupt what is a socially and culturally acceptable time marker, although these expectations have greatly relaxed over the last few decades (Elder, 1974, 1994). Examples of not conforming to societal expectations may be entering college in mid-life, becoming pregnant in early teens, and retiring in one's 40s. Another example is the impact the age in which individuals enlisted into service during World War II had on normal life development. Those who enlisted in their 30s vs. those who enlisted in their teens or 20s experienced a comparatively wide range of disruptions of multiple life course trajectories due to significant interruptions of career and family pathways.

The fifth theme of *linked lives* points to the fact that all family members are interconnected and interdependent. How one person in a family reacts and interprets a particular historical or personal event or role transition affects the development of all of the family members both within and across generations (Settersten, 2002). For example, an adult child's decision to have a child in their teens would immediately result in significant role changes and role additions as that person becomes a parent and her parent becomes a grandparent. The person becoming a grandparent did not choose this transition and may not feel ready for this responsibility at this stage in their lives. This example also reflects many of the life course themes discussed above. Please see the Charlie Case: Part A to apply the theoretical constructs discussed in this chapter to develop your understanding of families with older adults.

Identifying Issues in Families That Include Older Adults: Implications for Community-Based Assessment

As intergenerational, oftentimes involuntary and lifelong social groups, families change and morph over time as members age, develop, and are added. All family systems are complex; however, families that include older adult members provide distinct circumstances, challenges, and characteristics that are important for community-based professionals to understand and consider for practice. As community-based practitioners identify issues that impact health and participation of older adults and their families, it is important to consider the older adult and family members (e.g., grandchildren, children, siblings, informal caregivers) that make up a family system, as well as the home and community environment in which the family engages and the system-level policies and programs that impact families (Figure 18-1).

Furthermore, when creating an assessment plan for older adults and their families, it is important for community-based practitioners to consider many areas of assessment that may reflect their own professional perspective as well as assessments that other professionals in an interprofessional team can bring to a collective understanding of health and participation. Please see Table 18-1 for areas to assess when evaluating health and participation in older adults and their families.

System-level policies and programs that are available to older adults and their family are very important for interprofessional practitioners to consider as part of the assessment, intervention, and referral process in community-based practice. Furthermore, community-based practitioners have a critical role in identifying the needs of their clients (older adults and families) within populations they serve and advocating for, developing, and evaluating these system-level interventions. Oftentimes, system-level policies and programs are created and implemented to address specific family situations. The next section will describe key family situations that include older adults and discuss implications for community-based practice intervention in individual older adult–level, family-level, and population-level policies and programs.

Table 18-1

Assessments Available to Understand Health and Participation of Older Adults Within Families

AREAS TO ASSESS IN FAMILIES WITH OLDER ADULTS	EXAMPLES OF TYPES OF ASSESSMENTS*	SOURCES
Health status	Medical history, heart rate, blood pressure, hearing and vision screens, pain, balance and gait, strength, range of motion, fall risk, cognition (e.g., Observation and interview, Lighthouse Acuity Chart, Wong-Baker Pain Rating Scale, Berg Balance Test, Activity-Specific Balance Confidence Scale, Montreal Cognitive Assessment [MoCA])	Berg et al. (1995) Nasreddine et al. (2005) Powell & Myers (1995) Wong-Baker (2018)
Psychosocial status	Depression, anxiety, QOL, well-being (e.g., Geriatric Depression Scale, Zung Self-Rating Anxiety Scale (SAS), 36-Item Short-Form Health survey (SF-36), Zarit Burden Interview)	Brink et al. (1982) Hays et al. (1995) Zarit & Zarit (1983) Zung (1971)
Social support and family relationships	Social support and capital assessments (e.g., Interpersonal Support Evaluation List, Interview Schedule for Social Interactions, Lubben's Social Network Scale, Perceived Social Support for Caregivers and Social Conflict Scales)	Cohen et al. (1985) Goodman (1991) Henderson et al. (1980) Lubben (1988)
Activities of daily living (ADLs; e.g., bathing, dressing, toileting, eating)	Functional performance in ADLs (e.g., Functional Independence Measure [FIM], Barthel ADL Index, Performance Assessment of Self-Care Skills [PASS])	Collin et al. (1988) Dodds et al. (1993) Mahoney & Barthel (1965) Rogers & Holm (1989)
Instrumental activities of daily living (IADLs) (e.g., grocery shopping, laundry, housework, money management)	Functional performance in IADLs (e.g., Test of Grocery Shopping Skills, Lawton-Brody IADL Scale)	Brown et al. (2009) Graf (2008)
Driving and transportation management	Driving assessments, access to public transportation	Dickerson (2013)
Home accessibility and safety	Home safety and accessibility assessments (e.g., AARP Home Safety Checklist, Safety Assessment of Function and the Environment for Rehabilitation [SAFER Tool])	AARP (2009) Letts & Marshall (1995)
Community accessibility and safety	Community safety and accessibility assessments (e.g., Community Integration Measure, Community Participation Indicators, Late-Life Function and Disability Instrument)	Heinemann et al. (2011) Jette et al. (2002) McColl et al. (2001) Willer et al. (1993)

*These are not all encompassing but are included to provide a sample of options of assessments useful to understand key issues of older adults in their families.

Family Situations That Include Older Adults and Implications for Community-Based Practice

This chapter focuses on three major types of family situations that include older adults: grandparents raising grandchildren, caregiving, and care transitions. With these three types of family situations, community-based practice interventions will be discussed at the population level (i.e., policy and advocacy), family level, and older adult level. The Charlie case will be woven throughout this discussion in order to support the reader to apply concepts to consider as a community-based practitioner.

Grandparents Raising Grandchildren

Grandparents raising grandchildren is a unique family situation in which older adults play a vital role. It has been estimated that nationally, over 7 million grandparents are living with their grandchildren and about 2.7 million grandparents are "grandparent caregivers," whereby grandparents are primarily responsible for the needs of grandchildren under the age of 18 years (Ellis & Simmons, 2014). Furthermore, approximately 6 million children are cared for by a grandparent either full- or part-time in the United States (Generations United, 2015). Households with grandparents and grandchildren can include various arrangements, including 1) multigenerational households in which a grandparent may serve in supportive roles to the parent-child relationship or in a co-parenting role; 2) grandparent-maintained households where biological parents may or may not be living in the home and likely variations of parental involvement over time; and 3) skipped generation households where the parent generation is not present (Baker et al., 2008; Ellis & Simmons, 2014; Hayslip et al., 2019).

Those households with **custodial grandparents**, where grandparents are legally responsible for grandchildren, include grandparents who are typically under the age of 65 years, female, and heterogeneous in terms of race, ethnicity, LBGT grandparents, and rural/suburban/urban geographical location (Hayslip & Kaminski, 2005; Ellis & Simmons, 2014). However, Black individuals have a higher chance of becoming custodial grandparents and keeping their grandchildren in their homes longer and Mexican American grandparents who live below the poverty line are twice as likely to become grandparents raising grandchildren (Hayslip, et al., 2019). Grandparent raising grandchildren households make up a higher percentage of low-income households yet receive lower amounts of public assistance, experience difficulty obtaining health insurance for grandchildren, and are more likely to have inadequate housing conditions, including overcrowding (Baker et al., 2008; Hayslip et al., 2019). Oftentimes, children come under grandparent's care as a result of a family crisis and are more likely to have suffered a history of abuse, neglect, instability, and/or loss due to death, which may result in behavioral and/or emotional issues (Fruhauf et al., 2015; Hayslip et al., 2019; Sampson & Hertlein, 2015). Grandparents raising grandchildren tend to have lower rated health and well-being, higher level of physical health problems, and lower levels of mental health when compared to grandparents who are not raising grandchildren (Baker & Silverstein, 2008; Leder et al., 2007). Furthermore, grandparents raising grandchildren report conflict and strained relationships between themselves and adult children, strains on family social, financial and temporal resources, and difficulty managing multiple roles, including work (Leder et al., 2007; Sampson & Hertlein, 2015). It is important to recognize that the health of these grandparents is complex and can change over time. In research using National Health and Retirement Study data, Baker and Silverstein (2008) found that grandparents who recently began raising grandchildren reported lower levels of well-being than their counterparts but that grandparents with a longer history of raising grandchildren seem to experience increased well-being.

Despite the challenges faced by families in which grandparents are raising their grandchildren, many benefits exist. Baker et al. (2008) acknowledge the societal benefit of this family situation in that grandparent provided care is a public good, as they offer a preferable placement for children in the child welfare and foster care systems, and economic burden shifts from the government to families. Benefits to grandparents who are raising their grandchildren include maintaining close relationship with their grandchildren, having a sense of purpose in life, contributing to a family's sense of well-being, and having a "second chance" at parenting (Hayslip & Kaminski, 2005; Hayslip et al., 2019). There are also obvious benefits to grandchildren in this situation, as they receive familial care when parents are not physically or emotionally present.

Considering these benefits and challenges, community-based practitioners from various professional backgrounds have a critical role in maintaining the health and well-being of families that include grandparents raising grandchildren through the development of interventions at the population, family, and older adult levels. At a policy level and service access level, it is critical that grandparents raising grandchildren have access to financial and health resources regardless of custodial status (Baker et al., 2008; Chan et al., 2019). For example, programs such as the National Family Caregiver Support Program created out of the Older American's Act offer benefits to grandparents and other relatives raising children under the age of 18 years, yet carer age requirements and other eligibility parameters limit the provision of needed services. Furthermore, grandparents experience barriers in accessing services even if they are eligible. In a qualitative study of service providers to grandparents raising grandchildren, needed services to families included navigation within and between systems, such as that of a Kinship Care System Navigator, referral, counseling, education of benefits and legal issues, and assistance with completing paperwork (Fruhauf et al., 2015). Community-based interventions that target grandparents raising grandchildren are necessary to support the health, wellness, and quality of life (QOL) of both the grandparent and grandchildren within families. Specifically, social and educational components of grandparents raising grandchildren interventions suggest increases in social support and parentings skills while decreasing behavioral issues in children in these situations (Chan et al., 2019). As grandparents raising grandchildren encounter professionals in community-based settings, it is clear these professionals need to be prepared to meet the unique challenges confronting these families (Charlie Case: Part B). Please see Appendix B to reflect on needs and program development for grandparents raising grandchildren.

Charlie Case: Part B

Charlie and his daughter, Claire, have an especially close relationship. They have learned to rely on one another in recent years. Claire is a 47-year-old woman who is employed full time as a director of a nonprofit organization. She works long hours managing the organization, which oftentimes includes participating in fundraising events in the evenings. In addition, she has three teenage children, daughters aged 12 and 15 years, and a son who is in his first year of college. Charlie's granddaughters are involved in sports and after school activities, and the 12-year-old granddaughter has struggled academically in the past. Around the time Claire's mother passed away, she and her husband were separated and later divorced. The children primarily live with Claire and spend some weekends and holidays with their father. Charlie has increasingly become involved in the care of his grandchildren, assisting with homework after school, transporting them to and from various school and social activities, and attending sports events. Some of these responsibilities can become fatiguing for Charlie due to the cardiac issues he experiences. He has also expressed to his primary care physician that at times he feels overwhelmed but does not want to tell Claire, as he knows she relies on him, and he enjoys being needed by his family.

DISCUSSION QUESTIONS

1. Identify the benefits for Charlie's role in caring for his grandchildren: to Charlie, his daughter, Claire, and the grandchildren.
2. What are some barriers Charlie experiences while assisting his daughter in raising his grandchildren?
3. What community-based services or supports might be useful to Charlie and his family that you might provide, from your professional perspective? What might other professionals provide?

Caregiving of Older Adult Family Members

Family caregiving, or informal care, is defined as providing assistance and support to family members without payment (Behr & Tebb, 2016). Various types of caregiving relationships can take place in families that include older adults: spousal, adult child, or other relative caregiving of an older adult, older adults taking care of adult children with disabilities, and older adults taking care of parents and children at the same time (e.g., sandwich generation). Furthermore, two types of family caregivers have been identified: primary and secondary. **Primary caregivers**, typically spouses or daughters, provide the greatest number of hours per week of care and make major decisions regarding the older family member's care and treatment. **Secondary caregivers**, who are often men and nonrelatives, provide fewer hours of care and function more as supplemental care providers in such areas as financial support, home repairs, and yard work (although there has been a recent noticeable increase in the involvement of male caregivers; National Academies of Sciences, Engineering, and Medicine, 2016; Wolff et al., 2018).

Diversity of Family Caregivers

Approximately 30% of family caregivers of older adults self-identify as a racial/ethnic minority. It is expected that this percentage will increase in the future as the older adult population becomes more diverse (Rote et al., 2019). In fact, a significant increase among all racial and ethnic groups is predicted. For example, by 2050 Black older adult populations will quadruple, Hispanic and Asian American older adult populations will increase to 7 times their current number, and the older adult Native American population will increase 3.5 times (Dilworth-Anderson, et al., 2002).

Racial and ethnic older adults are generally poorer than their White counterparts. Households headed by older White people had a median net worth four and half times that of households headed by older Black individuals (Periyakoil, 2019). White older adults report more physical activity and lower levels of chronic diseases, such as hypertension and diabetes, than most racial and ethnic older adults, including Black, Asian American, and Hispanic populations (Periyakoil, 2019). The implications are that over the next few decades racial and ethnic families will be experiencing an increased need to provide caregiving for older family members. Further, it is clear that these responsibilities, due to the chronic nature of the older adults' conditions and the underuse of formal support systems, will grow in complexity and intensity.

There is a dearth of research available on LGBTQ people providing care for an older adult (Grossman et al., 2007) and the literature on the caregiving experience across this population is limited. What is known is that the caregiving experience for the LGBTQ community is similar to non-LGBTQ persons in terms of barriers and challenges. In addition, it is more likely for LGBTQ individuals to provide or receive care for or from a nonrelative than it is for non-LGBTQ people (National Academies of Sciences, Engineering, and Medicine, 2016).

Support is crucial when it comes to the caregiver's well-being. Formal support systems, such as paid in home care, help to reduce caregiver stress and provide important respite. Even so, ethnic and racial family caregivers underuse formal services and tend to rely more on family, fictive kin, and friends or neighbors for help than on formal services

(Dilworth-Anderson et al., 2002; Rote et al., 2019). This may be due, in part, to not having the funds to spend on costly in-home care and the caregiver's negative experience when seeking formal support services.

It is not uncommon for racial and ethnic minorities to encounter multiple and extensive barriers and racial disparities when attempting to access health care systems. One way health inequity is clearly evident is the great disparity in life expectancy. The cumulative impact of these inequities creates an overwhelming burden for older adults and their families (Periyakoil, 2019). Barriers experienced by racial and ethnic older adults and their families within the health care system may include "limited English proficiency, low health literacy, varying levels of acculturation, biases about Western health care and medicines, mistrust of clinicians, inability to navigate the complex health care systems, and cultural beliefs and taboos" (Periyakoil, 2019, p. S423). While some progress has been made in addressing racial disparities, such as efforts to provide staff with ethnogeriatric training, racial and ethnic older adults routinely experience unequal treatment compared to White older adults over a broad range of specialty care. Not surprisingly, research indicates that individuals prefer to be treated by health care professionals of the same racial or ethnic background as they are more apt to speak the same language (National Academies of Sciences, Engineering, and Medicine, 2016) thereby ensuring effective and meaningful communication. The affordability, accessibility, and availability of intervention services targeted to racial and ethnic older adults is in dire need of extensive policy and structural changes at both state and national levels. While this is true for services for older people of all races and ethnicities across the board, it is particularly true for Black and Mexican American caregivers (Rote et al., 2019).

Care Provision Activities and Roles

The older adult's inability to perform basic daily self-care tasks (such as bathing, dressing, eating, toileting, or mobility) occurs due to physical health and mental health functioning limitations (Table 18-2). These limitations are typically brought on by multiple factors including foreseeable life events, such as planned surgery, and unexpected life events, such as stroke and cardiac arrest. As would be expected, as a person ages it is more likely that they will experience physical and/or cognitive impairments that affect their ability to function independently (National Academies of Sciences, Engineering, and Medicine, 2016).

Family caregivers play a crucial role in their efforts to preserve the older adult family member's well-being and QOL, particularly during times of significant mental and physical decline. Notably, it is the family that provides the majority (80%) of home health care for aging relatives including assisting in activities of daily living (Behr & Tebb, 2016). The extent of family caregiver support is impressive. More than half of individuals between the ages of 85 and 89 years receive help and support from a family caregiver, and more than 75% of individuals over the age of 90 years report needing some assistance. At any one point in time 25% of adult children are providing care for an older relative and, of those, 20% have co-residence (Bonder, 2019). As of 2018, 95% of caregivers live within 30 minutes of a relative. It is common for spousal and adult children caregivers to provide intense and long-term caregiving averaging in the excess of 30 hours per week (Wolff et al., 2018).

Caregiving for older adults in the future will depend, in part, on the availability and capacity of their family members to assist them. In previous generations, older adults could often count on large, extended families for help with health and functioning needs—although in most cases the caregiver was either a wife or adult daughter, as they are today (Wolff & Kasper, 2006).

The Positive and Burdensome Aspects of Caregiving

Family members become informal caregivers for many reasons, including a sense of responsibility, a lack of available formal services due to financial or other constraints, and a desire to serve a loved one. While onerous, caregiving has been associated with a sense of meaning, joy, and happiness often experienced by the caregiver while caring for a loved one. Numerous studies describe the impact of what has been termed "uplifts" for caregivers' well-being (Cartwright et al., 1994; Motenko, 1989; Pinquart & Sörensen, 2004; Shim et al., 2012). Shim et al. (2012) define uplifts as events of short duration that evoke pleasure during caregiving and are associated with caregiver meaning and satisfaction. It has been suggested that the meaning of the caregiver's role in daily life has a considerable impact on the positive experiences of caregiving. In fact, meaning "helps to transcend the daily constraints and make sense of the caregivers' experience" (Carbonneau et al., 2010, p. 336). Furthermore, Noonan and Tennstedt (1997) discovered that meaning in informal caregiving explained a significant portion of the differences in psychosocial well-being indicators, such as depression and self-esteem.

In addition, there has been recognition in the literature that the relationship between the caregiver and receiver is a central element in positive caregiving. Positive prior relationships may be predictive of a deeper level of satisfaction while performing the caregiver role (Lloyd et al., 2016). The quality of the daily relationship between the caregiver and care recipient is associated with positive aspects of caregiving (Carbonneau et al., 2010). For instance, the presence of more positive aspects, such as a closer relationship with the care-receiver, has been associated with greater subjective well-being and fewer depressive symptoms in caregivers (Pinquart & Sörensen, 2004).

Table 18-2

What Family Caregivers Do for Older Adults

DOMAIN	CAREGIVERS' ACTIVITIES AND TASKS
Household tasks	• Help with bills, deal with insurance claims, and manage money • Home maintenance (e.g., install grab bars, ramps, and other safety modifications, repairs, yardwork) • Laundry and other housework • Prepare meals • Shopping • Transportation
Self-care, supervision, and mobility	• Bathing and grooming • Dressing • Feeding • Supervision • Management of behavioral symptoms • Toileting (e.g., getting to and from the toilet, maintaining continence, dealing with incontinence) • Transferring (e.g., getting in and out of bed and chairs, moving from bed to wheelchair) • Help getting around inside or outside
Emotional and social support	• Provide companionship • Discuss ongoing life challenges with care recipient • Facilitate and participate in leisure activities • Help care recipient manage emotional responses • Manage family conflict • Troubleshoot problems
Health and medical care	• Encourage healthy lifestyle • Encourage self-care • Encourage treatment adherence • Manage and give medications, pills, or injections • Operate medical equipment • Prepare food for special diets • Respond to acute needs and emergencies • Provide wound care
Advocacy and care coordination	• Seek information • Facilitate person and family understanding • Communicate with doctors, nurses, social workers, pharmacists, and other health care and long-term services and supports (LTSS) providers • Facilitate provider understanding • Locate, arrange, and supervise nurses, social workers, home care aides, home-delivered meals, and other LTSS (e.g., adult day services) • Make appointments • Negotiate with other family member(s) regarding respective roles • Order prescription medicines • Deal with insurance issues
Surrogacy	• Handle financial and legal matters • Manage personal property • Participate in advanced planning • Participate in treatment decisions

While family caregiving offers many rewards and benefits, it can be financially, physically, and emotionally difficult (Table 18-3). Persons caring for people with high intensity needs result in more difficulties for caregivers. Caregivers involved in high-intensity caregiving situations experience increased exhaustion, a sense of being overwhelmed, and little time for their own self-care (National Academies of Sciences, Engineering, and Medicine, 2016). Family members, particularly spouses, who spend more than 36 hours per week caregiving are six times more likely to experience depression or anxiety than noncaregivers (Behr & Tebb, 2016). This high rate may be due to a wide range of unmet needs, such as finding time for oneself, balancing work and family responsibilities, managing physical and emotional stress, developing skills to safely and effectively provide care, navigating the health system, and making informed end-of-life decisions (Behr & Tebb, 2016; Zakrajsek et al., 2013). However, a noted decline in caregiving-related emotional, financial, and physical difficulties experienced by the family caregiver, particularly spouses, occurred between 1999 and 2015. This decline is somewhat due to participation in community based supportive services such as respite and support groups (Wolff et al., 2018). An awareness of caregivers' risk factors is critical for interprofessional health care providers in developing an assessment strategy. Assessing risk factors will inform community-based interventions for the older adult and caregiver as well as create community-based programs, services, and policies to support health and community participation.

Notably, the positive aspects of caregiving can be experienced simultaneously with the more difficult aspects (National Academies of Sciences, Engineering, and Medicine, 2016). Furthermore, there are cultural complexities to family caregiving. Black and Latino family caregivers report lower levels of depression and higher levels of life and caregiver satisfaction in comparison to non-Latino White caregivers. This is due, to some extent, to cultural values that prioritize family support (Rote et al., 2019). However, this population reports worsening physical health over time, which may be a result of **caregiver intensity** and other burden factors. Caregiving intensity is defined as "the level of dependency on the older adult and amount of care provided by the caregiver" (Rote et al., 2019, p. 2).

Care Transitions

As older adults are living longer due to advances in medical care and prevention, they are experiencing an increase in chronic illness and health conditions that require health care services that span various providers across hospital-based and community-based settings (Centers for Disease Control and Prevention & Merck Company Foundation, 2007). This occurrence of older adults and their family members requiring care at multiple health care delivery points necessitates transitional care. **Care transitions** is defined as "a set of actions designed to ensure the coordination and continuity of health care as patients transfer between different locations or different levels of care within the same location" (Coleman & Berenson, 2004, p. 533). Care transitions of older adults may include a series of episodic events such as hospitalizations, rehabilitation services, stays in long-term care facilities, transitioning home with home care, and interactions with community-based agencies, like Area Agencies on Aging and Program of All-Inclusive Care for the Elderly (PACE) service delivery system. Furthermore, care transitions represent a critical moment in older adults' continuum of care between hospital and community when communication breakdown, lack of planning and follow-up, and major life adjustments without necessary supports have been found to pose serious threats to health and participation for older adults and their family members (Chernof, 2012; Coleman & Berenson, 2004; Coleman et al., 2002; Dedhia et al., 2009; Graham et al., 2009; Harrison & Verhoef, 2002; Weaver et al., 1998). These threats to successful care transitions can be challenging to all stakeholders in the care transition process, including the health care- and community-based providers, patients, and family caregivers.

It is often family caregivers of older adults transitioning between health service delivery systems who provide a critical role in supporting care transitions (Lavine et al., 2013). In addition, there is a recognition that caregiver roles and responsibilities change over time, indicating a critical need for community-based practitioners to understand the caregiver experience with care transitions at multiple points in time (National Academies of Sciences, Engineering, and Medicine, 2016). A number of studies (Bull, 1992; Bull & Jervis, 1997; Byrne et al., 2011; Dossa et al., 2012; Sundar et al., 2014; Young et al., 2014) have identified multiple and changing caregiver roles during the transition process. Caregiving responsibilities and tasks vary during phases of caregiving (Nahm et al., 2010), may be transitory based on care recipient need (Gitlin & Wolf, 2011), and may occur in phases (Byrne et al., 2011), such as role engaging, role negotiating, and role settling identified by Shyu (2000).

Community-based practitioners have a critical role in supporting older adults and their family caregivers in facilitating effective care transitions between health delivery systems in understanding and supporting information transfer across settings, ascertaining status, progression, and redundancies of services and care, and having knowledge of patient's actual experiences and preparedness for transition (Chernof, 2012; Coleman et al., 2002). However, the complicated task of coordinating care challenges the health care provider's ability to provide high-quality and cost-effective care (American Geriatrics Society, 2005; Coleman, 2003). In a qualitative exploratory study of community-based interprofessional practitioners working in a home health care setting, older adults, and their caregivers, positive or successful care transitions were described by participants as those that included planning and preparation by all stakeholders and included the following features:

Table 18-3

Risk Factors for Adverse Outcomes Due to Family Caregiving

RISK FACTOR	ADVERSE OUTCOME
Sociodemographic factors	• Lower income • Lower education (high school or less) • Older age (50 years or older) • Spouse of care recipient • Female • Living with care recipient • Intensity/type of caregiving
Intensity/type of caregiving	• More than 100 hours of care per month • High care recipient personal/mobility care needs • Dementia care (including management of behavioral symptoms) • Medical care (shots/injections, wound care) • Coordinating care (appointments, interacting with providers, dealing with health insurance)
Caregiver's perceptions of the care recipient's physical, psychological, and existential suffering	• Lack of choice in taking on the caregiving role • Caregiver's health and physical functioning
Caregiver's health and physical functioning	• Poor/fair self-rated health • Feeling stressed • Having three or more medical conditions • Sleep problems • Difficulty breathing • Pain • Limited leg/arm strength • Unwanted weight loss
Caregiver's social and professional supports	• No one to help with caregiving • No one to talk to • No time to socialize with others • No access or use of professional support/care services • Care recipient's home physical environment
Care recipient's home physical environment	• Lacks appropriate home modifications • Stairs, clutter

Reproduced with permission from Risk Factors for Adverse Outcomes Due to Family Caregiving. Reprinted from *Families caring for an aging America* (p. 109) by National Academies of Sciences, Engineering, and Medicine, Copyright 2016 by the National Academies Press.

> ... patients having and using strong social supports; patients having and understanding information in order to make decisions and anticipate issues that may arise in care; service providers sharing this information in an effective manner; and patients and their families given the opportunity to ask questions at the time of the care transition and, importantly, throughout the duration of the recovery process. (Zakrajsek et al., 2013, p. 339)

In the same study, negative care transitions were described as those in which information was poorly communicated and timed from service provider to service provider as well as between service providers and service recipients (older adults and their family caregivers). These findings indicate a need for coordination of health care service provision, including hospital-based and community-based, and a critical role for community-based practitioners to play in coordinating these services, providing resources to older adults and their family members, and ensuring relevant information is accessible to care recipients through health literacy efforts (Chesser et al., 2016; Coleman & Berenson, 2004; Weaver et al., 1998). Furthermore, evidence-based care transition models, such as the Care Transitions Intervention (Coleman Model; Coleman et al., 2002, 2006) the Transitional Care Model (Naylor Model; Naylor et al., 1999, 2004), Project RED (Jack et al., 2009), Bridge Model (Altfeld et al., 2013; Alvarez et al., 2016) and Project BOOST (Society of Hospital Medicine, 2008) offer effective strategies and programs that can guide health care providers in supporting older adults and their family caregivers during care transitions (Charlie Case: Part C).

Charlie Case: Part C

When Claire's youngest daughter was a junior in high school, she came over to Charlie's house after school to find him lying on the floor in the kitchen, unconscious. Charlie, who is now 75 years old, was immediately rushed to the hospital where he was diagnosed with a cerebrovascular accident (CVA). After his CVA, he received inpatient hospital services, including physiatry, nursing, social work, occupational therapy, physical therapy, and speech-language pathology. After a 3-week stay, Charlie is medically stable, able to complete ambulation and basic activities of daily living at a supervision level, and able to communicate with some strategies for memory issues. At his discharge planning meeting, Charlie, his family, and his interprofessional health care team decided he would be discharged home with home health care services. Charlie's adult grandson, Jared, who is in between jobs, has volunteered to move in with Charlie temporarily during his recovery to assist with basic and IADLs. Other family members are available to frequently provide support to Charlie as well.

DISCUSSION QUESTIONS

1. Assume you are a member of the interprofessional home health care team. What information would be important for you to know about Charlie, his family, and his care from his hospital stay?
2. What other information would be important for you to ask or assess from your professional perspective?
3. What other members of the home health care team do you expect would be on the home health care team? What are their roles and responsibilities?
4. How might you facilitate communication between Charlie, his family, and the rest of your home health care team?
5. What would be important information and education might you provide Jared to care for his grandfather?

Community-Based Programs and Interventions

Families that include older adults can become overwhelmed with roles and responsibilities (National Academies of Sciences, Engineering, and Medicine, 2016) and make the decision to engage formal community-based services. Also, it is not unusual for family caregivers to be proactive on their own behalf in order to avoid burden and burnout and take preventative action to develop a system of support. Table 18-4 describes various services that are available to families with links to examples and resources. These services are delivered by community-based professionals, such as social workers, nurses, occupational therapists, physical therapists, and others, who work collaboratively with families to address health and well-being issues of the older adult family member (Charlie Case: Part D).

Please see Appendix C to explore one community-based model.

Conclusion

Family structures are complex, existing for long periods of time, bound by stronger ties than other social groups, and made up of more than one generation. Families that include older adults are prevalent in family structures and provide unique challenges and opportunities. Older adult grandparents come to raise children typically in less than ideal circumstances where they take on a parental role with little preparation, support, and resources. Family caregivers of older adults provide selfless acts of caring and nurturing of members of our society who are often neglected, ignored, and made invisible due to ageist attitudes and an unwillingness to accept the inevitability of old age and death. In addition, racial, ethnic, and economic status disparities further contribute to the myriad of additional challenges families face. These disparities result in overwhelming barriers to adequate health care and access to services. Our society would be in dire straits were it not for family members who are, at times, forced to leave their jobs, juggle multiple roles as participants in the sandwich generations, take on financial burdens, and risk exhaustion and decline in health due to mounting responsibilities and tasks. And yet, family members will often speak of the great rewards of caring for a loved one, whether it be a grandchild or parent, of the ways in which lives that have been linked over generations benefit from the opportunity to be of service during this time of need. This deepening relationship between caregiver and care recipient is reciprocal, in that everyone benefits from what evolves into a meaningful and profound relationship. Community-based practitioners serve in critical roles by supporting families with older adults through the development and provision programs and services, enhancing health and QOL, and supporting meaningful engagement in roles, occupations, and activities.

Table 18-4

Community-Based Interventions, Program, and Services Available to Older Adults and Their Families

SERVICE	DESCRIPTION	EXAMPLES OR RESOURCES
Adult day care	Adult Day Care Centers offer social, recreational, and health-related services to individuals who cannot be alone during the day because of health and social needs, memory loss, or disability.	Alzheimer's Association Public and Private providers of Adult Day Care Centers
Area agencies on aging	Resource center for various services and programs for community dwelling older adults.	Area Agencies on Aging included in all 50 states and Washington D.C.
Caregiver programs	Provides programs and services for caregivers of older adults and limited services to grandparents raising grandchildren.	National Family Caregiver Support Program Alzheimer's Association
Community-based care transitions programs (CCTP)	Models to improve care transitions from hospital to community-based settings and reduce readmissions to hospitals.	Centers for Medicare and Medicaid Services CCTP: https://innovation.cms.gov/innovation-models/cctp Coleman's Care Transition Program: https://caretransitions.org/
Case management	Case managers work with older adults and family members, often within interprofessional teams, to assess, arrange, and evaluate supportive efforts to maintain independence.	Commonly found in various services and programs; positions are fulfilled by professionals from various backgrounds (e.g., nursing, social work, therapy).
Elder abuse prevention programs	Allegations of abuse, neglect, and exploitation of senior citizens are investigated by highly trained protective service specialists. Intervention is provided in instances of substantiated elder abuse, neglect, or exploitation.	National Center on Elder Abuse: https://ncea.acl.gov/
Grandparents raising grandchildren programs	Privates various services to grandparents who reside with children in kinship care, such as workshops, support groups, intergenerational activities, and other resources.	Varies by community. https://www.grandfamilies.org/
Home health care services	Home health care includes a range of health care services that are provided in one's home, such as wound care, patient and caregiver education, intravenous or nutrition therapy, and rehabilitation services to regain function and independence. Providers include skilled nursing care and other skilled services, such as occupational therapy, physical therapy, speech-language therapy, and medical social services.	Varies by community
Home repair	Programs that help older adults keep their homes in good condition before any problems become major. Volunteers may visit a home to patch a leaky roof, repair faulty plumbing, or insulate drafty walls.	Local, state, and federal organizations Rebuilding Together: https://rebuildingtogether.org/
Home modification	Programs that provide housing adaptations and/or renovations to increase ease of use, safety, security, and independence. Some local, state, federal, and volunteer programs provide special grants, loans, and other assistance for modifications.	Local, state, and federal organizations Rebuilding Together: https://rebuildingtogether.org/
Information, referral, and assistance services	Information Specialists are available to provide guidance and connections to available services and resources.	Area Agencies on Aging

(continued)

Table 18-4 (continued)

Community-Based Interventions, Program, and Services Available to Older Adults and Their Families

SERVICE	DESCRIPTION	EXAMPLES OR RESOURCES
Legal assistance	Legal advice and representation is available for certain legal matters, including government program benefits, tenant rights, and consumer problems.	Area Agencies on Aging Elder attorney
Medical equipment assistance and lending programs	Organizations that assist older adults and people with disabilities by providing free or long-term loans of durable medical equipment.	National Foundations, Local Organizations, and Faith-Based Networks
Nutrition services	Home-delivered nutritious meals delivered to older adults who are homebound. Congregate meals provide opportunities for people to enjoy a meal and socialize with other older adults in their communities.	Meals on Wheels Senior centers
Personal care	Personal care services assist individuals with functional impairments to bathe, dress, shop, walk, light housekeeping, and eating. Services also include general supervision, provision of emotional security, and assistance with chores and other activities.	Offered through the state Medicaid waiver system, state and local programs, and private organizations
PACE	Provide social and medical services primarily in an adult day health center, supplemented by in-home and referral services for individuals who meet Long-Term Care level of care criteria living at home in the community. Services provided by an interprofessional team of providers who assess the participants' needs, develop care plans and deliver all services, including acute care services, hospital services, and if necessary, nursing facility services.	Varies by community
Respite care	Respite is a specific period of relief or rest from the continual supervision, companionship, therapeutic, and/or personal care of a person with a functional impairment.	Medicaid waiver system, state and local programs, and private organizations
Senior housing options	Assisted living, retirement communities, nursing facilities, government-assisted housing, and shared housing.	Varies by community
Senior center programs	Senior Centers offer a variety of recreational and educational programs, seminars, events, and activities for older adults with varying activity levels.	Varies by community
State health insurance counseling and assistance	Paid professionals and trained volunteers offer unbiased, one-on-one counseling to help consumers understand their Medicare benefits and resolve billing problems. They also address issues related to supplemental insurance and long-term care insurance options.	PACE Programs Area Agencies on Aging
Support groups	A group of individuals, sometimes led by a therapist or other practitioner, who provide each other moral support, information, and advice on problems relating to some shared characteristic or experience.	Caregiver support groups Bereavement support groups Grandparents Raising Grandchildren support groups
Telephone reassurance and visiting programs	Provides regular contact and safety check by trained volunteers to reassure and support senior citizens and disabled persons who are homebound.	Varies by community
Transportation	Door-to-door transportation for older adults and people with disabilities who do not have private transportation and are unable to utilize public transportation.	Public transportation services offered by local transit authorities Private rideshare and carpooling services

Charlie Case: Part D

In the 6 months after Charlie's initial CVA, he experienced many functional gains and was able to complete ADLs independently, and returned to many IADLs, including paying his bills, cooking, and home maintenance. Jared has subsequently obtained a new position out of state and Charlie has been able to live alone with some support from his family, such as driving to medical appointments and social outings, grocery shopping and laundry. In the 2 years since this time, Charlie's overall health has continued to decline due to his cardiac issues and a subsequent minor CVA. It slowly became clear to family members that Charlie was losing strength and mobility, and that ADLs, such as dressing and toileting, were becoming more and more challenging. Charlie has been admitted to the hospital several times over the last year due to debility and falls at home. Due to his ongoing health issues and with this most recent hospital admission, the social worker suggested that Charlie and his family consider a more supportive living situation for him. Charlie's daughter is adamant that her father continue to live in the community and has volunteered to have Charlie live with her and Charlie has agreed. Charlie's other daughter, Rachel, helps with his care, bathing him two times each week, whereas Claire provides the majority of the care, including medication management, mobility around the house, dressing, and toileting. After 6 months of direct caregiving, Claire has realized she cannot manage her job and care for her father full-time.

DISCUSSION QUESTIONS

1. From your professional perspective, what are the key issues occurring with Charlie and his family that are impacting health, well-being, and QOL?
2. What community-based resources and programs would you recommend specifically for Charlie? (Please refer to Table 18-4.)
3. What community-based resources and programs would you recommend specifically for Claire and the rest of their family? (Please refer to Table 18-4.)

References

AARP. (2009). Home safety checklist. https://assets.aarp.org/external_sites/caregiving/checklists/checklist_homeSafety.html

Altfeld, S., Pavle, K., Rosenberg, W., & Shure, I. (2013). Integrating care across settings: The Illinois transitional care consortium's bridge model. *Generations Journal of the American Society on Aging, 36*, 98-101.

Alvarez, R., Ginsburg, J., Grabowski, J., Post, S., & Rosenberg, W. (2016). The social work role in reducing 30-day readmissions: The effectiveness of the Bridge Model of transitional care. *Journal of gerontological social work, 59*(3), 222–227. https://doi.org/10.1080/01634372.2016.1195781

American Geriatrics Society (2005). Caring for older Americans: The future of geriatric medicine. *Journal of the American Geriatrics Society, 53*, S245-256.

Baker, L. A., & Silverstein, M. (2008). Depressive symptoms among grandparents raising grandchildren: The impact of participation in multiple roles. Journal of Intergenerational *Relationships, 6*(3), 285-304. https://doi.org/10.1080/15350770802157802

Baker, L. A., Silverstein, M., & Putney, N. M. (2008). Grandparents raising grandchildren in the United States: Changing family forms, stagnant social policies. *Journal of Societal & Social Policy*, 7, 53-69.

Behr, S. K., & Tebb, S. C. (2016). Families and aging: The lived experience. In K. F. Barney & M. A. Perkinson (Eds.), *Occupational therapy with aging adults: Promoting quality of life through collaborative practice* (pp. 373-384). Elsevier.

Berg, K., Wood-Dauphinee, S., & Williams, J. I. (1995). The balance scale: Reliability assessment with elderly residents and patients with an acute stroke. *Scandinavian Journal of Rehabilitation Medicine, 27*(1), 27-36.

Brink, T. L., Yesavage, J. A., Lum, O., Heersema, P. H., Adey, M., & Rose, T. L. (1982). Screening test for geriatric depression. *Clinical Gerontologist, 1*, 37-43.

Bonder, B. R. (2019). Interactions and relationships. In B. R. Bonder & V. D. Bello-Haas (Eds.), *Functional performance in older adults* (3rd ed., pp. 386-408). F.A. Davis Company.

Bull, M. J. (1992). Managing the transition from hospital to home. *Qualitative Health Research, 2*, 27-41.

Bull, M. J., & Jervis, L. L. (1997). Strategies used by chronically ill older women and their caregiving daughters in managing post-hospital care. *Journal of Advanced Nursing, 25*, 541-547.

Brown, C., Rempfer, M., & Hamera, E. (2009). *The test of grocery shopping skills*. AOTA Press.

Byrne, K., Orange, J. B., & Ward-Griffin, C. (2011). Care transition experiences of spousal caregivers: From a geriatric rehabilitation unit to home. *Qualitative Health Research, 21*(10), 1371-1387.

Carbonneau, H., Caron, C., & Derosiers, J. (2010). Development of a conceptual framework of positive aspects of caregiving in dementia. *Dementia, 93*(3), 327-353. https://doi:10.1177/14713001210375316

Carter, B., & McGoldrick, M. (Eds.). (1988). *The changing family life cycle: A framework for family therapy* (2nd ed.). Gardner Press.

Cartwright, J. C., Archbold, P. G., Stewart, B. J., & Limandri, B. (1994). Enrichment processes in family caregiving to frail elders. *Advances in Nursing Science, 17*(1), 31-43. https://doi:10.1097/00012272-199409000-00006

Centers for Disease Control and Prevention & the Merck Company Foundation. (2007). *The state of aging and health in america 2007*. The Merck Company Foundation. https://www.cdc.gov/aging/pdf/saha_2007.pdf

Chan, K. L., Chen, M., Lo, K. M. C., Chen, Q., Kelley, S. J., & Ip, P. (2019). The effectiveness of interventions for grandparents raising grandchildren: A meta-analysis. *Research on Social Work Practice, 29*(6), 607-617. https://doi.org/10.1177/1049731518798470

Chernof, B. A. (2012). Synergy for senior care: Improving partnerships between medical services and community-based care. Health Policy Forum. http://www.altarum.org/forum/post/synergy-senior-care-improving-partnerships between-medical-services-and community-based-care

Chesser, A. K., Keene Woods, N., Smothers, K., & Rogers, N. (2016). Health literacy and older adults: A systematic review. *Gerontology and Geriatric Medicine*. https://doi.org/10.1177/2333721416630492

Cohen, S., & Hoberman, H. M. (1983). Positive events and social supports as buffers of life change stress. *Journal of Applied Social Psychology, 13*(2), 99–125. https://doi.org/10.1111/j.1559-1816.1983.tb02325.x

Coleman, E.A. (2003). Falling through the cracks: Challenges and opportunities for improving transitional care for persons with continuous complex care needs. *Journal of the American Geriatrics Society, 51*, 549–555.

Coleman, E. A., & Berenson, R. A. (2004). Lost in transition: Challenges and opportunities for improving the quality of transitional care. *Annals of Internal Medicine, 141*(7), 33-536.

Coleman, E. A., Parry, C., Chalmers, S., & Min, S. J. (2006). The Care Transitions Intervention: Results of a Randomized Controlled Trial. *Archives of Internal Medicine, 166*, 1822-8.

Coleman, E. A., Smith, J. D., Frank, J. C., Eilersten, T. B., Thiare, J. N., & Kramer, A. M. (2002). Development and testing of a measure designed to assess the quality of care transitions. *International Journal of Integrated Care, 2*, 1-9.

Collin C., Wade D. T., Davies S., & Horne V. (1988). The Barthel ADL Index: A reliability study. *International Disabilities Studies, 10*(2), 61-63. https://doi.org/10.3109/09638288809164103.

Dedhia, P., Kravet, S., Bulger, J., Hinson, T., Sridharan, A., Kolodner, K., et al. (2009). A quality improvement intervention to facilitate the transition of older adults from three hospitals back to their homes. *Journal of the American Geriatrics Society, 57*, 1540- 1546.

Dickerson, A. E. (2013). Driving assessment tools used by Driver Rehabilitation Specialists: Survey of use and implications for practice. *American Journal of Occupational Therapy, 67*(5), 564-573. https://doi.org/10.5014/ajot.2013.007823

Dilworth-Anderson, P., Burton, L. M., & Klein, K. M. (2004). Contemporary and emerging theories in studying families. In V. L. Bengtson, A. C. Acock, K. R. Allen, P. Dillworth-Anderson, & D. M. Klein (Eds.), *Sourcebook of family theory and research* (pp. 35-58). Sage Publishing.

Dilworth-Anderson, P., William, I. C., & Gibson, B. E. (2002). Issues of race, ethnicity and culture in caregiving research: A 20-year review (1980-2000). *The Gerontologist, 42*(2), 237-272.

Dodds, T. A., Martin, D. S., Stolov W. C., & Deyo, R. A. (1993). A validation of the Functional Independence Measure and its performance among rehabilitation inpatients. *Archives of Physical Medicine and Rehabilitation, 74*, 531-536.

Dossa, A., Bokhour, B., & Hoenig, H. (2012). Care transitions from the hospital to home for patients with mobility impairments: Patient and family caregiver experiences. *Rehabilitation Nursing, 37*(6), 277-285.

Elder, G. H. Jr. (1974). Age differentiation and the life course. *Annual Review of Sociology, 1*, 165-190.

Elder, G. H. Jr. (1985). Perspectives on life course. In G. H. Elder, Jr. (Ed.), *Life course dynamics: Transitions and trajectories* (pp. 23-49). Ithaca, NY: Cornell University Press.

Elder, G. H., Jr. (1994). Time, human agency, and social change: Perspectives on the life course. *Social Psychology Quarterly, 57*(1), 4-15.

Elder, G. H., Jr. & Johnson, M. K. (2003). The life course and aging: Challenges, lessons, and new directions. In R. H. Settersten Jr. (Ed.) *Invitation to the life course: Toward a new understanding of later life* (pp. 49-81). Baywood.

Ellis, R. R., & Simmons, T. (2014). Coresident grandparents and their grandchildren: 2012. Current Population Reports, P20-576, U.S. Census Bureau. https://www.census.gov/content/dam/Census/library/publications/2014/demo/p20-576.pdf

Fruhauf, C. A., Pevney, B., & Bundy-Fazioli, K. (2015). The needs and use of programs by service providers working with grandparents raising grandchildren. *Journal of Applied Gerontology, 34*(2), 138-157. https://doi.org/10.1177/0733464812463983

Generations United. (2015). The state of grandfamilies in America. https://www.gu.org/resources/the-state-of-grandfamilies-in-america-2015/

Gitlin. L. N., & Wolf, J. (2011). Family involvement if care transitions of older adults: What do we know and where do we go from here? *Annual Review of Gerontology and Geriatrics, 31*, 31-64.

Goodman, C. C. (1991). Perceived social support for caregiving measuring the benefit of self-help/support group participation. *Journal of Gerontological Social Work, 16*(3-4), 163-175.

Graf, C. (2008). The Lawton Instrumental Activities of Daily Living Scale. *American Journal of Nursing, 108*(4), 52-62.

Graham, C. L., Ivey, S. L. & Neuhauser, L. (2009). From hospital to home: Assessing the transitional care needs of vulnerable seniors. *The Gerontologist, 49*, 23-33.

Grossman, A. H., D'Augelli, A. R., & Dragowski, E. A. (2007). Caregiving and care receiving among older lesbian, gay and bisexual adults. *Journal of Gay and Lesbian Social Services, 18*(3-4), 15-38. https://doi.org/10.1300/J041v18n03_02

Harrison, A., & Verhoef, M. (2002). Understanding coordination of care from the consumer's perspective in a regional health system. *Health Services Research, 37*, 1031-1054.

Hays, V., Morris, J., Wolfe, C., & Morgan, M. (1995). The SF-36 health questionnaire: Is it suitable for use with older adults? *Age and Aging, 24*, 120-125.

Hayslip, B., Fruhauf, C. A., & Dolbin-MacNab, M. L. (2019). Grandparents raising grandchildren: What have we learned over the past decade? *The Gerontologist, 59*(3), e152-e163. https://doi.org/10.1093/geront/gnx106

Hayslip, B., & Kaminski, P. L. (2005). Grandparents raising their grandchildren: A review of the literature and suggestions for practice. *Gerontologist, 45*(2), 262-269, https://doi.org/10.1093/geront/45.2.26

Heinemann, A. W., Lai, J., Magasi, S., et al. (2011). Measuring participation enfranchisement. *Archives of Physical Medicine & Rehabilitation, 92*, 564-571.

Henderson, S., Duncan-Jones, P., Byrne, D. G., & Scott, R. (1980). Measuring social relationships: the Interview Schedule for Social Interaction. *Psychological Medicine, 10*, 723–734.

Jack, B. W., Chetty, V. K., Anthony, D., Greenwald, J. L., Sanchez, G. M., Johnson, A. E., Forsythe, S. R., O'Donnell, J. K., Paasche-Orlow, M. K., Manasseh, C., Martin, S., & Culpepper, L. (2009). A reengineered hospital discharge program to decrease rehospitalization: a randomized trial. *Annals of internal medicine, 150*(3), 178–187. https://doi.org/10.7326/0003-4819-150-3-200902030-00007

Jette, A. M., Haley, S. M., Coster, W. J., et al. (2002). Late life function and disability instrument. *Journal of Gerontology, Series A: Biological Sciences and Medical Sciences, 57*, M209-M216.

Lavine, C., Hapler, D. E., Rutburg, J. L., & Gould, D. A. (2013). Engaging family caregivers as partners in care transitions. A Special Report from the United Hospital Fund.

Leder, S., Grinstead, L. N., & Torres, E. (2007). Grandparents raising grandchildren: Stressors, social support, and health outcomes. *Journal of Family Nursing, 13*(3), 333-352. https://doi.org/10.1177/1074840707303841

Letts, L., & Marshall, L. (1995). Evaluation the validity and consistency of the SAFER tool. *Physical and Occupational Therapy in Geriatrics, 13*(4), 49-66.

Lloyd, J., Patterson, T., & Muers, J. (2016). The positive aspects of caregiving in dementia: A critical review of the qualitative literature. *Dementia, 15*(6), 1534-1561. https://doi:10.117/1471301214564792

Lubben, J. E. (1988). Assessing social networks among elderly populations. *Family and Community Health, 11*(3), 42–52

Mahoney, F., & Barthel, D. (1965). Functional evaluation: The Barthel Index. *Maryland Medicine Journal, 14*, 61-65.

McColl, M. A., Davies, D., Carolson, P., Johnston, J., & Minnes, P. (2001). The Community Integration Measure: Development and preliminary validation. *Archives of Physical Medicine and Rehabilitation, 82*, 429-434.

Moen, P., Elder, G. H. Jr., & Luscher, K. (1995). *Examining lives in context: Perspectives on the ecology of human development.* American Psychological Association.

Motenko, A. K. (1989). The frustrations, gratifications, and well-being of dementia caregivers. *The Gerontologist, 29*(2), 166-172. https://doi.org/10.1093/geront/29.2.166

Mortimer, J. T., & Shanahan, M. J. (Eds.). (2003). *Handbook of the life course.* Springer.

Nasreddine, Z. S., Philllips, N. A., Bédirian, V., et al. (2005). The Montreal Cognitive Assessment (MoCA): A brief screening tool for mild cognitive impairment. *Journal American Geriatric Society, 53*, 695-699.

Nahm, E., Resnick, B., Orwig, D., Magaziner, J., & DeGrezia, M. (2010). Exploration of informal caregiving following hip fracture. *Geriatric Nursing, 31*, 254-262.

National Academies of Sciences, Engineering, and Medicine (2016). *Families caring for an aging America.* The National Academies Press. https://doi.org/10.17226/23606.

Naylor et al. (1999). Comprehensive discharge planning and home follow-up of hospitalized elders: A randomized clinical trial. *The Journal of the American Medical Association, 281*, 613-620.

Noonan, A. E., & Tennstedt, S. (1997). Meaning in caregiving and its contribution to caregiver well-being. *The Gerontologist, 37*(6), 785-794.

Periyakoil, V. S. (2019). Building a culturally competent workforce to care for diverse older adults: Scope of the problem and potential solutions. *Journal of Applied Gerontology, 67*(52), S423-S432. https://doi.org/10.1111/jgs.15939

Pinquart, M., & Sörensen, S. (2004) Associations of caregiver stressors and uplifts with subjective well-being and depressive mood: A meta-analytic comparison. *Aging & Mental Health, 8*(5), 438-449. https://doi.org/10.1080/13607860410001725036

Powell, L. E., & Myers, A. M. (1995). The Activities-Specific Balance Confidence (ABS) scale. *Journals of Gerontology, Series A: Biological Sciences and Medical Sciences, 50A*(1), M28-M34.

Quadagno, J. S. (1999). *Aging and the life course.* McGraw-Hill.

Rogers, J. C., & Holm, M. B. (1989). *Performance Assessment of Self-Care Skills.* University of Pittsburgh.

Rote, S. M., Angel, J. L., Moon, H., & Markides, K. (2019). Caregiving across diverse populations: New evidence from the national study of caregiving and Hispanic EPESE. *Innovation in Aging, 3*(2), 1-11. https://doi.org/10.1093/geroni/igz033

Sampson, D., & Hertlein, K. (2015). The experience of grandparents raising grandchildren. Grandfamilies. *The Contemporary Journal of Research, Practice and Policy, 2*(1). https://scholarworks.wmich.edu/grandfamilies/vol2/iss1/4

Scott-Maxwell, F. (1968). *The measure of my days.* Penguin Books.

Settersten, R. A., Jr. (2002). *Invitation to the life course: Toward a new understanding of later life.* Baywood.

Settersten, R. A., Jr. (2005). Linking the two ends of life: What gerontology can learn from childhood studies. *The Journals of Gerontology, 60B*, S173-S180.

Shim, B., Barroso, J., & Davis, L. (2012). A comparative qualitative analysis of stories of spousal caregivers of people with dementia: Negative, ambivalent, and positive experiences. *International Journal of Nursing Studies, 49*, 220-229. https://doi.org/10.1016/j.ijnurstu.2011.003

Shyu, Y. I. (2000). The needs of family caregivers of frail elders during the transition from hospital to home: A Taiwanese example. *Journal of Advanced Nursing, 32*, 619-625.

Society of Hospital Medicine. (2008). BOOST implementation guide to improve care transitions. John A. Hartford Foundation. Available at: http://www.hospitalmedicine.org/Web/Quality_Innovation/Implementation_Toolkits/Project_BOOST/Web/Quality___Innovation/Implementation_Toolkit/Boost/First_Steps/Implementation_Guide.aspx

Sundar, V., Fox, S., & Phillips, K. (2014). Transitions in caregiving: Evaluating a person centered approach to supporting family caregivers in the community. *Journal of Gerontological Social Work, 57*, 750-765.

Weaver, F. M., Perloff, L., & Waters, T. (1998). Patients' and caregivers' transition from hospital to home: Needs and recommendations. *Home Health Care Services Quarterly, 17*, 27-49.

White, J. M., Martin, T. F., & Addamsons, K. (2019). *Family theories: An introduction* (3rd ed.). Sage Publications.

Willer, B., Rosenthal, M., Kreutzer, J., Gordon, W., & Rempel, R. (1993). Assessment of community integration following rehabilitation for traumatic brain injury. *Journal of Head Trauma Rehabilitation, 8*(2), 75-87.

Wolff, J. L., & Kasper, J. D. (2006). Caregivers of frail elders: Updating a national profile. *The Gerontologist, 46*(3), 344-356.

Wolff, J. L., Mulcahy, J., Huang, J., Roth, D. L., Kovinsky, K., & Kasper, J. D. (2018). Family caregivers of older adults, 1999-2015: Trends in characteristics, circumstances, and role-related appraisal. *The Gerontologist, 58*(6), 1021-1032. https://doi.org/10.1093/geront/gnx093

Wong-Baker, A. (2018). Wong-Baker FACES pain rating scale. http://www.WongBakerFACES.org

Young, M. E., Lutz, B. J., Creasy, K. R., Cox, K. J., & Martz, C. (2014). A comprehensive assessment of family caregivers of stroke survivors during inpatient rehabilitation. *Disability and Rehabilitation 36*(22), 1892-1902.

Zarit, S. H., & Zarit, J. M. (1983). Cognitive impairment. In P. M. Lewinsohn & L. Teri (Eds.). *Clinical geropsychology* (pp. 38-81). Pergamon Press.

Zakrajsek, A. G., Schuster, E., Guenther, D., & Lorenz, K. (2013). Exploring older adult care transitions from hospital to home: A participatory action research project. *Physical and Occupational Therapy in Geriatrics, 31*(4), 328-344.

Zung, W. K. (1971). A rating instrument for anxiety disorders. *Psychosomatics, 12*, 371-379.

Appendix A: Personal Reflections on Your Own Life Course

In enhancing your understanding of the life course perspective (Elder, 1994), please reflect on your own life experiences with the questions below:

1. What are two events that occurred during your lifetime and what impact did they have on the trajectory of your life course?
2. What are two transitions that have occurred during your lifetime and what impact did they have on the trajectory of your life course?
3. At what age were you first confronted with having to make the first big decision of your life? What was that decision?
4. What historical event had the greatest impact on your life course? Describe the impact the event had on at least one life course trajectory.

Appendix B: Grandparents Raising Grandchildren Program Development

A large role of community-based professionals is to understand needs of those who live in the community and develop programs and services that address these needs. As you develop your professional reasoning about grandparents raising grandchildren, please reflect on program development in this area by discussing the following questions upon reading about this unique family situation in the chapter:

1. What are the key needs of situations of grandparents raising grandchildren, or grandfamilies? Consider the needs of the grandparents and grandchildren.
2. Identify goals or outcomes of a program or service that would address these needs.
3. What activities would be involved in this program or service?
4. Which professional(s) would ideally carry out this program or service? Why?
5. Would other professionals play a role? How so?

Appendix C: Community-Based Practice in a PACE Model

The PACE is an evidence-based model of community-based care to support the needs of older adults who wish to live in the community and their families. Please visit the Centers for Medicare and Medicaid Services webpage describing PACE programs: https://www.cms.gov/Medicare-Medicaid-Coordination/Medicare-and-Medicaid-Coordination/Medicare-Medicaid-Coordination-Office/PACE/PACE

After you have reviewed this website, please discuss the following questions:

1. What services are offered through PACE Programs?
2. How might services provided by your profession be enacted in a PACE program?
3. Choose one profession outside your discipline. How might this profession provide services within a PACE that would be different from your own?
4. Search for a PACE program in your community. Does one exist? If so, what services does it provide?

Part VII

Promoting Spiritual Health

19

CHAPTER

Promoting Spiritual Health

Children and Youth

Tamera Keiter Humbert, DEd, OTR/L, FAOTA; Emmy Vadnais, OTR/L; and Deanna Waggy, OTR, MSA

Learning Objectives

At the end of this chapter, the reader will:

1. Identify and describe aspects of spirituality with children and youth (ACOTE B.1.1, B.1.2)
2. Articulate the various ways spirituality is explored, heightened, and pursued with children and youth (ACOTE B.3.4, B.3.6)
3. Consider various activities and intervention strategies used in daily life and through major life events that attend to spirituality (ACOTE B.4.3)
4. Consider an interprofessional approach focused on a strengths-based approach with children and youth (ACOTE B.4.19)

The ACOTE Standards used are those from 2018.

Key Words

Essence, Flourishing, Generous Purpose, Mindfulness, Progressive Muscle Relaxation, Spiritual Awakening, Spiritual Development, Spiritual Distress, Spiritual Formation, Thriving

Case Study

As part of your consideration in taking on the role of providing an after-school health and wellness program, you receive further information about the role and the organization. The after-school program is an urban, community-funded program offered through a local nonprofit organization. The program is provided to children (ages 8 to 12 years), youth (ages 12 to 15 years), and adolescents (ages 15

Pizzi, M. A., & Amir, M. (Eds.). *Interprofessional Perspectives for Community Practice: Promoting Health, Well-Being, and Quality of Life* (pp. 363-376).

to 18 years). Currently, membership in the after-school program averages 60 children and youth per day, with the majority of members attending in the 8 to 15 age group. The adolescents, ages 15 to 18, participate as volunteers to support the activities of the younger children and are typically older siblings. Some of the members have cognitive and physical developmental delays. The mission of the program is to provide opportunities for holistic development, including spiritual development. There has been a strong physical health and wellness program established but there is now a desire to promote spiritual health and well-being into the program. Structured activities are planned each day, Monday through Friday, for 1 hour. Additionally, there is unstructured time set aside for the children and youth to engage in play, crafts, games, and completing homework. Most of the members attend three to four times per week for 2 hours each day.

Reflective Questions: Part 1

Consider what additional information might be helpful to know about the organization, the members, and past goals and focus of the group. What are your immediate considerations and questions about your role and, in particular the role of promoting spiritual health and well-being?

The Development of Spirituality

Spiritual health and well-being, as well as all other aspects of human development (physical, social, cognitive, emotional) is established through engagement in occupations (including life activities), a nurturing environment, life events, and client factors (Humbert, 2016; James & Ward, 2019). Sometimes referred to as **thriving** or **flourishing**, spiritual health and well-being in childhood and adolescence entails movement toward the integration of roles and routines, spiritual practices in daily life, self-expression, and beliefs. It is the integration of the individual with others that facilitate and nurture a greater sense of love and purpose (Surr, 2011, 2012, 2014) and overall health and well-being (James & Miller, 2017), sometimes referenced as wholeness (Surr, 2014).

The terms thriving and flourishing are terms in spiritual health and well-being that indicate continuous personal and communal growth with the ability to share joy and love and handle life challenges (Allen & Stonehouse, 2021; Bennetts & Bone, 2019; Lee et al., 2019; Wagani & Golani, 2017; Wills, 2019). For some, there is also an understanding of a connection to a higher being, God, the Divine, or transcendence (Allen & Stonehouse, 2021; Boyd, 2017). Religious beliefs and practices may inform spirituality in children and youth; however, when there is no affiliation with religious groups or practices, spirituality still exists. What is important to remember is the various cultural and social considerations of children/youth and their family/communities and how those contexts impact spiritual health and wellness (Bennetts & Bone, 2019; Dillen, 2020; Haugen, 2018; Hong, 2018; King et al., 2017; Richert et al., 2017; Wagani & Golani, 2017).

Connections With Others at Birth and Throughout Infancy

It might be hard to imagine the idea of spirituality at birth and in infancy, as many of us consider spirituality developing later in life, especially when language emerges, and the conceptualization of thoughts and ideas develop. The intimate connection between child and caregiver, and the overall development of newborns toward infancy suggests an awareness of self and others, moving from necessary and strong bonds with others to the individuality of the child. There is an evolution of **spiritual formation** that starts at birth and continues throughout infancy, early childhood, and then adolescent development. Spiritual formation is defined as the process and practices that sets the foundation for ongoing spiritual development (Allen & Stonehouse, 2021).

There is a belief among many that we are all born with an inherent connection to spirituality, whether that connection is with those around us or something greater in the universe (sometimes referred to as the Divine/God) and expressed verbally, as well as, with unspoken language (Adams, 2010; Burgman, 2010; Lovelock & Adams, 2017). There is also some acknowledgement that infants and children have a connection to an intangible world, one that can be observed, engaged, and known (Adams, 2010, 2019). According to Surr (2011), spirituality is facilitated during infant attachment experiences and continues to develop over time through nurturing and safe environments. Surr states,

> For me spirituality is a human condition, not necessarily a religious characteristic. The spirit integrates, bringing together into a coherent whole what otherwise seems disconnected. What is brought together includes: the inner and outer, the known and unknown, the perceived and unacknowledged, the thought and the felt, the then and the now, the here and the there, the real and the imagined, the full and the empty, and the good and the evil (p. 129).

A Personal Reflection

I (Tam, first author) remember the time that I was playing with my young niece, before she could utter a word. We were sitting on the grass in her front yard on a sunny summer afternoon while I was blowing bubbles her way. She was actively engaged in following the bubbles visually and when one would come toward her, she would reach out to touch it. This was a familiar play task engaged many times in my role as a therapist working with children.

What was particularly profound that day was what happened next. At one point in our play, my niece put down her hands and looked up into the sky. I looked as well, trying to make out if there was something above that caught her attention. There were no birds, no planes, nothing observable to my eyes that would have disrupted our play.

I sat there quietly, just observing. I wanted to see what would occur next. I was curious to try to understand what was happening. Then my niece raised both hands above her head. Still looking toward the sky, she was reaching for something not there. She then broke out into a glorious smile, still holding her hands above her head and looking straight up. She maintained that position for at least 1 minute.

I had no idea what she was responding to back then, nor to this day can tell you what was happening in those few moments, but I believe she was responding to something spiritual, something not tangible, but within a greater connection to the universe.

Burgman (2010) shares several stories in her book about the children that she worked with during her time as an occupational therapist. The deep spiritual connections that she observed, many from children who were not verbal, were profound to her and incredibly helpful in understanding who the children were, their true **essence**. Burgman encourages therapists to make space for children to explore a sense of wonder and have the time to relate in different ways to one another. "Children draw upon spiritual qualities to meet life's challenges as well as to offer love and friendship to others" (Burgman, 2010, p. 99). Burgman focuses on three qualities she sees as foundational to spirituality: creating a sense of belonging, hope, and trust.

As a therapist, Burgman (2010) encourages us to approach all individuals with a physical, mental, and spiritual presence that emanates an attitude that all are welcome and enables how we express compassion to one another that is diverse and also welcomed. A sense of belonging references both a belonging to family/community and to one another. Hope entails the ability to imagine and see change and growth in all people, no matter the disability or extent of that disability. In order to promote belonging and hope, relationships and trust between the therapist and child need to be established and developed over time, allowing children to feel safe and allowing them to set the pace of therapy. The children whom we engage in therapy show us as therapists or practitioners who they are.

Ultimately, it is a child's self that we wish to see and relate to meaningfully, not a child's identity as prescribed by the world. When we are in this space, our therapeutic power is quieted, and we must be patient. This is not always easy as our acculturated professional self keeps wanting to resurface and take charge, giving prescriptive choices in the name of empowerment. When we succeed in remaining quiet, the relationship that develops is one of mutual respect and enjoyment. There is a deeper pleasure in being *with*, from a sense that this relationship will be a journey of discovery and sharing. For a little while we are his or her companion, establishing a meaningful relationship with a child within their world (Burgman, 2010, pp. 102-103)

A Reflection on a Spiritual Intervention

As I (Tam) read Burgman's stories, I was reminded of a time in my own practice. I was working with children in an early intervention classroom setting for children with significant physical and cognitive challenges. All of the children, ages 3 to 5 years, were nonverbal.

The relationships built over a period of years between the teachers, aids, therapists, and other children were easy to observe through facial expressions and vocalizations. We knew when the children were happy, irritated, upset, and calm. We could anticipate what activities would bring great joy to the children during playtime and often engaged them in their beloved activities.

One day, I took a child to a quiet part of the room in the attempt to initiate some therapy tasks. I sat there quietly beside the child, trying to collect my thoughts and ponder what to do. I had worked with this particular child for 3 months and had not seen any observable changes or movement toward the established therapy goals. I rationalized that I could sit for a time and not actively engage in any therapy task so I could consider some new activity while also hoping for some inspiration.

It may have only been a few moments that had passed until I felt the light touch of her hand on my shoulder, she was slowly making her way down my arm with her tender small fingers. I continued to sit quietly observing her movements through my sideways glance. When she got to my hand, she took my index finger into her delicate hand and held my finger for some time. Our relationship changed that day, not intentional on my part, other than inadvertently offering space and time to this beautiful child. That day, she had the time and space to share her compassion with me.

Spirituality moves from an unspoken connection, albeit a nonverbal sense, to one that is often externally driven through family and community roles and routines. The development of beliefs during early and middle childhood is often facilitated and reinforced through religious and

Table 19-1

Learning Styles and Prayer Forms

IF YOU LEARN BEST BY:	TRY PRAYING WITH:
Word Linguistic/auditory—Writing, reading, speaking, talking about it, listening to information/lectures	Journaling, blurts, spiritual memoirs, Scripture memory, letters to God, vision board with goals, Jesus prayer, Lectio Divina (meditation with scripture), poetry, haiku, names/metaphors for God
Number Logical/mathematical—reasoning, exploring patterns, conceptualize it	Life mapping, timeline, pros and cons list, Bible study, reading sacred Scriptures and comparing, Ignatian discernment process, hermeneutics (i.e., text interpretation)
Picture Visual/spatial—Visualizing, seeing, images and pictures, daydreaming, drawing, working with color, maps and charts	Mandalas, praying in color, artwork expressing spirituality, guided imagery, imagination with Scripture, creating an altar, collage, cartooning scriptures, discovery journal, online prayer sites, contemplative gazing, ZenTangles®, Visio Divina
Music Musical—Rhythm, melody, composing, sing, rap, instruments, listening to music	Meditating with music, singing, drum circles, playing instruments, sign language with music, writing poetry or lyrics, hum, whistle, music appreciation, concerts, chants
Body Bodily/kinesthetic—Touching, moving, building, acting, dance	Liturgical dance, tai chi, qigong, finger labyrinth, walking the labyrinth, focusing prayer, yoga, praying with clay/playdoh, prayer beads, fabric art, different prayer postures, knitting prayer shawl, sculpture
People Interpersonal—Relating, sharing with others, teaching others, collaborate	Small groups, group spiritual direction, group retreats, intercessory prayer, faith-based book club, discussion groups, praying out loud with others, spiritual friendship, sharing faith stories with others
Self Intrapersonal—Understanding self, working alone	Centering prayer, individual guided retreat, spiritual self-evaluation, silent contemplation, conscious examen, evening review, goal setting, practicing the presence of God, dream analysis, mediation, Yoga Nidra, guided imagery
Nature Natural world—Learning through immersion in nature	Walk in nature, wilderness trips, vision quests, praying through nature, senses prayer walk, gardening, photographing nature, camping, animals/pets, bird watching, food preparation, Zen gardens
Deep Questions Tackling questions about human existence such as the meaning of life	Silent contemplation, practicing the presence of God, asking God questions, What is the meaning of life? What is my calling? Why do we die? How did we get here?

Reproduced with permission from Waggy, D. (2013). *Learning styles and prayer forms.*

faith-based activities and our communities, religious or not. In adolescence, rituals and routines may become more selective and refined to the individual.

Alternative Forms of Spiritual and Religious Practices

The need for alternative and adaptive forms of spiritual and/or religious practices extends to those with different learning needs (Table 19-1). Rachel Brubaker (2017) looked at a small group of faith-based organizations in her local community to assess how individuals with intellectual developmental disabilities (IDD) were supported in their spiritual and religious roles and routines.

She found that the faith-based communities that she explored provided several approaches that complement the occupational therapy practice of modifying activities and environments to enable individuals to engage in select occupations. At times, a buddy system was employed to assist the individual through the activities of the community. Volunteers were trained by a disability ministry staff and the individual's parents/caregivers to provide necessary assistance and support to the individuals when engaging in church activities and to ensure safety during activities. Education was provided to church workers and volunteers regarding applicable sensory and behavioral approaches that could be utilized during activities. Church school curriculums and equipment were modified and the idea of flexibility and assessing the ongoing needs to individuals with intellectual disabilities was always evolving and needed to be specific to the individual.

The faith-based communities facilitated an ethos of inclusion welcoming individuals with disabilities into congregational life while also educating and encouraging members of the congregation to embrace diversity and challenge their own beliefs and stigmas related to disabilities. Rachel shared that the people she engaged in her discussion about disability ministries acknowledged the opportunities for congregants to be open to new ways of relating to others and the ability to show and share love with one another. Ultimately, it was about the many ways in which relationships are understood and built over time through church and community activities. These inclusive programs create and include interprofessional perspectives for community practice. Interprofessional practice does not have to incorporate other "health" professionals. In this case, professionals include church personnel and trained individuals.

Reflective Questions: Part 2

If we understand that spiritual development in early childhood and adolescence is often a significant part of family traditions and routines, and beliefs, religious or otherwise, what needs to be considered in providing activities for spiritual health and wellness? What are the ethical responsibilities that need to be thought through with your potential role in this after-school program? What additional information and resources are needed to remain person and family-centered?

Identity, Agency, Resiliency, and Meaningful Relationships

During early and later adolescence, spiritual development becomes internalized (Spurr et al., 2013) and is often shaped by others outside the family. **Spiritual development**, at times, may be observed as a period of questioning with attempts to integrate previous behaviors and routines with new identity or varying internalized beliefs systems. **Spiritual awakening**, or the heightened awareness of the value and importance of spirituality is often associated with adolescent development (Benson et al., 2012; Fraser, 2014). Struggles with religious beliefs and spirituality, including beliefs adopted in youth and then questioned in later adolescence continues during this life span development through emerging adulthood (Barkin et al., 2015).

Observable outcomes of spirituality entails *doing* (the engagement in select occupations, routines, activities, and roles), *being* (the formation of identity, compassion, wisdom, beauty, and hope) and *becoming* (the integration of agency, ethos, and worldview). Within this spiritual development of doing, being, and becoming, there is also a sense of *belonging* or connection with others (Table 19-2). The progression of spiritual health and wellness is lived out through relationships and continues to develop as relationships are expanded and diversified (King et al., 2011, 2014; Qinn, 2017; Wilcock, 1999).

Importantly, there are multiple cultural and social considerations of and for children and adolescents and how those contexts impact spiritual health and wellness. There is an intersection of culture and/or race, age, gender, and sexual identity that further represents the diversity in spiritual beliefs and practices that impact on health and well-being (Benavides, 2014; Daughtry, 2020; Jebreel et al., 2018; Lee et al., 2019; Michaelson et al., 2019; Pandya, 2015).

Discovery and Facilitation of Spiritual Thriving

Beyond an understanding of the developmental aspects of spirituality, there is an appreciation that spirituality is inherent in all humans (Benavides, 2014). The idea of essence provides an understanding that everyone has the capacity to experience and express spirituality. This notion also posits the idea that each of us knows this uniquely and expresses spiritual health and well-being differently.

Spirituality, influenced by parents and others, is a contributor to health and wellness (Spurr et al., 2013), the notion of thriving (James & Ward, 2019) and flourishing (Gill & Thomson, 2014) and ethical development (Herzog & Beadle, 2018). While spirituality is associated with personal development, spiritual health and wellness also promotes connection to others (people, nature, transcendence) and with the inner self (Michaelson et al., 2019). Spirituality is not only about understanding and embracing our essence, our uniqueness or feeling a sense of love and belonging. Spirituality must go beyond ourselves to help create a sense of purpose in and contribution to our world. It supports how we understand our fit into the larger context of love. Contexts, such as families, schools, and communities, that support **generous purpose**, or the notion of discovering ways in which our lives have meaning and can contribute to the world, are considered important to foster in spiritual well-being. In this process of spiritual health and development, generosity moves us from the focus of self to the expansive view of others and provokes a greater appreciation for the lived experiences of others and the acceptance and inclusion of others (Gill & Thomson, 2014).

Table 19-2

Spiritual Development in Children and Youth

OUTCOMES OF SPIRITUALITY	FOCUS OF SPIRITUALITY	DESCRIPTION/EXAMPLES	REFERENCES
Doing	Engaging in family rituals and routines or family-encouraged activities	• Participating in religious activities and educational activities, youth groups, volunteer activities, community leadership • Participating in spiritual/religious activities of prayer, reading sacred texts • Practicing dietary laws	Carter & Boehm (2019)
	Engaging in self-selected occupations and conscious interactions	• Volunteering or engaging in charitable events • Connecting with others and developing relationships • Connecting with others, nature, and transcendence (relational spirituality) • Developing confidence competence, character, connections, and caring	Benavides (2014) Fernandez et al. (2016) Fraser (2014) James & Ward (2019) Jebreel et al. (2018) King et al. (2011) Michaelson et al. (2019)
Being	Shaping identity	• Engaging a desire or longing to connect with something beyond ourselves • Discovering who I am or the essence of the person, accepting and affirming one's uniqueness • Developing congruence and agency, what one believes and lives out. This process is developed through reflection, opportunities to develop voice through the engagement in relationships	Daughtry (2020) Fraser (2014) Harris (2016) Jackson et al. (2010) Taplin (2014)
	Developing compassion and generosity, altruism	• Being concerned for and caring for others, giving beyond ourselves	Büssing et al. (2010) Byrnes (2012) Johnstone et al. (2016)
	Aspiring to beauty, awe, curiosity, and wisdom	• Making sense of the world and experiencing the goodness of and inspiration through the world	Harris (2016)
	Embracing hope for the future	• Seeing and understanding future possibilities	Hardy et al. (2019) James & Ward (2019) Rogers (2014)
Becoming	Developing a worldview and ethos	• Understanding my world and my place in the world; making sense of my culture	Daughtry (2020) Ekblad & Oviedo (2017) Mason et al. (2007)

Considering Spiritual Health and Well-Being as a Component of Awareness and Intervention

Life events and personal circumstances from infancy or acquired during childhood and adolescence, may disrupt spiritual development and health. If we understand the importance of relationships and the value connection with others have in the development of spirituality, then factors and circumstances that disrupt those relationships such as loss, abuse, and trauma may also disrupt spiritual health and well-being. **Spiritual distress** is the term used to describe when spiritual constructs or beliefs are in conflict with one another that diminishes one's meaning or purpose of life and a loss of connectedness with others (Hall et al., 2016). For example, a child might believe that they are loved and cared for and have embraced that understanding in their life but when a tragic accident takes away a parent's life and the resulting circumstances effects stress and conflict in the home, the idea of love may be challenged for the child. The long-term impact of spiritual distress may lead to further complex and compromising conditions such as substance use disorders (SUD), suicidality, homelessness, and incarceration, which ultimately further impacts health and wellness (Centers for Disease Control and Prevention [CDC], n.d.).

Approaches that support realigning and expanding relationships, and ultimately spiritual health, include recognizing where prosocial relationships may be encountered, building and strengthening a variety of relationships, and engaging with others in valued occupations and activities (Hennessy et al., 2019). This may include facilitating a relationship with another individual (peer or family member) and engaging in a valued activity (sport, game, craft, etc.) and then facilitating greater connections with small groups who have that same valued activity. It is within these relationships that more holistic and expanded roles may be engaged and allowed to flourish (Bryant-Davis et al., 2012; Hardy et al. 2019).

Beyond building trust and connection with others, spirituality has also been used to provide some sense of coping, hopefulness, and resiliency, either in the temporarily ordering of one's beliefs (Beckstead et al., 2015; Bryant-Davis et al., 2012; Hardy et al. 2019; James & Ward, 2019) or within the long-term process of dealing with life challenges (Clayton-Jones, 2019; Warner et al., 2020) and in providing renewal and healing (Jackson et al., 2010; Mirkovic et al., 2020).

Youth in foster care, incarcerated youths, and youths who have experienced trauma and abuse have utilized spirituality as a coping mechanism in dealing with their life events by wrestling with their own beliefs, coming to terms with situations beyond their control, and making sense of or further exploring their understanding of a higher being within their own pain and suffering and healing (Jackson et al., 2010; Rogers, 2014). Art and music-related activities may be used to allow the youth to initially express their feelings through drawings, collages, the selection or creation of lyrics, and then to discuss how those feelings are grounded in our beliefs and ultimately can be reconfigured or understood (Coholic et al., 2020; Forrest-Bank et al., 2016; Gambrel et al., 2020).

Additionally, the use of daily activities, such as prayer and meditation, have also been linked to the development of routines providing an internalizing of spiritual aspects, and thus, providing greater spiritual health and wellness (Stewart et al., 2019). It is in the process of doing (prayer, meditation) that we start to understand our own self (being) and what we are becoming, and how we belong. Routines and rituals that become integrated and helpful for our coping bring relief from spiritual distress.

Life events that surround acquired health or long-term, chronic conditions may also disrupt or have a significant impact on spiritual health and well-being in children and youth. Identity, hope for the future, and a changed world view shifts during these life events. Some examples of such events include the diagnosis of cancer and the impact on personal growth and hope for the future (Sodergren et al., 2017; Warner et al., 2020), the diagnosis of HIV and the challenges to one's personal beliefs (Smith et al., 2017), and the diagnosis of sickle cell disease with the understanding of self, the expectations of health care providers, and beliefs regarding health and wellness (Clayton-Jones et al., 2019). The intentional focus of spiritual care during such life events provides a way to cope with the physical and psychological challenges associated with medical treatment by producing a reduction in levels of anxiety (Vazifeh doust et al., 2020), an avenue to connect or reconnect with spiritual practices (Smith et al., 2017), and a mechanism to evaluate and challenge one's personal beliefs and assumptions (Clayton-Jones et al., 2019; Smith et al., 2017).

Beyond the perspective of life events and circumstances impacting spiritual development, the notion of spiritual development for all needs to be considered. When spiritual health and wellness is supported with cognitive and neurodiverse children and youth, new paradigms are established in understanding constructs of spirituality and the adaptation of roles and responsibilities. For example, an appreciation for or belief in the spiritual meaning of animals may provoke comfort when seen or experienced and facilitate care for the animals. There is an appreciation for the diversity in conceiving spiritual identity and understanding different world views (Ekblad & Oviedo, 2017; Gill & Thomson, 2014), and in ways to engage spiritual practices and routines. In one particular study, individualized approaches and activities to support the engagement in religious and spiritual practices with children and youth with IDD were identified (Carter & Boehm, 2019). The primary activities engaged tended to center around social activities and being invited to or incorporated into group activities; however, there were limited opportunities to actually engage in spiritual and religious

Table 19-3

Examples of Activities That Facilitate Spirituality in Children and Adolescence

ACTIVITY	EXAMPLES	REFERENCES
Culturally sensitive spiritual and/or religious practices	• Meditation • Prayer • Rituals	Daughtry (2020)
Mindfulness	• Breathing • Meditation • Mind-focused exercises	Byrnes (2012) Cobb et al. (2015a, 2015b)
Creativity	• Art • Play	Harris (2016)
Shared perspectives	• Self-narratives • Storytelling	Daughtry (2020) Smith et al. (2017)
Discovery of meaning and purpose (critical analysis of beliefs)	• Discussion groups	Daughtry (2020) Smith et al. (2017)
Project-driven events	• Charitable events • Leisure activities	Fernandez et al. (2016)
Inspiration and awe	• Nature activities	Harris (2016)
Connectedness	• Intergenerational activities • Holiday celebrations and rituals	Harris (2016)

practices. Recommendation by the authors included the need to modify tasks and environments to accommodate tasks that allow individualized contributions to the religious and spiritual community (Carter & Boehm, 2019).

Avenues to and Through Spirituality

Spiritual development that fosters health and wellness is promoted through the engagement of activities and/or occupations (activities with personal meaning; Humbert, 2016; Maley et al., 2016). While some activities lead us toward spirituality, other activities bring us into the realm of spirituality. It is not always easy to know what activities are leading to or producing spiritual growth, but it is in the experience of engaging activities or occupations that spirituality and spiritual health is promoted (Table 19-3). Such activities and occupations are generally understood as those that ultimately create or facilitate a greater awareness of the self and of others.

Beyond the doing of such activities, there is also an understanding of the internal sense of presence, or a state of "being" sometimes called mindfulness, that one brings to or gains through activities and occupations, further contributing to one's spiritual development. **Mindfulness**, described as an inborn trait, one that is personal and dispositional, augments the spiritual experience (Brown et al., 2013; Cobb et al., 2015a; Kabat-Zinn, 2018). Mindfulness, believed to exist in all humans at birth, is simply the ability to be present in the moment or to pay attention to what is occurring in the moment (remember the story of the first authors' niece earlier in this chapter). Babies need to be attentive to the moment to survive; they are aware when they are hunger or uncomfortable or in pain. Even though they do not conceptually understand mindfulness, they do it all of the time. Watch a child play and see how they observe and inspect and discover toys. Mindfulness tends to fade as we begin to develop language, cognition, thought, and anticipation of future events. However, it is in the practice of mindful exercises and activities that we rediscover the primal use of our mind.

Mindfulness decreases stress (Schussler et al., 2021) increases sensory awareness and perception (Ciesla et al., 2012) and spiritual awareness (Ciesla et al., 2012). Mindfulness activities, as an intentional practice, is about attending to the present moment through select activities such as breathing, meditation, and mind-focused tasks (Byrnes, 2012; Cobb et al., 2015b). The following section will highlight avenues in which a relaxation state may be achieved, thus facilitating a state of mindfulness and potentially greater spiritual awareness.

The Relaxation Response

According to the World Health Organization (WHO), stress is a significant problem that can affect both physical and mental health (WHO, 2020). Stress is defined as a situation where the organism's homeostasis is threatened or perceives a situation as threatening (Perry & Pollard, 1998). Progressive muscle relaxation, autogenic training, relaxation response, biofeedback, emotional freedom technique (EFT), guided imagery, diaphragmatic breathing, transcendental meditation, cognitive behavioral therapy, mindfulness-based stress reduction, and emotional freedom technique are all evidence-based techniques that are easy to learn and practice that have good results with people whether they have good health or those experiencing disease, illness, or disability (Varvogli & Darviri, 2011).

We need a certain amount of movement, energy, stress, or tension to move us forward in our lives. Stress can enhance performance to a point, but when a line is crossed, excessive stress impedes performance and can cause or exacerbate illness or disease. Stress can create negative cycles of fear, worry, anxiety, negative thought patterns, racing heart, high blood pressure, anger, greater vulnerability to pain, poor sleep and eating habits, and lifestyle choices that can impact health and wellness.

Prayer and meditation have been shown in research to be able to elicit the relaxation response of rest and digest (parasympathetic nervous system) that is opposite of the stress response of fight, flight, or freeze (sympathetic nervous system; Ciesla et al., 2012; Take Steps to Prevent or Reverse Stress-Related Health Problems, 2017). People who have elicited the relaxation response have also reported experiencing a connection with something greater than them, and they feel a more spiritual connection (Johnstone et al., 2016).

For some children, it may be difficult to achieve a deep relaxation response without other calming activities. Active play and physical exertion can be a way for children to initially release excess energy and to get ready for more techniques in developing relaxation and improving physical, mental, and spiritual resilience. Below are some examples of strategies for achieving a deep relaxation response for children and youth that may lead to a deeper link to their spiritual health and well-being.

Progressive Muscle Relaxation

One may be seated or lying or even standing to complete **progressive muscle relaxation (PMR)**. It does not require any equipment to complete, and the approach can be done in quiet or throughout daily activities when relaxation is needed. PMR helps children and youth to attend to their bodies and recognize the difference between tight and contracted muscles and relaxed ones. A regular practice of PMR helps tune our mind and body to quickly recognize periods of stress so that we can actively engage in relaxation.

- Starting with the feet and working up the body, contract a muscle group and hold for 10 to 30 seconds. For example, start by curling your toes and holding that position.
- After holding the position for 10 to 30 seconds, slowly release that hold, paying attention to how that body part feels.
- Rest the body part for another 10 to 30 seconds and then slowly move or rock that body part, again paying attention to how that movement feel on the body part.
- Repeat the same steps with the same body part(s) and then move up the body to the next area. From the feet, progress to the ankles by pulling your toes toward your stomach.
- Continue this process up through the legs, the buttocks and stomach, chest, arms, jaw, and eyes until you have reached the top of your head.

Breath Work

The quality of breath can impact a person's quality of life, the physical body, and mental and emotional states or mood. The body can become tense if not breathing well, and conversely, tension or poor body posture or positions can affect the breath. Shallow breathing limits the range of motion of the diaphragm. As a result, the lowest part of the lungs doesn't get a full amount of oxygenated air. This can make a person feel short of breath and anxious. Deep abdominal breathing encourages full oxygen exchange, that is, the beneficial trade of incoming oxygen for outgoing carbon dioxide. This can then slow the heartbeat and lower or stabilize blood pressure (Russo et al., 2017).

Breath work techniques are simple and effective. There are generally two types of breath-focused practices—those that emphasize focus on breathing, such as mindfulness, and those that require breathing to be controlled, such as deep breathing practices including diaphragmatic or abdominal breathing and pranayama. In cases when a person's attention is compromised, practices that emphasize concentration and focus, such as mindfulness, where the individual focuses on feeling the sensations of respiration but make no effort to control them, could possibly be most beneficial. In cases where a person's level of arousal is the cause of poor attention, for example, a pounding heart during an exam, or during a panic attack, it should be possible to alter the level of arousal in the body by controlling breathing. Both of these techniques have been shown to be effective in both the short and the long term (Cruz et al., 2020).

Table 19-4

Examples of and Resources for Breathing Techniques

Mindful breathing	https://ggia.berkeley.edu/practice/mindful_breathing
Diaphragmatic breathing	https://www.healthline.com/health/breathing-exercise
Lion's breath	https://www.healthline.com/health/breathing-exercise
Alternative nostril breath	https://www.verywellmind.com/abdominal-breathing-2584115
Box breathing	https://www.verywellmind.com/abdominal-breathing-2584115
4-7-8 breathing	https://www.healthline.com/health/4-7-8-breathing

With deep and slow breathing, breath work can stimulate the vagus nerve and induce the relaxation response (Table 19-4). Treatments that target the vagus nerve increase the vagal tone and inhibit cytokine production. Both are important mechanism of resiliency. Increased through meditation and yoga, breath work may likely contribute to resilience and the mitigation of mood and anxiety symptoms. Stimulation of vagal afferent fibers in the gut influences brain systems in the brain stem that play crucial roles in major psychiatric conditions such as mood and anxiety disorders (Breit et al., 2018; Hayes et al., 2019; Hashim & Zainol, 2015; Joy et al., 2014; Larson et al., 2014; Mandreş & Crăciun, 2015; Währborg et al., 2016).

Listening to our Heart—Creative Expressions and Relating to Others

In this avenue to and through spirituality, the focus is about developing the ability to listen, to hear deeply what others are saying and what our heart or intuition are saying to us. (This follows "Incorporated Spirituality" described in the introductory chapter). For many, including children and youth, this creative endeavor follows nicely after breath work and some relaxation activities. Examples of creative and expressive activities include:

- Telling our stories and listening to others' stories
- Creative writing
- Poetry exploration
- Nature walks
- Collages
- Listening to music and completing free flowing drawing
- Drama play
- Animal therapy, petting a dog or cat or other trained animal that is sensitive to children's touch

Reflective Questions: Part 3

Consider the suggested activities mentioned in the preceding section. How might you adapt these activities to the demands and needs of the children and youth in different age groups? What activities could be adapted to meet any physical or cognitive or social client factors of the children and youth?

An Interprofessional Approach to Spirituality: Implications for Health and Wellness

Interprofessional approaches integrate multiple voices and perspectives from various disciplines to maximize our understanding and application of a topic. Within the area of health and wellness, an interprofessional approach may be used to expand our understanding of concepts, to provide more comprehensive interventions, and to better appreciate an ethos or approach to support spiritual health and well-being.

As previously stated, the formative years of childhood are filled with activities, rituals, and routines, often provided by families and communities that influence and impact spiritual development. Sometimes, these communities can be religious or faith-based or not and also include schools, sports, or other social groups. The plurality of understanding spirituality in these multiple contexts is broad. What is needed to support spiritual development, health, and wellness is first a cultural appreciation for family rituals and routines, and cultural awareness, sensitivity, and humility when we do not have an understanding or an appreciation of the child and family's culture (Surr, 2014). Deep listening and respecting the narratives of children and youth plays another significant role in promoting human flourishing (Adams, 2010, 2019; Burgman, 2010; Rogers, 2014). In addition, we are encouraged in our contemporary understanding of spirituality to be more expansive of our understanding of spirituality.

> The spiritual dimension of life helps individuals create frameworks of meaning and provides individuals with a way of being in the world which influences their decisions and actions. It enables them to interpret their life experiences, which can help them to work through difficult and unhappy times, overcome challenges, and find purpose in being. … We have reached a stage in the transitional process of this discipline, then, where we can say that no particular form or expression of spirituality is superior to another, or which can be weighted more favourably than another. (de Souza et al., 2016, p. 346)

We are thus encouraged to embrace a concept of spirituality that is "sufficiently broad enough to be inclusive... that recognizes human rights and voice…and recognizes the whole person" with the message that every child matters (Watson, 2017, p. 14).

Conclusion

Spiritual health and well-being begins at birth and continue to develop throughout childhood. The ability to bond and connect with caregivers, and the ability for children to experience tangible and intangible worlds around them initially grounds their spiritual experiences. Later, family rituals and routines further support the child in ways of "doing," facilitating opportunities for developing the self and relating to others (being). Ultimately, spiritual health and well-being is marked by "becoming" as one's beliefs and resiliency are shaped and developed and "belonging" to groups with similar identities. Spiritual development is promoted through the engagement in meaningful activities and within a context of safety, support, and respect.

References

Adams, K. (2010). *Unseen worlds: Looking through the lens of childhood.* Jessica Kingsley Publishers.

Adams, K. (2019). Navigating the spaces of children's spiritual experiences: Influences of tradition(s), multidisciplinarity and perceptions. International *Journal of Children's Spirituality, 24*(1), 29-43. https://doi.org/10.1080/1364436X.2019.1619531

Allen, H. C., & Stonehouse, C. (2021). *Forming resilient children: The role of spiritual formation for healthy development.* IVP Books.

Barkin, S., Miller, L., & Luthar, S. (2015). Filling the void: Spiritual development among adolescents of the affluent. *Journal of Religion & Health, 54*(3). https://doi.org/10.1007/s10943-015-0048-z

Beckstead, D. J., Lambert, M. J., DuBose, A. P., & Linehan, M. (2015). Dialectical behavior therapy with American Indian/Alaska Native adolescents diagnosed with substance use disorders: Combining an evidence based treatment with cultural, traditional, and spiritual beliefs. *Addictive Behaviors, 51*, 84-87. https://doi.org/10.1016/j.addbeh.2015.07.018

Benavides, L. E. (2014). Spiritual journey from childhood to adolescence: Pathways to strength and healing. *Journal of Religion & Spirituality in Social Work, 33*(3/4), 201-217. https://doi.org/10.1080/15426432.2014.930628

Bennetts, K., & Bone, J. (2019). Adult leadership and the development of children's spirituality: Exploring Montessori's concept of the prepared environment. *International Journal of Children's Spirituality, 24*(4), 356-370. https://doi.org/10.1080/1364436X.2019.1685949

Benson, P., Scales, P., Syvertsen, A., & Roehlkepartain, E. (2012). Is youth spiritual development a universal developmental process? An international exploration. *Journal of Positive Psychology, 7*(6), 453-470. https://doi.org/10.1080/17439760.2012.732102

Boyd, J. P. (2017). *Imaginative prayer: A yearlong guide for your child's spiritual formation.* IVP Books.

Breit, S., Kupferberg, A., Rogler, G., & Hasler, G. (2018). Vagus nerve as modulator of the brain-gut axis in psychiatric and inflammatory disorders. *Frontiers in Psychiatry, 9*, 44. https://doi.org/10.3389/fpsyt.2018.00044

Brown, K., Goodman, R., & Inzlicht, M. (2013). Dispositional mindfulness and the attenuation of neural responses to emotional stimuli. *Social Cognitive and Affective Neuroscience, 8*(1), 93-99. https://doi.org/10.1093/scan/nss004

Brubaker, R. (2017). *The role of occupational therapy in developing and implementing Christian church ministries for adults and children with intellectual/developmental disabilities.* Unpublished manuscript. Elizabethtown College.

Bryant-Davis, T., Ellis, M. U., Burke-Maynard, E., Moon, N., Counts, P. A., & Anderso, G. (2012). Religiosity, spirituality, and trauma recovery in the lives of children and adolescents. *Professional Psychology: Research & Practice, 43*(4), 306-314. https://doi.org/10.1037/a0029282

Burgman, I. (2010). Enabling children's spirituality in occupational practice. In S. Roger (Ed.), *Occupation-centred practice with children: a practical guide for occupational therapists.* Wiley.

Byrnes, K. (2012). A portrait of contemplative teaching: Embracing wholeness. *Journal of Transformative Education, 10*(1), 22-41. https://doi.org/10.1177/1541344612456431

Carter, E. W., & Boehm, T. L. (2019). Religious and spiritual expressions of young people with intellectual and developmental disabilities. *Research & Practice for Persons with Severe Disabilities, 44*(1), 37-52. https://doi.org/10.1177/1540796919828082

Centers for Disease Control and Prevention. (n.d.). Adverse childhood experiences (ACEs). https://www.cdc.gov/violenceprevention/aces/index.html

Ciesla, J., Reilly, L., Dickson, K., Emanuel, A., & Updegraff, J. (2012). Dispositional mindfulness moderates the effects of stress among adolescents: Rumination as a mediator. *Journal of Clinical Child & Adolescent Psychology, 41*(6), 760-770. https://doi.org/10.1080/15374416.2012.698724

Clayton-Jones, D., Haglund, K. A., Schaefer, J., Koenig, H. G., & George Dalmida, S. (2019). Use of the Spiritual Development Framework in conducting spirituality and health research with adolescents. *Journal of Religion & Health, 58*(4), 1259-1271. https://doi.org/10.1007/s10943-018-00752-z

Cobb, E. F., Miller, L. J., & McClintock, C. (2015a). Mindfulness and spirituality in positive youth development. In I. Ivtzan & T. Lomas (Eds.), *Mindfulness in positive psychology: The science of meditation and wellbeing.* Routledge.

Cobb, E., Kor, A., & Miller, L. (2015b). Support for adolescent spirituality: Contributions of religious practice and trait mindfulness. *Journal of Religion & Health, 54*(3), 862-870. https://doi.org/10.1007/s10943-015-0046-1

Coholic, D., Schwabe, N., & Lander, K. (2020). A scoping review of arts-based mindfulness interventions for children and youth. *Child & Adolescent Social Work Journal, 37*(5), 511-526. https://doi.org/10.1007/s10560-020-00657-5

Cruz, M. Z., Fernandes de Godoy, M., Valenti, V. E., Pereira Jr, A., & Dias Cardoso, R. A. (2020). The effects of slow breathing exercise on heart rate dynamics and cardiorespiratory coherence in preschool children: A prospective clinical study. *Alternative Therapies in Health & Medicine, 26*(4), 14-21.

Daughtry, P. (2020). Portraits of the "Shy Hope": Engaging youth spiritualities in the Australian context. *International Journal of Religion & Spirituality in Society, 10*(1), 13-27. https://doi.org/10.18848/2154-8633/CGP/v10i01/13-27

de Souza, M., Bone, J., & J. Watson. (2016). *Spirituality across disciplines: Research and practice*. Springer.

Dillen, A. (2020). Children's spirituality and theologising with children: The role of "context." *International Journal of Children's Spirituality, 25*(3/4), 238-253. https://doi.org/10.1080/1364436X.2020.1843412

Ekblad, L. & Oviedo, L. (2017). Religious cognition among subjects with autism spectrum disorder (ASD): Defective or different? *Clinical Neuropsychiatry, 14*(4), 287-296.

Fernandez, N. A., Schnitker, S. A., & Houltberg, B. J. (2016). Charitable sporting events as a context for building adolescent generosity: Examining the tole of religiousness and spirituality. *Religions, 7*(3), 35. https://doi.org/10.3390/rel7030035

Forrest-Bank, S., Nicotera, N., Bassett, D., & Ferrarone, P. (2016). Effects of an expressive art intervention with urban youth in low-income neighborhoods. *Child & Adolescent Social Work Journal, 33*(5), 429-441. https://doi.org/10.1007/s10560-016-0439-3

Fraser, D. (2014). The eternal yearning. *International Journal of Children's Spirituality, 9*(1), 17-24. https://doi.org/10.1080/1364436X.2014.886559

Gambrel, L. E., Burge, A., & Sude, M. E. (2020). Creativity, acceptance, and the pause: A case example of mindfulness and art in therapy with an adolescent. *Journal of Creativity in Mental Health, 15*(1), 81-89. https://doi.org/10.1080/15401383.2019.1640151

Gill, S., & Thomson, G. (Eds.). (2014). *Redefining religious education: Spirituality for human flourishing*. Palgrave Macmillan,

Hall, E. J., Hughes, B. P., & Handzo, G. H. (2016). *Spiritual care: What it means, why it matters in healthcare*. Healthcare Chaplaincy Network. https://healthcarechaplaincy.org/docs/about/spirituality.pdf

Hardy, S. A., Nelson, J. M., Moore, J. P., & King, P. E. (2019). Processes of religious and spiritual influence in adolescence: A systematic review of 30 years of research. *Journal of Research on Adolescence, 29*(2), 254-275. https://doi.org/10.1111/jora.12486

Harris, K. I. (2016). Let's play at the park! Family pathways promoting spiritual resources to inspire nature, pretend play, storytelling, intergenerational play and celebrations. *International Journal of Children's Spirituality, 21*(2), 90-103. https://doi.org/10.1080/1364436X.2016.11646

Hashim, H. A., & Zainol, N. A. (2015). Changes in emotional distress, short term memory, and sustained attention following 6 and 12 sessions of progressive muscle relaxation training in 10-11 years old primary school children. *Psychology, Health & Medicine, 20*(5), 623-628. https://doi.org/10.1080/13548506.2014.1002851

Haugen, H. M. (2018). It is time for a general comment on children's spiritual development. *International Journal of Children's Spirituality, 23*(3), 306-322. https://doi.org/10.1080/1364436X.2018.1487833

Hayes, D., Moore, A., Stapley, E., Humphrey, N., Mansfield, R., Santos, J., Ashworth, E., Patalay, P., Bonin, E.-M., Moltrecht, B., Boehnke, J. R., & Deighton, J. (2019). Examining mindfulness, relaxation and strategies for safety and wellbeing in English primary and secondary schools: Study protocol for a multi-school, cluster randomised controlled trial (INSPIRE). *Trials, 20*(1), N.PAG. https://doi.org/10.1186/s13063-019-3762-0

Hennessy, E. A., Cristello, J. V., & Kelly, J. F. (2019). RCAM: A proposed model of recovery capital for adolescents. *Addiction Research & Theory, 27*(5), 429-436. https://doi.org/10.1080/16066359.2018.1540694

Herzog, P. S., & Beadle, D. A. T. (2018). Emerging adult religiosity and spirituality: Linking beliefs, values, and ethical decision-making. *Religions, 9*(3), 84. https://doi.org/10.3390/rel9030084

Hong, C. J. (2018). Cultivating Woori: The experience and formation of children and youth in Korean immigrant communities. *Practical Matters, 11*, 46-56.

Humbert, T. K. (2016). *Spirituality and occupational therapy: A model for practice and research*. AOTA Press.

Jackson, L. J., White, C. R., O'Brien, K., DiLorenzo, P., Cathcart, E., Wolf, M., Bruskas, D., Pecora, P. J., Nix, E. V., & Cabrera, J. (2010). Exploring spirituality among youth in foster care: Findings from the Casey Field Office Mental Health Study. *Child & Family Social Work, 15*(1), 107-117. https://doi.org/10.1111/j.1365-2206.2009.00649.x

James, A., & Ward, R. M. (2019). Temporal relation between youths' perceived spirituality and indicators of positive development. *Journal of Research on Adolescence, 29*(2), 345-356. https://doi.org/10.1111/jora.12448

James, A. G., & Miller, B. (2017). Revisiting Mahoney's "My Body Is a Temple…" study: Spirituality as a mediator of the religion-health interaction among adolescents. *International Journal of Children's Spirituality, 22*(2), 134-153. https://doi.org/10.1080/1364436X.2017.1301888

Jebreel, D. T., Doonan, R. L., & Cohen, V. (2018). Integrating spirituality within Yalom's group therapeutic factors: A theoretical framework for use with adolescents. *Group: Journal of the Eastern Group Psychotherapy Society, 42*(3), 225-244. https://doi.org/10.13186/group.42.3.0225

Johnstone, B., Cohen, D., Konopacki, K., & Ghan, C. (2016). Selflessness as a foundation of spiritual transcendence: Perspectives from the neurosciences and religious studies. *International Journal for the Psychology of Religion, 26*(4), 287-303. https://doi.org/10.1080/10508619.2015.1118328

Joy, F. E., Jose, T. T., & Nayak, A. K. (2014). Effectiveness of Jacobson's Progressive Muscle Relaxation (JPMR) technique on social anxiety among high school adolescents in a selected school of Udupi District, Karnataka State. *Nitte University Journal of Health Science, 4*(1), 86-90.

Kabat-Zinn, J. (2018). *The healing power of mindfulness: A new way of being*. Hachette Press.

King, P. E., Abo, Z. M. M., & Weber, J. D. (2017). Varieties of social experience: The religious cultural context of diverse spiritual exemplars. *British Journal of Developmental Psychology, 35*(1), 127-141. https://doi.org/10.1111/bjdp.12181

King, P. E., Carr, A., & Boitor, C. (2011). Spirituality, religiosity, and youth thriving. In R. M. Lerner, J. V. Lerner, & J. B. Benson (Eds.), *Advances in child development and behavior, Vol. 1: Positive youth development: Research and applications for promoting thriving in adolescence* (pp. 161-195). Elsevier.

King, P. E., Clardy, C. E., & Ramos, J. S. (2014). Adolescent spiritual exemplars: Exploring spirituality in the lives of diverse youth. *Journal of Adolescent Research, 29*(2), 186-212. https://doi.org/10.1177/0743558413502534

Larson, H. A., Kim, S. Y., McKinney, R., Swan, A., Moody, A., Offenstein, K. L., German, D., & Puschalski, S. (2014). This is just a test: Overcoming high-stakes test anxiety through relaxation and gum chewing when preparing for the ACT. *Eastern Education Journal, 42*. Faculty Research & Creative Activity. http://thekeep.eiu.edu/csd_fac/4

Lee, S., Jirásek, I., Veselský, P., & Jirásková, M. (2019). Gender and age differences in spiritual development among early adolescents. *European Journal of Developmental Psychology, 16*(6), 680-696. https://doi.org/10.1080/17405629.2018.1493990

Lovelock, P., & Adams, K. (2017). From darkness to light: Children speak of divine encounter. *International Journal of Children's Spirituality, 22*(1), 36-48. 10.1080/1364436X.2016.1268098

Maley, C. M., Pagana, N. K., Velenger, C. A., & Humbert, T, K. (2016). Dealing with major life events and transitions: A systematic literature review on and occupational analysis of spirituality. *American Journal of Occupational Therapy, 70*(4), 1-6. https://doi.org/10.5014/ajot.2016.015537

Mandreş, C. M., & Crăciun, A. (2015). The effectiveness of the relaxation techniques, in stress reduction and optimization strategies for coping in teenagers. *Romanian Journal of Cognitive-Behavioral Therapy & Hypnosis, 2*(4), 31-41.

Mason, M., Singleton, A., & Webber, R. (2007). *The spirit of generation Y—Young people's spirituality in a changing Australia*. John Garratt Publishing.

Michaelson, V., King, N., Inchley, J., Currie, D., Brooks, F., & Pickett, W. (2019). Domains of spirituality and their associations with positive mental health: A study of adolescents in Canada, England and Scotland. *Preventive Medicine, 125*, 12-18. https://doi.org/10.1016/j.ypmed.2019.04.018

Mirkovic, B., Cohen, D., Garny de la Rivière, S., Pellerin, H., Guilé, J.-M., Consoli, A., & Gerardin, P. (2020). Repeating a suicide attempt during adolescence: Risk and protective factors 12 months after hospitalization. *European Child & Adolescent Psychiatry, 29*(12), 1729-1740. https://doi.org/10.1007/s00787-020-01491-x

Pandya, S. P. (2015). Adolescents, well-being and spirituality: Insights from a spiritual program. *International Journal of Children's Spirituality, 20*(1), 29-49. https://doi.org/10.1080/1364436X.2014.999230

Perry, B. D., & Pollard, R. (1998). Homeostasis, stress, trauma, and adaptation: A neurodevelopmental view of childhood trauma. *Child and Adolescent Psychiatric Clinics of North America, 7*(1), 33-51. https://doi.org/10.1016/S1056-4993(18)30258-X

Quinn, B. P. (2017). Supporting generous purpose in adolescence: The roles of school climate and spirituality. *International Journal of Children's Spirituality, 22*(3/4), 197-219. https://doi.org/10.1080/1364436X.2017.1373077

Richert, R. A., Boyatzis, C. J., & King, P. E. (2017). Introduction to the British Journal of Developmental Psychology special issue on religion, culture, and development. *British Journal of Developmental Psychology, 35*(1), 1-3. https://doi.org/10.1111/bjdp.12179

Rogers, C. L. (2014). Search for transcendence revealed in childhood narratives of poverty, abuse and neglect, and social isolation. *Journal of Spirituality in Mental Health, 16*(3), 218-236. https://doi.org/10.1080/19349637.2014.925369

Russo, M. A., Santarelli, D. M., & O'Rourke, D. (2017). The physiological effects of slow breathing in the healthy human. *Breathe, 13*(4), 298-309. https://doi.org/10.1183/20734735.009817

Schussler, D. L., Oh, Y., Mahfouz, J., Levitan, J., Frank, J. L., Broderick, P. C., Mitra, J. L., Berrena, E., Kohler, K., & Greenberg, M. T. (2021). Stress and well-being: A systematic case study of adolescents' experiences in a mindfulness-based program. *Journal of Child & Family Studies, 30*(2), 431-446. https://doi.org/10.1007/s10826-020-01864-5

Smith, S., Blanchard, J., Kools, S., & Butler, D. (2017). Reconnecting to spirituality: Christian-Identified adolescents and emerging adult young men's journey from diagnosis of HIV to coping. *Journal of Religion & Health, 56*(1), 188-204. https://doi.org/10.1007/s10943-016-0245-4

Sodergren, S., Husson, O., Robinson, J., Rohde, G., Tomaszewska, I., Vivat, B., Dyar, R., & Darlington, A. S. (2017). Systematic review of the health-related quality of life issues facing adolescents and young adults with cancer. *Quality of Life Research, 26*(7), 1659-1672. https://doi.org/10.1007/s11136-017-1520-x

Spurr, S., Berry, L., & Walker, K. (2013). The meanings older adolescents attach to spirituality. *Journal for Specialists in Pediatric Nursing, 18*(3), 221-232. https://doi.org/10.1111/jspn.12028

Stewart, C., Rapp-McCall, L., & Drum, L. (2019). The relationship of spirituality and mental health to recidivism. *Social Work & Christianity, 46*(4), 67-86. https://doi.org/10.34043/swc.v46i4.105

Surr, J. (2011). Links between early attachment experiences and manifestations of spirituality. *International Journal of Children's Spirituality, 16*(2), 129-141. https://doi.org/10.1080/1364436X.2011.580725

Surr, J. (2012). Peering into the clouds of glory: Explorations of a newborn child's spirituality. *International Journal of Children's Spirituality, 17*(1), 77-87. https://doi.org/10.1080/1364436X.2012.677810

Surr, J. (2014). Children growing whole. *International Journal of Children's Spirituality, 19*(2), 123-132. https://doi.org/10.1080/1364436X.2014.924907

Take Steps to Prevent or Reverse Stress-Related Health Problems. (2017). *Harvard Health Letter, 42*(5), 1-7. https://www.health.harvard.edu/stress/take-steps-to-prevent-or-reverse-stress-

Taplin, M. (2014). A model for integrating spiritual education into secular curricula. *International Journal of Children's Spirituality, 19*(1), 4-16. https://doi.org/10.1080/1364436X.2013.873860

Varvogli, L., & Darviri, C. (2011). Stress management techniques: Evidence-based procedures that reduce stress and promote health. *Health Science Journal, 5*, 74-89.

Vazifeh doust, M., Hojjati, H., & Farhangi, H. (2020). Effect of spiritual care based on Ghalbe Salim on anxiety in adolescent with cancer. *Journal of Religion & Health, 59*(6), 2857-2865. https://doi.org/10.1007/s10943-019-00869-9

Wagani, R., & Golani, R. (2017). Effectiveness of association with spiritual missions on spiritual wellness among adolescence. Indian *Journal of Positive Psychology, 8*(3), 338-341.

Waggy, D. (2013). Learning styles and prayer forms. ot4peace@gmail.com

Währborg, P., Day, A. L., Andersson-Gäre, B., Golsäter, M., Rydå, U., Jansson, M., & Nilsson, M. (2016). An evaluation of daily relaxation training and psychosomatic symptoms in young children. *Health Behavior & Policy Review, 3*(3), 198-208. https://doi.org/10.14485/HBPR.3.3.2

Warner, E. T., Zhang, Y., Gu, Y., Taporoski, T. P., Pereira, A., DeVivo, I., Spence, N. D., Cozier, Y., Palmer, J. R., Kanaya, A. M., Kandula, N. R., Cole, S. A., Tworoger, S., & Shields, A. (2020). Physical and sexual abuse in childhood and adolescence and leukocyte telomere length: A pooled analysis of the study on psychosocial stress, spirituality, and health. *PLoS ONE, 15*(10), 1-24. https://doi.org/10.1371/journal.pone.0241363

Watson, J. (2017). Every child still matters: Interprofessional approaches to the spirituality of the child. *International Journal of Children's Spirituality, 22*(1), 4-13. https://doi.org/10.1080/1364436X.2016.1234434

Wilcock, A. A. (1999). Reflections on doing, being and becoming. *Australian Occupational Therapy Journal, 46*, 1-11. https://doi.org/10.1046/j.1440-1630.1999.00174.x

Wills, R. J. (2019). Creating the condition for doubt. How might questioning and critical thinking inspire children's spiritual development? International *Journal of Children's Spirituality, 24*(4), 341-355. https://doi.org/10.1080/1364436X.2019.1672628

World Health Organization. (2020). Doing what matters in times of stress: An illustrated guide. https://www.who.int/publications/i/item/9789240003927

CHAPTER 20

Promoting Spiritual Health
Adults

Tamera Keiter Humbert, DEd, OTR/L, FAOTA and Emmy Vadnais, OTR/L

Learning Objectives

At the end of this chapter, the reader will:

1. Identify and describe aspects of spirituality with adults (ACOTE B.1.1, B.1.2)
2. Articulate the various ways spirituality is explored, heightened, and pursued with adults (ACOTE B.3.4, B.3.6)
3. Consider various activities and intervention strategies used in daily life and through major life events that attend to spirituality (ACOTE B.4.3)
4. Consider an interprofessional approach focused on crisis intervention with adults (ACOTE B.4.19)

The ACOTE Standards used are those from 2018.

Key Words

Coherence, Conscientiousness, Contemplation, Distress, Emerging Adults, Evolved Altruism, Existential Well-Being, Flow and Spirituality, Guided Imagery, Individuation, Intuition, Intuitive Awareness, Resiliency, Transcendence, Transformative Coping, Universal Self, Wholeness

Case Study

As part of the anticipated role in delivering health and wellness programs, you are asked to consider developing a day-long retreat for women at a local, privately owned health and fitness organization. The organization provides wellness activities for the community with a focus on individuals, children, and families from the local area. Members come from a variety of racial and socioeconomic backgrounds. There has been an expressed interest by some of the women who attend exercise classes to offer retreats one time per

Pizzi, M. A., & Amir, M. (Eds.). *Interprofessional Perspectives for Community Practice: Promoting Health, Well-Being, and Quality of Life* (pp. 377-391).

month from 9 am to 3 pm with the focus on spiritual health and wellness. The women who are organizing the first event includes one woman in her mid-50s who is divorced, one woman in her 40s who is committed in a partnership and identifies as LGBQT, and one woman in her 30s that is married with one child, age 10 years. Two of the organizers are women of color, the other identifies as White.

Reflective Questions: Part 1

Consider what you know about spiritual health and wellness to this point. What questions do you have about designing a women's retreat focused on spirituality? What resources could be helpful in planning activities for the day retreat? What additional information is helpful to have as you consider this opportunity?

Spiritual Development in Adults—Moving to Wholeness

Spirituality in adulthood is further refined and developed from adolescence through the period identified as emerging adulthood through middle adulthood. The overall focus of spiritual health and wellness is on the integration and movement to wholeness, bringing disparate personal, social and cultural actions, beliefs, and perspectives together. The development of spirituality within this age group includes aspects of 1) self-discovery and awareness, 2) conscientiousness and individuation, 3) transformative coping and resiliency, 4) transcendence and renewal, 5) meaning, purpose, and existential well-being, 6) wholeness and the search for wisdom, 7) compassion and empathy, 8) values and beliefs, and 9) evolved altruism (see Table 20-1 for references and descriptions). These aspects are further developed or strengthened through the intentional engagement of attending to the spiritual through the engagement in select practices and/or by the impact of major life transitions (Reymann et al., 2015) and events including childbirth (Athan & Miller, 2013; Hansen et al., 2021) and parenting (Hyde, 2020; Watson, 2017), disease or illness (Maley et al., 2016), or trauma and loss (Barry et al., 2020; Karimi et al., 2019). Generally speaking, these aspects are developed internally and expressed or acted upon externally. For example, after going through a major break-up, someone may take time to evaluate what is most important to them, what values and beliefs about relationships still hold true, and what ideas no longer fit into their understanding of life. Through this internal "working" of spiritual constructs, the person may come to enlightenment about how they wish to pursue new relationships. This personal and spiritual growth is then observed in the outward "doing" of building new relationships. Spiritual development to wholeness is considered an ongoing process. With further reflection within this internal/external process, additional clarity and growth and development happens (Humbert, 2016).

Spirituality still exists even with no religious identification. Cultural and social considerations are contexts that impact spiritual health and wellness. There is an intersection of culture and/or race, age, gender, and sexual identity that further represents the diversity in spiritual beliefs and practices and which may impact on health and well-being (Barkin et al., 2015; Beagan & Hattie, 2015; Boro & Dhanalakshmi, 2015; Bryant et al., 2016; Kralovec et al., 2018; Ochoa et al., 2018; Reymann et al., 2015; Voisin et al., 2016; Waizbard-Bartov et al., 2019). There is also some recognition from authors that describe the great diversity needed in incorporating spirituality and religious beliefs and practices with those who have immigrated from their home country and culture to a new life experience in another county (Cuevas et al., 2010; Hall et al., 2019; Kim & Kim-Godwin, 2019)

The period of **emerging adults** (ages 18 to 25 years) demonstrates a significant period of discovery, choice, and often change in life perspectives that impact spiritual beliefs and practices (Barry et al., 2010; Burney et al., 2017; Koenig, 2015; Voisin et el., 2016) or religious beliefs and practices (Bryant et al., 2016). During the emerging adult phase, spirituality is frequently influenced by peers, older adults, parents, social media, and communities (Barry et al., 2010; Herzog & Beadle, 2018). Struggles with religious beliefs and spirituality, including beliefs adopted in youth and then questioned in emerging adulthood are understood as typical throughout the evolution of this development (Barkin et al., 2015; Krause & Hayward, 2013). In emerging adults, spiritual health and well-being is strengthened through the engagement in spiritual practices, the psychological adjustment to life events, personal reflection, and dialogue with others (Barry et al., 2020; Herzog & Beadle, 2018). Physical and psychological wellness is further impacted by spiritual wellness practices and the ability to attend to life events (Scalora et al., 2020).

Adults who have conflicting or varying differences between their beliefs, religious or otherwise, and spiritual practices speak about an ongoing process of bringing these disparate ideas and perspectives together or in alignment. It is a process that both requires and engenders contemplation, reflection or introspection, thoughtful dialogue, active doing or engaging in meaningful activities, and a community that will support this self-discovery (Beagan & Hattie, 2015; Bryant et al., 2016; Halkitis et al., 2009; Humbert, 2016; Maley et al., 2016; Martinez & Scott, 2014).

Table 20-1

Aspects of Spirituality in Adults

ASPECT	DESCRIPTION	REFERENCES
Self-discovery and awareness	A holistic experience in which understanding of the self and self-acceptance is developed or heightened.	Burney et al. (2017) Hall et al. (2019) Trama & Modi (2016) Waizbard-Bartov et al. (2019)
Conscientiousness and individuation	Becoming attuned to the present (mindfulness) and how we respond uniquely to the present.	Mudge (2018) Scalora et al. (2020)
Transformative coping and resiliency (sometimes expressed as hope)	The use of spiritual practices brings about new insights and ways to cope with ongoing life challenges.	Corry et al. (2014) Corry et al. (2015) Hiebler-Ragger et al. (2016) Sagan (2016)
Transcendence and renewal	Experiences of "other worldly" and finding a new sense of power, energy, and clarity.	Steffler & Murdoch (2017)
Meaning, purpose, and existential well-being	An awareness as to what is most important in this life, clarity as to one's role within their life.	Waizbard-Bartov et al. (2019)
Compassion and empathy	Expanding one's capacity to see and experience new perspective that brings about a deeper level of care for another (person or population).	Athan & Miller (2013) Waizbard-Bartov et al. (2019)
Wholeness and the search for wisdom	A feeling of integration of the self (aspects known and unknown) with all of the universe.	Beagon & Hattie (2015) Bryant et al. (2016) Surr (2014)
Values and beliefs	Guiding principles that inform how we carry out our daily life and how we respond to life.	Kobza & Salter (2016) Herzog & Beadle (2018) Trama & Modi (2016)
Evolved altruism	Giving back to others or a community as a direct response of one's life experiences.	Bryant et al. (2016)

Reflective Questions: Part 2

Based on the descriptions provided in Table 20-1, what aspects of adult spirituality do you most connect with, and which areas are the most unknown or unfamiliar to you? At this point in the planning, do you think it better to address multiple aspects of spirituality during the retreat or focus on one or two areas with greater depth? How would you determine how to make those decisions?

Use of Spirituality Within Intervention: A Populations Approach

Spiritual health and wellness can be addressed with adults, whether they have a medical or clinical diagnosis or not and has been addressed in the literature to include general health and wellness practices. In addition, spiritual health and wellness can be focused on specific adult populations facing changes in roles, physical and/or psychosocial client factors. A few examples are provided in the following section.

Adults With Cancer

The literature highlights attention to and the support of spirituality with those diagnosed with cancer (Ochoa et al., 2019; Whitney, 2019). Palliative care, a philosophical approach to attending to and alleviating suffering and promoting quality of life (QOL), is provided to individuals with or without a terminal illness (National Institute on Aging [NIA], n.d.). Hospice care is provided to those with a terminal illness in which life expectancy is limited to 6 months or less (NIA, n.d.). In both palliative care and hospice care, the focus of spirituality is addressed by investigating what is most meaningful for the individual and/or family/caregivers, clarifying goals and desires for daily life, and attending to end-of-life concerns (Pizzi, 2014). It is highly recommended that palliative care and hospice care be an integral part of the intervention plan for those diagnosed with end-stage cancer (NIA, n.d.). However, what is not as well investigated in the literature is the assessment and intervention with those with advanced cancer. The American Society of Clinical Oncology recommends that all patients with advanced cancer be referred for interprofessional palliative care early in their diagnosis (Ferrell et al., 2016); however, palliative care is frequently underutilized with this population. What is documented in the literature is the value of finding and upholding a sense of meaning in one's life and a feeling of peace during the end stages of cancer (Ferrell et al., 2016, 2020; Pizzi, 2014, 2015).

Adults Dealing With Trauma

Understanding the interconnection between trauma and spiritual and/or religious practices and beliefs is complex. Adverse childhood experiences (ACEs) are sometimes complicated by the child's and emerging adult's personal experiences conflicting with spiritual and/or religious beliefs and practices (Bryant-Davis & Wong, 2013; Easton et al., 2019; Glenn, 2014; McCormick et al., 2017; Prior & Petra, 2020; Waterman, 2020). Emerging adults and middle-aged adults who have experienced violence, sexual assault, loss of a parent or significant caregiver, serious illness or disability, either as a child or in their adult lives, are often faced with the need to make meaning of the event or trauma (Ashraf & Fatima, 2014; Jalote, 2016; Prior & Petra, 2020; Rogers, 2014; Shackle, 2017; Zhang et al., 2015a, 2015b).

Trauma-informed practice entails the awareness and sensitivity to how trauma impacts neurological, physical, cognitive, psychosocial, and spiritual function and development. Intervention practices include both direct mediation in promoting continued interpersonal development, along with implementing environments and activities to best adapt and support daily function (Treatment Improvement Protocol [TIP], 2014). Therapeutic intervention also entails a careful look at spiritual and religious practices that are or have been destructive and those that are protective. The recognition of resilient children and adults in breaking cycles of trauma highlights the ongoing work of attending to generational trauma and finding new meaning and life purpose (Anderson & Bernhardt, 2020).

Recovery from Violence, Women Supporting Women—A Personal Reflection

In my work with women overcoming violence, I (Tam, first author) have spent many hours listening to women's personal stories. This appears to be a form of spiritual healing when the women are ready to share their narratives, their lived experiences of violence and recovery.

On a trip to Kenya, visiting an organization that supported women learning and engaging in work and economic trades, I was met by a group of women who were part of this faith-based group. Some of the women were members of the group for a decade or longer, others just a few months. All the women experienced violence, whether through intimate partner violence, genocide, civil war, or poverty. Their ages ranged from early 20s through 60s. I was there to continue my research in understanding how women overcome violence. I invited any woman to come and share their insights and perspectives with me. Initially, I was planning to record the interviews, with their permission, so that I could transcribe and code the interviews for themes.

What I found out pretty quickly was that the women's stories were rich, unique, and very powerful. I made the decision to leave their narratives fully intact to better appreciate their wisdom. All of the women made meaning of their experiences, were able to talk about their own resiliency through the process of recovery, and were reclaiming their life purpose. Each woman's recovery was often challenging and frequently diverted due to other obligations and family responsibilities but is ongoing and present.

What grounded these women through their recovery was the support of one another, their care for others, and daily work and occupations. They considered this organization a spiritual home and community. They cooked for one another, shared meals together, taught one another work skills, and participated in singing and prayers. What was apparent in the women's stories was the love expressed and shared between them, with me, and the other guests to the organization. These values and beliefs of love and compassion were lived out, tested frequently, and reaffirmed through their daily lives.

Each of the women who shared their stories had a "mission," something that they felt called to do, share, or engage that brought healing to others.

Persons Living With HIV and AIDS

Persons living with HIV/AIDS (PLWHA) often experience stress and limited QOL in aspects of physical, emotional, environmental, and spiritual well-being that ultimately impacts independence (Brandt et al., 2017). The literature highlights PLWHA having significantly higher incidences of suicidal ideation than the general public (Serafini et al., 2015; Zarei & Joulaei, 2018). In a comparative study between adults with HIV-positive or HIV-negative indicators, both groups demonstrated compatible differences in spiritual and religious practices (Cuevas et al., 2010). In addition to these results, the comparison between older adults, ages 50 years and older, and younger adults, ages 21 to 49 years, from the HIV-positive group were similar in their spiritual and religious practices. The significant difference, as noted in the study, concluded that individuals who are HIV-positive and have higher indices toward spirituality and religious practices have greater health outcomes, a larger support system, and a more positive affect (Cuevas et al., 2010).

Populations Dealing With Suicidal Ideation

Suicidal ideation, or the thoughts and preoccupation about suicide, is a significant indicator for attempted and completed suicides. Two populations that experience greater incidence of suicidal ideation than their peers have been identified in extensive studies and include young adults dealing with substance addiction and mental health (Harris et al., 2020; Oh et al., 2021) and veterans suffering from post-traumatic stress disorder (PTSD; Florez et al., 2018; Kopacz et al., 2016; Lusk et al., 2018; Smigelsky et al., 2020). In these studies, one of the mediating factors to reduce or eliminate ideation is spiritual well-being and/or religious beliefs and practices (Sepala et al., 2014). The ability to explore existential perspective to life and to find meaning, hope, and resilience through protective spiritual health and well-being practices aids in the reduction of suicidal ideation and ultimately impacts greater health and life satisfaction (Lawrence et al., 2016; Lusk et al., 2018; Shinde & Wagani, 2019).

Parents of Children With Autism Spectrum Disorder

Within the general empirical literature, the focus of parents' reports of raising a child with autism has been to highlight this role as complicated, difficult, and stressful (Yehonatan-Schori et al., 2019). However, within the literature, there is also some indication that glimmers of hope or something positive may also come about or from that parenting relationship. What is now being better understood is that growth from both a psychological and spiritual perspective can result from this important parenting role. This perspective is supported by the idea that trauma, and other challenging life experiences, while stressful and often complex, can bring about personal growth (Waizbard-Bartov et al., 2019; Zhang et al., 2015a, 2015b). This may be experienced as a greater or more complete sense of self, a clearer understanding as to what is most important in life, and an appreciation of diverse ways to relate to one another. This growth, referenced as spiritual growth, is one that is ongoing, progressive, and constantly evolving throughout daily life and over time (Waizbard-Bartov et al., 2019; Zhang et al., 2015a, 2015b).

Spiritual Assessment

Spiritual assessment is important to conduct prior to suggesting and providing intervention goals and activities. There are several assessment guides that can be used within interprofessional practice. When working with adults, it is important to have an appreciation for how they understand spirituality, what they wish to accomplish in their spiritual lives, and what brings them closer to their understanding of spirituality.

Throughout this chapter it has been emphasized that spirituality is deeply connected to the meaningfulness of life activities in a person's life. Assessment of a person's activities of daily life, the meaning they have in their lives, and how it may be connected to one's sense of self, spirit, and participation in such would be an important first step in addressing interventions that make care client-centered. These interventions can then help support and promote one's health, well-being, and QOL, in particular, one's spiritual health. Several assessments are addressed in the "Introduction to Spiritual Health" chapter.

Intervention Practices to Support Spiritual Health and Well-Being in Adults

Interventions with adults and/or groups and populations that focus on spirituality may be direct and focused, with the goal of stabilization when attending to crisis or a major life challenge. Conversely, intervention may also entail general strategies that support an overall wellness perspective. Intervention strategies fall into categories of *Body Awareness*, *Mindfulness*, *Introspection*, and *Engagement*. All these strategies can be completed individually or taught and implemented in groups and within select populations and will be further described in the following section.

Practitioners often start with activities associated with body awareness and mindfulness as those are often considered the least intrusive. Practitioners then move to more intense activities associated with introspection and

Table 20-2

Body Awareness and Mindfulness Intervention Strategies

INTERVENTION STRATEGIES	PRIMARY PURPOSE	EXAMPLES OF THERAPEUTIC ACTIVITIES	REFERENCES
Body awareness	Relaxing the body and preparing for deeper levels of mindfulness and introspection	Breathing Progressive muscle relaxation Yoga	de Diego et al. (2021) Park et al. (2017) Pascoe et al. (2017) Riley et al. (2017) Wang & Szabo (2020) Saxena, et al. (2020) Yadav et al. (2015)
Mindfulness	Paying attention to what we are experiencing in the moment, directing our inner thoughts	Meditation Mindful activities	Amaro et al. (2010) Bin Abdullah et al. (2018) Carlson et al. (2016) Lifshitz et al. (2019) Trombka et al. (2018)

engagement. It is important to note, however, that all individuals, but particularly those who have experienced trauma, need to be an integral part of decision making in which activities they engage. Those who have experienced physical, psychological, and sexual trauma may have adverse effects from activities addressing body and mind.

Body Awareness and Mindfulness

As in the previous chapter, we will start by looking at ways to prepare the body for relaxation to facilitate further spiritual experiences and responses. The following section will highlight background information about the relaxation response and basic yoga principles. We will then transition to attending to the mind in bringing greater clarity and attention through mindfulness and meditation practices (Table 20-2).

The Relaxation Response

There is evidence that the more one elicits the relaxation response, the greater one's chances are of preventing and recovering from disease. Your genes can literally change to a positive expression that is the opposite of the stress response that can create disease (Benson & Proctor, 2011; Bhasin et al., 2013).

Benson updated the relaxation response method and created the *Benson-Henry Protocol* on how to induce the relaxation response and improve genetic expression to prevent and heal from disease (Benson, 2011). Regularly inducing the relaxation response through meditation, the Benson-Henry Protocol, or other relaxation activities are healthy lifestyle choices that can create health promotion and wellness (Mind-Body Medicine Research at Massachusetts General Hospital, n.d.).

In addition to the health benefits, Dr. Benson also found that people experienced increased spirituality from the relaxation response and described two aspects of the experience: 1) the presence of an energy, a force, a power—God—that was beyond themselves; and 2) this presence felt close to them. The people who felt a presence had the greatest health benefits.

> ...those who elicit the relaxation response regularly for more than one month had higher spirituality scores than those who did so less than one month. It didn't matter if you were novice or an old-timer, religious or nonreligious; the effects and rewards of the faith factor proved possible for very diverse individuals. (Benson & Stark, 1997)

Yoga

When you think of yoga, you may visualize the yoga poses or physical postures, also known as asanas. Yoga, however, goes beyond the physical postures and can produce significant changes in health and well-being (Griera, 2017). Asanas were believed to be developed to help us connect to the divine within and the divine seemingly outside of ourselves. Translations of yoga communicate union or to yoke your divine self and spiritual connection, that is, to be connected with your inner divine self simultaneously with the greater divine and be at one. Yet, yoga is not a religion.

There are eight limbs, or stages of yoga, that may help you with states of consciousness, including intuition, being healthy, and living a meaningful and purposeful life. The eighth limb is a state of absorption, known as samadhi (considered by many to be the goal of yoga), where intuition may be most easily experienced. The eight limbs of yoga are:

1. Yama: Universal morality
2. Niyama: Personal observances
3. Asanas: Body postures
4. Pranayama: Breathing exercises and control of prana
5. Pratyahara: Control of the senses
6. Dharana: Concentration and cultivating inner perceptual awareness
7. Dhyana: Devotion, meditation on the Divine
8. Samadhi: Union with the Divine (Sarbacker & Kimple, 2015)

Performing traditional yoga through the eight limbs entails paying attention to mind, body, and spirit with the ultimate goal of moving past the ego or self-consciousness to a collective or **Universal Self** that sees the visible and invisible, the tangible and intangible in all people and nature (Ram, 2010). It is a way of perceiving reality beyond our cognitive thinking, ultimately freeing the mind in grasping for answers or control (Ram, 2010). Practitioners of yoga who engage the eight limbs develop awareness of what is happening within their body (postures, breathing, senses, perceptions) and within the collective universe (mediation and union with the Divine; Sarbacker & Kimple, 2015).

Engaging in a more western yoga practice, particularly performing postures, breathing, and developing our perception and senses provides an opportunity to attend to how the body and mind feels, to relax the body and mind, and to attune the body and mind in response to stress (Tarkeshi, 2017). The increased state of body-mind relaxation then allows the person to be ready to engage in further practices of meditation and mindfulness (Tarkeshi, 2017).

Meditation

Meditation is a form of focused attention where a person can be present with a compassionate and nonjudgmental awareness where they can become quieter and freer from negative thoughts, worries, concerns, or emotions. This can allow a person to access greater insight, intuition, and spirituality (Lifshitz et al., 2019). In many cultures, meditation is a way to get into a state of awareness that the personal self and the Universal Self (a collective understanding or knowing) are one (Radin, 2018).

Structures of the brain can change just after 8 weeks of meditating regularly. A study by Hölzel et al. (2010) found that people who were new to meditation and went through an 8-week mindfulness-based stress reduction program had thickening in four regions of the brain (likely the result of the creation of new neuronal connections):

1. The posterior cingulate, which is involved in mind wandering and self-relevance
2. The left hippocampus, which assists in learning, cognition, memory, and emotional regulation
3. Thetemporo-parietal junction, which is associated with perspective taking, empathy, and compassion
4. The pons, an area of the brainstem where a lot of regulatory neurotransmitters are produced

In addition, an area that got smaller was the amygdala, the fight-or-flight part of the brain, which is important for anxiety, fear, and stress in general.

Meditation can also make your brain younger. However, long-term meditators have an increased amount of gray matter in the insula and sensory regions, as well as the auditory and sensory cortex. They have more gray matter in the frontal cortex, which is associated with working memory and executive decision making (Lazar et al., 2005). In one study, 50-year-old meditators had the same amount of gray matter in their prefrontal cortex as 25-year-olds (Schulte, 2015).

Meditation may:

- Regulate emotions
- Calm the mind and body
- Enhance spiritual states
- Assist you to quiet your mental chatter, creating space between thoughts, judgments, or worrying mind
- Help return the body back toward homeostatic balance
- Lower physical and emotional pain, stress, and tension
- Ease depression and insomnia
- Create clearer awareness and insight
- Improve compassion, sense of well-being, and QOL (Amaro et al., 2010; Bin Abdullah et al., 2018; Carlson et al., 2016; Lifshitz et al., 2019 Trombka et al., 2018).

There are many types of meditation (Table 20-3). While health care practitioners can teach others how to meditate, it is best that the health care practitioner has learned meditation skills and has implemented them into their lives with their own regular practice. Experience in meditation is necessary to be able to understand what can occur in meditation and to be able to help others navigate developing their own meditation practice. It is best to receive support when learning meditation to have a positive experience, allowing for a pleasurable experience and thus supporting people to look forward to meditation time.

Mindfulness can be practiced as a form of meditation or as a skill brought into ADLs.

Table 20-3

Examples of and Resources for Meditation/Mindfulness Practices

Mindful dialogue	https://www.wiseheartpdx.org/12-competencies-of-mcd
Mindful body scan	https://www.mindful.org/the-body-scan-practice/
Eating mindfulness/ meditation	https://www.thecenterformindfuleating.org/FREE-Meditations
Guided meditation	https://www.tarabrach.com/guided-meditations/
Heart meditation	https://healthy-heart-meditation.com/heart-meditation/
Mindful contemplative prayer	https://www.contemplative.org/contemplative-practice/centering-prayer/
Walking meditation	https://ggia.berkeley.edu/practice/walking_meditation
Writing mindfulness	https://www.developgoodhabits.com/mindful_writing/
Mindful yoga	https://www.mindful.org/yoga-poses-for-meditation/

Introspection and Engagement

As the body and mind are relaxed, our ability to attend to insights and expand perspectives (introspection) may be facilitated and our ability to engage with others, nature, and creativity can be increased, thereby expanding our spiritual health (Table 20-4). In the following section, we will further describe the use of guided imagery, prayer, energy healing, love, and heart work as approaches to introspection. Lastly, we will address the use of creativity and play and states of flow as it relates to engagement. It is our belief that these practices may certainly be used with adults during times of life transitions and dealing with major life events; however, the development of these practices over time produces daily life resilience and prepares people to better deal with life transitions and events through established body-mind-spirit connections embedded in daily routines.

Guided Imagery

Often, an image can convey a meaning or symbolism far greater than we can describe in words. Before we learned verbal language, we perceived the world with all our senses and saw in images or pictures. Carl Jung promoted active imagination. He stated in his book, *Jung on Active Imagination*,

> When you concentrate on a mental picture it begins to stir, the image becomes enriched by details, it moves and develops ... and so when we concentrate on an inner picture and when we are careful not to interrupt the natural flow of events, our unconscious will produce a series of images which make a complete story. (Jung & Chodorow, 1997, p. 145)

Guided imagery is a simple way to connect to intuition and spirituality. It is a healing approach that bridges the communication between the mind, the body, and the spirit (Table 20-5). It occurs in a relaxed, meditative state, and may also be referred to as creative visualization, mental imagery, therapeutic imagery, interactive guided imagery, guided meditation, and active imagination. It can assist in healing physical, emotional, mental, and spiritual disharmony (Mobini & White, 2020; Nooner et al., 2016; Schlesinger et al., 2014; Sharp et al., 2021).

Through guided imagery, you may discover parts of yourself you are now ready to see. This can be very enlightening, as it will give you the opportunity to connect more deeply with your essence or true self. In addition, there may be suppressed emotions and beliefs that need to come to the surface, which may need healing or will create new insights. Your own light and love may be suppressed as well. You may find you can transform your limitations into new opportunities.

A key component of guided imagery is its ability to help others connect to their inner wisdom, or intuition, that can then guide in ways that are not always accessible in normal waking states. Guided imagery encompasses all our senses. Jeanne Achterberg, PhD, a pioneer of imagery and mind, body, spirit medicine, states that imagery is,

> ... the thought process that invokes the senses: vision, audition, smell, taste, the sense of movement, position, and touch. It is the communication mechanism between perception, emotion, and bodily change. A major cause of both health and sickness, the image is the world's greatest healing resource. Imagery, or the stuff of the imagination, affects the body intimately on both seemingly mundane and profound levels. (Achterberg, 1985)

This is the main premise in the field of psychoneuroimmunology—how thoughts, feelings, emotions, and beliefs affect the body and the nervous and immune systems. When we experience prolonged stress or tension, we are more at risk of being unwell, as our immune systems can be compromised, and certain areas of our being may be negatively affected (Jessop, 2019; Littrell, 2019; Ravi et al., 2021; Vasile, 2020).

Table 20-4

Introspection and Engagement Intervention Strategies

INTERVENTION STRATEGIES	PRIMARY PURPOSE	EXAMPLES OF THERAPEUTIC ACTIVITIES	REFERENCES
Introspection	Preparing for greater insights and self-awareness; sometimes referred to as enlightenment	Guided imagery Prayer and contemplation	Johnson (2018) Lehmann et al. (2019) Mobini & White (2020) Nooner et al. (2016) Puchalska-Wasyl & Zarzycka (2020) Schlesinger et al. (2014) Sharp et al. (2021)
Engagement	Intentionally doing something that builds relationships, increases compassion for others and self, and/or promotes creativity (creation)	Prayer Energy healing Practices Art/poetry Dance Nature activities	Birocco et al. (2012) Corry et al. (2014) Corry et al. (2015) Illueca & Doolittle (2020) Johnson (2018) Krause & Hayward (2013) Lehmann et al. (2019) Puchalska-Wasyl & Zarzycka (2020) Ünal Aslan & Çetinkaya (2021)

Table 20-5

Introspection and Engagement Intervention Strategies

ORGANIZATION	RESOURCES
University of California, San Francisco Osher Center for Integrative Medicine	https://osher.ucsf.edu/guided-imagery-meditation-resources https://osher.ucsf.edu/patient-care/clinical-specialties/guided-imagery
University of Minnesota, Earl E. Bakken Center for Spirituality and Healing	https://www.takingcharge.csh.umn.edu/sources-guided-imagery
U.S. Department of Veteran Affairs, Whole Health Library	https://www.va.gov/WHOLEHEALTHLIBRARY/tools/guided-imagery.asp
Interactive Guided Imagery (IGI)	https://positivepsychology.com/interactive-guided-imagery-therapy/
Thomas More Center, Guided Imagery and Prayers	https://www.thomasmorecenter.org/resources/prayers/guided-imagery/
Benson-Henry Institute Mind-Body Medicine at Massachusetts General Hospital	https://bensonhenryinstitute.org/meditation-cd-and-dvd/

Energy Healing

Energy healing has been used in all cultures for many years. In some cultures, it has its root in healing temples where "laying on of hands" was practiced: a person receives divine life force channeled through the energy healer (Vadnais, 2020). Energy healing, such as qigong, reiki, or laying on of hands may be considered a form of prayer, mental intention, or psychokinesis—a mental ability that affects physical reality (Chandran, 2019; Dunn, 2019). Energy healing is noninvasive with little risk. During energy healing a person often naturally begins contemplating the nonphysical reality and their minds turn to the spiritual realm (Meredith, 2020; Vadnais, 2020). Energy healing has been shown in research studies to decrease stress, anxiety, pain, depression, and insomnia (Beseme et al., 2020; Gonella et al., 2014; Jauregui et al., 2012; Rafii et al., 2020; Siegel, 2018).

Love and the Heart

Throughout history, ancient societies, philosophers, poets, and prophets have regarded the heart as the source of love, wisdom, intuition, the soul, and positive emotions (Dunn, n.d.). The Egyptians believed that the heart was connected to spiritual dimensions. After death, the heart was weighed to see how much good and evil it contained, and it was put in special urns for burial, and the brain was discarded. Thus, there is a disparity between what ancient traditions believed and modern predominant science's teaching that the heart solely provides a physical function (Noetic Systems International, n.d.).

Images of the heart can be seen in religious iconography and are elevated, imploring us to contemplate what it represents, the highest values. Most spiritual or religious practices teach the importance of the heart and being loving and kind to the self and others. Adages such as "listen to your heart," "follow your heart," or "lead from the heart" must derive from a physical feeling of well-being in the body when we take direction from that organ or its location in the chest. The positive effect of doing so is likely why these sayings have survived so long. As we connect with our heart center, we shift into a loving, compassionate awareness. From a neutral, nonjudgmental place we may switch into our **intuitive awareness**. When we are more coherent—not emotional, thinking, confused, and so on—we are able to listen to our heart more clearly (Vadnais, 2020).

Heart rate variability is associated with resilience, better health and fitness, and mental clarity. It is the amount of variability your heart has in between your heartbeats. It is a marker of physiological resilience and behavioral flexibility, how well your mind and body can handle stressors and environmental demands (HeartMath Institute, 2017; Tyagi et al., 2016).

The HeartMath Institute has created simple steps to achieve what they term a "coherent state" or "**coherence**." This is when there is more heart rate variability allowing you to feel better and have more mental clarity. The more relaxed and positive you feel, the more heart rate variability you will have, and the more your heart and brain will function in a coherent state. This coherent state practice, Quick Coherence Technique, can be achieved in about 1 minute. Connecting with the heart and feeling more positive echoes the compassion, mindfulness, and lovingkindness meditations. The more that we are in a coherent state, the more easily we can listen to the higher intelligence of intuition (heartmath.org). Therefore, the more you abide in these states of consciousness, the better you will feel, with a stronger ability to cope with and respond to what may come your way in life.

Creativity and Play

Creativity, or the ability to make something out of seemingly nothing, reflects a process of longing for something missing and intuitively seeking something to answer the missing link (Rodrigues et al., 2019). It is a process of moving between intuition and conscious awareness as building blocks are developed overtime and the creation is being formed (Lucchesi, 2017; Nelson & Rawlings, 2007). There is a sense of the process beyond one's control, a sense of joy and flow, and being in the moment, aspects frequently referenced as spiritual (Nelson & Rawlings, 2007). An aspect of creativity is also described as play in which potential and possibilities are discovered through openness and engaging in activity. In addition, the use of creativity can build spiritual health and well-being by allowing the expression of the human spirit to be generated. and with that engagement, insights may be expanded, feelings of gratitude and joy may be evoked (Corry et al., 2014, 2015).

A State of Flow

Spirituality is often synonymous with joy and peace. When a person is immersed in the moment with whatever activity they're engaging in, not thinking of the past or the future but being in the now, the subsequent **flow** can create the most exhilarating, joyful, or serene feelings. This, ancient wisdom sages have said for millennia, is the path to enlightenment. Modern health care research shows that this flow state may help people prevent, recover from, or cope with disease.

Mihaly Csikszentmihalyi says in his informative book, *Flow: The Psychology of Optimal Experience* (2008),

> In our studies, we found that every flow activity, whether it involved competition, chance, or any other dimension of experience, had this in common: It provided a sense of discovery, a creative feeling of transporting the person into a new reality. It pushed the person to higher levels of performance and led to previously undreamed-of states of consciousness. In short, it transformed the self by making it more complex. In this growth of the self lies the key to flow activities. (2008, p. 74)

Reflective Questions: Part 3

After reviewing the examples of activities that may be used to highlight spiritual health and well-being, what activities do you feel most comfortable leading and which activities would be a challenge for you? Which activities would require additional training and/or certification to provide? Are there additional considerations and information that you need to ponder before planning a retreat day? Are there additional activities that you may consider for spiritual health and wellness?

An Interprofessional Approach in Crisis Intervention

In this chapter's focus of an interprofessional approach, we look at spirituality incorporated into intervention. Crisis Intervention Teams (CIT) are employed to address individuals within a community who are in psychiatric distress and crisis. The unique challenges for those experiencing the **distress**, as well as family and community members (and those responding to the crisis) have frequently led to ineffective and sometimes unsafe and violent reactions from those attending to the crisis.

Alternative options are being promoted in the literature that uses a compassionate and spiritual approach to intervention where the responding CIT personnel take on a very intuitive approach that integrates heightened awareness of safety concerns along with compassionate approach to the individual (Chopko, 2011). Specific training aimed at deconstructing beliefs about mental health, psychiatric, and spiritual distress, and control is the first step in transforming integrated, and often long-term approaches to such crisis scenarios. In addition, training looks at developing narratives and images from Native spirituality that encompass warrior strength with awareness, compassion, and intuition (Chopko, 2011).

Reflection and developing an understanding of compassion to those that are in psychological pain and crisis and exploring morality as it relates to one's responsibility to protect and serve enhances the ability to better relate to those in crisis. In addition, an appreciation for our interconnectedness to one another and a calling to the greater good of all humanity is highlighted in a spiritual approach to such intervention (Chopko, 2011).

Conclusion

Emerging and middle adulthood is a time for developing and refining spiritual practices, integrating beliefs with identity, purpose, and meaning, developing greater resiliency and intuition, recognizing transcendence and the start of wisdom. It is through the personal and communal journeys that one may heal after trauma or major life events. Spiritual health and well-being encompass an ongoing choice toward wholeness.

References

Achterberg, J. (1985). *Imagery in healing: Shamanism in modern medicine*. Shambhala.

Amaro, H., Magno-Gatmaytan, C., Meléndez, M., Cortés, D., Arevalo, S., & Margolin, A. (2010). Addiction treatment intervention: An uncontrolled prospective pilot study of spiritual self-schema therapy with Latina women. *Substance Abuse, 31*(2), 117-125. https://doi.org/10.1080/08897071003641602

Anderson, K. M., & Bernhardt, C. (2020). Resilient adult daughters of abused women: Turning pain into purpose. *Violence Against Women, 26*(6/7), 750-770. https://doi.org/10.1177/1077801219842946

Ashraf, R., & Fatima, I. (2014). Role of personality and spirituality in nonviolent behavior in young adults. *Journal of Behavioural Sciences, 24*(1), 57-70.

Athan, A. M., & Miller, L. (2013). Motherhood as opportunity to learn spiritual values: Experiences and insights of new mothers. *Journal of Prenatal & Perinatal Psychology & Health, 27*(4), 220-253.

Barkin, S., Miller, L., & Luthar, S. (2015). Filling the void: Spiritual development among adolescents of the affluent. *Journal of Religion & Health, 54*(3), 844-861. https://doi.org/10.1007/s10943-015-0048-z

Barry, C. M., Christofferson, J. L., Boorman, E. P., & Nelson, L. J. (2020). Profiles of religiousness, spirituality, and psychological adjustment in emerging adults. *Journal of Adult Development, 27*(3), 201-211. https://doi.org/10.1007/s10804-019-09334-z

Barry, C. M., Nelson, L., Davarya, S., & Urry, S. (2010). Religiosity and spirituality during the transition to adulthood. International Journal of Behavioral Development, 34(4), 311-324. https://doi.org/10.1177/0165025409350964

Beagan, B. L., & Hattie, B. (2015). Religion, spirituality, and LGBTQ identity integration. *Journal of LGBT Issues in Counseling, 9*(2), 92-117. https://doi.org/10.1080/15538605.2015.1029204

Benson, H. (2011). *Relaxation revolution: The science and genetics of mind body healing*. Scribner.

Benson, H., & Proctor, W. (2011). *Relaxation revolution: The science and genetics of mind body healing*. Scribner.

Benson, H., & Stark, M. (1997). *Timeless healing: The power and biology of belief* (Reprint ed.). Fireside.

Beseme, S., Fast, L., Bengston, W., Turner, M., Radin, D., & McMichael, J. (2020). Effects induced in vivo by exposure to magnetic signals derived from a healing technique. *Dose-Response, 18*(1), 1-10. https://doi.org/10.1177/1559325820907741

Bhasin, M. K., Dusek, J. A., Chang, B. H., Joseph, M. G., Denninger, J. W., Fricchione, G. L., Benson, H., & Libermann, T.A. (2013). Relaxation response induces temporal transcriptome changes in energy metabolism, insulin secretion and inflammatory pathways. *PLoS One, 8*, e62817. https://doi.org/10.1371/journal.pone. 0062817

Bin Abdullah, M. F. I. L., & Bin Mohamad, M. A. (2018). Does psychosocial interventions enhance posttraumatic growth and spirituality in cancer patients and survivors? A narrative review of the literature. *Malaysian Journal of Medicine & Health Sciences, 14*, 164-172.

Birocco, N., Guillame, C., Storto, S., Ritorto, G., Catino, C., Gir, N., Balisra., L., Tealdi, G., Orecchia, C., De Vito. G., Giaretta, L. Donadio. M., Bertetta, O., Schena, M., Ciuffreda L. (2012). The effect of Reiki therapy on pain and anxiety in patients attending a day oncology and infusion services unit. *American Journal of Hospice and Palliative Care, 29*, 290-294. https://doi.org/10.1177/1049909111420859

Boro, J., & Dhanalakshmi, D. (2015). Spirituality, personality and general health among college students. *Indian Journal of Health & Wellbeing, 6*(5), 475-479.

Brandt, C. P., Jardin, C., Sharp, C., Lemaire, C., & Zvolensky, M. J. (2017). Main and interactive effects of emotion dysregulation and HIV symptom severity on quality of life among persons living with HIV/AIDS. *AIDS Care, 29*(4), 498-506. https://doi.org/10.1080/09540121.2016.1220484

Bryant, L., Bowman, L., & Paulette Isaac, S. E. (2016). Adult education and spirituality: A "Liberatory Spaces" for black gay men. *New Directions for Adult & Continuing Education, 150*, 59-69. https://doi.org/10.1002/ace.20186

Bryant-Davis, T., & Wong, E. C. (2013). Faith to move mountains: Religious coping, spirituality, and interpersonal trauma recovery. *American Psychologist, 68*(8), 675-684.

Burney, N., Osmany, M., & Khan, W. (2017). Spirituality and psychological well-being of young adults. *Indian Journal of Health & Wellbeing, 8*(12), 1481-1484.

Carlson, L. E., Tamagawa, R., Stephen, J., Drysdale, E., Zhong, L., & Speca, M. (2016). Randomized-controlled trial of mindfulness-based cancer recovery versus supportive expressive group therapy among distressed breast cancer survivors (MINDSET): Long-term follow-up results. *Psycho-Oncology, 25*(7), 750-759. https://doi.org/10.1002/pon.4150

Chandran, S. (2019). Integrating transactional analysis and Tai Chi for synergy and spirituality. *Transactional Analysis Journal, 49*(2), 114-130. https://doi.org/10.1080/03621537.2019.1577336

Chopko, B. (2011). Walk in balance: Training crisis intervention team police officers as compassionate warriors. *Journal of Creativity in Mental Health, 6*(4), 315-328. https://doi.org/10.1080/15401383.2011.630304

Corry, D. A. S., Lewis, C. A., & Mallett, J. (2014). Harnessing the mental health benefits of the Creativity–spirituality construct: Introducing the theory of transformative coping. *Journal of Spirituality in Mental Health, 16*(2), 89-110. https://doi.org/10.1080/19349637.2014.896854

Corry, D. A. S., Lewis, C. A., & Tracey, A. P. (2015). Spirituality and creativity in coping, their association and transformative effect: A qualitative enquiry. *Religions, 6*(2), 499-526. https://doi.org/10.3390/rel6020499

Csikszentmihalyi, M. (2008). *Flow: The psychology of optimal experience*. Harper Perennial Modern Classics.

Cuevas, J., Vance, D., Viamonte, S., Lee, S., & South, J. (2010). A comparison of spirituality and religiousness in older and younger adults with and without HIV. *Journal of Spirituality in Mental Health, 12*(4), 273-287. https://doi.org/10.1080/19349637.2010.518828

de Diego, C. R., Lopez, Z. M. P., Vargas, M. A. M., Lucchetti, G., & Vega, E. J. (2021). The effectiveness of spiritual interventions in the workplace for work-related health outcomes: A systematic review and meta-analysis. *Journal of Nursing Management*, 1. https://doi.org/10.1111/jonm.13315

Dunn, J. (n.d.). *The ancient Egyptian heart*. http://www.touregypt.net/featurestories/heart

Dunn, J. (2019). There's something about energy healing. *Health, 33*(8), 92-95.

Easton, S. D., Leone-Sheehan, D. M., & O'Leary, P. J. (2019). "I will never know the person who I could have become": Perceived changes in self-identity among adult survivors of clergy-perpetrated sexual abuse. *Journal of Interpersonal Violence, 34*(6), 1139-1162. https://doi.org/10.1177/0886260516650966

Ferrell, B., Chung, V., Koczywas, M., Borneman, T., Irish, T. L., Ruel, N. H., Azad, N. S., Cooper, R. S., & Smith, T. J. (2020). Spirituality in cancer patients on phase 1 clinical trials. *Psycho-Oncology, 29*(6), 1077-1083. https://doi.org/10.1002/pon.5380

Ferrell, B. R., Temel, J. S., Temin, S., Alesi, E. R., Balboni, T. A., Basch, E. M., Firn, J. I., Paice, J. A., Peppercorn, J. M., Phillips, T., Stovall, E. L., Zimmermann, C., & Smith, T. J. (2016). Integration of palliative care into standard oncology care: American Society of Clinical Oncology clinical practice guideline update. *Journal of Clinical Oncology, 35*(1), 96-112. https://doi.org/10.1200/JCO.2016.70.1474

Florez, I. A., Allbaugh, L. J., Harris, C. E., Schwartz, A. C., & Kaslow, N. J. (2018). Suicidal ideation and hopelessness in PTSD: Spiritual well-being mediates outcomes over time. *Anxiety, Stress & Coping, 31*(1), 46-58. https://doi.org/10.1080/10615806.2017.1369260

Glenn, C. T. (2014). A bridge over troubled waters: Spirituality and resilience with emerging adult childhood trauma survivors. *Journal of Spirituality in Mental Health, 16*(1), 37-50. https://doi.org/10.1080/19349637.2014.864543

Gonella, S., Garrino, L., & Dimonte, V. (2014). Biofield therapies and cancer-related symptoms: A review. *Clinical Journal of Oncology Nursing, 18*(5), 568-576. https://doi.org/10.1188/14.CJON.568-576

Griera, M. (2017). Yoga in penitentiary settings: Transcendence, spirituality, and self-improvement. *Human Studies, 40*(1), 77-100. https://doi.org/10.1007/s10746-016-9404-6

Halkitis, P. N., Mattis, J. S., Sahadath, J. K., Massie, D., Ladyzhenskaya, L., Pitrelli, K., Bonacci, M., & Cowie, S. A. E. (2009). The meanings and manifestations of religion and spirituality among lesbian, gay, bisexual, and transgender adults. *Journal of Adult Development, 16*(4), 250-262. https://doi.org/10.1007/s10804-009-9071-1

Hall, P., Bacheller, L. L., & Desir, C. (2019). Spirituality and psychological well-being in adults of Haitian descent. *Mental Health, Religion & Culture, 22*(5), 453-466. https://doi.org/10.1080/13674676.2019.1581151

Hansen, L. B., Hvidt, N. C., Mortensen, K. E., Wu, C., & Prinds, C. (2021). How giving birth makes sense: A questionnaire study on existential meaning-making among mothers giving birth preterm or at term. *Journal of Religion & Health, 60*(1), 335-353. https://doi.org/10.1007/s10943-020-01106-4

Harris, K., Haddock, G., Peters, S., & Gooding, P. (2020). Psychological resilience to suicidal thoughts and behaviours in people with schizophrenia diagnoses: A systematic literature review. *Psychology & Psychotherapy: Theory, Research & Practice, 93*(4), 777-809. https://doi-org.proxy-etown.klnpa.org/10.1111/papt.12255

HeartMath Institute. (2017). The science of HeartMath. https://www.heartmath.com/science/.

Herzog, P. S., & Beadle, D. A. T. (2018). Emerging adult religiosity and spirituality: Linking beliefs, values, and ethical decision-making. *Religions, 9*(3), 84. https://doi.org/10.3390/rel9030084

Hiebler-Ragger, M., Falthansl-Scheinecker, J., Birnhuber, G., Fink, A., & Unterrainer, H. F. (2016). Facets of spirituality diminish the positive relationship between insecure attachment and mood pathology in young adults. *PLoS ONE, 11*(6), 1-9. https://doi.org/10.1371/journal.pone.0158069

Hölzel, B. K., Carmody, J., Evans, K. C., Hoge, E. A., Dusek, J. A., Morgan, L., Pitman, R. K., & Lazar, S. W. (2010). Stress reduction correlates with structural changes in the amygdala. *Social Cognitive & Affective Neuroscience, 5*(1), 11-17. https://doi.org/10.1093/scan/nsp034

Humbert, T. K. (2016). *Spirituality and occupational therapy: A model for practice and research.* AOTA Press.

Hyde, B. (2020). Evoking the spiritual through phenomenology: Using the written anecdotes of adults to access children's expressions of spirituality. International *Journal of Children's Spirituality, 25*(3/4), 197-211. https://doi.org/10.1080/1364436X.2020.1843006

Illueca, M. & Doolittle, B. R. (2020). The use of prayer in the management of pain: A systematic review. *Journal of Religion & Health, 59*(2), 681-699. https://doi.org/10.1007/s10943-019-00967-8

Jalote, S. (2016). Experiencing life post childhood physical abuse: Some case studies. *Indian Journal of Health & Wellbeing, 7*(1), 157-160.

Jauregui, M., Schuster, T. L., Clark, M. D., & Jones, J. P. (2012). Pranic healing: Documenting use, expectations, and perceived benefits of a little-known therapy in the United States. *Journal of Scientific Exploration, 26*(3), 569-588.

Jessop, D. S. (2019). The power of positive stress and a research roadmap. Stress: *The International Journal on the Biology of Stress, 22*(5), 521-523. https://doi.org/10.1080/10253890.2019.1593365

Johnson, K. A. (2018). Prayer: A helpful aid in recovery from depression. *Journal of Religion & Health, 57*(6), 2290-2300. https://doi.org/10.1007/s10943-018-0564-8

Jung, C. G., & Chodorow, J. (1997). *Jung on active imagination.* Princeton University Press.

Karimi, Z., Haghshenas, L., Mohtashami, T., & Dehkordi, M. A. (2019). Investigating the role of attachment styles, dysfunctional attitudes, and spirituality in predicting membership in addicted and non-addicted groups. *PsyCh Journal, 8*(2), 169-179. https://doi.org/10.1002/pchj.254

Kim, S. S., & Kim-Godwin, Y. S. (2019). Cultural context of family religiosity/spirituality among Korean-American elderly families. *Journal of Cross-Cultural Gerontology, 34*(1), 51-65. https://doi.org/10.1007/s10823-019-09363-x

Kobza, M., & Salter, N. P. (2016). Young adults' expectations about the values of religious and spiritual people. *Psi Chi Journal of Psychological Research, 21*(2), 70-79. https://doi.org/10.24839/2164-8204.JN21.2.70

Koenig, L. B. (2015). Change and stability in religiousness and spirituality in emerging adulthood. *Journal of Genetic Psychology, 176*(6), 369-385. https://doi.org/10.1080/00221325.2015.1082458

Kopacz, M. S., Currier, J. M., Drescher, K. D., Pigeon, W. R. (2016). Suicidal behavior and spiritual functioning in a sample of veterans diagnosed with PTSD. *Journal of Injury and Violence Research, 8*(1), 6-14. 10.

Kralovec, K., Kunrath, S., Fartacek, C., Pichler, E., Plöderl, M., & Pichler, E.-M. (2018). The gender-specific associations between religion/spirituality and suicide risk in a sample of Austrian psychiatric inpatients. *Suicide & Life-Threatening Behavior, 48*(3), 281-293. https://doi.org/10.1111/sltb.12349

Krause, N., & Hayward, R. (2013). Prayer beliefs and change in life satisfaction over time. *Journal of Religion & Health, 52*(2), 674-694. https://doi.org/10.1007/s10943-012-9638-1

Lawrence, R. E., Oquendo, M. A., & Stanley, B. (2016). Religion and suicide risk: A systematic review. *Archives of Suicide Research, 20*(1), 1-21. https://doi.org/10.1080/13811118.2015.1004494

Lazar, S. W., Kerr, C. E., Wasserman, R. H., Gray, J. R., Greve, D. N., Treadway, M. T., McGarvey, M., Quinn, B. T., Dusek, J. A., Benson, H., Rauch, S. L., Moore, C. I., & Fischl, B. (2005). Meditation experience is associated with increased cortical thickness. *Neuroreport, 16*(17), 1893-1897. https://doi.org/10.1097/01.wnr.0000186598.66243.19

Lehmann, O. V., Kardum, G., & Klempe, S. H. (2019). The search for inner silence as a source for eudemonia. *British Journal of Guidance & Counselling, 47*(2), 180-189. https://doi.org/10.1080/03069885.2018.1553295

Lifshitz, M., van Elk, M., & Luhrmann, T. M. (2019). Absorption and spiritual experience: A review of evidence and potential mechanisms. *Consciousness & Cognition, 73*, 102760. https://doi.org/10.1016/j.concog.2019.05.008

Littrell, J. L. (2019). The importance of psychoneuroimmunology for social workers. *Families in Society: Journal of Contemporary Social Services, 100*(1), 17-33. https://doi.org/10.1177/1044389418802515

Lucchesi, M. (2017). Religious and spiritual function of the artistic creative process. *International Journal of Arts & Sciences, 10*(2), 163-185.

Lusk, J., Dobscha, S. K., Kopacz, M., Ritchie, M. F., & Ono, S. (2018). Spirituality, religion, and suicidality among veterans: A qualitative study. *Archives of Suicide Research, 22*(2), 311-326. https://doi.org/10.1080/13811118.2017.1340856

Maley, C. M., Pagana, N. K., Velenger, C. A., & Humbert, T, K. (2016). Dealing with major life events and transitions: A systematic literature review on and occupational analysis of spirituality. *American Journal of Occupational Therapy, 70*(4), 1-6. https://doi.org/10.5014/ajot.2016.015537

Martinez, C. T., & Scott, C. (2014). In search of the meaning of happiness through flow and spirituality. *International Journal of Health, Wellness & Society, 4*(1), 37-49. https://doi.org/10.18848/2156-8960/CGP/v04i01/41088

McCormick, W. H., Carroll, T. D., Sims, B. M., & Currier, J. (2017). Adverse childhood experiences, religious/spiritual struggles, and mental health symptoms: Examination of mediation models. *Mental Health, Religion & Culture, 20*(10), 1042-1054. https://doi.org/10.1080/13674676.2018.1440544

Meredith, E. (2020). *The language your body speaks: Self-healing with energy medicine.* New World Library.

Mind-Body Medicine Research at Massachusetts General Hospital. (n.d.). Benson-Henry Institute. https://bensonhenryinstitute.org/

Mobini, S., & White, R. (2020). The immediate and delayed effects of mindfulness guided imagery and progressive muscle relaxation in patients with acquired brain injury. *Clinical Psychology Forum, 336*, 22-27.

Mudge, P. J. P. (2018). 'Re-souling daily life'—Towards a restored spirituality of the Sabbath as a cure for 'societal madness.' *International Journal of Children's Spirituality, 23*(3), 260-274. https://doi.org/10.1080/1364436X.2018.1460332

National Institute on Aging. (n.d.). What are palliative care and hospice care? https://www.nia.nih.gov/health/what-are-palliative-care-and-hospice-care

Nelson, B., & Rawlings, D. (2007). Its own reward: A phenomenological study of artistic creativity. *Journal of Phenomenological Psychology, 38*(2), 217-255. https://doi.org/10.1163/156916207X234284

Noetic Systems International. (n.d.). Thinking from the heart: Heart brain science. http://noeticsi.com/thinking-from-the-heart-heart-brain-science/

Nooner, A. K., Dwyer, K., DeShea, L., & Yeo, T. P. (2016). Using relaxation and guided imagery to address pain, fatigue, and sleep disturbances: A pilot study. *Clinical Journal of Oncology Nursing, 20*(5), 547-552. https://doi.org/10.1188/16.CJON.547-552

Ochoa, C. Y., Haardörfer, R., Escoffery, C., Stein, K., & Alcaraz, K. I. (2018). Examining the role of social support and spirituality on the general health perceptions of Hispanic cancer survivors. *Psycho-Oncology, 27*(9), 2189-2197. https://doi.org/10.1002/pon.4795

Oh, H. Y., Marinovich, C., Jay, S., Zhou, S., & Kim, J. H. J. (2021). Abuse and suicide risk among college students in the United States: Findings from the 2019 Healthy Minds Study. *Journal of Affective Disorders, 282*, 554-560. https://doi.org/10.1016/j.jad.2020.12.140

Park, C. L., Riley, K. E., Braun, T. D., Jung, J. Y., Suh, H. G., Pescatello, L. S., & Antoni, M. H. (2017). Yoga and cognitive-behavioral interventions to reduce stress in incoming college students: A pilot study. *Journal of Applied Biobehavioral Research, 22*(4). https://doi.org/10.1111/jabr.12068

Pascoe, M. C., Thompson, D. R., & Ski, C. F. (2017). Yoga, mindfulness-based stress reduction and stress-related physiological measures: A meta-analysis. *Psychoneuroendocrinology, 86*, 152-168. https://doi.org/10.1016/j.psyneuen.2017.08.008

Pizzi, M. (2014). Promoting health, wellness and quality of life at the end of life: Hospice interdisciplinary perspectives on creating a good death. *Journal of Allied Health, 43*(4), 214-223

Pizzi, M. A. (2015). Promoting health and well-being at the end of life through client-centered care. *Scandinavian Journal of Occupational Therapy, 22*(6), 442-449. https://doi.org/10.3109/11038128.2015.1025834

Prior, M. K., & Petra, M. (2020). Assessing the effects of childhood multitype maltreatment on adult spirituality. *Journal of Child & Adolescent Trauma, 13*(4), 469-480. https://doi.org/10.1007/s40653-019-00288-8

Puchalska-Wasyl, M. M., & Zarzycka, B. (2020). Internal dialogue as a mediator of the relationship between prayer and well-being. *Journal of Religion & Health, 59*(4), 2045-2063. https://doi.org/10.1007/s10943-019-00943-2

Radin, D. I. (2018). *Real magic: Ancient wisdom, modern science, and a guide to secret power of the universe*. Harmony.

Rafii, F., Eisavi, M., & Safarabadi, M. (2020). Explaining the process of spiritual healing of critically-ill patients: A grounded theory study. *Ethiopian Journal of Health Sciences*. https://doi.org/10.4314/ejhs.v30i4.13

Ram, B. (2010). *The eight limbs of yoga: Pathway to liberation*. Lotus Press.

Ravi, M., Miller, A. H., & Michopoulos, V. (2021). The immunology of stress and the impact of inflammation on the brain and behaviour. *BJPsych Advances, 27*(3), 158-165. https://doi.org/10.1192/bja.2020.82

Reymann, L. S., Fialkowski, G. M., & Stewart, S. J. A. (2015). Exploratory study of spirituality and psychosocial growth in college students. *Journal of College Counseling, 18*(2), 103-115. https://doi.org/10.1002/jocc.12008

Riley, K. E., Park, C. L., Wilson, A., Sabo, A. N., Antoni, M. H., Braun, T. D., Harrington, J., Reiss, J., Pasalis, E., Harris, A. D., & Cope, S. (2017). Improving physical and mental health in frontline mental health care providers: Yoga-based stress management versus cognitive behavioral stress management. *Journal of Workplace Behavioral Health, 32*(1), 26-48. https://doi.org/10.1080/15555240.2016.1261254

Rodrigues, A. P., Jorge, F. E., Pires, C. A., & António, P. (2019). The contribution of emotional intelligence and spirituality in understanding creativity and entrepreneurial intention of higher education students. *Education + Training, 61*(7/8), 870-894. https://doi.org/10.1108/ET-01-2018-0026

Rogers, C. L. (2014). Search for transcendence revealed in childhood narratives of poverty, abuse and neglect, and social isolation. *Journal of Spirituality in Mental Health, 16*(3), 218-236. https://doi.org/10.1080/19349637.2014.925369

Sagan, O. (2016). The intersubjectivity of spiritual experience in the art practice of people with histories of mental distress: A phenomenological study. *Mental Health, Religion & Culture, 19*(2), 138-149. https://doi.org/10.1080/13674676.2015.1126704

Sarbacker, S. R., & Kimple, K. (2015). *The eight limbs of yoga: A handbook for living yoga philosophy*. North Point Press.

Saxena, K., Verrico, C. D., Saxena, J., Kurian, S., Alexander, S., Kahlon, R. S., Arvind, R. P., Goldberg, A., DeVito, N., Baig, M., Grieb, A., Bakhshaie, J., Simonetti, A., Storch, E. A., Williams, L., & Gillan, L. (2020). An evaluation of yoga and meditation to improve attention, hyperactivity, and stress in high-school students. *Journal of Alternative & Complementary Medicine, 26*(8), 701-707. https://doi.org/10.1089/acm.2020.0126

Scalora, S., Anderson, M., Crete, A., Drapkin, J., Portnoff, L., Athan, A., & Miller, L. (2020). A spirituality mind-body wellness center in a university setting; A pilot service assessment study. *Religions, 11*(9), 466. https://doi.org/10.3390/rel11090466

Schlesinger, I., Benyakov, O., Erikh, I., & Nassar, M. (2014). Relaxation guided imagery reduces motor fluctuations in Parkinson's Disease. *Journal of Parkinson's Disease, 4*(3), 431-436. https://doi.org/.3233/JPD-130338

Schulte, B. (2015). Harvard neuroscientist: Meditation not only reduces stress, here's how it changes your brain. https:// www.washingtonpost.com/news/inspired-life/wp/2015/05/26 /harvard-neuroscientist-meditation-not-only-reduces-stress-it- literally-changes-your-brain/

Seppala, E. M., Nitschke, J. B., Tudorascu, D. L., Hayes, A., Goldstein, M. R., Nguyen, D. T. H., Perlman, D., & Davidson, R. J. (2014). Breathing-based meditation decreases posttraumatic stress disorder symptoms in U.S. military veterans: A randomized controlled longitudinal study. *Journal of Traumatic Stress, 27*, 397-405. https://doi.org/10.1002/jts.21936

Serafini, G., Montebovi, F., Lamis, D. A. (2015). Associations among depression, suicidal behavior, and quality of life in patients with human immunodeficiency virus. *World Journal of Virology, 4*(3), 303-312.

Shackle, E. (2017). The contribution of Donald Kalsched to the understanding of the relationship of early childhood trauma to spirituality. *Transpersonal Psychology Review, 19*(1), 9-11.

Sharp, D. M., Walker, A. A., Green, V. L., Greeman, J., Russell, D., Russell, I. T., Walker, M. B., & Walker, L. G. (2021). Psychosocial effects of relaxation therapy and guided imagery: A pragmatic randomized controlled trial. *Contemporary Hypnosis & Integrative Therapy, 35*(1), 21-36.

Shinde, F., & Wagani, R. (2019). Does spirituality work as a buffer in suicide: A systematic review. *Journal of Psychosocial Research, 14*(2), 249-256. https://doi.org/10.32381/JPR.2019.14.02.1

Siegel, D. J. (2018). *Aware: The Science and Practice of Presence*. TarcherPerigee.

Smigelsky, M. A., Jardin, C., Nieuwsma, J. A., Brancu, M., Meador, K. G., Molloy, K. G., Elbogen, E. B., & VA Mid-Atlantic MIRECC Workgroup. (2020). Religion, spirituality, and suicide risk in Iraq and Afghanistan era veterans. *Depression & Anxiety, 37*(8), 728-737. https://doi.org/10.1002/da.23013

Steffler, D. J., & Murdoch, K. C. (2017). Meaning and spirituality: A thematic analysis. *International Journal of Existential Psychology & Psychotherapy, 7*(1), 1-22.

Surr, J. (2014). Children growing whole. *International Journal of Children's Spirituality, 19*(2), 123-132. https://doi.org/10.1080/1364436X.2014.924907

Tarkeshi, J. (2017). *Yoga body and mind handbook: Easy poses, guided meditations, perfect peace wherever you are*. Sonoma Press.

Trama, S., & Modi, S. (2016). Impact of self-enhancement on spiritual orientation in young adults: An intervention study. *Indian Journal of Health & Wellbeing, 7*(6), 585-593.

Treatment Improvement Protocol Series, No. 57. (2014). Trauma-informed care in behavioral health sciences. Center for Substance Abuse Treatment. Substance Abuse and Mental Health Services Administration.

Trombka, M., Demarzo, M., Bacas, D. C., Antonio, S. B., Cicuto, K., Salvo, V., Claudino, F. C. A., Ribeiro, L., Christopher, M., Garcia-Campayo, J., & Rocha, N. S. (2018). Study protocol of a multicenter randomized controlled trial of mindfulness training to reduce burnout and promote quality of life in police officers: The POLICE study. *BMC Psychiatry, 18*(1). https://doi.org/10.1186/s12888-018-1726-7

Tyagi, A., Cohen, M., Reece, J., Telles, S., & Jones, L. (2016). Heart rate variability, flow, mood and mental stress during yoga practices in yoga practitioners, non-yoga practitioners and people with metabolic syndrome. *Applied Psychophysiology & Biofeedback, 41*(4), 381-393. https://doi.org/10.1007/s10484-016-9340-2

Ünal Aslan, K. S., & Çetinkaya, F. (2021). The effects of therapeutic touch on spiritual care and sleep quality in patients receiving palliative care. *Perspectives in Psychiatric Care, 1*. https://doi.org/10.1111/ppc.12801

Vadnais, E. (2020). *Intuitive development: How to trust your inner knowing for guidance with relationships, health, and spirituality*. Author.

Vasile, C. (2020). Mental health and immunity (review). *Experimental & Therapeutic Medicine, 20*(6). https://doi.org/10.3892/etm.2020.9341

Voisin, D. R., Corbin, D. E., & Jones, C. (2016). A conceptualization of spirituality among African American young adults. *Western Journal of Black Studies, 40*(1), 14-23.

Waizbard-Bartov, E., Yehonatan-Schori, M., & Golan, O. (2019). Personal growth experiences of parents to children with autism spectrum disorder. *Journal of Autism and Developmental Disorders. 49*(4), 1330-1341. https://doi.org/10.1007/s10803-018-3784-6.

Wang, F., & Szabo, A. (2020). Effects of yoga on stress among healthy adults: A systematic review. *Alternative Therapies in Health & Medicine, 26*(4), 58-64.

Waterman, A. S. (2020). "Now what do I do?": Toward a conceptual understanding of the effects of traumatic events on identity functioning. *Journal of Adolescence, 79*, 59-69. https://doi.org/10.1016/j.adolescence.2019.11.005

Watson, J. (2017). Every child still matters: Interprofessional approaches to the spirituality of the child. *International Journal of Children's Spirituality, 22*(1), 4-13. https://doi.org/10.1080/1364436X.2016.1234434

Whitney, R. V. (2019). An intimate conversation about cervical cancer: Ten lessons along the journey. *Journal of Palliative Medicine, 22*(7), 865-867. https://doi.org/10.1089/jpm.2018.0565

Yadav, R. K., Sarvottam, K., Magan, D., & Yadav, R. (2015). A two-year follow-up case of chronic fatigue syndrome: Substantial improvement in personality following a yoga-based lifestyle intervention. *Journal of Alternative & Complementary Medicine, 21*(4), 246-249. https://doi.org/10.1089/acm.2014.0055

Yehonatan-Schori, M., Golan, O., & Waizbard-Bartov, E. (2019). Personal growth experiences of parents to children with autism spectrum disorder. *Journal of Autism & Developmental Disorders, 49*(4), 1330-1341. https://doi.org/10.1007/s10803-018-3784-6

Zarei, N., & Joulaei, H. (2018). The impact of perceived stigma, quality of life, and spiritual beliefs on suicidal ideations among HIV-positive patients. *AIDS Research & Treatment*, 1-7. https://doi.org/10.1155/2018/6120127

Zhang, H., Pittman, D. M., Lamis, D. A., Fischer, N. L., Schwenke, T. J., Carr, E. R., Shah, S., & Kaslow, N. J. (2015a). Childhood maltreatment and PTSD: Spiritual well-being and intimate partner violence as mediators. *Journal of Aggression, Maltreatment & Trauma, 24*(5), 501-519. https://doi.org/10.1080/10926771.2015.1029182

Zhang, W., Yan, T. T., Barriball, L. K., While, A. E., & Liu, X. H. (2015b). Post-traumatic growth in mothers of children with autism: A phenomenological study. *Autism, 19*(1), 29-37. PMID: 24216071.

21

CHAPTER

Promoting Spiritual Health

Older Adults

Tamera Keiter Humbert, DEd, OTR/L, FAOTA; Priscilla Denham, MDiv, D.Min.; and Emmy Vadnais, OTR/L

Learning Objectives

At the end of this chapter, the reader will:

1. Identify and describe aspects of spirituality with older adults (ACOTE B.1.1, B.1.2)
2. Analyze differences between spirituality and religion (ACOTE B.2.1)
3. Articulate the various ways spirituality is explored, heightened, and pursued with older adults (ACOTE B.3.4, B.3.6)
4. Consider various activities and intervention strategies used in daily life and through major life events that attend to spirituality (ACOTE B.4.3)
5. Consider an interprofessional approach focused on a strengths-based approach with older adults (ACOTE B.4.19)

The ACOTE Standards used are those from 2018.

Key Words

Abiding, Altruism, Elderhood, Elders, Generativity, Interdependence, Resilient Aging, Sacred, Valorization of Age and Time

Pizzi, M. A., & Amir, M. (Eds.). *Interprofessional Perspectives for Community Practice: Promoting Health, Well-Being, and Quality of Life* (pp. 393-403).

Case Study

As part of your consideration of providing a health and wellness program to the community, you are considering the opportunity to offer a weekly series of topics on spiritual health and wellness to the senior citizen's group. Members in this group range in age from 58 to 95 years with varying levels of physical ability. At least two of the members utilize a wheelchair for mobility and three members have significant visual impairments. Some of the members are in cognitive decline. The average daily attendance to the center is 25 community-dwelling, older adults. Most members come two to three times per week. There is a set schedule of planned activities that range from 9 am till 2 pm and your group would be offered one morning every week for 1 hour.

Reflective Questions: Part 1

Consider your image of older adults. What do believe are the needs and challenges of older adults and what are the strengths that they bring to their lives and others? Consider what it might feel like working with a group of elders that might be three or four times your age. What hesitations might you have? What excites you about this possibility?

Spirituality and Elders

There is an understanding that spirituality is an ongoing evolutionary process for individuals, communities, and populations. Our life experiences and the contexts in which we live provide opportunities for ongoing spiritual health, growth, and well-being. Moving into later life provides opportunities not afforded to others in different life stages. The unique aspect of spirituality and **Elders** connects with the perspective of time and reflection (Martinson, 2019; Stanford & Stearns, 2019). The term Elders is being used in the chapter as a sign of respect, recognizing a group of individuals who have moved into a stage of enlightenment or Elderhood (Aronson, 2019; Martinson, 2019). During this life stage, we are able to have a broader understanding of our life journey, have richer and deeper perspectives of the world and others, and we often have the luxury of more time to devote to spiritual health and wellness (Martinson, 2019). The many different life events that are experienced during this life span, including death of loved ones and friends, illness, limitations in what we are able to accomplish and do, decreased financial resources, and tragic world events play a significant role in how individuals attend to spirituality and utilize it in daily life.

Evolution of Spirituality and Elders

The evolution of spirituality within this age group includes 1) capacity for awe and gratitude, 2) generosity, 3) trust in providence and hope, 4) resting in beauty and goodness, 5) a sense of belonging and interconnectedness, 6) wisdom and perspective, and 7) humility (Table 21-1). There is an understanding that spirituality may be a continuation of our spiritual development in youth and adulthood or one that may be activated or further explored through major life events (Maley et al., 2016).

A Personal Reflection of My Father

I (Tam, first author) remember my father, who in his last years of life would take his time to complete his daily routines. His frequent comment was "I have all of the time in the world." It did not matter if he was taking a bath or making a meal, he would luxuriate in completing the activity. His sense of timing and schedule did not fit into what most of us have and do, a list of tasks or chores that need to be accomplished, in a particular order, and within an allotted time frame. Gardening would take hours that stretched into days and weeks and months. He would spend at least 1 hour each day outside in his vegetable and flower beds. This was one of the activities that brought him great joy and meaning. When he would have visitors to his home, he would go to his garden and pick whatever was ripe and offer it as a gift.

He also was quite wise about his gardening practices having and tending to some form of a vegetable garden most of his life. He was an organic farmer before that term or idea was ever known in the public domain. He cross-pollinated vegetables and grew them in various pots and environments. He once grew a pumpkin hanging from a clothesline to see if the traction would produce a different shape, texture, and flavor. His wisdom of what worked and didn't in the garden allowed him the luxury to take time to further experiment and add new knowledge to his beloved occupation.

Time for my father changed in other ways too during his later years. He realized his time on earth was limited and spent some of his days and weeks going through his house and garage, paring down items no longer needed, wanted, or necessary. He would go to the grocery store whenever necessary, no longer part of a weekly task. He did not want to have an abundance of food on hand that would not be needed. He gave more of his money away to charities and organizations that he believed in. His priorities about what was needed in life, within the time that we have left in this world, shifted. I do not remember when this actually happened, but seemed to be a gradual change over time but especially after the death of my mother. Some might look at these changes as part of a grief process, and it may have been. It was also a spiritual shift in his own understanding of purpose, time, happiness, and joy.

Table 21-1

Aspects of Spirituality With Elders

ASPECT	DEFINITION	REFERENCES
Capacity for awe and gratitude	Recognizing amazing events, small or large, and expressing gratitude.	Lepherd et al. (2020a, 2020b) Manning (2012)
Generosity	Being generous with time, resources, insights, and knowledge. Terms may also include **altruism, generativity, valorization of time.**	Adams-Price et al. (2018) Von Humboldt et al. (2014)
Trust in providence/hope	Believing that life happens for a purpose or reason and hope may be experienced even through tragedy.	Allison & Smith (2020) Lepherd et al. (2020a, 2020b)
Resting in beauty and goodness	Delighting in the beauty seen in nature, in others, in life events. Seeking and facilitating harmony, QOL satisfaction and inner peace.	Allison & Smith (2020) Lepherd et al. (2020a, 2020b) Von Humboldt et al. (2014)
Sense of belonging/ interconnectedness	Understanding and appreciating how our actions impact others and nature, being sensitive to our interconnectedness. Feeling a sense of belonging with others.	Cornwell (2011) Lepherd et al. (2020a, 2020b)
Wisdom and perspective	Having insights and perspectives that have developed over time that puts the everyday events into a larger understanding of personal or communal history. May include meaning of life and death and an overall sense of life satisfaction.	Adams-Price et al. (2018) Janus & Smrokowska-Reichmann (2019) Wright et al. (2018)
Humility	Recognizing and accepting our own limitations in knowledge, ability while also celebrating what we do have to offer to others.	Barclay (2016) Wright et al. (2018)

Spirituality and Elderhood—A Deeper Look at Maturity

In the previous chapters focused on youth, adolescents, emerging adults, and middle adults, the notion that spirituality is developed over time, with the engagement of religious and/or spiritual practices, and through life experiences is well supported in the literature. Conversely, the idea of **Elderhood**, a resurgence of constructs associated with indigenous cultures (Elder, 2014; Kahn-John et al., 2021; Lisson et al., 2018; Nakasone, 2013; Nie, 2021) or lost cultures (Brause, 2010; DeConick, 2019; Jenkinson, 2018; Walsh, 2019) has gained attention in the last decade. The primary idea in Elderhood is the embrace of wisdom and maturity with the obligation to pass along that understanding to generations while also being honored by those generations for these contributions (Ambrogi, 2017; Bouchard et al., 2021; Jenkinson, 2018). Elderhood is seen as a desirable part of life; it is the "summit of a lifelong journey" (Nie, 2021, p. 316).

In Elderhood, spirituality is much more nuanced in one's understanding of self, culture, relationships, and world views (Elder, 2014; Kane, 2016; Lisson et al., 2018). It is the embodiment of decades of spiritual practice and beliefs that is ripe to address the needs of current and future generations (Jenkinson, 2018). Elderhood is seen as a process of coming into one's truest identity, of becoming fully human (Ambrogi, 2017; Kahn-John et al., 2021; Nie, 2021; Zweig, 2021). In particular, there is the integration of cultural wisdom, deep reflection, and self-critique that produces acceptance of uncertainty and immortality, generativity and relational interdependence, deep values, and shared worldviews (Dandaneau & East, 2011; Elder, 2014; Jenkinson, 2018; Kahn-John et al., 2021).

Cultural Wisdom

In communities in which Elderhood is embraced, there is a cultural shift in understanding the value and need for Elders who have developed spiritual practices and embody wisdom (Kahn-John et al., 2021; Reynolds et al., 2021). Not only is there great respect given to Elders, but they are also looked to as vital members within their communities (Brause, 2010; Reynolds et al., 2021) and an integral part of the collective community wisdom (da Silva, 2010; Jenkinson, 2018). Aging is not viewed in negative terms but seen as approaching infinity, the Divine, ultimate wisdom (DeConick, 2019; Jenkinson, 2018; Kahn-John et al., 2021; Nie, 2021). The role of older adults is then the intergenerational transfer of wisdom. Generativity is directed to humanity and the needs of the community (Jenkinson, 2018). It is in the giving away of self that produces spiritual growth in others. According to Martinson (2019), "In the new frontier of aging, theirs is a generative presence, being available, being with, being for [others]" (p. 262).

Deep Reflection

Part of Elderhood also includes the wider perspectives of accepting uncertainty, immortality, and embracing loss as part of the aging process and life in general. Movement away from gathering, controlling, and productivity found in our younger lives is not only welcomed but seen as a process of deep and transformative growth and an avenue to thriving (Weber & Orsborn, 2015). Instead of fighting or denying physical, cognitive, financial decline, or loss, Elders understand the strength found in letting go, embracing the moment, and honoring the spiritual connections with one another (Ambrogi, 2017; Elder, 2014; Khodarahimi et al., 2021; Weber & Orsborn, 2015; Zweig, 2021).

Deep reflection is also referred to as a "process discernment and translation" (Jenkinson, 2018, p. 209). It entails discerning what is most important to pay attention to in life and being able to communicate those ideas to others, particularly younger generations, in a way that addresses their needs. Deep reflection not only brings enlightenment to the individual but to the larger community (Jenkinson, 2018).

Death (physical, metaphysical, or symbolic) is viewed as not only natural and part of the life cycle but something transformative for both the self and the community (Elder, 2014). An appreciation for the life cycle and the nearing of one's self brings about a greater sense of love for self, others, the world, and humanity with the desire to carefully and thoughtfully attend to the end of life (Gawande, 2014; Weber & Orsborn, 2015).

Self-Critique and Living Into Valued Beliefs

Elderhood requires the continuous evaluation of personal and shared values and beliefs (Ambrogi, 2017; Dandaneau & East, 2011; Kane, 2016). It entails deep listening and being opened to discovering new insights and developing new paradigms of knowing oneself and the world (Brause, 2010; Cera, 2020; Dandaneau & East, 2011, Zweig, 2021). The time afforded to Elders (when not having or needing to be productive) is not to generate luxury or self-indulgence but to invest in the internal and sacred space of self (Ambrogi, 2017; Zweig, 2021) and of the world around us (Jenkinson, 2018; Lisson et al., 2018). Valued beliefs are further developed and embodied and often transcend religious affiliations and/or rituals (Cera, 2020; Kim & Kim-Godwin, 2019; Orr et al., 2020).

Reflective Questions: Part 2

Having read this perspective of spirituality and Elderhood, do you now have a different way of understanding the aging process? What parts of Elderhood intrigued you or brought new meaning to you? What additional questions may you now have about spirituality and the older population? If you had the ability to ask a chaplain or spiritual guide more about the topic of death and dying, what might you ask?

Resilient Aging and Interdependence of Older Adults: Perspectives, Social Structures, and Resources

Beyond a varied cultural understanding of Elderhood, spirituality in older adults is often perceived as a coping mechanism for the reality of life events. The term **resilient aging** is used in multiple ways to describe the mindset and the practices used to remain at our very best physically, mentally, cognitively, and spiritually (Avelar-González et al., 2020; Fastame et al., 2017; Fry, 2000). This not only includes a lifetime of developed routines that maximize functioning, but it also entails the ability to take on new or adapt to current lifestyles and habits (Avelar-González et al., 2020; McDougall, 2020; Shaw et al., 2016; van Leeuwen et al., 2019). The notion of resiliency, or the ability to cultivate the body-mind-spirit connection to overcome or deal with crisis, challenges, illness, disease, and other life events and hardships, continues throughout our lifetime and is called upon in old age (Hagerty, 2017). In this particular perspective of resiliency, our past experiences in dealing with adversity prepares us to deal with more challenges in our later years (Hagerty, 2017).

From an alternative viewpoint, resiliency while aging continues with the acknowledgement that we may lose a portion of our ability to adapt to life or not be able to regain physical, cognitive, emotional, or social abilities that we had in our youth. Ultimately, it is the acceptance of aging as a natural process, a universal phenomenon, not as a disease that needs to be cured or overcome (Aronson, 2019; Gawande, 2014) and this acceptance is no longer connected with the idea of social desirability (Fastame et al., 2017) but universal care and quality of life (QOL) for all humanity (Gawande, 2014; Jenkinson, 2018).

Interdependence is the capacity to accept when help, assistance, or adaptation is needed to maximize our health and/or QOL (Ludlow et al., 2021; Stanford & Stearns, 2019). When personal independence may not be achievable or desirable, interdependence is embraced by the individual and caregiver(s). There is recognition that levels of cultural awareness, sensitivity, and humility are needed by the health care community in understanding and supporting this interdependence (Fahlberg et al., 2016; Gawande 2014; Johnson & Hasan, 2021; McGovern et al., 2016) and respecting the rights, choices, and dignity of the elderly (Ludlow et al., 2021; Nie, 2021). Marginalized older adults may be more vulnerable during this life period and interdependence, along with great respect and humility provided by the health care members is vital (especially when Elderhood is not part of community understanding), but how that is supported needs to be culturally relevant (Johnson & Hasan, 2021; McGovern et al., 2016; Mengting et al., 2020; Nelson-Becker & Thomas, 2020, Nie, 2021). Intergenerational interdependence promotes the idea that there is reciprocity in that relationship. Care, support, and love is not only received by the older adult but is reciprocally given back to others (Nie, 2021).

Spirituality and Select Populations

The literature highlights a variety of spiritual approaches with select populations of older adults including those who are adjusting to aging (Kumari & Sangwan, 2020; Von Humboldt et al., 2014), those dealing with a major life event, past or present, (McCormack & Joseph, 2014), those with frail health (Andreasen et al., 2015; Thauvoye et al., 2020), and those approaching death (Ebenau et al., 2017). As stated in the previous chapters, the context of the individual or group needs to be part of this discussion. The intersection of age, gender, race, ethnicity, and sexual orientation (Bailey & Gordon, 2016; McGovern et al., 2016; Mengting et al., 2020; Reich et al., 2020; Sharma et al., 2019; Von Humboldt et al., 2014), cognitive abilities (Bolton et al., 2019), and spirituality and/or religious beliefs and practices (Johnson & Hasan, 2021; Kapri & Kathpalia, 2019; Sessanna, 2008; Sullivan & Beard, 2014; Thompson et al., 2020) produces nuanced understanding of the topic of spiritual health and well-being and how spirituality is lived out daily.

Advanced Directive Decision Making and Independent Community Dwellers

In one study, Sessanna (2008) described an understanding of spiritualty as a process of contributing to others, supporting individuals and communities, and believing in others to reciprocally care for them in need. Participants in the study described this process in connection with both everyday activities and with Advanced Directive decision making. As part of their understanding and practice of spirituality, these Elders expressed the need and desire to contribute to their communities (family, friends, or a larger sense of community), to support their communities, and believed that their contributions and support were valued and important. They also believed that there would be support for them in their end-of-life needs. This interconnection of contributing, supporting, and believing follows or mirrors the process of Advanced Directive decision making. How one sees their particular life in terms of these spiritual attributes ultimately influences their desires and decisions about end-of-life care.

Spirituality and Cognitive Impairment

What is shared in the literature is the value and importance of spirituality in maintaining overall health and well-being (Cohen-Mansfield, 2016; Tiwari et al., 2016; Zimmer et al., 2016), including cognitive abilities (Datta & Newberg, 2020). What is not well reported is the challenges and concerns for those who have experienced neurodegenerative and functional declines and their engagement in spiritual and/or religious activities (Datta & Newberg, 2020). The movement from extrinsic, or observable behaviors and religious and/or spiritual practices, to an intrinsic or inward approach in attending to our beliefs shifts for those with cognitive challenges. The interpersonal aspects or focus of spirituality and/or religious practices during cognitive decline become even more profound and valued (Bolton et al., 2019; Sullivan & Beard, 2014). The embodiment of spiritual and/or religious practices that have been cultivated for generations becomes instinctual even when cognitive decline is noted (Sullivan & Beard, 2014; Swinton, 2014).

Reflection of an Adapted Church Service for Those With Severe Dementia

Several years ago, I (Tam) completed a 12-week chaplaincy internship at a faith-based extended-living community. My primary role was to provide chaplaincy services to the residents in the long-term care and the dementia units. This learning opportunity offered me the ability to use my occupational therapy knowledge and experiences along with expanding my interests in providing opportunities for spiritual health and wellness to the residents and those in end-of-life care.

One of my tasks was to be part of a team that would create and design a sensory-based church service for those with significant dementia. Many of the residents in this service would have been regular church attendees for decades. Some of the residents were still part of the regular church services held every Sunday for the community. They may have been wheeled into the service in their gerichair and placed at the back of the room to sit and listen, and possibly observe, what was going on. The other alternative was to have the resident remain in their personal room and have the television station set to the broadcasted service. There was really no opportunity to engage in the service beyond being a passive participant.

It was also unclear how much of the service the residents could actually take in as the weekly service took 1 hour to deliver at the regular speed and with much sensory stimulation in the service and lots of information to process from the sermon.

In the redesign of the church service, we took a look at the structure and routines of a regular service and broke down the major components to include prayer, music, greetings with one another, reading of sacred texts, a sermon or message from the minister or leader, and then Eucharist or a form of communion.

This particular faith-based community had a predominately protestant presence and so it was fairly easy for us to consider the past experiences of the residents and determine what characteristics of the service would or could be remembered and tapped into. We adapted the service in length and the amount of sensory stimulation provided. We allowed time between activities, allowing the experience to sink into their being. We provided therapeutic touch while greeting and saying prayers. We choose songs with care and sang together one-on-one in a circle and allowed any vocalizations of the members to join in.

What was the most significant part of the adapted service was the Eucharist. Because many of the members were no longer able to eat and swallow well, they were often bypassed in this part of the regular service. For our adapted service we decided to incorporate the speech-language pathologists in designing the type and amount of wafer/bread and the wine to use. Each person would be given what was appropriate for their diet. We took our time, slowly moving from person to person offering the sacrament in different ways. Quiet and soft music (without words) played in the background. We stayed with each person as long as it was needed to provide spiritual nourishment. For many of the attendees that day, we saw emotions not typically or otherwise noticed. They were smiling. They were calm. They squeezed our hands. And even some of the attendees that day had tears flowing down their cheeks.

End of Life

Anxiety around death is found throughout the literature including those with a terminal illness (Emafti et al., 2019; Sprik et al., 2019), the aged, and frail elderly (Khormaei et al., 2017); however, there are disputes about what death anxiety actually means and what contributes to or reduces this anxiety (Newberg et al., 2019). Some individuals approaching death indicate that they are accepting of death and yet seem to have significant anxiety through the death process. While others, religious or not, may have significant anxiety around death (Bengtson et al., 2015; French et al., 2017).

Accepting death, vs. denying or fighting the death process, and then living into the final and active process of dying seems to be a strong indicator of having and demonstrating less anxiety about death (Surall & Steppacher, 2020). There is some evidence to indicate that engaging in spirituality, being a part of a group that focuses on spirituality, and deep spiritual practices may reduce death anxiety (Emafti et al., 2019; Khormaei et al., 2017; Newberg et al., 2019; Sharma et al., 2019). Lessons from the literature is that anticipating and living through the death process is a unique experience for all (French et al., 2017). For those experiencing anxiety prior to the final, end stage and during the active dying process, spiritual and religious attention may be warranted. Chaplains and others trained in the process of **abiding** with someone during death is found to be helpful (Gordon et al., 2020; Sprik et al., 2019; Vahrmeyer & Cassar, 2017).

The Use of Reiki in End-Stage Dementia: A Personal Reflection

As part of my role as a volunteer chaplain, I (Tam) was often referred to various nursing homes and hospitals to provide care to women in late-stage dementia. Most of the time this meant spending time with them in a variety of tasks such as listening to music, reading poetry, or just sitting beside them and being a presence for them.

I always felt very honored to be with a woman over the course of months or a year through their journey. This gave me the opportunity to get to know them and what activities and occupations were most meaningful to them in their life and now in their later life. When the time came when the woman was no longer able to communicate their desires or wishes, I could pull from our experiences together and select the activities that were previously expressed as important.

That is what happened with Bea, a woman with a robust life of music, artistry, and creativity. I spent time with her in the assisted living facility, at times in the hospital when she needed medical care and her family was too far to come for the short hospitalization, and then later when she was in the skilled nursing, dementia care facility.

We would spend time listening to classical, choir, and organ music. We would listen to short clips of operas she loved. I would read poetry, some of which she penned. Our time together was important and, I believe, meaningful for Bea. We had established a bound, a deep relationship.

In the later month of her life, Bea would often be very agitated when I came. She was often moaning, as in pain, and unsettled in her body, moving continuously. I had not known what the cause was but tried my best, with the help of the nursing staff, to provide some comfort. Some of the time this worked but the frequency in her agitation and not being able to provide some calm increased in the last month of her life.

It was at that time that I spoke with the chaplain about her care. In that conversation, it was revealed that the chaplain used healing energy through Reiki and was a master Reiki practitioner. I was certified as a Reiki 1 healer. We decided that we would try Reiki with Bea and scheduled a visit after receiving permission from the family to do so. The nursing staff reported that Bea had been agitated all day and nothing seemed to bring relief. We approached Bea, as we would anyone else, letting her know what we were offering. Of course, she could not provide verbal consent, but we both knew Bea and felt that she would be open to receive such support. Within 1 minute, Bea started to relax and within 5 minutes of providing Reiki, Bea was fully relaxed, able to breath at a regular rate, and had a smile on her face. This intervention produced results that lasted several days.

The chaplain and I completed three more sessions of Reiki over the next several weeks. Each session producing the same results but lasting longer with each intervention until her death been. It was also a spiritual shift in his own understanding of purpose, time, happiness, and joy.

Widowhood and Singleness

Those who have lost a spouse or significant partner and women who have always been single speak about the challenges of aging and the spiritual disconnect when relationships are altered or no longer exist (Pandya, 2020; Rudaz et al., 2020). Within bereavement group sessions, both men and women speak about the death through the lens of spirituality as making meaning of the death, engaging in religious and spiritual practices to deal with the grief, and finding resilience in moving forward in their own life (Damianakis & Marziali, 2012; Rudaz et al., 2020).

Reflective Questions: Part 3

Consider the topics of loss, death, and cognitive decline. What is your own comfort level in understanding, talking about, or addressing any of these issues if they should arise within your intervention sessions? What resources would you utilize to assist individuals or groups in attending to these issues? What other health care disciplines could you call upon to assist with these topics? What ethical dilemmas may arise through attending to the spiritual needs of those with cognitive challenges?

Select Examples of Activities to Support Spiritual Health and Wellness With Older Adults

As in the previous chapters, the primary focus in presenting these intervention samples is to direct the body and mind to a relaxation state, to encourage the art of creativity, and then attending to aspects of spirituality. In the case of older adults, activities are related to focusing on relationships, current and lost, and through grief.

Meditation and Yoga

Both meditation (Jackson et al., 2016; Pandya, 2020) and yoga (Kumari & Sangwan, 2020; Von Humboldt et al., 2014) practices have contributed to a greater sense of health, connection to oneself, others, and the sacred during old age. Meditation can be learned and incorporated into daily routines at any age and ability (see Chapter 20 for more information). Yoga not only supports health and wellness throughout the life span, but it can also be modified or adapted to achieve well-being and spiritual connection. Yoga poses for older adults with physical limitations can be adapted while seated. Working collaboratively with a yoga instructor can create a powerful interprofessional team for older adults.

Creative Activities

As with children, adolescents, and adults, creative expression can be used to support spiritual health and wellness. Adams-Price et al. (2018) provide another way to understand creativity and spirituality with adults and older adults through the concept of "serious leisure." This is more than picking up a new craft or hobby, but instead, taking on the vocation of a leisure or volunteer pursuit that produces a sense of meaning and purpose, life satisfaction, and generativity. It often entails extensive learning, skill development, and much time and energy to achieve. Example of such might be becoming a gourmet chef, writing, starting a blog, or joining a community group such as a choir or theater.

Relationships

There are many types of love. They include friendship, family, romantic, universal, or spiritual love (Burton, 2019). Universal love or agape (ah-gah-pay), is the love for strangers, nature, or God/divine (Diessner et al., 2018). This encompasses the concept of altruism, unselfish concern for the welfare of others. Within all of these kinds of relationships, we can learn how to give and receive unconditional love and self-love (Diessner et al., 2018; McCarthy et al., 2019). In addition, many older adults have the time, wisdom, and experience to explore, seek, and develop deeper intimate relationships (Damianakis et al., 2020).

Love is the greatest healer. It can open the doorway for us to heal old wounds and to learn to love and accept ourselves. Through relationships, we can learn how to love others and ourselves (Diessner et al., 2018; McCarthy et al., 2019). This may be a relationship with people, a pet, animal, or higher power. Activities such as creating and sending cards, developing a memory book, or imagery can assist with building and sustaining relationships.

Grief and Loss

Grief is always about loss. Whether it is the loss of future dreams, the loss of current capacity, or the loss of past opportunities. Whether it is a sudden life event that pushes us into grief or a slow and progressive loss, there is a need to recognize and appreciate that loss, that difference. Grief is also about clinging onto or forming new images for the present and the future. If one gets stuck in grieving the loss without embracing something different or something new, spiritual health and wellness are impacted. The real issue here is how to do both. Grieve the loss and embrace newness (Hall, 2014; McClocklin & Lengelle, 2018; Smit, 2015). It often feels like a balancing act, or at least a reciprocal response, but the grief journey is an individual one with many twists and turns and approaches. Spirituality can assist in that journey from grief to newness, and the life event can precipitate the need for and use of spirituality in one's daily routines (Rudaz et al., 2020).

Grief and loss can often be catalysts for a person to seek deeper meaning in life, question their beliefs, and possibly seek new ones (McClocklin & Lengelle, 2018). When people have had major life challenges or changes, they often report that they learned a lot from their experience, and many describe developing new healthy habits and routines, including spirituality. Examples of activities used through the grief process can be:

- Journaling
- Memory boxes—a collection of memorabilia that reminds you of that person
- Creating a playlist of favorite songs that you shared with the person or remind you of that person
- Life narratives—writing stories about your experience with the person
- Life line—Create a life line of your relationship, highlighting significant events and turning points in the relationship

Reflective Questions: Part 4

Consider some of the activities mentioned earlier. What activities do you think would be able to be completed at the senior center? What adaptations might be needed for those with physical limitations or visual limitations?

An Interprofessional Strengths-Based Approach to Spiritual Health and Wellness

It may be easy for many of us to dwell on what is lost during our later years. It also may be easy for the practitioner to identify what are challenges and limitations for clients and/or populations. The strengths-based approach to spiritual health and well-being shifts that thinking into ways in which we focus on what is still present in our lives, what beauty remains, and what relationships may still be cultivated, and how we might embrace death (Chapin et al., 2016; Rajeev & Jenna, 2020). A sense of wonder, possibility, awe, and gratitude can come from new and possible perspectives. It does not minimize the challenges or loss but instead focuses on what is not lost and what is still present today. This approach also offers a problem-solving strategy where both the person and the practitioner work together to find ways to adapt to daily activities and valued occupations (Chapin et al., 2016; Hesamzadeh et al., 2017). The focus moves away from attending solely to what is lost to embracing QOL, present beauty, and the spiritual practice of acceptance and wisdom.

Conclusion

Spiritual health and wellness in the later stages of life continues to focus on carrying out valued and meaningful roles and routines, assessing what is most helpful in our lives and with others, engaging in meaningful relationships, and learning how to let go of our lives. It is a profound time that can be full of grace, compassion, interdependence, gratitude, and wisdom. Spirituality can evolve through the process of understanding and accepting loss and valuing the importance of grief.

References

Adams-Price, C. E., Nadorff, D. K., Morse, L. W., Davis, K. T., & Stearns, M. A. (2018). The Creative Benefits Scale. International *Journal of Aging & Human Development, 86*(3), 242-265. https://doi.org/10.1177/0091415017699939

Allison, T. A., & Smith, A. K. (2020). "Now I write songs": Growth and reciprocity after long-term nursing home placement. *Gerontologist, 60*(1), 135-144. https://doi.org/10.1093/geront/gnz031

Ambrogi, D. M. (2017). On the way to the fullness of elderhood. *Generations, 41*(4), 136-143.

Andreasen, J., Lund, H., Aadahl, M., Gobbens, R. J. J., & Sorensen, E. E. (2015). Content validation of the Tilburg Frailty Indicator from the perspective of frail elderly. A qualitative explorative study. *Archives of Gerontology & Geriatrics, 61*(3), 392-399. https://doi.org/10.1016/j.archger.2015.08.017

Aronson, L. (2019). *Elderhood: Redefining aging, transforming medicine, reimagining life*. Bloomsbury Publishing.

Avelar-González, A. K., Bureau-Chávez, M., Durón-Reyes, D., Mondragón-Cervantes, M. I., Jiménez-Acosta, Y. del C., Leal-Mora, D., & Díaz-Ramos, J. A. (2020). Spirituality and religious practices and its association with geriatric syndromes in older adults Attending to a geriatric's clinic in a university hospital. *Journal of Religion & Health, 59*(6), 2794-2806. https://doi.org/10.1007/s10943-020-00990-0

Bailey, W. A., & Gordon, S. R. (2016). Family caregiving amidst age-associated cognitive changes: Implications for practice and future generations. *Family Relations, 65*, 225-238.https://doi.org/10.1111/fare.12176

Barclay, A. (2016). Lost in Eden: Dementia from paradise. *Journal of Religion, Spirituality & Aging, 28*(1/2), 68-83. https://doi.org/10.1080/15528030.2015.1028696

Bengtson, V. L., Silverstein, M., Putney, N. M., & Harris, S. C. (2015). Does religiousness increase with age? Age changes and generational differences over 35 years. *Journal for the Scientific Study of Religion, 54*(2), 363-379. https://doi.org/10.1111/jssr.12183

Bolton, C., Lane, C., Keezer, R., & Smith, J. (2019). The transformation of religiosity in individuals with cognitive impairment. *Journal of Religion, Spirituality & Aging, 31*(4), 360-368. https://doi.org/10.1080/15528030.2018.1534706

Bouchard, L., Manning, L., Perton, C., & Flanagan, M. (2021). Connection, inclusion, support, and transition: The contextual significance of aging within faith communities. *Journal of Religion, Spirituality & Aging*, 1-19. https://doi.org/10.1080/15528030.2021.1938341

Brause, D. G. (2010). Elderhood, in and out of community. *Communities, 149*, 18-26.

Burton, N. (2019, June 19). These are the 7 types of love. https://www.psychologytoday.com/blog/hide-and-seek/201606/these-are-the-7-types-love

Cera, R. (2020). Education, spirituality, religion and transformative learning in aged adults: A qualitative study. *Rivista Di Scienze Dell'Educazione, 58*(2), 222-237.

Chapin, R., Nelson-Becker, H., Macmillan K., & Sellon, A. (2016). Strengths-based and solution-focused practice with older adults: New applications. In D. Kaplan & Berkman, B. (Eds.). *The Oxford handbook of social work in health and aging* (2nd ed., pp. 63-71). Oxford University Press.

Cohen-Mansfield, J., Shmotkin, D., & Hazan, H. (2016). Changes in religiosity in old age: An exploratory study. *The International Journal of Aging & Human Development, 83*(3), 256-273. https://doi.org/10.1177/0091415016651883

Cornwell, B. (2011). Independence through social networks: Bridging potential among older women and men. *Journal of Gerontology Series B: Psychological Sciences and Social Sciences,66B*, 782-794. https://doi.org/10.1093/geronb/gbr111

da Silva, A. (2010). On becoming elders. *Communities, 149*, 24-26.

Damianakis, T., Coyle, J. P., & Stergiou, C. L. (2020). Searching for more: Spirituality for older adult couples seeking enhanced relationship quality. *Journal of Religion, Spirituality & Aging, 32*(1), 25-44. https://doi.org/10.1080/15528030.2018.1555780

Damianakis, T., & Marziali, E. (2012). Older adults' response to the loss of a spouse: The function of spirituality in understanding the grieving process. *Aging & Mental Health, 16*(1), 57-66. https://doi.org/10.1080/13607863.2011.609531

Dandaneau, S., & East, E. (2011). Listening to sociological elders: An interview with Maurice R. Stein. *American Sociologist, 42*(1), 129-144. https://doi.org/10.1007/s12108-011-9123-4

Datta, S., & Newberg, A. (2020). The relationship between the brain and spirituality with respect to aging and neurodegenerative diseases: Clinical and research implications. *Journal of Religion, Spirituality & Aging, 32*(4), 357-380. https://doi.org/10.1080/15528030.2020.1773372

DeConick, A. (2019). *The Gnostic new age: How a countercultural spirituality revolutionized religion from antiquity to today*. Columbia University Press.

Diessner, R., Pohling, R., Stacy, S., & Güsewell, A. (2018). Trait appreciation of beauty: A story of love, transcendence, and inquiry. *Review of General Psychology, 22*(4), 377-397. https://doi.org/10.1037/gpr0000166

Ebenau, A., van Gurp, J., & Hasselaar, J. (2017). Life values of elderly people suffering from incurable cancer: A literature review. *Patient Education & Counseling, 100*(10), 1778-1786. https://doi.org/10.1016/j.pec.2017.05.027

Elder, A. (2014). Zhuangzi on friendship and death. *Southern Journal of Philosophy, 52*(4), 575-592. https://doi.org/10.1111/sjp.12086

Emafti, M. F., Hedayatizadeh-Omran, A., Noroozi, A., Janbabai, G., Tatari, M., & Modanloo, M. (2019). The effect of group logotherapy on spirituality and death anxiety of patients with cancer: An open-label randomized clinical trial. *Iranian Journal of Psychiatry & Behavioral Sciences*, 1-8. https://doi.org/10.5812/ijpbs.93572

Fahlberg, B., Foronda, C., & Baptiste, D. (2016). Cultural humility: The key to patient/family partnerships for making difficult decisions. *Nursing, 46*(9), 14-16. https://doi.org/10.1097/01.NURSE.0000490221.61685.e1

Fastame, M. C., Hitchcott, P. K., & Penna, M. P. (2017). Does social desirability influence psychological well-being: perceived physical health and religiosity of Italian elders? A developmental approach. *Aging & Mental Health, 21*(4), 348-353. https://doi.org/10.1080/13607863.2015.1074162

French, C., Greenauer, N., & Mello, C. (2017). A multifactorial approach to predicting death anxiety: Assessing the role of religiosity, susceptibility to mortality cues, and individual differences. *Journal of Social Work in End-of-Life & Palliative Care, 13*(2/3), 151-172. https://doi.org/10.1080/15524256.2017.1331181

Fry, P. S. (2000). Religious involvement, spirituality and personal meaning for life: existential predictors of psychological wellbeing in community-residing and institutional care elders. *Aging & Mental Health, 4*(4), 375-387. https://doi.org/10.1080/713649965

Gawande, A. (2014). *Be mortal: Medicine and what matters in the end.* Metropolitan Books.

Gordon, C. S., Jones, S. C., Taylor, M., McInerney, M., & Wegener, J. (2020). An Australian study on the benefits of pastoral care to aged care residents in Christian affiliated homes. *Health & Social Care in the Community, 28*(2), 366-375. https://doi.org/10.1111/hsc.12868

Hagerty, B. B. (2017). *Life reimagined: The science, art, and opportunity of middle life.* Riverhead Books.

Hall, C. (2014). Bereavement theory: Recent developments in our understanding of grief and bereavement. *Bereavement Care, 33*(2014), 7-12. https://doi.org/10.1080/02682621.2014.902610

Hesamzadeh, A., Dalvandi, A., Bagher Maddah, S., Fallahi Khoshknab, M., Ahmadi, F., & Mosavi Arfa, N. (2017). Family caregivers' experience of activities of daily living handling in older adult with stroke: A qualitative research in the Iranian context. *Scandinavian Journal of Caring Sciences, 31*(3), 515-526. https://doi.org/10.1111/scs.12365

Jackson, D., Doyle, C., Capon, H., & Pringle, E. (2016). Spirituality, spiritual need, and spiritual care in aged care: What the literature says. *Journal of Religion, Spirituality & Aging, 28*(4), 281-295. https://doi.org/10.1080/15528030.2016.1193097

Janus, E., & Smrokowska-Reichmann, A. (2019). Level of happiness and happiness-determining factors perceived by women aged over 60 years. *Journal of Women & Aging, 31*(5), 403-418. https://doi.org/10.1080/08952841.2018.1485387

Jenkinson, S. (2018). *Come of age: The case of elderhood in a time of trouble.* North Atlantic Books.

Johnson, J., & Hasan, L. (2021). Paddling together for culturally safe emergency care for elders. *International Journal of Indigenous Health, 16*(1), 146-164. https://doi.org/10.32799/ijih.v16i1.33051

Kahn-John, M., Badger, T., McEwen, M. M., Koithan, M., Arnault, D. S., & Chico-Jarillo, T. M. (2021). The Diné (Navajo) Hózhó Lifeway: A focused ethnography on intergenerational understanding of American Indian cultural wisdom. *Journal of Transcultural Nursing, 32*(3), 256-265. https://doi.org/10.1177/1043659620920679

Kane, M. (2016). My journey with Annemarie Roeper: Lessons learned along the way. *Roeper Review, 38*(4), 237-244. https://doi.org/10.1080/02783193.2016.1220866

Kapri, A., & Kathpalia, J. (2019). Impact of spirituality on well-being of old aged people. *Indian Journal of Health & Wellbeing, 10*(4-6), 129-131. B00338V2I32015

Khodarahimi, S., Ghadampour, E., & Karami, A. (2021). The roles of spiritual well-being and tolerance of uncertainty in prediction of happiness in elderly. *Anales de Psicología, 37*(2), 371-377. https://doi.org/10.6018/analesps.446871

Khormaei, F., Dehbidi, F. A., & HassanZehi, E. (2017). Prediction of death anxiety based on demographic characteristics and spirituality components in the elderly. *Health, Spirituality & Medical Ethics Journal, 4*(2), 21-26. 841b3f8beb5745c3a8ea6f586ca7e24c

Kim, S. S., & Kim-Godwin, Y. S. (2019). Cultural context of family religiosity/spirituality among Korean-American elderly families. *Journal of Cross-Cultural Gerontology, 34*(1), 51-65. https://doi.org/10.1007/s10823-019-09363-x

Kumari, A., & Sangwan, S. (2020). Importance of spirituality in the life of elderly. *Indian Journal of Health & Wellbeing, 11*(4-6), 173-175.

Lepherd, L., Rogers, C., Egan, R., Towler, H., Graham, C., Nagle, A., & Hampton, I. (2020a). Exploring spirituality with older people: (1) Rich experiences. *Journal of Religion, Spirituality & Aging, 32*(4), 306-340. https://doi.org/10.1080/15528030.2019.1651239

Lepherd, L., Rogers, C., Egan, R., Towler, H., Graham, C., Nagle, A., & Hampton, I. (2020b). Exploring spirituality with older people: (2) A rigorous process. *Journal of Religion, Spirituality & Aging, 32*(3), 288-304. https://doi.org/10.1080/15528030.2019.1672236

Lisson, K., Elders, N., Walley, R., & Pettersen, C. (2018). Tapping into the sacred place, plant, and energy. *Sufi, 95*, 12-21.

Ludlow, K., Churruca, K., Mumford, V., Ellis, L. A., & Braithwaite, J. (2021). Aged care residents' prioritization of care: A mixed-methods study. *Health Expectations, 24*(2), 525-536. https://doi.org/10.1111/hex.13195

Maley, C. M., Pagana, N. K., Velenger, C. A., & Humbert, T. K. (2016). Dealing with major life events and transitions: A systematic literature review on and occupational analysis of spirituality. *The American journal of occupational therapy: official publication of the American Occupational Therapy Association, 70*(4), 7004260010p1–7004260010p6. https://doi.org/10.5014/ajot.2016.015537

Manning, L. K. (2012). Spirituality as a lived experience: Exploring the essence of spirituality for women in late life. *International Journal Aging Human Development, 75*(2), 95-113. https://doi.org/10.2190/AG.75.2.a

Martinson, R. (2019). Elderhood: Aging's new frontier. *Dialog: A Journal of Theology, 58*(4), 260-268. https://doi.org/10.1111/dial.12516

McCarthy, V. L., Bowland, S., Nayar, E., Connelly, J., & Woge, A. (2019). Developing a new perspective in late life: The PATH Program. *Journal of Adult Development, 26*(4), 304-320. https://doi.org/10.1007/s10804-018-9319-8

McClocklin, P. A., & Lengelle, R. (2018). Cures for the heart: A poetic approach to healing after loss. *British Journal of Guidance & Counselling, 46*(3), 326-339. https://doi.org/10.1080/03069885.2017.1381665

McCormack, L. & Joseph, S. (2014). Psychological growth in aging Vietnam veterans: Redefining shame and betrayal. Journal of Humanistic *Psychology, 54*(3), 336-355. https://doi.org/10.1177/0022167813501393

McDougall, E. E. (2020). Past or present spirituality? Predicting mental health outcomes in older adults. *Journal of Religion, Spirituality & Aging, 32*(1), 70-87. https://doi.org/10.1080/15528030.2019.1663772

McGovern, J., Brown, D., & Gasparro, V. (2016). Lessons learned from an LGBTQ senior center: A Bronx tale. *Journal of Gerontological Social Work, 59*(7/8), 496-511. 10.1080/01634372.2016.1255692

Mengting, L., Ruijia, C., & XinQi, D. (2020). Elder mistreatment across diverse cultures. *Generations, 44*(1), 20-25.

Nakasone, R. Y. (2013). Spiritual genealogy: Interfaith and multicultural reflections on spirituality and aging with an introduction to the articles. *Journal of Religion, Spirituality & Aging, 25*, 2-11. https://doi.org/10.1080/15528030.2013.738578

Nelson-Becker, H., & Thomas, M. (2020). Religious/spiritual struggles and spiritual resilience in marginalized older adults. *Religions, 11*(9), 431. https://doi.org/10.3390/rel11090431

Newberg, A., Wintering, N., & Waldman, M. (2019). Comparison of different measures of religiousness and spirituality: Implications for neurotheological research. *Religions, 10*(11), 637. https://doi.org/10.3390/rel10110637

Nie, J.-B. (2021). The summit of a moral pilgrimage: Confucianism on healthy ageing and social eldercare. *Nursing Ethics, 28*(3), 316-326. https://doi.org/10.1177/0969733020944446

Orr, J., Kenny, R. A., & McGarrigle, C. A. (2020). Longitudinal associations of religiosity and physical function in older Irish adults. *Journal of the American Geriatrics Society, 68*(9), 1998-2005. https://doi.org/10.1111/jgs.16470

Pandya, S. P. (2020). Meditation to improve the quality of life of community-dwelling ever-single older adults: A multi-city five-year follow-up experiment. *Journal of Religion, Spirituality & Aging, 32*(1), 45-69. https://doi.org/10.1080/15528030.2019.1600631

Rajeev, S. P., & Jenna, A. V. (2020). Strengths perspective in working with elderly. *Indian Journal of Gerontology, 34*(3), 377-393.

Reich, A. J., Claunch, K. D., Verdeja, M. A., Dungan, M. T., Anderson, S., Clayton, C. K., Goates, M. C., & Thacker, E. L. (2020). What does "Successful Aging" mean to you?—Systematic review and cross-cultural comparison of lay perspectives of older adults in 13 countries, 2010-2020. *Journal of Cross-Cultural Gerontology, 35*(4), 455-478. https://doi.org/10.1007/s10823-020-09416-6

Reynolds, J., Bernard, M., & Ray, M. (2021). Being a gerontologist: Intersections between the professional and the personal in the Ageing of British Gerontology project. *Ageing & Society, 41*(5), 1051-1071. https://doi.org/10.1017/S0144686X1900151X

Rudaz, M., Ledermann, T., & Grzywacz, J. G. (2020). The role of private religious practices, spiritual mindfulness, and years since loss on perceived growth in widowed adults. *Journal of Religion & Health, 59*(6), 2819-2832. https://doi.org/10.1007/s10943-020-00986-w

Sessanna, L. (2008). The role of spirituality in advance directive decision making among independent community dwelling older adults. *Journal of Religion & Health, 47*(1), 32-44. https://doi.org/10.1007/s10943-007-9144-z

Sharma, P., Asthana, H. S., Gambhir, I. S., & Ranjan, J. K. (2019). Death anxiety among elderly people: Role of gender, spirituality and mental health. *Indian Journal of Gerontology, 33*(3), 240-254.

Shaw, R., Gullifer, J., & Wood, K. (2016). Religion and spirituality: A qualitative study of older adults. *Ageing International, 41*(3), 311-330. https://doi.org/10.1007/s12126-016-9245-7

Smit, C. (2015). Theories and models of grief: Applications to professional practice. *Whitireia Nursing & Health Journal, 22*, 33-37.

Sprik, P. J., Walsh, K., Boselli, D. M., & Meadors, P. (2019). Using patient-reported religious/spiritual concerns to identify patients who accept chaplain interventions in an outpatient oncology setting. *Supportive Care in Cancer, 27*(5), 1861-1869. https://doi.org/10.1007/s00520-018-4447-z

Stanford, B. H., & Stearns, R. N. (2019). Perspectives of elders in thriving marriages on why their marriages thrive. *Educational Gerontology, 45*(3), 227-243. https://doi.org/10.1080/03601277.2019.1602373

Sullivan, S. C., & Beard, R. L. (2014). Faith and forgetfulness: The role of spiritual identity in preservation of self with Alzheimer's. *Journal of Religion, Spirituality & Aging, 26*(1), 65-91. https://doi.org/10.1080/15528030.2013.811462

Surall, V., & Steppacher, I. (2020). How to deal with death: An empirical path analysis of a simplified model of death anxiety. *Omega: Journal of Death & Dying, 82*(2), 261-277. https://doi.org/10.1177/0030222818808145

Swinton, J. (2014). What the body remembers: Theological reflections on dementia. *Journal of Religion, Spirituality & Aging, 26*(2/3), 160-172. https://doi.org/10.1080/15528030.2013.855966

Thauvoye, E., Vanhooren, S., Vandenhoeck, A., & Dezutter, J. (2020). Spirituality among nursing home residents: A phenomenology of the experience of spirituality in late life. *Journal of Religion, Spirituality & Aging, 32*(1), 88-103. https://doi.org/10.1080/15528030.2019.1631939

Thompson, E. H., Futterman, A. M., & McDonnell, M. O. (2020). The legacy of the Black church: Older African Americans' religiousness. *Journal of Religion, Spirituality & Aging, 32*(3), 247-267. https://doi.org/10.1080/15528030.2019.1611521

Tiwari, S., Singh, R., & Chand, H. (2016): Spirituality and psychological wellbeing of elderly of Uttarakhand: A comparative study across residential status. *Journal of Psychology, 7*(2), 112-118.

Vahrmeyer, M., & Cassar, S. (2017). The paradox of finitude in the context of infinitude: Is death denial an essential aspect of being in the world? *Existential Analysis: Journal of the Society for Existential Analysis, 28*(1), 151-165.

van Leeuwen, K. M., van Loon, M. S., van Nes, F. A., Bosmans, J. E., de Vet, H. C. W., Ket, J. C. F., Widdershoven, G. A. M., & Ostelo, R. W. J. G. (2019). What does quality of life mean to older adults? A thematic synthesis. *PLoS ONE, 14*(3), 1-39. https://doi.org/10.1371/journal.pone.0213263

Von Humboldt, S., Leal, I., & Pimenta, F. (2014). Does spirituality really matter? A study on the potential of spirituality for older adult's adjustment to aging. *Japanese Psychological Research, 56*(2), 114-125. https://doi.org/10.1111/jpr.12033

Walsh, L. (2019). The lady as elder in the Shepherd of Hermas. *Journal of Early Christian Studies, 27*(4), 517-547. https://doi.org/10.1353/earl.2019.0050

Weber, R. L., & Orsborn, C. (2015). *The spirituality of age: A seeker's guide to growing older*. Park Street Press.

Wright, S. T., Breier, J. M., Depner, R. M., Grant, P. C., & Lodi-Smith, J. (2018). Wisdom at the end of life: Hospice patients' reflections on the meaning of life and death. *Counselling Psychology Quarterly, 31*(2), 162-185. https://doi.org/10.1080/09515070.2016.1274253

Zimmer, Z., Jagger, C., Chiu, C. T., Ofstedal, M. B., Rojo, F., & Saito, Y. (2016). Spirituality, religiosity, aging and health in global perspective: A review. *SSM—Population Health*. https://doi.org/10.1016/j.ssmph.2016.04.009

Zweig, C. (2021). *The inner work of age: Shifting From role to soul*. Park Street Press.

Part VIII

Developing Interprofessional Practice

CHAPTER 22

Building Community Capacity From an Interprofessional Perspective Using Small Grants

Gail Whiteford, PhD; Michael A. Pizzi, PhD, OTR/L, FAOTA; Amy Sawyer, B.Bus; B.Soc.Sc; Jane Evans, MSc; and Andrew Bailey, D Psych (Clinical)

Learning Objectives

At the end of this chapter, the reader will:

1. Develop understandings of the concept of community capacity (ACOTE B.4.7)
2. Stimulate consideration of how health professionals can strengthen community capacity in sustainable ways (ACOTE B.4.7)
3. Describe what co-design is and the principles that underpin it (ACOTE B.4.7)
4. Discuss community perceptions of using small grants to undertake health promoting activities generated through multimethod evaluation (ACOTE B.6.4)
5. Consider use of small grants for health promotion activities in communities as supporting contextually relevant forms of self-determination (ACOTE B.6.4)

The ACOTE Standards used are those from 2018.

Key Words

Co-Design, Community, Community Capacity, Community Capacity Building, Empowerment, Health Equity, Health Promotion, Human Capital, Small Grants Programs, Social Capital, Sustainability

Pizzi, M. A., & Amir, M. (Eds.). *Interprofessional Perspectives for Community Practice: Promoting Health, Well-Being, and Quality of Life* (pp. 407-414).

Table 22-1

Community and Community Capacity Building

COMMUNITY AND COMMUNITY CAPACITY CONCEPT	DEFINITION
Client-centered approach	"Promotes participation, exchange of information, client-decision making, and respect for choice" (Law, 1998, preface)
Social capital	Connections and relationships between people and their communities
Human capital	Attributes of people such as health, knowledge, and skills that can be harnessed for community development and capacity building
Health equity	When all members of society enjoy a fair and just opportunity to be as healthy as possible (CDC, 2019, p. 1)
Social determinants of health	"The non-medical factors that influence health outcomes. They are the conditions in which people are born, grow, work, live, and age, and the wider set of forces and systems shaping the conditions of daily life. These forces and systems include economic policies and systems, development agendas, social norms, social policies and political systems" (WHO, n.d., p. 1)
Strengths-based approach	An approach that examines and utilizes a persons' or community's strengths, abilities and capabilities and not what is missing

Defining Community and Community Capacity

In order to understand building and strengthening community capacity, one needs to understand the concept of community. Community can be a geographic area, a shared commitment to a common idea or goal, or interactions among people through mutual participation. Fazio (2017) cites Hillery (1955) who focused on locale as central to a definition of community.

> .... he proposed that groups of people differing in terms of place and time may also differ in their interpretations of meaning surrounding locale. He distinguished between community and *the* community. His distinction separated the idea of common ties and social interactions from locale. In his view, community is the most powerful of the two concepts, emphasizing moral commitment, social cohesion and continuity in time... (Fazio, 2017, p. 4)

From a health perspective, Kniepmann defines it as "... more than a geographic location for practice, but includes an orientation to collective health, social priorities, and different modes of service provision" (1997, p. 540) while the World Health Organization (WHO, n.d.) defines **community** as "groups of people that may or may not be spatially connected, but who share common interests, concerns or identities. These communities could be local, national or international, with specific or broad interests" (para. 1).

Community and community capacity building utilize many different concepts that may be unfamiliar to many health professionals. Table 22-1 describes these concepts and defines them.

When working from and within a community perspective, understanding these concepts will help health professionals optimize the development and implementation for community programming. For example, knowing the social determinants of health of a community, and the human and social capital that health professionals encounter, can determine the types of programs that a community can implement to promote positive community health, well-being, and quality of life (QOL) for all in the community. In building and strengthening community capacity, it is essential to also understand the concepts of community empowerment and sustainability.

Community Capacity

Thus far we have explored the concept of community and defined concepts related to community. However, it is important to also understand the building and strengthening of **community capacity** and its relationship to community programming. "Community capacity is the combined influence of a community's commitment, resources and skills that can be deployed to build on community strengths and address community problems and opportunities" (Aspen Institute, 1996). Rogers et al. (1995) define it as "the cultivation and use of transferable knowledge, skills, systems, and resources that affect community- and individual-level changes consistent with public health-related goals and objectives."

While **community capacity building** is "about promoting the 'capacity' of local communities to develop, implement and sustain their own solutions to problems in a way

Table 22-2

Three-Dimensional Model of Community Empowerment

DIMENSIONS OF EMPOWERMENT	DEFINED AS
Three levels of empowerment: individual, organization, and community	The impact of empowerment occurs at the individual, organization and community levels. Each of the levels have both internal and external locus of empowerment.
Locus empowerment can either be internal or external	Internal for individuals is a belief in oneself to enact change. External is "being able to use that capacity to bring about change for oneself or one's community (Wiggins, 2012, p. 359).
Components of empowerment are both processes and outcomes	The process of empowerment is nonlinear and includes the level of participation of the community. The outcomes are the final community health change enabled by empowerment.

Adapted from Wiggins, N. (2012). Popular education for health promotion and community empowerment: a review of the literature. *Health Promotion International, 27*(3), 356-371. https://doi.org/10.1093/heapro/dar046

that helps them shape and exercise control over their physical, social, economic and cultural environments" (Stuart, 2014, p. 1).

The case in the second section of this chapter describes community and community capacity building in more depth and offers insight how grants and funding sources empower communities for capacity building. The case is built on the concept of community-based participatory research (CBPR).

CBPR is increasingly utilized to engage community stakeholders in addressing public health priorities. In its purest form, CBPR is a collaborative process that equitably involves community members in the research process. For communities, the value of CBPR is manifested by increased capacity and sustainable adoption of evidence-based practices for social change (Hacker et al., 2012, p. 349).

Involving community members in strategy development to improve health and health conditions for their own community yields greater involvement and participation.

Empowerment

For community capacity building, it is important that communities feel and experience that they are in control.

> "Empowerment" refers to the process by which people gain control over the factors and decisions that shape their lives. It is the process by which they increase their assets and attributes and build capacities to gain access, partners, networks and/or a voice, in order to gain control. Community empowerment refers to the process of enabling communities to increase control over their lives. (WHO, 2010, p. 1)

From a public health context, it "is conceptualized as including perceived control at the individual, organizational and community levels; sense of community; critical awareness of the social context (critical consciousness) and participation in change" (Wiggins, 2012, p. 358). Wiggins has conceptualized a three-dimensional model of community empowerment (Table 22-2).

Community empowerment relies on the self-described needs of a community and working with that community to effect positive change in health and well-being. Social and political change can and should also occur, which then can optimize the enablement of the promotion of health and well-being.

> Power is a central concept in community empowerment and health promotion invariably operates within the arena of a power struggle. Community empowerment necessarily addresses the social, cultural, political and economic determinants that underpin health, and seeks to build partnerships with other sectors in finding solutions. (WHO, 2010, p. 1)

When communities themselves participate in capacity building, there are eight outcomes identified:

1. Expanding, diverse, inclusive community participation
2. Expanding leadership base
3. Strengthening individual skills
4. Encouraging a shared understanding and vision
5. Strategic community agenda
6. Facilitating consistent, tangible progress toward goals
7. Creating effective community organizations and institutions
8. Promoting resource utilization by the community (The Aspen Institute, 1996)

Empowerment needs to be an inclusive concept, with the ultimate goal being social, political, cultural, and economic change and positive health outcomes in communities in order to enable the promotion of health, well-being, and QOL for all.

Table 22-3

Elements of a Sustainability Plan

1.	Methods and plan for collection of data to demonstrate program effectiveness. (Important for newer programs)
2.	How will activities and infrastructure be sustained once initial funding ends? (Also important for newer programs)
3.	Will the target population be enlarged? (Particularly for experienced programs)
4.	Will you transfer best practices to other programs? (Particularly for experienced programs)
5.	Will you build relationships with other agencies?
6.	How will you build more efficient mechanisms for funding (such as repurposing of existing resources through improved alignment, and coordination of complementary activities and resources)?
7.	Will you collect additional data that demonstrate program efficiencies and effectiveness, community advocacy, funding diversification, and collaborative partnerships that can maximize resources?
8.	What are your plans for developing community assets through staff/volunteer training and programming?
9.	Do you have other plans for developing community assets?

Adapted with permission from Fazio, L. S. (2017). *Developing occupation-centered programs with the community* (3rd ed.). SLACK Incorporated.

Sustainability

When interprofessional teams focus on the development of community programming, the process and outcomes of that program development requires that the program be sustainable. Once a program is implemented, it is the building of community capacity that allows for sustainability to occur. Sustainability occurs when a community's needs are being met and there is ongoing evaluation of the program in order to adapt according to changing needs of a community. Hence, **sustainability** is defined as a continuous process of community partnerships that can be viewed from an individual, organizational, and community level; it is a way of thinking to build strong coalitions among community members and the external environment in order for the health, well-being, and QOL of individuals and the community to be enabled.

The descriptive research of Hacker et al. (2012) related to a community-academic conference exploring concepts of community capacity and sustainability, revealed the following: "(1) the concepts of capacity and sustainability were considered interconnected; (2) partnership was perceived as both a facilitator and an outcome of community-based participatory research (CBPR); (3) sustainability was linked to "transfer of knowledge" from one generation to another within a community; and (4) capacity and sustainability were enhanced when goals were shared and health outcomes were achieved" (p. 349).

Development of a sustainability plan is important during program development and building community capacity. Table 22-3 are questions to be answered for building a sustainability plan.

Summary

Community capacity building is a proactive and necessary approach when promoting the health, well-being, and QOL of a community. It is essential that interprofessional teams and researchers consider the potential of a community to optimize health outcomes through concepts such as empowerment. It is also crucial to build in sustainability plans for the ongoing and changing health needs of a community, while also attending to the social determinants of health, health equity, and social justice needs of communities. The following example, using development of a grant to build community capacity, utilizes all of these concepts.

The Healthy Communities Small Grants in Health Promotion Program and Recipient Feedback

The *Healthy Communities* Accord is an initiative of a local health government agency/health district on the Mid North Coast of NSW (MNCLHD), Australia, working in partnership with other government agencies, academic institutions, and community organizations. Its overarching aim has been to build capacity (see previous section) for preventive health with partners and communities in the belief that, first, communities are the experts when it comes to their own health and, second, that health promotion processes can be vehicles for empowerment and self-determination (WHO, 1986). The MNCLHD is classified as a *rural* Health District within NSW (Figure 22-1) and has some unique demographic features, including a higher than national and state average aging community, a higher than national and state average of Aboriginal persons, and the existence of some geographically isolated areas with limited access to mainstream health services.

Acknowledging this unique demography, the *Healthy Communities* small grants were developed through a co-designed (see next section) process with the input of all partners. From the outset, it has been orientated to addressing the burden of chronic disease through innovative preventive health strategies, especially those that prioritized healthy eating and/or active living.

Since 2018, *Healthy Communities* has offered competitive small grants of up to $3000 AUD (about $2300 in the United States) to community-based organizations to implement healthy eating and/or active living preventive health innovations. Three rounds of small grants have been undertaken at the time of writing. Round 1 funding was predominantly awarded to strategies that addressed the burden of child obesity, whereas Round 2 funding expanded to ensure Aboriginal communities and cultural perspectives could be recognized and supported. Across the three rounds of grants, there has been a diverse mix of the types of community groups who were successful in receiving a small grant including:

- Schools
- Support groups for specific conditions (e.g., Parkinson's disease)
- Child care centers
- Aboriginal health and well-being organizations/groups
- Refugee support groups

The grants supported activities that included growing vegetable gardens, dancing for well-being, preparing nutritious meals in groups, setting up a healthy menu school cafeteria, and the creation of walking and swimming groups. What has been noteworthy about the small grants program is the fact that while each organization had to meet core objectives about what specific aspect of health promotion it addressed in the program implementation, each small grant recipient went about it in their own culturally and contextually relevant and appropriate way based on the feedback we have received. This is an important dimension that underpins both capacity and sustainability, which we will discuss in subsequent sections.

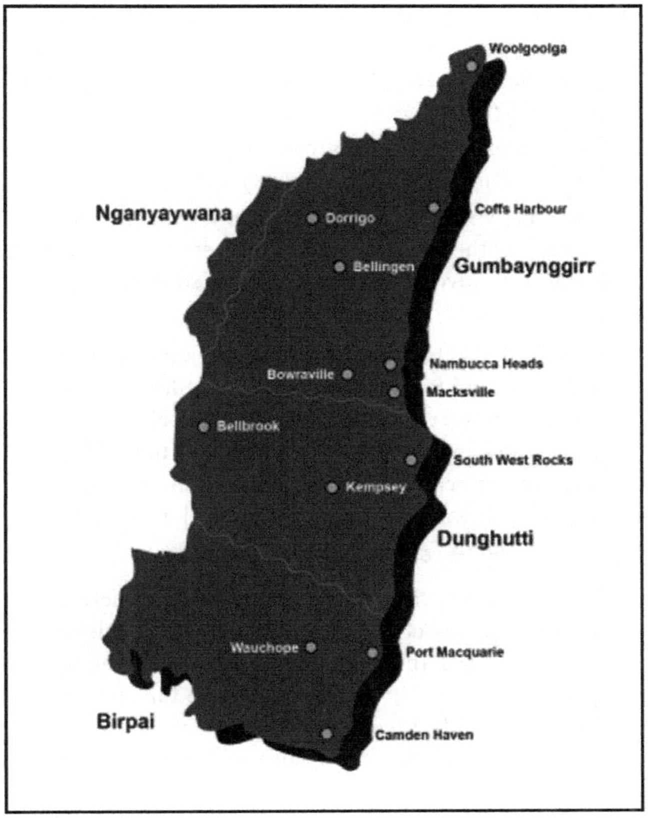

Figure 22-1. Map of mid north coast local health district within NSW, Australia.

What the Grant Recipients Said

In terms of feedback, the researchers (Gail Whiteford, Amy Sawyer, Jane Evans, and Andrew Bailey) sought to gather evaluative data systematically from the grant recipients through use of a purpose designed survey and through undertaking qualitative interviews with people from the organizations who volunteered. In our evaluation, we wanted to give the recipients a "voice" so that we could:

1. Determine the effectiveness and impact from recipient perspectives
2. Illuminate factors that prevented or enabled sustainability from recipient perspectives
3. Understand the process of knowledge generation and identify strategies that were utilized by the grant recipients as they implemented their respective projects
4. Provide a platform for the identification of other issues relevant in the organization, management, or delivery of the grant

Overall, the feedback from the participating grant recipients was very positive. In response to six key questions on the survey, they indicated the following:

- Did the grant enable you to meet your project objectives? *Completely, 75%, Exceeded, 10%*
- Was the grant money sufficient to meet the needs of the project? *Partially, 46%, Completely, 54%*
- To what extent has the project been sustained? *Somewhat, 39%, Completely, 57%*
- If your project was sustainable, what contributed to this? *Embedded in everyday work, 63%, Capacity developed, 33%*

- To what extend did your project raise knowledge of health promotion principles and/or preventive health strategies, for example, primary and secondary prevention? *Partially, 58%, Completely, 42%*
- To what extent did your project impact on the target audience? *Partially, 50%, Completely, 50%*

The following are some strong commentaries reflecting the "voice" of the recipients, which covered issues relating to participant involvement through to sustainability and impact:

> We used the health promotion literature and its great, I've got to say it's really great…I felt because we saw them every week it was quite social. It was habitual change and they really did get the understanding of health promotion…it wasn't just about the food, it was about screen time and everything. They certainly "got it."

> I mean I know that people can isolate themselves, depression, anxiety as well as movement problems they have, but this sort of thing is just bringing people together…in a community like this, people become friends, I feel very fulfilled that people are feeling better about their quality of life. That's what it's all about.

> …it's good actually because we have a lot of families that may not be as active as some others. The kids go home and tell them they want to go and do such a thing at the park or something. Then it's sort of encouraging them to get out and do that sort of thing…it definitely all starts with the kids.

What Is Community Capacity and Why Use Small Grants in Community Health Promotion?

When we refer to a community, we are basically referring to a group of people who have something in common. It may be that they have a location in common (a geographic community), a belief system or heritage (e.g., a cultural or religious community), or that they share an interest/occupation or profession (e.g., organic gardening or farming), or as summarized by Mohamad et al. (2012), communities can be considered as place, social system, or interest base. In everyday life, people belong to multiple communities simultaneously and move between them relative to what they want, need, and aspire to do on a daily basis.

When it comes to community capacity, and the idea of building community capacity to increase the health status of populations through health-promoting activity, there is a long history of such a focus that was captured formally in the WHO's Jakarta Accord of 1997 (1997). A recent definition of community capacity has been developed by Ubert et al. (2017) that draws upon this early work of the WHO suggesting it is the "local promotion of knowledge, skills, commitments, structures and leadership" (p. 1). They also point out that this is best done through network development, training, competence development, and the allocation of financial resources (the latter two of which apply to the project described in this chapter).

Considering the earlier definition a little more closely, it is possible to see that, if knowledge and skills of people within communities are built effectively, people and communities are less reliant on professional input. In this way it is much like the old adage of "If you give a man a fish, you feed him for a day, if you teach him how to fish, you feed him for life." In this regard, developing/building community capacity is most essentially about sustainability. However, building community capacity, especially in health promotion is also about the development and implementation of activities that are culturally and contextually relevant and appropriate, and the people who understand this best are the members of distinct communities (Hyett at al., 2019). The best method for developing initiatives aimed at building community capacity is, quite obviously, by involving community members in the planning and design of activities a process known as co-design, which discussed in the next section. Providing the financial resources, in the form of a small grants program, was a way in which the community groups in the researchers' region could develop and implement health promotion programs, which encouraged healthier eating and more movement in the ways that fit best—and were most appropriate and relevant as perceived by them.

Why Is a Co-Design Approach Important in Working With Communities?

Co-design has been described as essentially being about the process of collaboratively designing services with the involvement of key stakeholders including service-users, service-deliverers, and service-procurers (WACOSS, 2017) and may be seen as representing a moral and ethical commitment to transformation-based collaborative action (Whiteford, 2020).

The five principles of co-design are that co-design is always:

1. *Inclusive*—The process includes representatives from critical stakeholder groups who are involved in the co-design project from framing the issue to developing and testing solutions. It utilises feedback, advice and decisions from people with lived or work experience, and the knowledge, experience and skills of experts in the field.
2. *Respectful*—All participants are seen as experts and their input is valued and has equal standing. Strategies are used to remove potential or perceived inequality. Partners manage their own and others' feelings in the interest of the process. Co-design requires everyone to negotiate personal and practical understandings at the expense of differences.
3. *Participative*—The process itself is open, empathetic and responsive. Co-design uses a series of conversations and activities where dialogue and engagement generate new, shared meanings based on expert knowledge and lived experience. Major themes can be extracted and used as the basis for co-designed solutions. All participants are responsible for the effectiveness of the process.
4. *Iterative*—Ideas and solutions are continually tested and evaluated with the participants. Changes and adaptations are a natural part of the process, trialling possibilities and insights as they emerge, taking risks and allowing for failure. This process is also used to fine-tune potential outcomes or solutions as it reaches fruition and can later be used to evaluate its effectiveness.
5. *Outcomes focused*—The process can be used to create, redesign or evaluate services, systems or products. It is designed to achieve an outcome or series of outcomes, where the potential solutions can be rapidly tested, effectiveness measured and where the spreading or scaling of these solutions can be developed with stakeholders and in context (NCOSS, 2016, pp. 3-4).

Similar to co-design, co-creation is the systematic process of creating new solutions with people, not for them (Bason, 2010). Underpinning these concepts is the idea that collaborative, cooperative, and community-centered approaches to creating transformed social conditions can lead to more effective services, which, as a corollary, can have greater social impact. For interprofessional teams, this represents the most valid, powerful, and sustainable way in which they can work in and with communities.

Key Learnings in, and Recommendations for, Developing a Community Small Grants Program in Health Promotion

There are several reasons why the small grants projects, as perceived by community members who actually received and utilized them, were successful. Based on the experiential process of the interdisciplinary team involved (including psychologists, dieticians, occupational therapists, Aboriginal health workers, and health service managers) and the feedback and data generated through the evaluation process, the key learnings have been that:

- Co-designed processes are important *from outset to implementation*
- Focusing on *community self-determination and empowerment counts*
- Being philosophically oriented to *health and well-being as being best understood relative to social, cultural, and geographic contexts* is a respectful basis for collaboration
- *Capacity development* can be understood as a form of *knowledge co-production* that represents a work in progress
- *Making sustainability a key focus at all stages* of the grant orientates grant recipients to its importance in planning and implementation

Based on this, the following is recommended for health professionals considering developing and using a small grants program to promote healthy living in communities:

- Be clear from the outset what you are hoping to achieve, where, how, and with whom
- Ensure you have the recurrent funds to support the small grant program, for at least 3 years, if possible
- Consult widely within the community who you are going to be working with, making sure you seek diverse views
- Create a co-design team drawn from the community to establish foci and criteria
- Make the grant application process straightforward and available through multiple channels (not just online that disadvantages some communities/community members)
- Build in a requirement for sustainability planning in the grants
- Check in with grant recipients in terms of progress against their objectives regularly

- Gather feedback continuously
- Celebrate successes in terms of outcomes and communicate these as widely as possible

In conclusion, small grants programs such as what we have described in this chapter can be powerful and effective in strengthening the capacity of communities to design and deliver health promotion activities that are culturally and contextually relevant and, most importantly, get results. Even small amounts of money make a difference to community groups, especially when, alongside accountability, they are empowered to be autonomous and self-determining in their unique, context-oriented actions to create stronger, healthier subcommunities. Such an approach represents an investment in sustainable change as well as a platform from which interprofessional teams and groups can work "shoulder to shoulder" with diverse people in diverse settings to co-create those communities we collectively imagine.

References

The Aspen Institute. (1996). *Measuring community capacity building: A workbook in progress for rural communities*. https://www.aspeninstitute.org/wp-content/uploads/files/content/docs/csg/Measuring_Community_Capactiy_Building.pdf

Bason, C. (2010). *Leading public sector innovation: Co-creating for a better society*. Bristol University Press

Centers for Disease Control and Prevention. (2019). Health equity considerations and racial and ethnic minority groups. https://www.cdc.gov/coronavirus/2019-ncov/community/health-equity/race-ethnicity.html

Fazio, L. S. (2017). *Developing occupation-centered programs with the community* (3rd ed.). SLACK Incorporated.

Hacker, K., Tendulkar, S.A., Rideout, C., Bhuiya, N., Trinh-Shevrin, C., Savage, C. P., Grullon, M., Strelnick, H., Leung, C., & DiGirolamo, A. (2012). Community capacity building and sustainability: Outcomes of community-based participatory research. *Progress in Community Health Partnerships: Research, Education and Action, 6*(3), 349-360. https://doi.org/10.1353/cpr.2012.0048

Hillery, G. (1955). Definitions of community: Areas of agreement. *Rural Sociology, 20*, 194-204.

Hyett, N., Kenny, A., & Dickson-Swift, V. (2019). Reimagining occupational therapy clients as communities: Presenting the community centred practice framework. *Scandinavian Journal of Occupational Therapy, 26*(4), 246-260. https://doi.org/10.1080/11038128.2017.1423374

Kniepmann, K. (1997). Prevention of disability and maintenance of health. In C. Christiansen & C. Baum (Eds.), *Occupational therapy: Enabling function and well-being* (pp. 531-555). SLACK Incorporated.

Law, M. (1998). *Client-centered occupational therapy*. SLACK Incorporated.

Mohamad, N., Talib, N., Ahmad, M., Shah, I., Leong, F. & Ahmad, M. (2012). Role of community capacity building construct in community development. *International Journal of Academic Research, 4*(1), 172-176.

New South Wales Council of Social Services. (2016). Principles of co-design. https://www.ncoss.org.au/wp-content/uploads/2017/06/Codesign-principles.pdf

Rogers, T., Howard-Pitney, B., & Lee, H. (1995). *An operational definition of local community capacity for tobacco prevention and education*. Stanford Center for Research in Disease Prevention.

Stuart, G. (2014). Sustaining community. https://sustainingcommunity.wordpress.com/2014/03/10/ccb/

Ubert, T., Forbenger, S., Ganesfort, D., Zeeb, H., & Brand, T. (2017). Community capacity building for physical activity promotion among older adults: A literature review. *International Journal of Environmental Research and Public Health, 14*, 1058. https://doi.org/103390ijerph.14091058

West Australian Council of Social Services. (2017). Co-design toolkit. https://www.wacoss.org.au/wp-content/uploads/2017/07/co-design-toolkit-combined-2-1.pdf

Whiteford, G. (2020). Sylvia Docker Memorial Lecture. Together we go further: Service co-design, knowledge co-production and radical solidarity. *Australian Occupational Therapy Journal 66*(6) 682-689. https://doi.org/10.111114440-1630.12628

Wiggins, N. (2012). Popular education for health promotion and community empowerment: a review of the literature. *Health Promotion International, 27*(3), 356-371. https://doi.org/10.1093/heapro/dar046

World Health Organization. (n.d.). Social determinants of health. https://www.who.int/health-topics/social-determinants-of-health#tab=tab_1

World Health Organization. (1986). Ottawa Charter for Health Promotion: First International Conference on Health Promotion Ottawa, 21 November 1986. https://www.healthpromotion.org.au/images/ottawa_charter_hp.pdf

World Health Organization. (1997). Leading health promotion into the 21st century: proceedings of the 4th International Conference on Health Promotion, Jakarta, Indonesia. = https://www.who.int/publications/i/item/WHO-HPR-HEP-41CHP-98.1

World Health Organization. (2010). 7th Global Conference on Health Promotion. https://www.who.int/teams/health-promotion/enhanced-wellbeing/seventh-global-conference/community-empowerment

23

CHAPTER

Community Program Planning, Design, and Evaluation

Joy Doll, OTD, OTR/L, FNAP

Learning Objectives

At the end of this chapter, the reader will:

1. Describe the best practices in needs and assets assessments (ACOTE B.4.4)
2. Understand the fundamentals of program design using an interprofessional approach (ACOTE B.4.25, B.4.27)
3. Recognize approaches to program evaluation appropriate to different types of programs including logic models (ACOTE B.4.27)

The ACOTE Standards used are those from 2018.

Key Words

Active Recruitment, Appreciative Inquiry, Community Need, Cost-Benefit Analysis, Environmental Factors, External Evaluation, Formative Evaluation, Impact Evaluation, Implementation Plan, Internal Evaluation, Mission Statement, Needs and Assets Assessment, Outcome Evaluation (Or Effectiveness Evaluation), Participatory Evaluation, Passive Recruitment, Population Description, Primary Data, Process Evaluation (Or Implementation Evaluation), Program Activity, Program Evaluation, Program Goal, Program Objective, Program Planning, Secondary Data, SMART, SWOT Analysis, Vision Statement

Pizzi, M. A., & Amir, M. (Eds.). *Interprofessional Perspectives for Community Practice: Promoting Health, Well-Being, and Quality of Life* (pp. 415-431).

Case Study: Expanding Care for Older Adults

The older adult population continues to grow and expand with older adults desiring to age in place. The John A. Hartford Foundation presents the opportunity to support older adults by supporting age-friendly care (Cacchione, 2020). One way to support this concept is to design programs focused on the 4Ms Framework for Age Friendly Health Systems: what Matters, Medications, Mobility, and Mentation (Fulmer, 2019). In this case scenario, a local home care company is interested in implementing programs that support the model to enhance age-friendly care.

The "Home Care Company," specializing in nonmedical caregiving, is interested in exploring how to maximize the use of technology to support older adults to safely age in their home and prevent social isolation. The organization hires an interprofessional team of consultants to help them design and implement the program, including a home care nurse, an occupational therapist, and a physical therapist. The charge by the home care company is to design a relevant program that can bring value to older adults and is also sustainable.

The team starts with a **needs and assets assessment** to explore the health needs of the local older adult population. In addition, the team explores which technologies might be appropriate and whether older adults will adopt these technologies. Through the needs and assets assessment, the interprofessional team recommends the company explore ways to implement a program combining in-person caregiving with remote patient monitoring technology. The team also conducts a Strengths, Weaknesses, Opportunities, and Threats (SWOT) Analysis, which is included below (Helms & Nixon, 2010; Kash & Deshmukh, 2013; Holmes & Scaffa, 2009):

STRENGTHS	WEAKNESSES
• Continuous care at home • Peace of mind for individuals and family members • Allows one to stay in their home longer • Early intervention capability	• Not typically reimbursed, so private pay is most likely needed, which could be prohibitive for some • Technology does not connect to health system which means patient has to report any health issues
OPPORTUNITIES	**THREATS**
• Potential to address social isolation • Can prevent serious health incidents	• Cost • Lack of adoption • Barriers in technology access (i.e., digital divide) • Regulation (professional practice act)

The interprofessional team shares the needs and assets assessment with the home care company. Together, the interprofessional consultant team (i.e., the nurse, occupational therapist, and physical therapist) and company leaders brainstorm goals and objectives for the program along with metrics. It is decided based on this program plan that the organization can develop a business plan to support the developing program. Through this planning, the team recognizes that this type of care might not be accessible to those who cannot privately pay and a recommendation to develop a fund to support those eligible is also added to the program plan.

Case Questions

1. Review the **SWOT Analysis**. What do you believe is missing in this needs and assets assessment?
2. Consider the consultant team. Who else would you add to this team to enhance the program design?
3. What metrics would you suggest are added to the evaluation plan to demonstrate the value of this program?

Introduction

Communities are inherently collaborative. The skills of teamwork and bringing voice to diverse perspectives are foundational to community program development (Hosny et al., 2013; Kurowski-Burt et al., 2017; Luebbers et al., 2017). In this chapter, the focus on program planning, design, and evaluation are discussed from the lens and bias that community programming, when successful, is interprofessional (Coats et al., 2017; Howell et al., 2020). In most cases, community programs are designed and implemented to address community-identified concerns that may be addressed through multiple solutions (Doll, 2009). The intent of community program design is to bring together the minds and voices of many to develop impactful and sustainable solutions to a community need. In fact, interprofessional approaches have been as bold as to discuss the approach as an opportunity to dismantle systemic racism, a structure that silences, discounts, or ignores the voices of some community members (Cahn, 2020).

This chapter provides a high-level overview of program planning, design, and evaluation in the context of interprofessional community and population health approaches. Each element of program planning, design, and evaluation could exist as its own chapter or even textbook. The intent here is to give the best practice considerations when developing a community program from an interprofessional perspective to assist a team in program design and implementation.

Program Planning

Programs exist for many reasons and are often created to address a perceived community need. How needs are identified and flow into a meaningful program requires intention and thoughtfulness. The first step in any **program planning** is to deeply understand the need and ensure that the community members are ready to address the need. It is easy for clinicians, who are trained in identifying problems, to point out potential program development opportunities. The true success of many community programs is based upon the interprofessional approach where stakeholders, community champions, and experts all come together to discuss challenges and potential solutions to community needs.

A structured way to understand the needs of communities is through a formal needs and assets assessment (LeClair, 2010; Talmage et al., 2021). A needs assessment can be defined as "systematic identification of a population's needs or the assessment of individuals to determine the proper level of services needed" (National Library of Medicine, 2018, p. 1). However, a focus on needs alone is limited and adding a focus on strengths and assets ensures that a community's abilities are as important as its challenges. Program development can be more successful when built on the capacities and assets of the community and not just the needs. One strategy for conducting a needs and assets assessment is to complete a SWOT analysis (Helms & Nixon, 2010; Holmes & Scaffa, 2009; Kash & Deshmukh, 2013). This approach can easily be coordinated with multiple stakeholders and can expose both the opportunities and challenges of a community need. Other strategies exist and can be viable in the discovery phase. Whatever the approach, the intent should be to include and encourage the voice of as many stakeholders as are available to ensure a broad perspective of the community and its needs.

Table 23-1

Population Description for Needs and Assets Assessment

DATA CATEGORY	EXAMPLES
Demographics	• Age • Race • Gender
Health issues and risk factors	• Rates of obesity • Socioeconomic status • Food insecurity
Priority health needs	• Obesity rates of school age children are high in a community
Values and beliefs about health	• Family decision maker • Ideal body weight

In some cases, writing a formal needs and assets assessment can be a critical first step in program planning (Brownson, 2008; Janssen et al., 2020). When identifying needs, it is important to regard the community as a population through a clear description. A **population description** typically focuses on four different components about a population: demographic information about the community members, health issues and risk factors, priority health needs and disparities, and values and beliefs about health (Doll, 2009). Although therapists, especially occupational therapists, have a long history of community-based practice, work in population health is evolving and being defined in both occupational therapy and physical therapy (Domholdt et al., 2020; Bass & Baker, 2017). When understanding community needs, having multiple data elements are consequential to gaining a holistic picture of the community (Table 23-1). In the case provided earlier, the age-friendly approach uses a population health structure where the system and program are designed to support the population and not just an individual. Age-friendly care is identified by a focus on the 4Ms: what matters, medications, mobility, and mentation. It exists to ensure needs are met as people age and to ensure quality of life is a focus of health care (Mate et al., 2018). This kind

Professional Reasoning Box A

Think about a community or population with which you are familiar. Brainstorm the following information commonly included in a population description in a needs and assets assessment of this community or population.

Demographic information about the community members	
Health issues	
Risk factors	
Priority health needs	
Health disparities	
Values and beliefs about health	

of systems thinking helps when engaging in community program development (Professional Reasoning Box A).

Environment also plays a significant role in community needs and assets (Pizzi & Richards, 2017; Hammell, 2019). A comprehensive needs and assets assessment values how **environmental factors** impact health. The environmental factors include the following: physical environment, social environment, and socioeconomic/sociopolitical contexts (Pereira, 2017; Crawford et al., 2017; Petruseviciene et al., 2018). Examples of physical environmental assets include parks and playgrounds. An example of an environmental need is a food desert, or a community or neighborhood with low access to healthy foods that impacts health status (Fong et al., 2021). Social environmental assets include the opportunities to interact socially through neighborhood associations. A social environmental need example includes social isolation from a global pandemic or a local high crime neighborhood. Socioeconomic and sociopolitical factors directly impact health and communities. One example of a sociopolitical factor that can influence communities is Medicaid expansion. Medicaid expansion is a state-based policy decision and can directly influence a community's ability to access health care. When examining the case, an environmental influencer is one's socioeconomic status that can indicate whether a family can financially support caregiving for their loved one. One way to think about these aspects is to identify social determinants of health that directly acknowledge one's health is dictated by where they work, live, and play (County Health Rankings Model, 2021).

Needs and assets assessments are critical to establish the clear focus and approach of a program (Leclair et al., 2019). The assessment should include public health data infused with community perspectives. A wide and broad assessment, inclusive of multiple perspectives and foci, ensures that a program can be designed to be comprehensive and truly impact community health. There are many ways to collect data for such an assessment and different approaches to community assessment exist (Hyett et al., 2019). For example, demographic data can be collected through the U.S. Census Bureau. To understand the community perspective, data can be collected via surveys, focus groups, interviews, community forums, and asking key community stakeholders. The method for data collection should be chosen based on community needs and the team conducting the assessment as each approach comes with strengths and limitations. Typically, a needs and assets assessment is a combination of primary data and secondary data. **Secondary data** is existing data collected and collated in an existing report (Carman, 2007; Olatunji et al., 2019). **Primary data** is new data that must be obtained and added to the assessment profile. In the case example of the program for older adults, a demographic profile of older adults in local zip codes along with statistics from a local community health assessment retrieved from the local health department can be critical secondary data sources to help establish community need for the program.

Communities have diverse needs. In a needs and assets assessment, it is critical that the intent is to recognize gaps and prioritize the health needs of the population. As previously mentioned, the needs and assets assessment is community-driven and not simply identified by a practitioner wanting to partner in a community (Akintobi, 2018). A strong needs and assets assessment integrates facts and evidence with the experience of the community to define clear opportunities and areas for growth when doing program design. It sets the state for program design and implementation.

Program Design

Program design can be an iterative and complicated process where many factors interact to determine the plausible steps to ensure a program's success (Olson & Brennan, 2017). In addition to visioning, program design requires pragmatic and structural planning that includes detailed approaches and considerations that broadly impact program implementation. Multiple experts can support the program design process. Using an interprofessional team that includes diverse community members to support program design can ensure a broad and comprehensive approach.

Professional Reasoning Box B

Imagine you are developing a program for a day facility for people with mild dementia. Identify who you might want to include on your interprofessional team to design a comprehensive and effective program.

Professional Reasoning Box C

Based on the case and exemplars provided, write your own Goal, Objective, and Activity for the proposed program.

When designing a program, it is best to start broadly considering the vision and mission of the program, analyzing who it will impact and how (Pandey et al., 2017). A **vision statement** is aspirational. It is intended to be what an organization or program desires to accomplish. A **mission statement** is more focused, identifying why a program exists and its purpose. A mission statement helps to keep a program on track and ensure that the program along with its elements support the vision. If the program is being designed as part of an existing organization, the vision and mission statements may already be clearly established and not a necessary step in program design. If brand new, then a program should consider starting with establishing a clear vision and mission statement as the first step in program design (Professional Reasoning Box B).

A critical success factor to any program is a well-designed program **implementation plan**. The implementation plan should include the program's goals, objectives, and activities. Unlike clinical practice, goals in program development are typically broad and focused on overall outcomes. Goals identify the future state to be accomplished by the program. For example, a **program goal** may be to reduce falls among individuals 65 years and older in the Grace Village Independent Living Community. In program implementation plans, three to five goals are a common structure with objectives and activities in complement to each goal. Objectives tend to be measurable and specific while activities are the actions needed to accomplish both the objectives and goals of the program. Unlike goals, objectives include clear timelines for completion. Depending on the goal, three to five objectives may be needed for each.

When writing program goals and objectives, it is best to follow the **SMART** pneumonic (Bjerke & Renger, 2017). SMART recommends that goals and objectives be specific to the program; measurable by a clear outcome; attainable by aligning with budgeting and resources, such as staffing; relevant to align with the needs and assets assessment; and timely (Ogbeiwi, 2017). When writing goals, objectives, and activities in the implementation plan, it is important to recognize the intended program outcomes, the evaluation plan, and the roles and responsibilities of the team (Professional Reasoning Box C).

In acknowledgment of the case provided at the beginning of the chapter, the following could be an appropriate program goal, objective, and activity.

Goal: By the end of Year 1, the program will implement the 4Ms of Age Friendly care as a foundation for its home care program.

Objective 1: Within 2 months, the program team will identify 10 to 15 participants for a 6-month pilot project using remote patient monitoring and nonmedical caregiving to support aging in place.

Activity 1: The program manager will recruit older adults with the established program eligibility for the pilot program.

A program implementation plan should include a budget. Depending on the focus of the program, the budget may include a business proposal. Whatever the context and approach, cost and revenue need to be considered and are critical to any implementation plan. Like program evaluation, budget planning and writing a business proposal could exist as its own chapter. Some programs are not-for-profit, and others are for-profit.

The implications when considering a not-for-profit vs. for-profit depends on many factors especially the mission and vision of the program. No matter the financial structure, a business plan is important as both types of organizations need financial viability. A budget must be multiyear and include aspects like start-up costs, salaries, fees for aspects like technology or other needed services, rent, income, and so on. The approach to the budget is formatted differently in a grant vs. a formal business request. Grant proposals follow the guidelines outlined in a request for proposal and still require both a budget and sustainability plan. A business proposal focuses more on costs and revenue and will align with the financial approach of the program (i.e., not-for-profit vs. for-profit). Sustainability planning from a financial perspective should be considered from the beginning including start-up costs and ongoing expenses along with opportunities for future revenue. One effective strategy is to include an accountant, grant writer, or other experts in financial planning on the interprofessional team to support the program design and implementation. Whatever the program, a budget is a critical component to any program design.

Program Recruitment

A program can only make impact if there are people enrolled or participating in the program. Any program design should include recruitment and retention of participants. Programs often have a defined target population. The target population is the subset of a population or community that the program plans to serve. When thinking about program design, identifying the target population is a critical step, delving into who is eligible for the program and how the program will accept referrals. The uniqueness of the program needs to be recognized as well when thinking about recruitment and retention. Cultural, equitable, and inclusive approaches should be examined and adapted to support the target population. Eligibility should be designed to establish whether services are offered for free or for cost. Cost may be on a sliding scale, where the fee is based on additional eligibility criteria like a person's income. Program eligibility should be unique to the program, the results of the needs and assets assessment, and the budgeting for the program along with a fit with the needs of the target population.

People cannot participate or benefit from a program of which they are not aware. Program recruitment can take on both passive and active approaches. **Active recruitment** is a direct contact approach. An active recruitment strategy for the case provided at the beginning of the chapter would be to do a presentation at a local senior center. **Passive recruitment** is indirect, with some examples including flyers, advertisements, and mailings. Flyers posted at a senior center would be an example of passive recruitment based on the chapter case example. Each program must identify their approach and may combine approaches (Estabrooks et al., 2017). Snowball recruiting might also be used. This is a word-of-mouth approach, that can be culturally appropriate in some communities especially when engaging leaders in those communities. When choosing an approach or approaches, considerations should at least recognize that various demographics may require different considerations. Gender, ethnicity, racial identity, culture, religious affiliation, literacy level, language, and education level are some to consider (Davis et al., 2018). These factors directly influence where, when, and how recruitment is done. For example, in some communities, a faith-based community may be an appropriate place for recruitment and engaging religious leaders, yet it might be ineffective in other communities. How a recruitment strategy is presented may increase or decrease its effectiveness. Certain groups of people may not feel welcome to a program based on its approach. One example is to use engendered language. This may prevent someone who identifies as gender fluid not to participate even if they are welcome. Being thoughtful in how recruitment is performed and presented is an important step in any program design.

To support the variety of recruitment approaches, a critical factor in program recruitment is a marketing plan that focuses on the target population. Marketing approaches will vary based on the population. Factors to consider in marketing include literacy levels, health literacy, language, and inclusive representation in visuals or photos. In addition, where and when the marketing materials will be distributed should be determined based on the population. The concepts of diversity and inclusivity discussed in the recruitment section are also vital with marketing. Marketing may include paper flyers or social media, depending on the type of target population. The amount and frequency of marketing also needs to be identified. The effectiveness of the marketing plan should also be studied and measured to ensure the strategies meet the intended population (Hamby et al., 2017). An intentional marketing plan is an integral aspect of program implementation.

In the recruitment plan, retention in a program may be critical. If a program is longitudinal, meaning it will exist over time, then retaining participants is a significant strategy to contemplate. Participants may need to make a program commitment and should understand all the requirements up front. Incentives may be used to ensure retention if appropriate to the program. Unique factors like peer mentors or support groups, again, if appropriate to the program, may help increase retention as building social connections can support retention (Estreet et al., 2017). It is important to try to develop a proactive retention plan and not blame a target population for a lack of program participation and retention. Typically, multi-prong approaches are most successful, and retention should be an ongoing metric included in the program's evaluation plan (Grape et al., 2018). Each program will have its own retention targets based on the program design and evaluation plan. Planning for program retention is central in program design to ensure the success of the program.

Location and Space

Programs often need location and space to successfully implement. When identifying space and location, multiple factors should be explored. When thinking of location, accessibility is critical, including both building accessibility and transportation accessibility. For example, if a community program targets individuals who need to use public transportation, then being on a bus line might be essential for people to be able to access the organization. In addition, a ramp and close parking will also be important additions. The type of space and equipment should also be considered.

Making a list of equipment needs for the program will ensure the space matches the programmatic needs. Some spaces will come with furniture and in other times, these items will need to be purchased. Understanding these needs up front can help with discerning an ideal space and location along with the program budget. The type of space within a location is also important to examine. For example, office space and conference rooms are common spaces but facilities that have the need to hang a swing or other heavy equipment may require unique structural adjustments to an existing space. When identifying space, clear needs for the program are critical to ensure the space is a match to support the program. Involving the community or target population also can be an asset in choosing an appropriate location and space (Anderson et al., 2017). Some areas of community may be viewed as undesirable or unsafe by some and may prohibit program access. Community member input can help discern a safe and accessible location. Input can be gathered in multiple ways including focus groups, stakeholder interviews, or through community events like neighborhood association meetings or community town hall meetings.

Other considerations in space are insurance liability protection for the space utilization along with compliance of building and zoning code and other local regulations. A legal consultation when signing a lease is important. The terms of the lease and opportunities for early termination without penalties should be strongly considered, especially for a new program without a proven history. In addition, space requires maintenance with cleaning and management of equipment. When budgeting for the program, fixed costs such as rent can be budgeted, and variable costs such as maintenance may need to be estimated. In some cases, space can be donated by a community organization like a faith community. In other cases, communities have space for community programs that offer start-ups low rent and space at no or a reduced cost. When choosing a space, it is imperative to be comprehensive in detailing location, budget, and the unique programmatic needs. Part of space design should include a growth plan and consideration when building fixed structures such as shelves and walls need to be weighed against using mobile furniture such as cabinets and workstations.

Staffing and Personnel

Each program will have staffing and personnel needs to ensure the program can be implemented as intended. Some programs have unique staffing needs and others are broader on what type of professional can implement a program. When considering staff and personnel, the first step is to define necessary roles and responsibilities with each position. Even for volunteers, a job description can be helpful to match people with an appropriate opportunity to support the program. If staff need to be hired, a formal hiring process should be put in place with plans to evaluate and potentially promote staff. Standard operating procedures and guidelines might need to be developed to support employees. Adding human resource experts to the interprofessional team can be a way to ensure these processes follow regulation, policy, and legal aspects. Clear policies and procedures ensure employees know what is expected of them and can protect the entity with compliance requirements.

Programs that are nonprofit and community-based often benefit from volunteers. Local resources like university, high school students, or corporate volunteer benefits can help supplement a staffing. The types and skills of volunteers may be unique to a program and a volunteer job description can help ensure a good match between volunteers interested in the program and the expectations. Volunteer sign ups and tracking hours of service may be required to ensure a good experience for volunteers (Einoff, 2018). In addition, volunteers often need training and accountability. For example, a master gardener volunteer program requires extensive training and maintenance of knowledge. In this example, training can be detailed, prolonged, and extensive and these expectations need to be clear to those considering volunteering (Henley & Traunfeld, 2021). Considering the case of the older adults presented in the chapter, training will be critical for the nonmedical caregivers whether these positions are paid or voluntary. Identifying who will provide training and tracking attendance will be important to plan. Developing a mentorship and train the trainer programs would help tier upward mobility opportunities at every level and minimize staff dropouts.

If a volunteer position is long term, incentives for volunteer retention should be included in program planning. Research shows that volunteers return or continue if roles are clear and the volunteers perceive their work makes a meaningful impact on the community (Harp et al., 2017). Evaluating the experience of the volunteers should be included in the program evaluation to ensure a positive experience for all involved (Pesut et al., 2018). Volunteers can truly support a program, but it is not without work and management. Training, tracking, and recognizing volunteers are all integral aspects of **program planning**.

Program Evaluation

Program evaluation is a field of study that means that this section will give a high-level overview of the topic. Additionally, program evaluation may go by a different name in clinical contexts often called quality improvement or process improvement. In business situations, evaluation metrics may be referred to as objectives and key results (OKRs) or key performance indicators (KPIs; Doerr, 2018). The important thing to remember is that no matter what they are called, planning to evaluate success and improve upon implementation should be done in every program. This section will focus on the best practices typically used in community program evaluation.

The goal of all program evaluation is to improve the delivery of the program to meet community needs (Janzen et al., 2017). When designing a program, the evaluation aspect is critical to demonstrate program successes both along the way in implementation and at the conclusion of a program. All programs should include evaluation to be able to develop evidence and demonstrate programmatic value. Evaluation

Professional Reasoning Box D

Imagine you are implementing a day program for older adults at a local community center. What would you evaluate to demonstrate the impact of your program?

does not have to be complex and should match the skills of those involved in the program.

In program evaluation, there are multiple aspects to consider in the design phase. The first is whether to do internal or external evaluation. **Internal evaluation** occurs when a member or members of the program team conducts the evaluation (Muir & Dean, 2017). This approach can be cost-effective if a team member is equipped to perform the evaluation. The challenge can be that internal evaluation typically holds more bias than an external approach. In some cases, this might not be problematic but in other cases, it can cause barriers to improving program delivery.

External evaluation occurs when a person outside the program or organization conducts the evaluation aspect of the program (Muir & Dean, 2017). Typically, external evaluators hold expertise in evaluation and only support that aspect of the program. The challenge with external evaluation is often the cost to hire an experienced evaluator. The opportunities with an external evaluator include expertise and tends to be viewed as less biased. In some cases, an external evaluator may be required by a funder like a grant. Whether evaluation is internal or external should be based on the expertise of the team, the budget, and the needs of the program (Professional Reasoning Box D).

Other approaches to program evaluation exist including **participatory evaluation** and **appreciative inquiry**. A participatory approach occurs when the evaluation is decided by the program participants or target population. It often follows the guidelines of action research and community-based participatory research (Scarinci et al., 2009). The intent is that the program should be for and supported by the community. In participatory evaluation, the community identifies what it wants to measure, when it is measured, and how it is measured. The focus is on a democratic process and the community determines through much discussion and facilitation the evaluation strategy. Although participatory evaluation is a very community-centered approach to program evaluation, it can be challenging in the feasibility of evaluation to meet community member expectations and it can be a time intensive process (Chouinard & Milley, 2018). Additionally, community members may not hold the expertise to understand evaluation, especially when implementing more complicated evaluation and barriers may emerge to meet community desires with budget and program expertise.

Appreciative inquiry is an approach to program evaluation that is asset focused. It recognizes that many potential solutions to a problem exist. The focus of appreciative inquiry is on strengths and opportunities. Appreciate inquiry is an "affirmative, learning- and strengths-based evaluation tool used to understand and promote transformational change when faced with challenging circumstances" (Paige et al., 2015, p. 2). In this approach, those designing the program evaluation lead with big picture dreaming, discovering, exploring destiny, and then follow with designing. The intent is to appreciate what is, what might be, and what should be. Appreciative inquiry is embedded in the values of participatory evaluation. The intent of the approach is to build trust and engage in dialogue about opportunity (Paige et al., 2015). Additionally, the evaluation approach centers on what is working well and how to expand those aspects to their fullest potential.

Multiple types of program evaluation exist and matching the correct type with the program depends on the program outcomes. It is important to remember, there is no one "right way" to evaluate a program. Instead, being informed on the options and choosing what is optimal based on community needs and programmatic sustainability is the best way to approach program evaluation. A variety of evaluation metrics are possible, and a mix of the following often ensures an ideal approach. **Formative evaluation** focuses on improving the program implementation as it is being implemented (Elwy et al., 2020). An example would be to send a survey to a volunteer to assess if the onboarding and training process met their needs and using the results to tweak the process for improved delivery. **Process evaluation**, also known as **implementation evaluation**, is focused on ensuring program activities meet participant needs and are implemented as planned (Sharma et al., 2017). For example, if program participants are dropping out, process evaluation can help develop understanding around this issue and develop a potential solution. **Outcome evaluation**, also known as **effectiveness evaluation**, explores the impact of a program on its participants (Belizan et al., 2019). An example would be if a diabetes lifestyle improvement program lowers hemoglobin A1C levels. **Impact evaluation** focuses on the overall program and if it met its intended goals (Olfert et al., 2018). Programs often can benefit from using multiple evaluation metrics to demonstrate impact and should include the best match for the program.

Recently, especially related to health care outcomes, metrics around cost and cost savings have become increasingly valued. Financial-related evaluation can include a return-on-investment (ROI) metric, which looks at upfront investment and the results from that investment on a community or target population. ROI is often a metric used to show that the initial investment improved health status or avoided unnecessary downstream costs to a target population. Another example of a financial metric would be to conduct a **cost-benefit analysis**, which analyzes the impact of financial investments vs. the program outcomes (Choy, 2018). Whether focused on cost savings or program revenue, financial metrics consider how the benefits of the program compare to the cost to implement. Financial responsibility and impacting cost reductions are important aspects in programmatic evaluation to ensure a program is cost effective and a good steward of resources.

Multiple evaluation methods are commonly used. Two signature frameworks for evaluation are the Centers for Disease Control and Prevention (CDC) Framework for Program Evaluation in Public Health and the Re-AIM Model. The CDC Framework offers robust resources on the internet and is meaningful to explore when engaging in program evaluation. The Framework follows a process to engage stakeholders, describe the program, focus on evaluation design, gather credible evidence, justify conclusions, ensure use, and share lessons (CDC, 1999).

Designing and implementing an evaluation is a collaborative venture. The first stage in the process is to engage as many stakeholders as are available. Engaging stakeholders involves bringing together perspectives from those involved in program operation, the representative target population and other community members impacted by the program, and the individuals conducting the evaluation. The stakeholders are critical to help describe the program, which includes identifying the need for the program, how the program will obtain success, program activities, resources, and context. Familiarizing community stakeholders with the program vision and mission are important as part of this process to ensure useful feedback is generated. Next, the design of the evaluation is identified recognizing purpose, evaluation questions, evaluation methods, and who will agree to support the evaluation. Whatever methods and questions are decided, credible evidence must be considered including indicators or metrics, data sources, data quality, data quantity, and logistics of the evaluation. Once this has been accomplished, it is important to justify conclusions of the evaluation plan with a clear plan to analyze and interpret findings along with making recommendations from the findings to improve or modify the program to optimize outcomes. Lastly, in the CDC Framework, the plan should include how the evaluation results will be used and how lessons learned will be shared. This process should all occur grounded in an evaluation that has utility, is feasible, and is performed ethically and accurately. The CDC Framework offers a comprehensive structure to follow when designing and implementing program evaluation (Kidder & Chapel, 2018). It can act as a guide when designing and implementing community program evaluation.

A structure common in the CDC Framework is to utilize a logic model (Kaplan & Garrett, 2005; Savaya & Waysman, 2005; Helitzer et al., 2010). A logic model provides a clear roadmap from goals to outputs. Logic models may be formatted in different ways but typically include program goals, assumptions, inputs, activities, outputs, and outcomes. Assumptions include aspects that could influence the goals. For example, an assumption may be that participants will be retained in a program for a set timeline. Inputs are what infrastructure or aspect is needed to ensure the program goals are met. For example, an input may be volunteers or funding needed to support the program. Activities are the specific actions that will be taken to ensure goals are met and outputs are the measures of those activities. An example may be a training program as an activity and the output is the number of people who attended the training. Outcomes are the ultimate occurrence if the program goal is met. In a fall prevention program, the outcome would often be to reduce falls among older adults. The CDC website offers a plethora of forms and examples for those wanting to draft a logic model for a program design and evaluation. The literature also has extensive resources on logic models that can support anyone embarking on creating one (Jones et al., 2020; Peyton & Scicchitano, 2017). Logic models can be an easy way to think through the components of an evaluation and provide a clear roadmap to ensure the evaluation is completed. Another benefit of the logic model is it offers a snapshot of the evaluation plan in one document, which can be helpful to team members and others involved in program implementation that should include program evaluation.

Another common evaluation framework is the RE-AIM Framework. RE-AIM stands for reach, effectiveness, adoption, implementation, and maintenance (Gaglio et al., 2013; Kwan et al., 2019; Harden et al., 2018). Reach is focused on identifying the intended impact. This is usually centered on the target population of the program. In a fall prevention program, it would include the number of older adults participating in the program. Effectiveness centers on the impact the program has made on the program participants. Related to fall prevention, effectiveness would identify if the program decreased falls. Adoption explores how the participants became engaged in the program, meaning how they learned about it and enrolled as participants. In the fall prevention example, it could include adoption of participants in a Tai Chi program or changes to the home environment to prevent falls. Implementation focuses on the "how" and "what" of the program including when and where it occurred. Maintenance is attentive to how the program participants enacted what they learned at the program's completion. For example, if older adults in the fall prevention program decreased their falls through exercise, do they maintain those activities and decrease fall risk over time? If the intent was to reduce falls, the exploration into if the number of falls remained at a reduced rate is important to consider. Significant literature exists with programs using the RE-AIM Framework to support program evaluation (Shaw et al., 2019; Glasgow et al., 2019).

When putting together a program evaluation, no singular approach is best. However, it is appropriate to recognize the context of the program and the purpose of the evaluation. If a framework is required by a funding agency, it should be followed. Otherwise, choosing approaches that feel feasible and comfortable are a good place to begin. Once an approach is determined, the program evaluation plan must identify what to measure, how to measure it, and what tools can support the measurement. Program evaluation methods can include quantitative and qualitative metrics. Every program should plan to demonstrate its value and there are many ways to do this. If a project is grant funded, the expectations of the funding agency may drive the metrics. In some cases, the community will drive the metrics. Whatever the drivers, the metrics should be identified with tools and strategies that complement one another and ultimately explicate the program's outcomes and value proposition (Guyadeen & Seasons, 2018; Olfert et al., 2018).

As with program design, program evaluation should be designed and implemented using an ethical focus. Evaluation should be well planned and intentional to support the program and target population. Results should be shared with the appropriate stakeholders, participants, and community to optimize outcomes. A poorly designed program evaluation plan can result in issues with wasting time and funds. When designing the program evaluation, it is important to consider the program needs around evaluation, resources, and the intended use of the results (Glennerster, 2017; Jacob, 2018). Keep in mind that even an initial poorly designed program plan is better than no plan at all, as it can be modified and improved when updated information is assessed.

Program evaluation offers rich opportunities to share the challenges, opportunities, and benefits of a program. Many stakeholders are often involved in program development, design, and implementation. These stakeholders can advocate and support a program well when they understand its impact. In addition, programs are not perfect even with the best of intentions, because information may be misinterpreted or lacking. Program evaluation offers the opportunity to explore ways to improve program implementation as new and relevant data is considered to meet community needs. Community-based programs and population health also require evidence, metrics, and ongoing data analysis to demonstrate value. Programs need to be replicated and supported from one community to the next in order to transform the health and quality of life of those it was intended to serve. Program evaluation offers the opportunity to explore ways to deliver better health outcomes which is always important to the community served.

Conclusion

Solving complex health issues in a community requires the voices and perspectives of many (Cahn, 2020; Cano, 2020). Considering all stakeholder views is a naturally interprofessional and inclusive endeavor when done comprehensively and well. Additionally, the challenges and opportunities of community-based work is often best tackled by a team of individuals willing to come together bringing their knowledge and qualities to ensure community needs are met. In this chapter, the basics of program planning, design and evaluation are discussed. The intent and hope are to lay a foundation for thought and intention around community-based program development that can improve population health. When engaging in program design, implementation, and evaluation, involving a passionate and compassionate team willing to tackle challenges, ask questions, and evaluate their impact will lead to many lessons learned and ultimately improvements in the lives of many.

ACOTE Objectives

1. Demonstrate use of the consultative process with groups, programs, organizations, or communities. MOT - Understand when and how to use the consultative process with groups, programs, organizations, or communities. OTA - Understand when and how to use the consultative process with specific consumers or consumer groups as directed by an occupational therapist (B.5.26 OTD).
2. Analyze the trends in models of service delivery, including, but not limited to, medical, educational, community, and social models, and their potential effect on the practice of occupational therapy (B.6.5).
3. Demonstrate knowledge of and the ability to write program development plans for provision of occupational therapy services to individuals and populations (B.7.9).
4. Demonstrate an understanding of the process of locating and securing grants and how grants can serve as a fiscal resource for scholarly activities (B.8.9).
5. Discuss and justify the varied roles of the occupational therapist as a practitioner, educator, researcher, policy developer, program developer, advocate, administrator, consultant, and entrepreneur. MOT - Discuss and justify the varied roles of the occupational therapist as a practitioner, educator, researcher, consultant, and entrepreneur. OTA - Identify and appreciate the varied roles of the occupational therapy assistant as a practitioner, educator, and research assistant (B.9.7 OTD).

References

Akintobi, T. H., Lockamy, E., Goodin, L., Hernandez, N. D., Slocumb, T., Blumenthal, D., ... & Hoffman, L. (2018). Processes and outcomes of a community-based participatory research-driven health needs assessment: A tool for moving health disparity reporting to evidence-based action. *Progress in Community Health Partnerships: Research, Education, and Action, 12*(Suppl. 1), 139.

Anderson, J., Ruggeri, K., Steemers, K., & Huppert, F. (2017). Lively social space, well-being activity, and urban design: Findings from a low-cost community-led public space intervention. *Environment and Behavior, 49*(6), 685-716.

Bass, J. D., & Baker, N. A. (2017). Occupational therapy and public health: Advancing research to improve population health and health equity. *OTJR: Occupation, Participation and Health, 37*(4), 175-177.

Belizan, M., Chaparro, R. M., Santero, M., Elorriaga, N., Kartschmit, N., Rubinstein, A. L., & Irazola, V. E. (2019). Barriers and facilitators for the implementation and evaluation of community-based interventions to promote physical activity and healthy diet: A mixed methods study in Argentina. *International Journal of Environmental Research and Public Health, 16*(2), 213.

Bjerke, M. B., & Renger, R. (2017). Being smart about writing SMART objectives. *Evaluation and Program Planning, 61*, 125-127.

Brownson, C. A. (2008). Occupational therapy services in the promotion of health and the prevention of disease and disability. *American Journal of Occupational Therapy, 62*(6), 694.

Cacchione, P. Z. (2020). Age-friendly health systems: The 4Ms framework. *Clinical Nursing Research, 29*(3), 139-140.

Cahn, A. (2020). How interprofessional collaborative practice can help dismantle systemic racism. *Journal of Interprofessional Care, 34*(4), 431-434. https://doi.org/10.1080/13561820.2020.1790224

Cano, M. (2020). Diversity and inclusion in social service organizations: Implications for community partnerships and social work education. *Journal of Social Work Education, 56*(1), 105-114.

Carman, J. G. (2007). Evaluation practice among community-based organizations: Research into the reality. *American Journal of Evaluation, 28*(1), 60-75.

Centers for Disease Control and Prevention. (1999). Framework for program evaluation in public health. *Morbidity and Mortality Weekly Report, 48*(RR-11), 1-42.

Chouinard, J. A., & Milley, P. (2018). Uncovering the mysteries of inclusion: Empirical and methodological possibilities in participatory evaluation in an international context. *Evaluation and Program Planning, 67*, 70-78.

Choy, Y. K. (2018). Cost-benefit analysis, values, wellbeing, and ethics: An indigenous worldview analysis. *Ecological Economics, 145*, 1-9.

Coats, H., Paganelli, T., Starks, H., Lindhorst, T., Starks Acosta, A., Mauksch, L., & Doorenbos, A. (2017). A community needs assessment for the development of an interprofessional palliative care training curriculum. *Journal of Palliative Medicine, 20*(3), 235-240.

County Health Rankings Model. (2021). County Health Rankings & Roadmaps. https://www.countyhealthrankings.org/explore-health-rankings/measures-data-sources/county-health-rankings-model.

Crawford, E., Aplin, T., & Rodger, S. (2017). Human rights in occupational therapy education: A step towards a more occupationally just global society. *Australian Occupational Therapy Journal, 64*(2), 129-136.

Davis, S. N., Govindaraju, S., Jackson, B., Williams, K. R., Christy, S. M., Vadaparampil, S. T., Quinn, G. P., Shibata, D., Roetzheim, R., Meade, C. D. & Gwede, C. K. (2018). Recruitment techniques and strategies in a community-based colorectal cancer screening study of men and women of African ancestry. *Nursing Research, 67*(3), 212.

Doerr, J. (2018). *Measure what matters: How Google, Bono, and the Gates Foundation Rock the World with OKRs.* Penguin.

Doll, J. D. (2009). *Program Development and Grant Writing in Occupational Therapy: Making the Connection.* Jones & Bartlett Publishers.

Domholdt, E., Cooper, S. K., & Kleinhoff, R. J. (2020). Population health content in entry-level occupational therapy programs. *American Journal of Occupational Therapy, 74*(3), 7403205160p1-7403205160p9.

Einolf, C. J. (2018). Volunteers in community organizations. In *Handbook of community movements and local organizations in the 21st century* (pp. 229-242). Springer, Cham.

Elwy, A. R., Wasan, A. D., Gillman, A. G., Johnston, K. L., Dodds, N., McFarland, C., & Greco, C. M. (2020). Using formative evaluation methods to improve clinical implementation efforts: Description and an example. *Psychiatry Research, 283*, 112532.

Estabrooks, P., You, W., Hedrick, V., Reinholt, M., Dohm, E., & Zoellner, J. (2017). A pragmatic examination of active and passive recruitment methods to improve the reach of community lifestyle programs: The Talking Health Trial. *International Journal of Behavioral Nutrition and Physical Activity, 14*(1), 1-10.

Estreet, A., Apata, J., Kamangar, F., Schutzman, C., Buccheri, J., O'Keefe, A. M., Wagner, F. & Sheikhattari, P. (2017). Improving participants' retention in a smoking cessation intervention using a community-based participatory research approach. *International Journal of Preventive Medicine, 8*, 106-123.

Fong, A. J., Lafaro, K., Ituarte, P. H., & Fong, Y. (2021). Association of living in urban food deserts with mortality from breast and colorectal cancer. *Annals of Surgical Oncology, 28*(3), 1311-1319.

Fulmer, T. (2019). Age-friendly health systems transform care for older adults. Modern Healthcare. Retrieved July 2, 2019.

Gaglio, B., Shoup, J. A., & Glasgow, R. E. (2013). The RE-AIM framework: A systematic review of use over time. *American Journal of Public Health, 103*(6), e38-e46.

Glasgow, R. E., Harden, S. M., Gaglio, B., Rabin, B., Smith, M. L., Porter, G. C., Ory, M. G., & Estabrooks, P. A. (2019). RE-AIM planning and evaluation framework: Adapting to new science and practice with a 20-year review. *Frontiers in Public Health, 7*, 64.

Glennerster, R. (2017). The practicalities of running randomized evaluations: Partnerships, measurement, ethics, and transparency. In *Handbook of economic field experiments, Vol. 1* (pp. 175-243). North-Holland.

Grape, A., Rhee, H., Wicks, M., Tumiel-Berhalter, L., & Sloand, E. (2018). Recruitment and retention strategies for an urban adolescent study: Lessons learned from a multi-center study of community-based asthma self-management intervention for adolescents. *Journal of Adolescence, 65*, 123-132.

Guyadeen, D., & Seasons, M. (2018). Evaluation theory and practice: Comparing program evaluation and evaluation in planning. *Journal of Planning Education and Research, 38*(1), 98-110.

Hamby, A., Pierce, M., & Brinberg, D. (2017). Solving complex problems: Enduring solutions through social entrepreneurship, community action, and social marketing. *Journal of Macromarketing, 37*(4), 369-380.

Hammell, K. W. (2019). Building globally relevant occupational therapy from the strength of our diversity. *World Federation of Occupational Therapists Bulletin, 75*(1), 13-26.

Harden, S. M., Smith, M. L., Ory, M. G., Smith-Ray, R. L., Estabrooks, P. A., & Glasgow, R. E. (2018). RE-AIM in clinical, community, and corporate settings: Perspectives, strategies, and recommendations to enhance public health impact. *Frontiers in Public Health, 6*, 71.

Harp, E. R., Scherer, L. L., & Allen, J. A. (2017). Volunteer engagement and retention: Their relationship to community service self-efficacy. *Nonprofit and Voluntary Sector Quarterly, 46*(2), 442-458.

Helitzer, D., Hollis, C., de Hernandez, B. U., Sanders, M., Roybal, S., & Van Deusen, I. (2010). Evaluation for community-based programs: The integration of logic models and factor analysis. *Evaluation and Program Planning, 33*(3), 223-233.

Helms, M. M., & Nixon, J. (2010). Exploring SWOT analysis–where are we now? A review of academic research from the last decade. *Journal of Strategy and Management, 3*(3), 215-251.

Henley, S., & Traunfeld, J. (2021). Assessing master gardener volunteers' involvement in and knowledge of food preservation. *Journal of Human Sciences and Extension, 9*(1), 84-93.

Holmes, W. M., & Scaffa, M. E. (2009). An exploratory study of competencies for emerging practice in occupational therapy. *Journal of Allied Health, 38*(2), 81-90.

Hosny, S., Kamel, M. H., El-Wazir, Y., & Gilbert, J. (2013). Integrating interprofessional education in community-based learning activities: Case study. *Medical Teacher, 35*(Suppl.), S68-S73.

Howell, B. M., Redmond, L. C., & Wanner, S. (2020). "I learned that I am loved": Older adults and undergraduate students mutually benefit from an interprofessional service-learning health promotion program. *Gerontology & Geriatrics Education*, 1-16.

Hyett, N., Kenny, A., & Dickson-Swift, V. (2019). Re-imagining occupational therapy clients as communities: Presenting the community-centred practice framework. *Scandinavian Journal of Occupational Therapy, 26*(4), 246-260.

Jacob, S. (2018). Knowledge, framing, and ethics in programme design and evaluation. In: *Ethics in public health practice in India* (pp. 45-61). Springer.

Janssen, S. L., Klug, M., Johnson Gusaas, S., Schmiesing, A., Nelson-Deering, D., Pratt, H., & Lamborn, B. (2020). Community-based health promotion in occupational therapy: Assess before you assess. *Journal of Applied Gerontology*, 0733464820921320.

Janzen, R., Ochocka, J., Turner, L., Cook, T., Franklin, M., & Deichert, D. (2017). Building a community-based culture of evaluation. *Evaluation and Program Planning, 65*, 163-170.

Jones, N. D., Azzam, T., Wanzer, D. L., Skousen, D., Knight, C., & Sabarre, N. (2020). Enhancing the effectiveness of logic models. *American Journal of Evaluation, 41*(3), 452-470.

Kaplan, S. A., & Garrett, K. E. (2005). The use of logic models by community-based initiatives. *Evaluation and Program Planning, 28*(2), 167-172.

Kash, B. A., & Deshmukh, A. A. (2013). Developing a strategic marketing plan for physical and occupational therapy services: A collaborative project between a critical access hospital and a graduate program in health care management. *Health Marketing Quarterly, 30*(3), 263-280.

Kidder, D. P., & Chapel, T. J. (2018). CDC's program evaluation journey: 1999 to present. *Public Health Reports, 133*(4), 356-359.

Kurowski-Burt, A. L., Evans, K. W., Baugh, G. M., & Utzman, R. R. (2017). A community-based interprofessional education fall prevention project. *Journal of Interprofessional Education & Practice, 8*, 1-5.

Kwan, B. M., McGinnes, H. L., Ory, M. G., Estabrooks, P. A., Waxmonsky, J. A., & Glasgow, R. E. (2019). RE-AIM in the real world: Use of the RE-AIM framework for program planning and evaluation in clinical and community settings. *Frontiers in Public Health, 7*, 345.

Leclair, L. L. (2010). Re-examining concepts of occupation and occupation-based models: Occupational therapy and community development. *Canadian Journal of Occupational Therapy, 77*(1), 15-21.

Leclair, L. L., Lauckner, H., & Yamamoto, C. (2019). An occupational therapy community development practice process. *Canadian Journal of Occupational Therapy, 86*(5), 345-356.

Luebbers, E. L., Dolansky, M. A., Vehovec, A., & Petty, G. (2017). Implementation and evaluation of a community-based interprofessional learning activity. *Journal of Interprofessional Care, 31*(1), 91-97.

Mate, K. S., Berman, A., Laderman, M., Kabcenell, A., & Fulmer, T. (2018, March). Creating age-friendly health systems: A vision for better care of older adults. In *Healthcare Vol. 6, No. 1* (pp. 4-6). Elsevier.

Muir, S., & Dean, A. (2017). Evaluating the outcomes of programs for Indigenous families and communities. Family Matters, (99), 56-65.

National Library of Medicine. (2018). *Needs Assessment MeSH Descriptor Data 2018*. Retrieved from https://meshb.nlm.nih.gov/record/ui?name=Needs%20Assessment

Ogbeiwi, O. (2017). Why written objectives need to be really SMART. *British Journal of Healthcare Management, 23*(7), 324-336.

Olatunji, E. K., Oladosu, J. B., Odejobi, O. A., & Olabiyisi, S. O. (2019). A needs assessment for indigenous African language-based programming languages. *Annals of Science and Technology, 4*(2), 1-5.

Olfert, M. D., Hagedorn, R. L., White, J. A., Baker, B. A., Colby, S. E., Franzen-Castle, L., Kattelmann, K. K., & White, A. A. (2018). An impact mapping method to generate robust qualitative evaluation of community-based research programs for youth and adults. *Methods and Protocols, 1*(3), 25.

Olson, B., & Brennan, M. (2017). From community engagement to community emergence: The holistic program design approach. *The International Journal of Research on Service-Learning and Community Engagement, 5*(1), 5-19.

Paige, C., Peters, R., Parkhurst, M., Beck, L. L., Hui, B., May, V. T. O., & Tanjasiri, S. P. (2015). Enhancing community-based participatory research partnerships through appreciative inquiry. *Progress in Community Health Partnerships: Research, Education, and Action, 9*(3), 457.

Pandey, S., Kim, M., & Pandey, S. K. (2017). Do mission statements matter for nonprofit performance? Insights from a study of US performing arts organizations. *Nonprofit Management and Leadership, 27*(3), 389-410.

Pereira, R. B. (2017). Towards inclusive occupational therapy: Introducing the CORE approach for inclusive and occupation-focused practice. *Australian Occupational Therapy Journal, 64*(6), 429-435.

Pesut, B., Duggleby, W., Warner, G., Fassbender, K., Antifeau, E., Hooper, B., Greig, M. & Sullivan, K. (2018). Volunteer navigation partnerships: Piloting a compassionate community approach to early palliative care. *BMC Palliative Care, 17*(1), 1-11.

Petruseviciene, D., Surmaitiene, D., Baltaduoniene, D., & Lendraitiene, E. (2018). Effect of community-based occupational therapy on health-related quality of life and engagement in meaningful activities of women with breast cancer. *Occupational Therapy International, 2018*, 1-13.

Peyton, D. J., & Scicchitano, M. (2017). Devil is in the details: Using logic models to investigate program process. *Evaluation and Program Planning, 65*, 156-162.

Pizzi, M. A., & Richards, L. G. (2017). Promoting health, well-being, and quality of life in occupational therapy: A commitment to a paradigm shift for the next 100 years. *American Journal of Occupational Therapy, 71*(4), 7104170010p1-7104170010p5.

Savaya, R., & Waysman, M. (2005). The logic model: A tool for incorporating theory in development and evaluation of programs. *Administration in Social Work, 29*(2), 85-103.

Scarinci, I. C., Johnson, R. E., Hardy, C., Marron, J., & Partridge, E. E. (2009). Planning and implementation of a participatory evaluation strategy: A viable approach in the evaluation of community-based participatory programs addressing cancer disparities. *Evaluation and Program Planning, 32*(3), 221-228.

Sharma, S., Adetoro, O. O., Vidler, M., Drebit, S., Payne, B. A., Akeju, D. O., Adepoju, A., Jaiyesimi, E., Sotunsa, J., Bhutta, Z.A., Magee, L.A., von Dadelszen, P. & Dada, O. (2017). A process evaluation plan for assessing a complex community-based maternal health intervention in Ogun State, Nigeria. *BMC Health Services Research, 17*(1), 1-10.

Shaw, R. B., Sweet, S. N., McBride, C. B., Adair, W. K., & Ginis, K. A. M. (2019). Operationalizing the reach, effectiveness, adoption, implementation, maintenance (RE-AIM) framework to evaluate the collective impact of autonomous community programs that promote health and well-being. *BMC Public Health, 19*(1), 1-14.

Talmage, C., Mercado, M., Yoder, G., Hamm, K., & Wolfersteig, W. (2021). Critiquing indicators of community strengths in community health needs assessments. *International Journal of Community Well-Being*, 1-22.

Appendix A: Logic Model Sample

Logic models follow multiple formats. The following is an exemplar from a grant application that required a logic model.

PROJECT HOPE EVALUATION PLAN

Activity	*Desired Outcome*	*Indicators*	*Data Source*	*Person Responsible*	*Time*	*Evaluation Description*
Media campaign	• Decrease stigma associated with suicide and mental illness • Increase suicide and mental health awareness	• More contacts for information about suicide/mental illness • Posters and information cards • Presentations and trainings • PSAs, skits, DVD/ video creation • Resource directory	• Mental health data • Product prepared and # disseminated • # of trainings conducted (tracking system) • Short post-program questionnaire • Sign-in sheet • PSI • Existing referral network • Agencies/persons requesting resource directory			• Observation • Pre/post tests • Point System Tracking • Comment sheet

(continued)

PROJECT HOPE EVALUATION PLAN (CONTINUED)

Activity	*Desired Outcome*	*Indicators*	*Data Source*	*Person Responsible*	*Time*	*Evaluation Description*
Community forums	• Increased community knowledge • Increased community readiness for suicide prevention programs • Increased support for family and friends of those with suicidal ideation, gestures/ attempts, or completions	• # awareness trainings held • # of persons attending awareness trainings • Knowledge levels • Quality of training reported by attendees • # of persons completing community assessment • Community plan in place • Community Response Plan implemented • # persons on Community Response Team • # families referring family members to Project Hope or Mental Health • # persons wishing to be trained as Gatekeepers	• Sign-in sheet • Surveys, focus groups • # of trainings conducted (tracking system) • Sign-in sheet • Short pre/ post-program questionnaire • Survey (TEPS?) • Community readiness training • Community Response Plan in place • EIRF • Centralized database for tracking; • # calls for information • reporting system in place • Gatekeeper Training implemented			• Observations • Pre/post tests • Item analysis of forum trainings minutes and meetings • Satisfaction and client surveys • Community member interviews
Cultural knowledge	• Increase cultural knowledge • Increase awareness of culture as mental health benefit	• Participants attending cultural events (e.g., handgames, gourd dance, war dance, pow-wows, Native American Church, etc.) • Participants reporting decreased stress, depression, suicidal ideation	• Sign-in sheet; • Surveys (Culture Survey); Pre and post test; interviews			• Observation • Surveys • Pre/post tests • Mental health/ suicide screens (TeenScreen) • Focus groups of select participants

(continued)

PROJECT HOPE EVALUATION PLAN (CONTINUED)						
Activity	*Desired Outcome*	*Indicators*	*Data Source*	*Person Responsible*	*Time*	*Evaluation Description*
School-based suicide prevention	• Increase suicide and mental health awareness of students • Increase staff • Increase staff development • Increase communication among project team • Increase school personnel preparedness & ability to respond to suicide threats or completions	• Implementation of curriculum • Implementation of AILS curriculum • Staff hired • Training • Seamless delivery of project services • School Suicide Protocol in place • Suicide Crisis Response Intervention Team in place at the schools	• Columbia TeenScreen • AILS assessments • Personnel Records • Training Evaluations • Informal peer evaluations • Regular meetings • Team Covenant • EIRF • Portland Model Survey • School Personnel reports increased use of School Suicide Protocol			• Suicide & Mental Health screens • Focus group interviews • Surveys and evaluation tools • Record of minutes of meetings • Regular review of team covenant
Implement sensory room activities	• Increase stress management techniques used by youth • Increase awareness of physiological benefits management of stress	• # of uses of sensory room • # of youth reporting decreased stress • Stress levels – pre and post • Training on use of sensory room items • # of persons attending training • Quality of training	• Log of use (sign in sheet) • Surveys, focus groups • Pre and post stress test • # of trainings conducted (tracking system) • Sign-in sheet • Short post-program questionn-aire	• School representatives • Student research group supervised by Joy Doll • Student research group • Joy Doll • Joy Doll • Joy Doll	• Ongoing • Beginning Fall 2010 • Beginning Fall 2010 • May of Year 1 then ongoing • May of Year 1 then ongoing • J Doll will create a monitor reporting to J Begay PRN	• This will be a sign in and out sheet monitored by the school. • Students will complete IRB and assess activities. • J Doll will create a monitor reporting to J Begay PRN • J Doll will create a monitor reporting to J Begay PRN • J Doll will create a monitor reporting to J Begay PRN

Appendix B: Glossary

active recruitment: Direct interaction with targeted audience including phone calls, text messages, or presentations to community groups.

appreciative inquiry: An approach to evaluation that is asset-focused recognizing that many potential solutions to a problem exist.

community need: An issue identified by a community that potentially can be addressed.

cost-benefit analysis: An analysis of investments made vs. the program outcomes to identify program impact.

environmental factors: A focus in a needs and assets assessment on the opportunities and challenges with physical environment, social environment, and socioeconomic/sociopolitical contexts.

external evaluation: When a person outside the program or organization, typically an expert in evaluation, conducts the evaluation aspect of the program.

formative evaluation: An evaluation plan metric focused on improving the program as it is being implemented.

impact evaluation: An evaluation plan metric focused on the overall program and if it met its intended goals.

implementation plan: A clear roadmap or plan for implementing a program.

internal evaluation: When a member of the program team conducts the evaluation.

mission statement: Describes why a program exists and its purpose.

needs and assets assessment: The "systematic identification of a population's needs or the assessment of individuals to determine the proper level of services needed" (National Library of Medicine, 2018, p. 1).

outcome evaluation (or effectiveness evaluation): An evaluation plan metric focused on the impact of a program on its participants.

participatory evaluation: A type of program evaluation that is decided by the program participants or target population often following the guidelines of action research and/or community-based participatory research.

passive recruitment: Outbound indirect strategies for potential participants with examples including flyers, advertisements, and mailings.

population description: This section of a needs and assets assessment typically focuses on four different components about a population: demographic information about the community members, health issues and risk factors, priority health needs and disparities, and values and beliefs about health.

primary data: Data that is currently unavailable on a topic and must be collected to add to the needs and assets assessment.

process evaluation (or implementation evaluation): An evaluation plan metric focused on ensuring program activities meet participant needs and are implemented as planned.

program activity: A written statement describing the actions needed to accomplish both the objectives and goals of a program.

program evaluation: A structured assessment focused on identifying the impact of the program.

program goal: A written statement identifying the broad intent of a program.

program objective: A written statement identifying measurable and specific outcomes of the program.

program planning: The development of a plan to design and implement a program that will address an identified community need.

secondary data: Existing data collected and collated in a report as part of a needs and assets assessment.

SMART: A strategy for writing goals and objectives that is specific to the program, measurable including a clear outcome, attainable aligning with budgeting and resources including staffing, relevant to align with the needs and assets assessment; and timely.

SWOT analysis: An approach to explore and identify the Strengths, Weaknesses, Opportunities and Threats (SWOT) of an issue to generate potential solutions to a community need.

vision statement: An aspirational statement that identifies what a program hopes to accomplish and why the program exists.

Additional Readings

The following are a list of supplemental readings you can seek out to complement their corresponding chapters.

Chapter 1

Interprofessional Education Collaborative Expert Panel. (2016). *Core competencies for interprofessional collaborative practice: Report of an expert panel.* Interprofessional Education Collaborative.

National Highway Transportation and Safety Administration, U.S. Department of Transportation (2021). Walkability checklist. https://www.nhtsa.gov/document/walkability-checklist

Pizzi, M. A., Reitz, S. M., & Scaffa. M. (2010). Assessments for health promotion practice. In M. E. Scaffa, S. M. Reitz, & M. A. Pizzi (Eds.), *Occupational therapy in the promotion of health and wellness* (pp. 173-194). F.A. Davis.

Chapter 2

Accreditation Council for Occupational Therapy Education (ACOTE®) standards and interpretive guide (effective July 31, 2020). *American Journal of Occupational Therapy, 72*(Suppl. 2), 7212410005. https://doi.org/10.5014/ajot.2018.72S217

Credentialing Commission of Physical Therapy Education. (2020). Standards and required elements for accreditation of physical therapist education programs. https://www.capteonline.org/globalassets/capte-docs/capte-pt-standards-required-elements.pdf

New York Department of State. (2021). New Americans. https://dos.ny.gov/office-new-americans

Poirier, J. M., Francis, K. B., Fisher, S. K., Williams-Washington, K., Goode, T. D., & Jackson, V. H. (2008). Practice brief 1: Providing services and supports for youth who are lesbian, gay, bisexual, transgender, questioning, intersex, or two-spirit. National Center for Cultural Competence, Georgetown University Center for Child and Human Development. https://www.samhsa.gov/sites/default/files/lgbtqi2-s-practice-brief.pdf

Tan, T. Q. (2019). Principles of inclusion, diversity, access, and equity. *The Journal of Infectious Diseases, 220*(220 Suppl 2), S30-S32. https://doi.org/10.1093/infdis/jiz198

The MedEdPORTAL, Journal of Teaching and Learning Resources (2021). Diversity, inclusion, and health equity collection. https://www.mededportal.org/diversity- inclusion-and-health-equity

U.S. Department of Health and Human Services. (2021). Office of Refugee Resettlement. https://www.acf.hhs.gov/orr

Wilcock, A. & Townsend, E. (2000). Occupational justice: Occupational terminology interactive dialogue. *Journal of Occupational Science, 7,* 84-86.

Chapter 3

Labonte, R., & Laverack, G. (2001). Capacity building in health promotion, Part 1: For whom? And for what purpose? *Critical Public Health, 11*(2), 111-127. https://doi.org/10.1080/09581590110039838

Liberato, S. C., Brimblecombe, J., Ritchie, J., Ferguson, M., & Coveney, J. (2011). Measuring capacity building in communities: A review of the literature. *BMC Public Health, 11*(1), 850. https://doi.org/10.1186/1471-2458-11-850

Chapter 4

2018 Accreditation Council for Occupational Therapy Education (ACOTE®) Standards and Interpretive Guide (effective July 31, 2020). (2018). *American Journal of Occupational Therapy, 72*(Suppl. 2), 7212410005p1–7212410005p83. doi: https://doi.org/10.5014/ajot.2018.72S217

Allvin, R. E. (2021). https://www.naeyc.org/resources/blog/compensation-ece

Alves, J. G. (2019). Effects of physical activity on children's growth. *Jornal de Pediatria, 95*(1), 72-78. https://doi.org/10.1016/j.jped.2018.11.003.

American Physical Therapy Association (APTA, 2020). Standards of Practice for Physical Therapy. https://www.apta.org/siteassets/pdfs/policies/standards-of-practice-pt.pdf

Brown, W. H., Pfeiffer, K. A., McIver, K. L., Dowda, M., Joao, Almeida, C. A., & Pate, R. R. (2006). Assessing preschool children's physical activity. *Research Quarterly for Exercise and Sport, 77*(2), 167-176. https://doi.org/10.1080/02701367.2006.10599351

Centers for Disease Control and Prevention. (2022). Inclusive school physical education and physical activity. Atlanta, GA: Centers for Disease Control and Prevention, U.S. Department of Health and Human Services. https://www.cdc.gov/healthyschools/physicalactivity/inclusion_pepa.htm

Flanders, J. L., Leo, V., Paquette, D., Pihl, R. O., & Séguin, J. R. (2009). Rough-and-tumble play and the regulation of aggression: an observational study of father-child play dyads. *Aggressive Behavior, 35*(4), 285-295. https://doi.org/10.1002/ab.20309

Guedes, C., Cadima, J., Aguiar, T., & Barata, C. (2020). Activity settings in toddler classrooms and quality of group and individual interactions. *Journal of Applied Developmental Psychology, 67.* https://doi.org/10.1016/j.appdev.2019.101100

Guidance document. (n.d.). https://convention.shapeamerica.org/Common/Uploaded%20files/uploads/pdfs/Instructional-Framework-for-Fitness-Education-in-Physical-Education.pdf

Institute of Medicine (2011). *Early childhood obesity prevention policies.* The National Academies Press.

Pizzi, M. A., & Amir, M. (Eds.). *Interprofessional Perspectives for Community Practice: Promoting Health, Well-Being, and Quality of Life* (pp. 433-437).

Making Connections: Unlocking Compensation and Benefits for Early Childhood Educators. (2021). National Association for the Education of Young Children. https://www.naeyc.org/

McBee, K., Craft, A., Leiby, R., Steinberger, J. (2021) Children's Hospital of Richmond at VCU. Gross motor skills: Birth to 5 years. https://www.chrichmond.org/therapy-services/occupational-therapy/developmental-milestones/gross-motor-skills-birth-to-5-years

McIver, K. L., Brown, W. H., Pfeiffer, K. A., Dowda, M., & Pate, R. R. (2016). Development and testing of the observational system for recording physical activity in children: Elementary school. *Research Quarterly for Exercise and Sport, 87*(1), 101-109. https://doi.org/10.1080/02701367.2015.1125994

Moore, L. L., et al (2003). Does early physical activity predict body fat change throughout childhood? *Preventive Medicine, 37*(4), 10-17.

Puhl, J., Greaves, K., Hoyt, M., & Baranowski, T. (1990). Children's activity rating scale (CARS): Description and calibration, *Research Quarterly for Exercise and Sport, 61*(1), 26-36. https://doi.org/10.1080/02701367.1990.10607475

Repko, A. S. (2014). *Introduction to Interprofessional Studies.* Sage Publications, Inc.

Rowlands, A. V. & Eston, R. G. (2007). The measurement and interpretation of children's physical activity. *Journal of Sports Science & Medicine, 6*(3), 270-276.

Slot, P. L., Boom, J., Verhagen, J., & Leseman, P. P. M. (2017). Measurement properties of the class toddler in ECEC in the Netherlands. *Journal of Applied Developmental Psychology, 48*, 79-91. https://doi.org/10.1016/j.appdev.2016.11.008

Trot, S., et al (2003). Physical activity in overweight and non-overweight preschool children. *International Journal of Obesity, 27*(3), 834-839.

U.S. Department of Health and Human Services (2021). Social determinants of health. Healthy People 2020. https://www.healthypeople.gov/2020/topics-objectives/topic/social-determinants-of-health

U.S. Department of Health and Human Services, U.S. Department of Agriculture. (2005). Dietary Guidelines for Americans 2005. https://www.healthierus.gov/dietaryguidelines. https://health.gov/sites/default/files/2020-01/DGA2005.pdf

Verbruggen S. W. (2018). Stresses and strains on the human fetal skeleton during development. *Journal of the Royal Society Interface*, 1-11. https://doi.org/10.1098/rsif.2017.0593

Welk, G. J., Corbin, C. B., & Dale, D (2000). Measurement issues in the assessment of physical activity in children. *Research Quarterly for Exercise and Sport, 71*(2), 59-73. https://doi.org/10.1080/02701367.2000.11082788

Wells, J. & Ritz, P. (2001). Physical activity at 9-12 months and fatness at 2 years of age. *American Journal of Human Biology, 13*(2), 384-389.

Chapter 6

Canepari, M., Pellegrino, M. A., D'Antona, G., & Bottinelli, R. (2010). Single muscle fiber properties in aging and disuse. *Scandinavian Journal of Medicine & Science in Sports, 20*(1), 10-19. https://doi.org/10.1111/j.1600-0838.2009.00965.x

Jones, C. L., Jensen, J. D., Scherr, C. L., Brown, N. R., Christy, K., & Weaver, J. (2015). The Health Belief Model as an explanatory framework in communication research: Exploring parallel, serial, and moderated mediation. *Health Communication, 30*(6), 566-576. https://doi.org/10.1080/10410236.2013.873363

Merriam-Webster.com Dictionary, Merriam-Webster, Wellness. https://www.merriam-webster.com/dictionary/wellness.

President and Fellows of Harvard College. Medical Dictionary of Health Terms. https://www.health.harvard.edu/q-through-z#S-terms

Rogina, B., Reenan, R. A., Nilsen, S. P., & Helfand, S. L. (2020). Extended life-span conferred by cotransporter gene mutations in Drosophila. *Science, 290*(5499), 2137-2140. https://doi.org/10.1126/science.290.5499.2137

Stark, S. L., Somerville, E. K., & Morris, J. C. (2010). In Home Occupational Performance Evaluation (I-HOPE). *American Journal of Occupational Therapy, 64*(4), 580-589.

Wallace, R. B. (2006). Primary prevention. In L. Breslow, L. & G. Cengage, (Eds.), *Encyclopedia of public health.*

World Health Organization. (2020). Physical Activity. https://www.who.int/news-room/fact-sheets/detail/physical-activity

World Health Organization. (2021). Falls. https://www.who.int/news-room/fact-sheets/detail/falls.

Chapter 7

2018 Accreditation Council for Occupational Therapy Education (ACOTE®) Standards and Interpretive Guide (effective July 31, 2020). *American Journal of Occupational Therapy, 72*(Suppl. 2), 7212410005. https://doi.org/10.5014/ajot.2018.72S217

Chapter 8

American Stroke Association. (2021). *Support group.* https://www.stroke.org/en/stroke-groups/aim-high-support-group

Council for Higher Education Accreditation. (2001). *Statement on good practices and shared responsibility in the creation and application of specialized accreditation standards.* Author.

Council on Social Work Education. (2011). *Recovery to practice: Developing mental health recovery in social work.* Author.

Council on Social Work Education. (2022). 2022 Educational policy and accreditation standards for baccalaureate and master's social work programs. *CSWE Commission on Educational Policy, CSWE Commission on Accreditation.* https://www.cswe.org/getmedia/bb5d8afe-7680-42dc-a332-a6e6103f4998/2022-EPAS.pdf

Chapter 9

Fidanza, N., Baker, A., Bastos, S., DiGiacinto, J., & Scotto, M. (2021). Frailty Education of Older Adults in a Senior Housing Complex. Submitted for publication.

Fischl, C., Asaba, E. & Nilsson, I. (2017) Exploring potential in participation mediated by digital technology among older adults, *Journal of Occupational Science, 24*(3), 314-326, https://doi.org/10.1080/14427591.2017.1340905

National Association for Continence. (n.d.). What is a urologist? https://www.nafc.org/bhealth-blog/what-is-a-urologist

Park, S. Smith, J., Dunkle, R. E., Ingersoll-Dayton, B., & Antonucci, T. C. (2019). Health and social–physical environment profiles among older adults living alone: Associations with depressive symptoms. *The Journals of Gerontology: Series B, 74*(4), 675-684, https://doi.org/10.1093/geronb/gbx003

Schulman, K. I., Hermann, N., Brodaty, H., Chui, H., & Lawlor, B. (2006). IPA survey of brief cognitive screening instruments. *International Psychogeriatrics, 18*(2), 281-294.

Taylor, L. J., Harris, J., Epps, C., & Herr, K. (2005). Psychometric evaluation of selected pain intensity scales for use in cognitively impaired and cognitively intact older adults. Reh*abilitation Nursing, 30*(2), 55-61. https://doi.org/10.1002/j.2048-7940.2005.tb00360.x

United States Census Bureau. (2017). An aging nation: Projected number of children and older adults. https://www.census.gov/library/visualizations/2018/comm/historic-first.html

Wallace, R. B. (2006). Secondary prevention. In: L. Breslow & G. Cengage (Eds.), *Encyclopedia of public health*. https://www.encyclopedia.com/medicine/divisions-diagnostics-and-procedures/medicine/secondary-prevention

Chapter 10

American Academy of Pediatrics. (2002). The medical home. Medical home initiatives for children with special needs project advisory committee. *Pediatrics, 110*, 184-186.

Case-Smith, J., & Clifford O'Brien, J. (2014). *Occupational therapy for children and adolescents* (7th ed.). Elsevier Health Sciences.

Center for Advanced Studies in Child Welfare. (2015) *Well-being indicator tool for youth (WIT-Y)*. University of Minnesota.

Dunn, W., Little, L., Dean, E., Robertson, S., & Evans, B. (2016). The state of the science on sensory factors and their impact on daily life for children: A scoping review. *OTJR: Occupation, Participation and Health, 36*(Suppl. 2), 3S-26S. https://doi.org/10.1177/1539449215617923

Hirai, A. H., Kogan, M. D., Kandasamy, V., Reuland, C., Bethell, C. (2018). Prevalence and variation of developmental screening and surveillance in early childhood. *JAMA Pediatrics, 172*(9), 857-866.

Hurd, A. R. & Anderson, D. M. (2011). *The park and recreation professional's handbook*. Human Kinetics.

Matin, B. K., Karyani, A. K., Rezaei, S., Soofi, M., & Soltani, S. (2019). Do countries with higher GDP spend more on disabilities? New evidence in OECD countries. *Medical Journal of the Islamic Republic of Iran, 33*, 22-122.

McSpadden, C., Therrien, M., & McEwen, I. R. (2012). Care coordination for children with special health care needs and roles for physical therapists. *Pediatric Physical Therapy, 24*(1), 70-77.

United Nations. (2006) Convention on the Rights of Persons with Disabilities: Article 30 – Participation in cultural life, recreation, leisure and sport. https://www.un.org/development/desa/disabilities/convention-on-the-rights-of-persons-with-disabilities/article-30-participation-in-cultural-life-recreation-leisure-and-sport.html

U.S. Department of Education. (2017). Individuals with Disabilities Education Act: Sec. 300.34 Related services. https://sites.ed.gov/idea/regs/b/a/300.34

Chapter 11

Human Factors and Ergonomics Society. (n.d.). What is human factors and ergonomics. https://www.hfes.org/About-HFES/What-is-Human-Factors-and-Ergonomics

World Health Organization. (2016). Human factors: Technical series of safer primary care. https://apps.who.int/iris/bitstream/handle/10665/252273/9789241511612-eng.pdf;sequence=1

Chapter 12

AARP. (n.d.). AARP livability index. https://livabilityindex.aarp.org/

American Therapeutic Recreation Association. (2019). Who we are. https://www.atra-online.com/page/WhoWeAre

Centers for Disease Control and Prevention. (2021). Health literacy basics. https://www.cdc.gov/healthliteracy/basics.html

Chapter 13

Center for Disease Control and Prevention. (n.d.). Maternal, infant and child health. https://www.healthypeople.gov/2020/topics-objectives/topic/maternal-infant-and-child-health

Eismann, E., Theuerling, J., Maguire, S., Hente, E., Shapiro, R. (2018). Integration of the Safe Environment for Every Kid (SEEK) model across primary care settings. *Clinical Pediatrics, 58*(2), 166-176. https://doi.org/10.1177/0009922818809481

Goodman R., Meltzer H., & Bailey V. (1998) The Strengths and Difficulties Questionnaire: A pilot study on the validity of the self-report version. *European Child and Adolescent Psychiatry, 7*, 125-130.

King, G., Yukari, S., Chiarello, L., Thompson, L. & Hartman, L. (2020). Building blocks of resiliency: A transactional framework to guide research, service design, and practice in pediatric rehabilitation. *Disability and Rehabilitation, 42*(7), 1031-1040, https://doi.org/10.1080/09638288.2018.1515266

Lutton, S. S. & Swank, J. (2018). The importance of intentionality in untangling trauma from severe mental illness. *Journal of Mental Health Counseling, 40*, 113-128.

Sandel, M., Sheward, R., & Sturtevant, L. (2015). Compounding stress: The timing and duration effects of homelessness on children's health. Insights from Housing Policy Research. https://www.childrenshealthwatch.org/wp-content/uploads/Compounding-Stress_2015.pdf

Scaffa, M. E. & Reitz, S. M. (2020) *Occupational therapy in community and population health practice* (3rd ed.). F.A. Davis.

U.S. Department of Health and Human Services. (n.d.). 2030 Health People Framework. https://health.gov/healthypeople/about/healthy-people-2030-framework

World Health Organization. (2019). *International Statistical Classification of Diseases and Related Health Problems* (11th ed.). https://icd.who.int/

Chapter 14

American Occupational Therapy Association (2020). Occupational Therapy Practice Framework, 4th ed. *American Journal of Occupational Therapy, 74*(Suppl. 2), 7412410010p1-7412410010p87. https://doi.org/10.5014/ajot.2020.74S2001

Miller, E., Stanhope, V., Restrepo-Toro, M., & Tondora, J. (2017) Person-centered planning in mental health: A transatlantic collaboration to tackle implementation barriers. *American Journal of Psychiatric Rehabilitation, 20*(3), 251-267. https://doi.org/10.1080/15487768.2017.1338045.

Saxena, S. & Garrison, P. J. (2004). Mental health promotion—Case studies from countries: A joint publication of the World Federation for Mental Health and the World Health Organization. https://www.who.int/publications/i/item/9241592176

Wellness Recovery Action Plan. (2021). *What is WRAP*. https://www.wellnessrecoveryactionplan.com/what-is-wrap/

Chapter 15

Brown, L. L., Mitchell, U. A., & Ailshire, J. A. (2018). Disentangling the stress process: Race/ethnic differences in the exposure and appraisal of chronic stressors among older adults. *The Journals of Gerontology: Series B, 75*(3), 650-660. https://doi.org/10.1093/geronb/gby072

Centers for Disease Control and Prevention. (n.d.). About mental health. https://www.cdc.gov/mentalhealth/about/index.htm.

Centers for Disease Control and Prevention. (2021a). Preventing elder abuse. https://www.cdc.gov/violenceprevention/elderabuse/fastfact.html.

Centers for Disease Control and Prevention. (2021b). Coping with stress. https://www.cdc.gov/mentalhealth/stress-coping/cope-with-stress/index.html.

Kwong, J., Bockting, W., Gabler, S., Abbruzzese, L. D., Simon, P., Fialko, J., … Hall, P. (2017). Development of an Interprofessional Collaborative Practice Model for Older LGBT Adults. *LGBT Health, 4*(6), 442-444. https://doi.org/10.1089/lgbt.2016.0160

National Council on Aging. (n.d.). https://www.ncoa.org/article/covid-19-resource-guide-terminology-for-virtual-programming

Substance Abuse and Mental Health Services Administration. (2011). *The treatment of depression in older adults: Depression and older adults: Key issues.* Center for Mental Health Services, Substance Abuse and Mental Health Services Administration, U.S. Department of Health and Human Services.

U.S. National Library of Medicine. (2020, May 5). Older adult mental health. MedlinePlus. https://medlineplus.gov/olderadultmentalhealth.html

Village to Village Network, Inc. (n.d.). What is a village? https://www.vtvnetwork.org/

Whitson, H. E., Duan-Porter, W., Schmader, K. E., Morey, M. C., Cohen, H. J., & Colón-Emeric, C. S. (2016). Physical resilience in older adults: Systematic review and development of an emerging construct. *The Journals of Gerontology Series A: Biological Sciences and Medical Sciences, 71*(4), 489-495. https://doi.org/10.1093/gerona/glv202

World Health Organization Quality of Life Assessment. (1995). Position paper from the World Health Organization. *Social Science & Medicine, 41*(10), 1403-1409. https://doi.org/10.1016/0277-9536(95)00112-k

Chapter 16

Ahn, R. (2016). Building resilience in a child with SPD. STAR Institute. https://www.spdstar.org/sites/default/files/file-attachments/Building%20Resilience%20Tip%20Sheet_1.pdf

Anaby, D., Law, M., Teplicky, R., & Turner, L. (2015). Focusing on the environment to improve youth participation: experiences and perspectives of occupational therapists. *International Journal of Environmental Research and Public Health, 12*(10), 13388-13398.

Bekhet, A K., Johnson, N. L., & Zauszniewski, J. A. (2012). Resilience in family members of persons with autism spectrum disorder: A review of literature. *Issues in Mental Health Nursing, 33*(10), 650-656.

Black, K., & Lobo, M. (2008). Family resilience factors. *Journal of Family Nursing, 14*(1), 33-55. https://doi.org/10.1177/1074840707312237

Emerson, E. (2013). Commentary: Childhood exposure to environmental adversity and the well-being of people with intellectual disabilities. *Journal of Intellectual Disability Research, 57*(7), 589-600. https://doi.org/10.1111/j.1365-2788.2012.01577.x

Masten, A. S. (2018). Resilience theory and research on children and families: Past, present, and promise. *Journal of Family Theory and Review, 10*(1), 12-31. https://doi.org/10.1111/jftr.12255

Stahmer, A. C., Rieth, S. R., Dickson, K. S., Feder, J., Burgeson, M., Searcy, K., & Brookman-Frazee, L. (2020). Project ImPACT for toddlers: Pilot outcomes of a community adaptation of an intervention for autism risk. *Autism: The International Journal of Research & Practice, 24*(3), 617-632.

Ungar, M. (n.d.). What works: A manual for designing programs that build resilience. https://resilienceresearch.org/wp-content/uploads/2024/01/What-Works-Manual-Michael-Ungar-November-2023.pdf

World Health Organization. (2017). Policy options on mental health: A WHO-Gulbenkian mental health platform collaboration.

Chapter 17

Center for Interprofessional Practice and Education. (n.d.) Core competencies for Interprofessional Collaborative Practice/ Center for Health Interprofessional Practice and Education. https://healthipe.utexas.edu/core-competencies-interprofessional-collaborative-practice

Frisch, M. B. (1994). Quality of Life Inventory. NCS Pearson.

National Child Traumatic Stress Network. (n.d.). Family assessment device. https://www.nctsn.org/measures/family-assessment-device

U.S. Census Bureau. (2017). Grandparents and grandchildren. https://www.census.gov/newsroom/blogs/random-samplings/2016/09/grandparents-and-grandchildren.html

U.S. Census Bureau. (2020). Unmarried partners more diverse than 20 years ago. https://www.census.gov/library/stories/2019/09/unmarried-partners-more-diverse-than-20-years-ago.html?utm_campaign=20190923msacos1ccstors&utm_medium=email&utm_source=govdelivery

Chapter 19

Büssing, A., Föller, M. A., Gidley, J., & Heusser, P. (2010). Aspects of spirituality in adolescents. *International Journal of Children's Spirituality, 15*(1), 25-44. https://doi.org/10.1080/13644360903565524

Gardner, H. (1994). *Frames of mind: The theory of multiple intelligences*. Basic Books.

Gardner. H. E. (2006). *Multiple intelligences: New horizons in theory and practice*. Basic Books.

Spurr, S., Bally, J., Ogenchuk, M., & Walker, K. (2012). A framework for exploring adolescent wellness. *Pediatric Nursing, 38*(6), 320-326. PMID: 23362631.

Chapter 20

Benson, H., & Klipper, M. (1975). *The relaxation response* (Reissue ed.) HarperTorch.

Bhakt, R. (2019). *A seeker's guide to the yoga sutras: Modern reflections on the ancient journey*. Rockridge Press.

Miller, M., & Chavier, M. (2013). Clinicians' experiences of integrating prayer in the therapeutic process. *Journal of Spirituality in Mental Health, 15*(2), 70-93. https://doi.org/10.1080/19349637.2013.776441

Chapter 22

Abildso, C., Dyer, A., & Daily, S. M. (2019) Evaluability assessment of "growing healthy communities," A mini-grant program to improve access to healthy foods and places for physical activity. *BMC Public Health, 19*, 779-784. https://doi.org/10.1186/s12889-019-7156-8

Alderwick, H., Ham, C., & Buck, D. (2015). *Population health systems: Going beyond integrated care*. The King's Fund. https://www.kingsfund.org.uk/publications/population-health-systems

Australian Institute of Health and Welfare. (2015). *Australian Burden of Disease Study: Impact and causes of illness and death in Australia*. Author.

Caperchione, C., Mummery, W., & Joyner, K. (2010) WALK Community Grants Scheme: Lessons learned in developing and administering a health promotion micro grants program. *Health Promotion Practice, 5*(1), 637-44. https://doi.org/10.1177/1524839908328996

Council of Australian Governments Health Council, Australian Health Ministers' Advisory Council. (2017). *National strategic framework for chronic conditions*. Author.

Hartwig, K., Dunville, R., Kim, M., Levy, B., Zaharek, M., Njike, V., & Katz, D. (2009). Promoting healthy people 2010 through small grants. *Health Promotion Practice, 10*(1), 24-33. https://doi.org/10.1177/1524839906289048

Jacob-Arriola, K. R., Hermstad, A., & St. Clair Flemming, S. (2016) Promoting policy and environmental change in faith-based organizations: Outcome evaluation of a mini-grants program. *Health Promotion Practice, 17*(1), 146-155. https://doi.org/10.1177/1524839915613027

Johnson H. H., Bobbitt-Cooke, M., Schwarz, M., & White, D. (2006) Creative partnerships for community health improvement: A qualitative evaluation of the Healthy Carolinians community micro-grant project. *Health Promotion Practice, 7*(2), 162-169. https://doi.org/10.1177/1524839905278898

Moore, J. B., Brinkley, J., Morris, S., Oniffrey, T., & Kolbe M. (2016). Effectiveness of community-based minigrants to increase physical activity and decrease sedentary time in youth. *Journal of Public Health Management Practice, 22*(4), 370-378. https://doi.org/10.1097/PHH.0000000000000274

Owens, J., Riehm, A., & Lilly, F. (2019). Social innovation micro-grants as catalysts to community development in economically marginalized urban communities. *Journal of Race, Religion, Gender and Class, 18*(2), 352-358.

Porter, C., McCrackin, P., & Naschold, F. (2015). Minigrants for community health: A randomized controlled trial of their impact on family food gardening. *Journal of Public Health Management and Practice, 22*(1), 10-16.

Schmidt, M., Plochg, T., Harting, J., Klazinga, N., & Stronks, K. (2009). Micro-grants as a stimulus for community action in residential health programmes: A case study. *Health Promotion International 24*(3), 234-242.

Tamminen, K., Faulkner, G., Witcher, C., & Spence, J. (2014). A qualitative examination of the impact of microgrants to promote physical activity among adolescents. *BMC Public Health*, Nov 22. https://doi.org/10.1186/1471-2458-14-1206

University of Edinburgh. (2016). Mobility, mood and place: The A-Z of co-design: A brief introduction to participatory design. https://blogs.ed.ac.uk/mmp-journal/wp-content/uploads/sites/8294/2016/06/WEBSITE-PDF-VERSION.pdf

Financial Disclosures

Dr. Laurel D. Abbruzzese is on the APTA-Geriatrics faculty for "Certified Exercise Experts for Aging Adults."

Dr. Lucinda Acquaye-Doyle reported no financial or proprietary interest in the materials presented herein.

Dr. Mark Amir reported no financial or proprietary interest in the materials presented herein.

Ashleigh Augello reported no financial or proprietary interest in the materials presented herein.

Holly Putnam Bacasa reported no financial or proprietary interest in the materials presented herein.

Dr. Kerryn Bagley reported no financial or proprietary interest in the materials presented herein.

Dr. Andrew Bailey reported no financial or proprietary interest in the materials presented herein.

Dr. Pamela Bartlo reported no financial or proprietary interest in the materials presented herein.

Dr. Catherine Cavaliere reported no financial or proprietary interest in the materials presented herein.

Dr. Tina Champagne reported no financial or proprietary interest in the materials presented herein.

Jennifer Crews is an employee at the Summit Center for Child Development.

Dr. Ann Marie Dale reported no financial or proprietary interest in the materials presented herein.

Dr. Deirdre Daley is the Director of Clinical Practice for WorkWell Prevention & Care.

Dr. Priscilla Denham reported no financial or proprietary interest in the materials presented herein.

Dr. Joy Doll reported no financial or proprietary interest in the materials presented herein.

Dr. Ayse Ozcan Edeer reported no financial or proprietary interest in the materials presented herein.

Jane Evans reported no financial or proprietary interest in the materials presented herein.

Dr. Nicole A. Fidanza reported no financial or proprietary interest in the materials presented herein.

Dr. Kelle DeBoth Foust reported no financial or proprietary interest in the materials presented herein.

Dr. Avi Friedman reported no financial or proprietary interest in the materials presented herein.

Katie J. Galezniak reported no financial or proprietary interest in the materials presented herein.

Dr. Cheryl A. Hall reported no financial or proprietary interest in the materials presented herein.

Dr. Lisa Hanson reported no financial or proprietary interest in the materials presented herein.

Dr. Brad Hodge reported no financial or proprietary interest in the materials presented herein.

Sharon Holt reported no financial or proprietary interest in the materials presented herein.

Dr. Tamera Keiter Humbert reported no financial or proprietary interest in the materials presented herein.

Dr. Nerida Hyett reported no financial or proprietary interest in the materials presented herein.

Dr. Michele Karnes reported no financial or proprietary interest in the materials presented herein.

Dr. Jacqueline Kendona reported no financial or proprietary interest in the materials presented herein.

Dr. Julie Kugel reported no financial or proprietary interest in the materials presented herein.

Alexander Lopez reported no financial or proprietary interest in the materials presented herein.

Melissa Neagles reported no financial or proprietary interest in the materials presented herein.

Dr. Michael A. Pizzi reported no financial or proprietary interest in the materials presented herein.

Dr. Sandra M. Ribeiro reported no financial or proprietary interest in the materials presented herein.

Dr. Nadia Rust reported no financial or proprietary interest in the materials presented herein.

Amy Sawyer reported no financial or proprietary interest in the materials presented herein.

Dr. John M. Schaefer reported no financial or proprietary interest in the materials presented herein.

Dr. Elizabeth Oates Schuster reported no financial or proprietary interest in the materials presented herein.

Dr. Phyllis Simon reported no financial or proprietary interest in the materials presented herein.

Kathleen Tithof reported no financial or proprietary interest in the materials presented herein.

Dr. Christine Urish reported no financial or proprietary interest in the materials presented herein.

Emmy Vadnais reported no financial or proprietary interest in the materials presented herein.

Deanna Waggy reported no financial or proprietary interest in the materials presented herein.

Dr. Madalynn Wendland reported no financial or proprietary interest in the materials presented herein.

Dr. Erica K. Wentzel reported no financial or proprietary interest in the materials presented herein.

Dr. Gail Whiteford reported no financial or proprietary interest in the materials presented herein.

Dr. Andrea Gossett Zakrajsek reported no financial or proprietary interest in the materials presented herein.

INDEX

For Product Safety Concerns and Information please contact our EU representative GPSR@taylorandfrancis.com Taylor & Francis Verlag GmbH, Kaufingerstraße 24, 80331 München, Germany

Batch number: 10793341

Printed by Printforce, the Netherlands